FIRST AID FOR THE® Family Medicine Boards

Third Edition

TAO LE, MD, MHS
Assistant Clinical Professor of Medicine and Pediatrics
Chief, Section of Allergy and Clinical Immunology
Department of Medicine
University of Louisville

MICHAEL D. MENDOZA, MD, MPH, MS, FAAFP
Commissioner of Public Health
Monroe County Health Department
Associate Professor
Departments of Family Medicine, Public Health Sciences, and Nursing
University of Rochester Medical Center

DIANA COFFA, MD
Associate Professor
Residency Program Director
Department of Family and Community Medicine
University of California, San Francisco

LAMERCIE SAINT-HILAIRE, MD
Assistant Clinical Professor
Department of Family and Community Medicine
University of California, San Francisco

Mc
Graw
Hill
Education

New York / Chicago / San Francisco / Athens / London / Madrid / Mexico City
Milan / New Delhi / Singapore / Sydney / Toronto

First Aid for the® Family Medicine Boards, Third Edition

5 6 7 8 9 0   LMN   22

ISBN 978-1-25-983501-8
MHID 1-25-983501-4

NOTICE

Medicine is an ever-changing science. As new research and clinical experience broaden our knowledge, changes in treatment and drug therapy are required. The authors and the publisher of this work have checked with sources believed to be reliable in their efforts to provide information that is complete and generally in accord with the standards accepted at the time of publication. However, in view of the possibility of human error or changes in medical sciences, neither the authors nor the publisher nor any other party who has been involved in the preparation or publication of this work warrants that the information contained herein is in every respect accurate or complete, and they disclaim all responsibility for any errors or omissions or for the results obtained from use of the information contained in this work. Readers are encouraged to confirm the information contained herein with other sources. For example and in particular, readers are advised to check the product information sheet included in the package of each drug they plan to administer to be certain that the information contained in this work is accurate and that changes have not been made in the recommended dose or in the contraindications for administration. This recommendation is of particular importance in connection with new or infrequently used drugs.

This book was set in Electra LT Std by Rainbow Graphics.
The editors were Bob Boehringer and Cindy Yoo.
The production supervisor was Jeffrey Herzich.
Project management was provided by Rainbow Graphics.
The designer was Tara Price.
LSC Communications was printer and binder.

This book is printed on acid-free paper.

Library of Congress Cataloging-in-Publication Data
Names: Le, Tao, editor. | Mendoza, Michael D., editor. | Coffa, Diana,
   editor. | Saint-Hilaire, Lamercie, editor.
Title: First aid for the family medicine boards / [edited by] Tao Le, Michael
   D. Mendoza, Diana Coffa, Lamercie Saint-Hilaire.
Description: Third edition. | New York : McGraw-Hill Education, [2018]
Identifiers: LCCN 2017046989| ISBN 9781259835018 (pbk. : alk. paper) | ISBN
   1259835014 (pbk. : alk. paper)
Subjects: | MESH: Family Practice | Specialty Boards | United States |
   Outlines
Classification: LCC R834.5 | NLM WB 18.2 | DDC 610.76—dc23
LC record available at https://lccn.loc.gov/2017046989

DEDICATION

To our families, friends, and loved ones, who endured and assisted in the task of assembling this guide, and to the contributors to this and future editions, who took the time to share their knowledge, insight, and humor for the benefit of residents.

Contents

CONTRIBUTING AUTHORS

Mary Bonnet, MD
Resident Physician
University of Rochester, New York

Marina Fomina-Nazarova, MD, MBA
Resident Physician
University of Rochester, New York

Richard Giovane, MD
Resident Physician
University of Alabama, Tuscaloosa

Michael Heller, MD
Image Editor
Chief Resident Physician, Diagnostic Radiology
University of California, San Francisco

Anna Jack, MD
Chief Resident Physician
University of Rochester, New York

Jennifer Karlin, MD, PhD
Resident Physician
University of California, San Francisco

Jolie LeBlanc, MD
Clinical Fellow
Los Angeles County + University of Southern California
    Medical Center

Sky Lee, MD
Hospitalist
Adventist Health St. Helena Hospital
St. Helena, California

Emilia H. De Marchis, MD
Clinical Fellow
University of California, San Francisco

Lisa Moore, MD
Practicing Physician
LaFamilia Medical Center
Santa Fe, New Mexico

Caroline Morgan, MD
Clinical Fellow
Boston University, Boston Medical Center, Massachusetts

Amanda Ashcraft Pannu, MD
Chief Resident Physician
University of Rochester, New York

Nicole Person-Rennell, MD, MPH
Chief Resident Physician
University of California, San Francisco

Amber Robins, MD, MBA
Assistant Professor of Family Medicine
Georgetown University, Washington, DC

Hannah Snyder, MD
Clinical Fellow, Primary Care Addiction Medicine
University of California, San Francisco

Sarah Stombaugh, MD
Resident Physician
NorthShore University HealthSystem, Glenview, Illinois
The University of Chicago Pritzker School of Medicine

N. Kenji Taylor, MD, MSc
Resident Physician
University of California, San Francisco

Jocelyn Young, DO, MS
Resident Physician
University of Rochester, New York

SENIOR REVIEWERS

Erica Brode, MD
Family Practice Physician
University of California, San Francisco

Magdalen Edmunds, MD
Assistant Professor, Department of Family and Community
  Medicine
University of California, San Francisco

Monica Hahn, MD
Assistant Clinical Professor, Women's Health Primary Care
University of California, San Francisco

David Holub, MD
Assistant Program Director, Family Medicine Residency
University of Rochester, New York

Ronald H. Labuguen, MD
Associate Clinical Professor, Department of Family and Community
  Medicine
University of California, San Francisco

Lydia Leung, MD
Associate Professor, Department of Family Medicine and
  Community Medicine
University of California, San Francisco

Susan H. McDaniel, PhD
Dr Laurie Sands Distinguished Professor of Families & Health in the
  Departments of Family Medicine and Psychiatry
University of Rochester, New York

Pooja Mittal, MD
Associate Physician, Department of Family Medicine and
  Community Medicine
University of California, San Francisco

Elizabeth H. Naumburg, MD
Professor (Part-Time), Department of Family Medicine
Associate Dean/Student Advising, Department of Offices of Medical
  Education
University of Rochester, New York

Christine Pecci, MD
Professor, Department of Family Medicine and Community
  Medicine
University of California, San Francisco

Suzanne Marie Piotrowski, MD
Associate Professor of Clinical Family Medicine, Department of
  Family Medicine
Associate Professor of Clinical Center for Community Health,
  Center for Community Health
University of Rochester, New York

Lealah Pollock, MD, MS
Assistant Clinical Professor, Department of Family and Community
  Medicine
University of California, San Francisco

Manuel Tapia, MD, MPH
Assistant Professor, Department of Family and Community
  Medicine
University of California, San Francisco

J. Chad Teeters, MD, MS, RPVI, FACC
Chief of Cardiology
Associate Professor of Clinical Medicine
Cardiology Division, Highland Hospital, Rochester, New York
Cardiology Faculty, University of Rochester, New York

Kristen Thornton, MD, FAAFP, AGSF, CWSP
Assistant Professor of Family Medicine, Highland Family Medicine
Assistant Professor of Medicine, Monroe Community Hospital,
  Division of Geriatrics & Aging
Co-Director Aging Theme
University of Rochester, New York

Ariel P. Zodhiates, MD
Associate Physician, Department of Family and Community
  Medicine
University of California, San Francisco

Preface

First Aid for the® Family Medicine Boards provides residents and clinicians with the most useful and up-to-date preparation guide for the American Board of Family Medicine (ABFM) certification and recertification examinations. This edition represents an outstanding effort by a talented group of authors and includes the following:

- An updated full-color design for more effective study.
- A practical exam preparation guide with resident-tested test-taking and study strategies.
- Concise summaries of thousands of board-testable topics.
- Hundreds of high-yield tables, diagrams, and color illustrations.
- Key facts in the margins, highlighting "must know" information for the boards.
- Mnemonics throughout, making learning memorable and fun.
- Timely updates and corrections through the First Aid Team's blog at **www.firstaidteam.com.**

We invite you to share your thoughts and ideas to help us improve *First Aid for the® Family Medicine Boards.* See How to Contribute, p. xiii.

Tao Le
Louisville

Michael Mendoza
Rochester

Diana Coffa
San Francisco

Lamercie Saint-Hilaire
San Francisco

Acknowledgments

This has been a collaborative project from the start. We gratefully acknowledge the thoughtful comments, corrections, and advice of the residents, international medical graduates, and faculty who have supported the authors in the revision of the third edition of *First Aid for the® Family Medicine Boards*. Also, we would like to acknowledge Khaled Al Bishi.

For support and encouragement throughout the process, we are grateful to Thao Pham.

Thanks to our publisher, McGraw-Hill, for the valuable assistance of their staff. For enthusiasm, support, and commitment to this challenging project, thanks to Bob Boehringer. For outstanding editorial support, we thank Linda Geisler, Emma Underdown, Catherine Johnson, and Louise Petersen. We also want to thank Artemisa Gogollari, Susan Mazik, Virginia Abbott, Marvin Bundo, and Hans Neuhart for superb illustration work. A special thanks to Rainbow Graphics, especially David Hommel, for remarkable editorial and production work.

Tao Le
Louisville

Michael Mendoza
Rochester

Diana Coffa
San Francisco

Lamercie Saint-Hilaire
San Francisco

How to Contribute

To continue to produce a high-yield review source for the ABFM exam, you are invited to submit any suggestions or corrections. We also offer **paid internships** in medical education and publishing, ranging from three months to one year (see below for details). Please send us your suggestions for:

- Study and test-taking strategies for the ABFM
- New facts, mnemonics, diagrams, and illustrations
- Low-yield topics to remove

For each entry incorporated into the next edition, you will receive up to a $10 gift certificate as well as personal acknowledgment in the next edition. Diagrams, tables, partial entries, updates, corrections, and study hints are also appreciated, and significant contributions will be compensated at the discretion of the authors. Also, let us know about material in this edition that you feel is low yield and should be deleted. Please submit entries, suggestions, or corrections to the First Aid Team's blog at:

www.firstaidteam.com

Please include your name, address, institutional affiliation, phone number, and e-mail address (if different from the address of origin). You can also e-mail us directly at:

firstaidteam@yahoo.com

NOTE TO CONTRIBUTORS

All entries become the property of the authors and are subject to editing and review. Please verify all data and spellings carefully. In the event that similar or duplicate entries are received, only the first entry received will be used. Include a reference to a standard textbook to facilitate verification of the fact. Please follow the style, punctuation, and format of this edition if possible.

INTERNSHIP OPPORTUNITIES

The author team is pleased to offer part-time and full-time paid internships in medical education and publishing to motivated physicians. Internships may range from three months (eg, a summer) up to a full year. Participants will have an opportunity to author, edit, and earn academic credit on a wide variety of projects, including the popular *First Aid* series. Writing/editing experience, familiarity with Microsoft Word, and Internet access are desired. For more information, submit a résumé or a short description of your experience, along with a cover letter, to **firstaid@usmlerx.com**.

Guide to the ABFM Examination

Introduction

For residents, the American Board of Family Medicine (ABFM) certification exam represents the culmination of 3 years of hard work, and for those taking the recertification exam, 7 to 10 years after that. However, the process of certification and recertification does not merely represent yet another in a series of expensive tests. To your patients and their families, it means that you have attained the level of clinical knowledge and competency required to provide up-to-date and high quality clinical care.

In this chapter, we talk more about the ABFM exam and provide you with proven approaches to conquering the exam. For details about the exam, visit **www.theabfm.org.** The ABFM also provides information about specific strategies for exam preparation, available at **www.theabfm.org/cert/exampreparation.aspx.**

KEY FACT

The majority of patients will be aware of your certification status.

ABFM—The Basics

WHEN IS THE EXAM OFFERED?

The exam is offered during 2 months each year, typically in April and in November. Applicants must register for one of the limited dates that are offered in each of those months. Generally, more dates are available in the spring session than in the winter session.

HOW DO I REGISTER TO TAKE THE EXAM?

KEY FACT

Register before mid-January to avoid late fees.

You can register for the ABFM exam online at **www.theabfm.org.** Individuals who are finishing residency on June 30 are eligible to take the April exam before graduation. Those who complete residency training after June 30 or who do not pass the exam in the spring may be eligible to take the test during the winter.

Those who are certifying for the first time must have a user name and password supplied by their residency program. The registration deadline is typically January, with increasing late fees for each subsequent month. The latest date to register is generally in March. The registration fee in 2017 was $1300.

Prior to registering for the exam, applicants must be up to date on their required Maintenance of Certification (MOC) training. Specifically, they must have completed 50 points of approved CME through the ABFM within the last 3 years. Of these 50 points, at least 15 must be from a Knowledge Self Assessment module on the ABFM Web site and another 15 must be from an ABFM approved Performance Improvement module. This applies to people who are still in residency as well as to those who have graduated. You can check the ABFM Web site to find modules that qualify for MOC points and to confirm that you have accrued enough points to be eligible to apply for the exam.

Check the ABFM Web site for the latest information on registration deadlines, fees, and policies. Note that the deadlines and schedules for the Certificates of Added Qualifications vary.

KEY FACT

Completing a Performance Improvement project can take a month. Be sure to start your MOC requirements months before you intend to apply for the exam.

WHAT IF I NEED TO CANCEL THE EXAM OR CHANGE TEST CENTERS?

The ABFM currently provides partial refunds if a cancellation is received a certain number of days before the scheduled exam (in 2017, there was no cancellation fee

30 days before the exam). You can also change your test center and test dates before a specific deadline. Check the ABFM Web site for the latest on refund and cancellation policies as well as current procedures.

HOW IS THE ABFM TEST STRUCTURED?

The ABFM certification/recertification exam is currently a 1-day computer-based test administered at approximately 350 test centers around the country. For information about the computer-based format and an online exam tutorial, see the "Cognitive Expertise" section of the ABFM Web site. The exam content is available at www.theabfm.org/moc/examcontents.aspx. The exam itself is divided into four equal sections of 100 minutes, with 80 multiple choice questions in each. In the second section, 40 of the multiple choice questions will be dedicated to your selected module. The module topics are described in detail on the Web site; briefly, they are Ambulatory Family Medicine, Child and Adolescent Care, Geriatrics, Women's Health, Maternity Care, Emergent/Urgent Care, Hospital Medicine, and Sports Medicine. You will have 100 minutes of total break time that you can use between sections. The examinee can decide how to divide up the time throughout the day. Twenty of the exam questions are being tested and are not included in the scoring—but you will not know which questions these are! Overall, you will have approximately 1 minute to answer each question.

WHAT TYPES OF QUESTIONS ARE ASKED?

All questions are **single-best-answer** type only. You will be presented with a scenario and a question followed by five options. Most questions on the exam are vignette based. A substantial amount of extraneous information may be given, or a clinical scenario may be followed by a question that could be answered without actually requiring that you read the case. As with other board exams, there is no penalty for guessing. Questions can pertain to the diagnosis, treatment, or prevention of disease.

> **KEY FACT**
>
> Most questions on the ABFM exam are case based.

HOW ARE THE SCORES REPORTED?

Both the scoring and the reporting of test results have varied, but may take up to 3 months. Your score report will give you a "pass/fail" decision, the overall number of questions answered correctly with a corresponding percentile, and the number of questions answered correctly with a corresponding percentile for more than 40 different subject areas. Results from all candidates who took the test on the same date are presented alongside your results for each subject area. In 2016 for first-time and repeat exam takers in the United States, the pass rate for the certification exam was 96%; for the recertification exam, the pass rate was 89%.

The Recertification Exam

The recertification exam is one part of the Maintenance of Certification for Family Physicians (MC-FP). The exam must be completed every 7 or 10 years, depending on your situation. Additional components of the MC-FP include Self-Assessment Modules (SAMs), Performance Improvement (PI) activities, called Performance in Practice Modules (PPMs), and continuing medical education. Please check the ABFM Web site for additional details.

Test Preparation Advice

The good news about the ABFM exam is that it tends to focus on the diagnosis and management of diseases and conditions that you have likely seen as a resident—and that you should expect to see as a family physician in practice. Assuming that you have performed well as a resident, *First Aid* and a good source of practice questions (such as from the ABFM mobile app and the in-service exams on the ABFM Web site) may be all you need to pass. However, you might also consider using *First Aid* as a **guide** and using multiple resources, including a standard textbook, journal review articles, and a concise electronic text such as *UpToDate*, as part of your studies. Original research articles are low yield, and very new research (ie, research conducted less than 1-2 years before the exam) will not be tested. In addition, a number of high-quality board review courses are offered around the country. Such courses are costly, but can help those who need some focus and discipline.

Ideally, you should start your preparation early in your **last year of residency.**

As you study, concentrate on the **nuances of management,** especially for difficult or complicated cases. For **common diseases,** learn both common and **uncommon presentations;** for **uncommon diseases,** focus on the **classic presentations** and manifestations. Draw on the experiences of your residency training to anchor some of your learning. When you take the exam, you will realize that you've seen most of the clinical scenarios during your 3 years of clinic and hospital medicine.

Depending on the module you choose in the morning session, you may want to focus on specific chapters and sections in the *First Aid for the Family Medicine Boards:*
- **Ambulatory Family Medicine:** Community Medicine, Cardiology (hypertension, dyslipidemia, heart failure), Endocrinology (diabetes), Gastroenterology, Pulmonary Medicine, Dermatology, Reproductive Health (gynecology), and Behavioral Health.
- **Child and Adolescent Care:** Pediatric and Adolescent Medicine, Reproductive Health (gynecology), and Hematology and Oncology (anemia, leukemias).
- **Geriatrics:** Geriatrics, Community Medicine, Cardiology, Neurology (cerebrovascular disease), Dermatology (herpes zoster), and Psychiatry.
- **Women's Health:** Reproductive Health, Geriatrics (osteoporosis, incontinence), Psychiatry, Pediatric and Adolescent Medicine (eating disorders, female athletic triad), Surgery (breast cancer), and Community Medicine (domestic violence).
- **Maternity Care:** Reproductive Health (obstetrics), Psychiatry, and Community Medicine (domestic violence).
- **Emergent/Urgent Care:** Emergency/Urgent Care, Psychiatry, Surgery, Pediatric and Adolescent Medicine (common acute conditions), and Community Medicine (bioterrorism).
- **Hospital Medicine:** Cardiology, Pulmonary Medicine, Endocrinology (DKA, HHNS), Gastroenterology (GI bleeding, end-stage liver disease, diverticulitis, pancreatitis), Hematology and Oncology (oncology), Infectious Disease, Pulmonary (lower respiratory disease), Nephrology (acute renal failure), Neurology (cerebrovascular disease, seizure, syncope), Surgery, and Emergency/Urgent Care.
- **Sports Medicine:** Sports Medicine.

OTHER HIGH-YIELD AREAS

Focus on topic areas that may not be emphasized during residency training but are board favorites. These include the following:
- Basic biostatistics (eg, sensitivity, specificity, positive predictive value, negative predictive value).
- Adverse effects of drugs.

KEY FACT

The ABFM tends to focus on the horses, not the zebras.

KEY FACT

Use a combination of *First Aid*, textbooks, journal reviews, and practice questions.

Test-Taking Advice

By this point in your life, you have probably gained more test-taking expertise than you care to admit. Nevertheless, here are a few tips to keep in mind when taking the exam:

- Arrive 30 minutes early for your test. You want to be relaxed and ready to start on time, not rushed and stressed by traffic. Bring snacks and dress in layers so that you will be comfortable all day.
- Avoid a heavy lunch! Many test-takers have reported that it can be difficult to focus on the exam after a heavy meal.
- For long vignette questions, read the question stem and scan the options, and **then** go back and read the case. You may get your answer without having to read through the whole case.
- There's no penalty for guessing, so you should **never** leave a question blank. If you aren't sure, ask yourself, *What would I do if this clinical situation really presented itself to me and I was alone managing it?* Your gut instinct is often right.
- Good pacing is key. You need to leave adequate time to get to all the questions. Even though you have 1 minute per question on average, you should aim for a pace of 45 seconds per question. If you don't know the answer within a short period of time, make an educated guess and move on. You can flag that question to come back to if you have time at the end.
- It's okay to **second-guess** yourself. Research shows that our "second hunches" tend to be better than our first guesses.
- Don't panic over "impossible" questions. These may be **experimental questions** that won't count in your score. Again, take your best guess and move on.
- Note the age and race of the patient in each clinical scenario. When race or ethnicity is given, it is often relevant. Know these well, especially for more common diagnoses.
- Questions often describe clinical findings instead of naming eponyms (eg, they cite "tender, erythematous bumps in the pads of the finger" rather than "Osler nodes" in a febrile adolescent).
- As noted above, visit **www.theabfm.org/cert/exampreparation.aspx** for study strategies specific to the ABFM certification/recertification exam.

KEY FACT

Never, ever leave a question blank! There is no penalty for guessing.

Testing and Licensing Agencies

American Board of Family Medicine
1648 McGrathiana Parkway, Suite 550
Lexington, KY 40511
859-269-5626 or 888-995-5700
Support Center: 877-223-7437
www.theabfm.org

Educational Commission for Foreign Medical Graduates (ECFMG)
3624 Market Street, Fourth Floor
Philadelphia, PA 19104-2685
215-386-5900
Fax: 215-386-9196
www.ecfmg.org

Federation of State Medical Boards (FSMB)
400 Fuller Wiser Road
Euless, TX 76039
817-868-4000
Fax: 817-868-4099
www.fsmb.org

NOTES

CHAPTER 2

Community and Preventive Medicine

Amanda Ashcraft Pannu, MD

Preventive Medicine

- **1° prevention:** Disease prevention measures such as counseling for at-risk behaviors, immunizations, and chemoprevention that are taken **before the disease develops.**
- **2° prevention:** Defined as **early detection and treatment of asymptomatic disease,** including risk assessment.
- **3° prevention:** Management of chronic diseases to **prevent or minimize complications.**
- Characteristics that make a disease appropriate for screening include:
  - Disease leads to **significant morbidity and mortality.**
  - **Effective treatment** is available.
  - Disease is **detectable** in the asymptomatic period.
  - Testing is accurate and simple.
  - Treatment administered during the asymptomatic period yields a better outcome than treatment in the symptomatic period.
- Characteristics of risk factors that would be appropriate for screening are:
  - **High prevalence** of the risk factor in the population to be screened.
  - Large portions of those with the risk factor are unidentified.
  - Associated **disease** should have a **high incidence** in the population to be screened.
  - Disease should have **serious consequences.**
  - Readily available treatment that can modify the risk factor.
  - **Risk modification should ↓ disease incidence.**

ADULT IMMUNIZATIONS

Table 2.1 outlines common adult immunizations and their indications. For information on immunization of pediatric populations, refer to the Child and Adolescent Medicine chapter.

CANCER SCREENING

The following guidelines are based on recommendations from the United States Preventive Services Task Force (USPSTF) and the American Academy of Family Physicians (AAFP). The USPSTF describes their strengths of recommendation as grades (Table 2.2) that communicate both the importance of the recommendation and how it should be incorporated into practice. Remember that these recommendations are updated annually.

Skin Cancer

- Insufficient evidence (grade I) for whole-body skin examination by a primary care clinician or patient skin self-examination for the early detection of cutaneous melanoma, basal cell cancer, or squamous cell skin cancer in the adult general population.
- However, there is grade B evidence recommending counseling children adolescents and young adults (ages 10-24) who have fair skin about minimizing their exposure to ultraviolet radiation to reduce risk for skin cancer.

Cervical Cancer

- Routinely screen for cervical cancer with a Papanicolaou smear all women 21 years of age who have been sexually active and have a cervix (**grade A strongly recommended**).
- Repeat screening at least every 3 years, but this interval can be lengthened to every 5 years in women aged 30 to 65 years if they are being screened with a combination of cytology and HPV testing.

TABLE 2.1.　**Recommended Adult Immunization Schedule**

VACCINE	SCHEDULE
Td/Tdap	Give the complete 1° series if the patient has not been previously vaccinated (first dose, Tdap; second dose, Td 4 weeks later; third dose, Td 6 months later) Tdap can substitute for only one of the three Td doses in the series Booster doses of Td should be given every 10 years thereafter
Human papillomavirus	Vaccinate girls and boys at 11 or 12 years (or as early as 9 years) with catch-up vaccination for young women and young men between 13 and 26 years, and for men aged 22-26 years if immunocompromised (including HIV) and men who have sex with men (MSM)
Varicella	If the patient has a history of chickenpox, consider immune; otherwise, vaccinate with two doses given 1-2 months apart
Herpes zoster	Single dose recommended for adults ≥60 years regardless of whether they report a prior episode of herpes zoster
Measles, mumps, rubella	If the patient was born before 1957, consider immune If the patient was born after 1957, two doses should be given at least 1 month apart For rubella specifically, ensure that women of childbearing potential have immunity
Influenza	One dose annually recommended for all persons aged ≥6 months, including all adults
Pneumococcal (polysaccharide): PPSV23 (older) PCV13 (newer)	Give to all adults ≥65 years: PCV13, then PPSV23 12 months later Adults 19-64 years with comorbid conditions (chronic pulmonary disorders excluding asthma, CVD, DM, chronic liver or renal disease): PPSV23 vaccine only, give second dose ≥5 years later Adults with asplenia or immunosuppression: Both vaccines (PCV13 first, then PPSV23 8 weeks later)
Hepatitis A	Vaccinate any person seeking protection or people of the following indications: MSM, chronic liver disease, persons traveling or working in endemic areas Two doses 6-12 months apart or three doses at 0, 1, and 6 months
Hepatitis B	Vaccinate any person seeking protection or people of the following indications: persons at high risk for STIs, health care personnel, end-stage liver disease patients, HIV-infected patients, chronic liver disease patients Three doses (0, 1-2 months, 4-6 months)
Meningococcal: 4-valent conjugate meningococcal B	Give to adults with asplenia, first-year college students in dormitories, military personnel 1-3 doses depending on type of vaccine and indication; consider a second dose at 5 years for those given polysaccharide vaccine

Data from the CDC.

■ Routine screening is **not** recommended for women >**65 years of age** with a history of adequate ⊖ screening and who are otherwise **not at high risk**. The evidence is insufficient to recommend for or against the routine use of new technologies or HPV testing alone to screen for cervical cancer.

Ovarian Cancer

Do not routinely screen for ovarian cancer by ultrasound, measurement of tumor markers, or pelvic examination. Although the specificity for screening strategies is high, the positive predictive value is low because of the low prevalence of ovarian cancer in the general population. Further, the invasive nature of testing that follows a ⊕ screening test led the USPSTF to conclude that the potential risks outweigh the potential benefits (grade D, against recommendation).

Breast Cancer

■ **Breast self-examination:** General consensus among expert groups is **not** to recommend breast self-examination.

TABLE 2.2.　**Definition of USPSTF Grades**

A—Strongly recommends service
B—Recommends service
C—Recommends selectively offering service based on professional judgment and patient preference
D—Recommends against service
I—Insufficient evidence

- **Mammography:**
  - Women aged 50 to 74 years: **Screen for breast cancer** every 2 years with mammography (grade B recommendation).
  - Women <50 years: **Individualize** your decision to start regular, biennial screening mammography based on patient context, including the patient's values regarding specific benefits and harms. (Grade C recommendation to screen women aged 40-49 years.)
  - Women ≥75 years: **Do not routinely screen** with mammography.
- **Germline predisposition (*BRCA1* or *BRCA2*):** Although a family history of breast cancer is common in women who develop breast cancer, only 5% to 6% of all breast cancers are associated with germline (inherited) genetic mutations. The majority of these involve two genes, *BRCA1* and *BRCA2.* Affected patients who meet the National Comprehensive Cancer Network (NCCN) criteria for *BRCA1* and *BRCA2* screening include:
  - Female breast cancer diagnosed <50 years old.
  - Triple-negative breast cancer diagnosed <60 years old.
  - Invasive ovarian or fallopian tube cancer or 1° peritoneal cancer.
  - Male breast cancer.
  - Ashkenazi Jewish descent with breast, ovarian, or pancreatic cancer diagnosed at any age.
  - Patients with breast cancer (any age) who have first-, second-, or third-degree relatives with breast cancer diagnosed <50 years old in one or more relatives; invasive ovarian, fallopian tube, or 1° peritoneal cancer in one or more relatives; breast, prostate, or pancreatic cancer diagnosed in two or more relatives.
- Women who test ⊕ for *BRCA1* or *BRCA2* mutations are at ↑ risk for both breast and ovarian cancer. Such women should be referred for appropriate counseling to consider options for reducing risk and intensified surveillance.
- The NCCN guidelines recommend that *BRCA* carriers be offered prophylactic bilateral mastectomy; however, that decision is made based on patient preference. Also, bilateral salpingo-oophorectomy should be offered to women who have completed childbearing. In women who opt not to have prophylactic bilateral mastectomy, annual mammogram (starting at age 30 years) and annual breast MRI (starting at age 25 years) is recommended. Additionally, selective estrogen receptor modulators (tamoxifen or raloxifene) can be used to ↓ the risk of invasive breast cancer in high-risk women who opt against surgical options. In postmenopausal women, an aromatase inhibitor (such as anastrozole) may also be used.

Prostate Cancer

The USPSTF recommends informed, individualized decision-making about screening for prostate cancer in men ages 55 to 69 years based on the man's values and preferences (grade C). PSA-based screening is not recommended for men 70 years and older (grade D). With early detection of asymptomatic disease, very few, if any, patients have improved survival and there will be more harm done by falsely elevated PSA levels and the subsequent additional testing and treatment.

Colon Cancer

- **Screen adults 50 to 75 years of age** for colon cancer with an annual fecal occult blood test, sigmoidoscopy every 3 to 5 years, or colonoscopy every 10 years (**grade A recommendation**). Screening adults aged 76 to 85 years is a grade C recommendation.
- Screen **earlier if there is ↑ risk** for colorectal cancer—eg, if the patient has a personal or strong family history of colorectal cancer, adenomatous polyps, or a family history of a hereditary syndrome (familial adenomatous polyposis, hereditary nonpolyposis colon cancer).
- Do not screen for colorectal cancer in adults >85 years of age (grade D recommendation).

Lung Cancer

There are currently differing opinions regarding lung cancer screening.

- USPSTF recommends (grade B) annual screening for lung cancer with low-dose CT in adults ages 55 to 80 with a 30-pack year smoking history and currently smoke, or have quit in the last 15 years. Screening should be stopped when that patient has ceased smoking for 15 years or develops a life-limiting condition or the willingness to have curative lung surgery.
- AAFP finds that there is insufficient evidence to support this recommendation, citing high number needed to screen, lack of reproducibility of these results in all settings, and high cost.

QUESTION

A 30-year-old woman who is otherwise healthy presents to you for the first time because she wants to be tested for the "breast cancer gene." She is concerned because her 52-year-old mother was diagnosed with metastatic breast cancer at 38 years of age. How would you answer this patient?

ADULT HEALTH MAINTENANCE

Tables 2.3 lists recommended clinical preventive services for different adult populations based on the grade A and B recommendations from the USPSTF and the AAFP. Male- and female-specific screening recommendations are discussed below. Table 2.4 lists clinical preventive services for pregnant woman. See cancer screening and immunization recommendations above.

TABLE 2.3.   Recommended Clinical Preventive Services for All Adults

AGE	CONDITION	RECOMMENDATION
≥18	Alcohol misuse	Screen and counsel behavior to ↓ alcohol misuse
	Depression	Screen all adults, including pregnant and postpartum women; implement screening with adequate systems in place to ensure accurate diagnosis, effective treatment, and appropriate follow-up
	HBV/HCV	Screen adults at high risk for infection; one-time screening for HCV infection to adults born between 1945 and 1965
	HIV infection	Screen adolescents and adults aged 18-65 years
	Hypertension	Screen for high BP; obtain measurements outside of the clinical setting for diagnostic confirmation before starting treatment
	Obesity	Refer patients with BMI ≥30 kg/m^2 for intensive, multicomponent behavioral interventions
	Physical inactivity/ unhealthy diet	Offer or refer adults who are overweight or obese and have additional CVD risk factors to intensive behavioral counseling interventions to promote a healthful diet and physical activity; clinicians may choose to selectively counsel patients about the benefits of a healthful diet rather than incorporate counseling into the care of all adults in the general population
	STIs	Counsel sexually active adolescents and counsel all adults at ↑ risk for STIs
	Tobacco use	Ask all adults about tobacco use, advise them to stop using tobacco, and provide behavioral interventions and FDA-approved pharmacotherapy for cessation to adults who use tobacco
	TB	Screen for latent TB infection in populations at ↑ risk
40-70	Type 2 DM	Screen for abnormal blood glucose as part of cardiovascular risk assessment in those who are overweight or obese; clinicians should offer or refer patients with abnormal blood glucose to intensive behavioral counseling interventions to promote a healthful diet and physical activity
40-75	Lipid disorders	Adults without a history of CVD (ie, symptomatic CAD or ischemic stroke) use a low- to moderate-dose statin for the prevention of CVD events and mortality when the following criteria are met: • They are aged 40-75 years • They have one or more CVD risk factors (ie, dyslipidemia, diabetes, hypertension, or smoking) • They have a calculated 10-year risk of a cardiovascular event of 10% or greater Identification of dyslipidemia and calculation of 10-year CVD event risk requires universal lipids screening in adults aged 40-75 years
50-59	CVD and colorectal cancer	Low-dose aspirin is recommended for adults with ≥10% 10-year CVD risk who are not at ↑ risk for bleeding, have a life expectancy of at least 10 years, and are willing to take low-dose aspirin daily for at least 10 years
≥65	Falls	Exercise or physical therapy and vitamin D supplementation in community-dwelling adults who are at ↑ risk for falls

Screening in Men

Abdominal Aortic Aneurysm: Offer one-time screening by ultrasonography for **men 65 to 75 years of age** who have ever smoked.

Screening in Women

Chlamydia and gonorrhea: Screen sexually active **women age 24 years and younger and older women** who are at ↑ risk for infection.

Intimate partner violence: Screen women of childbearing age for intimate partner violence (grade B). There was insufficient data to recommend for or against screening other populations (grade I). See the Domestic Violence section below for more information.

Osteoporosis: Screen in **women aged ≥65 years** and in younger women whose fracture risk is ≥ that of a 65-year-old white woman who has no additional risk factors. The FRAX (Fracture Risk Assessment) tool can be used to estimate 10-year risks for fractures for all racial and ethnic groups in the United States.

Screening for STI

- **Chlamydia and gonorrhea:** Screen sexually active **women ≤24 years and older women** who are at ↑ risk for infection.
- The USPSTF recommends that all **pregnant women** be screened for hepatitis B, HIV, and syphilis.

TABLE 2.4.   Recommended Clinical Preventive Services for Pregnant Women

CONDITION	RECOMMENDATION
Bacteriuria, asymptomatic	Screen with urine culture at 12-16 weeks' gestation or at the first prenatal visit
Breastfeeding	Provide interventions during pregnancy and after birth to promote and support breastfeeding
Depression	Screen pregnant and postpartum women, implement screening with adequate systems in place to ensure accurate diagnosis, effective treatment, and appropriate follow-up
Gestational DM	Screen asymptomatic pregnant women after 24 weeks of gestation
HBV infection	Screen at the first prenatal visit
HIV infection	Screen all pregnant women, including those who present in labor whose HIV status is unknown
Neural tube defects	All women planning or capable of pregnancy should take a daily supplement containing 0.4-0.8 mg (400-800 µg) of folic acid
Preeclampsia	Low-dose aspirin (81 mg/d) as preventive medication after 12 weeks of gestation in women who are at high risk for preeclampsia
Rh(D) incompatibility	Order Rh(D) blood typing and antibody testing at the first prenatal visit; repeat antibody testing for all Rh(D)-negative women at 24-28 weeks' gestation
Syphilis	Screen all pregnant women
Tobacco use	Provide smoking cessation behavioral interventions for all pregnant smokers

- **MSM:** The CDC recommends screening for HBsAg, syphilis (annually), gonorrhea, chlamydia, and HIV. Hepatitis C screening should be done when other risk factors are present. Anal Papanicolaou testing is available, but evidence and guidelines for its use are inconsistent.
- Additional screening for STI such as HIV and syphilis are recommended for all men and women (regardless of sexual orientation) engaging in high-risk sexual behavior. A thorough sexual history to assess patient sexual behavior is important. When determining patients at risk for STIs, also consider demographics of the population served (eg, if there is a high community prevalence of syphilis).

PREVENTION OF DENTAL CARIES IN PRESCHOOLERS

A total of 19% of children 2 to 5 years of age and 52% of children 5 to 9 years of age experience dental caries. Ethnic minority and economically disadvantaged children are at ↑ risk. Despite recommendations, few preschool-aged children ever visit a dentist.

Guidelines for the dental care of preschool children are as follows:
- Prescribe currently recommended doses of **oral fluoride supplementation** to preschool children >6 months of age whose 1° water source is fluoride deficient (USPSTF grade B recommendation).
- You may use **topical fluoride varnishes,** which are easier to use, accepted widely by patients, and have ↓ potential for toxicity, as adjuncts to oral supplementation. These can be applied every 3 to 6 months from the time of first tooth eruption until the age of 5 (USPSTF grade B recommendation).
- Monitor for dental fluorosis, a mild adverse effect of fluoride supplementation primarily of cosmetic significance.

ENDOCARDITIS PROPHYLAXIS

Offer antimicrobial prophylaxis for dental and other procedures to patients with cardiac conditions with the highest risk of adverse outcome from infective endocarditis.

Endocarditis prophylaxis is recommended for the following cardiac conditions:
- **Cardiac valvulopathy** in a cardiac transplant recipient.
- **Congenital heart defect completely repaired** within the previous 6 months with prosthetic material or device, whether placed by surgery or by catheter.
- **Repaired congenital heart disease** with residual defects at the site or adjacent to the site of a prosthetic patch or device.
- **Unrepaired cyanotic congenital heart disease,** including palliative shunts and conduits.
- Previous history of **infective endocarditis.**
- **Prosthetic heart valves.**

Do not offer antimicrobial prophylaxis to patients with any other form of congenital or acquired heart disease such as bicuspid aortic valve, acquired aortic or mitral valve disease (including mitral valve prolapse with regurgitation), or hypertrophic cardiomyopathy.

Offer antimicrobial prophylaxis to patients with the cardiac lesions cited above when they undergo procedures, such as the following, likely to result in bacteremia with a microorganism that has the potential to cause endocarditis:
- All **dental procedures** that involve manipulation of gingival tissue or the periapical region of teeth or that perforate the oral mucosa.
- **Procedures of the respiratory tract** that involve incision or biopsy of the respiratory mucosa.
- Procedures in patients with **ongoing GI or GU tract infection.**
- Procedures on infected skin, skin structure, or musculoskeletal tissue.

 QUESTION

A 45-year-old male nonsmoker presents for a routine annual physical exam. He is generally healthy and of a normal weight with no current medical complaints. He exercises by jogging 30 minutes two times a week, on average. His family history includes high blood pressure (BP) and an older brother with MI at age 48 years. He is worried that this might happen to him. What preventive services can you offer this patient?

KEY FACT

Three years after smoking cessation, the risk of recurrent MI ↓ to that of a nonsmoker.

MNEMONIC

The "5 A's" approach to tobacco cessation advocated by the National Cancer Institute:

- **A**sk about smoking habits
- **A**dvise all smokers to quit
- **A**ssess patient's readiness to quit
- **A**ssist with nonpharmacologic measures such as counseling and pharmacotherapy (as appropriate)
- **A**rrange follow-up and support

SMOKING CESSATION

Prevalence of cigarette smoking among adults in the United States was estimated by the CDC to be 17% in 2014. Smoking causes as many as 480,000 deaths/year and is the most common preventable cause of death (Figure 2.1).

Smoking cessation is known to confer the following **health benefits:**
- **MI:** ↓ mortality risk. The risk of recurrent coronary events is progressively ↓ to near that of a nonsmoker by 3 years after quitting.
- **Stroke:** Associated with a ↓ risk over time.
- **Pulmonary disease:** Slowed progression in the decline of FEV_1 in patients with COPD. Also associated with a ↓ risk of pulmonary infections such as bacterial pneumonia and TB.
- **Malignancy:** ↓ risk of lung, kidney, bladder, stomach, and cervical cancers, among others.
- **PUD:** ↓ risk of developing PUD; accelerated rate of healing.
- **Osteoporosis:** ↓ risk of bone loss and fracture (begins 10 years after quitting).

Cessation Methods

- Evaluate the patient's cigarette use, assess his or her interest in quitting, and find out about previous attempts at quitting.
- Once the patient is ready, offer strategies such as setting a "quit day" and help define alternative oral behaviors to substitute for the cigarette (eg, gum, throat lozenges).
- Many behavioral methods have been advocated to encourage patients to work toward quitting. Discuss and agree upon methods for cessation (Table 2.5) in advance of the quit day.

ANSWER

In addition to checking BP as part of his physical exam, you order a lipid panel and discuss the benefits of a healthy diet. Evidence is insufficient for recommending low-dose aspirin to prevent CVD in adults <50 years.

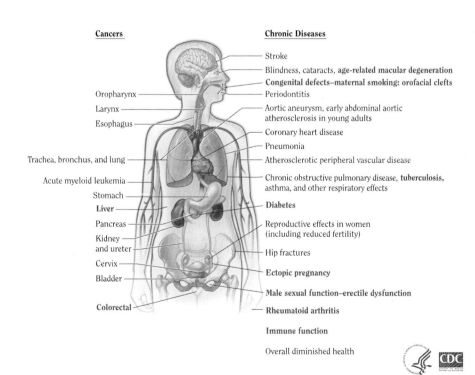

Risks from Smoking
Smoking can damage every part of your body

Cancers
- Oropharynx
- Larynx
- Esophagus
- Trachea, bronchus, and lung
- Acute myeloid leukemia
- Stomach
- **Liver**
- Pancreas
- Kidney and ureter
- Cervix
- Bladder
- **Colorectal**

Chronic Diseases
- Stroke
- Blindness, cataracts, **age-related macular degeneration**
- **Congenital defects–maternal smoking: orofacial clefts**
- Periodontitis
- Aortic aneurysm, early abdominal aortic atherosclerosis in young adults
- Coronary heart disease
- Pneumonia
- Atherosclerotic peripheral vascular disease
- Chronic obstructive pulmonary disease, **tuberculosis,** asthma, and other respiratory effects
- **Diabetes**
- Reproductive effects in women (including reduced fertility)
- Hip fractures
- **Ectopic pregnancy**
- Male sexual function–erectile dysfunction
- **Rheumatoid arthritis**
- Immune function
- Overall diminished health

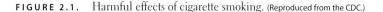

FIGURE 2.1. Harmful effects of cigarette smoking. (Reproduced from the CDC.)

TABLE 2.5. Methods for Smoking Cessation

METHOD	DESCRIPTION	EFFICACY
Group counseling	Lectures, groups, exercises, strategies	Associated with a 20% 1-year quit rate
Nicotine replacement (gum, patch, nasal spray, inhaler)	Suppresses withdrawal symptoms: depressed mood, insomnia, irritability, restlessness, weight gain	When used with a behavioral program, gum and patch methods double the quit rate
Bupropion	Enhances central noradrenergic and dopaminergic function when administered at a dosage of 150 mg twice daily	Greater efficacy than nicotine replacement Bupropion used together with nicotine patches has been shown to have >50% efficacy
Varenicline	Partial agonist of the nicotinic acetylcholine receptor Case reports of suicidal thoughts and aggressive and erratic behavior have been reported	As effective as or more effective than bupropion
Hypnosis, acupuncture, and electric cigarettes		No evidence to support the efficacy of these procedures

QUESTION 1

A 32-year-old 5-ft, 4-in, 203-lb woman presents for her annual physical exam. She would like to lose some weight and asks about use of guar gum for weight loss. What is the next step in the management of this patient?

QUESTION 2

A 47-year-old homeless man presents to your clinic to establish care. His known medical conditions include diabetes, hypertension, and a recently ⊕ purified protein derivative (PPD), for which he is currently taking isoniazid (INH). He complains of some cough, diarrhea, and tingling in his feet. On exam, his BP is 156/97 mm Hg, and you note that he smells of alcohol. He has pale conjunctivae, a red tongue, and fissures at the corners of his mouth. He also appears to have some loss of sensation to light touch in his feet bilaterally. How do you proceed?

Obesity

In the United States, the prevalence of obesity is now about 34% in adults and 17% in children. Screen all adult patients for obesity and offer intensive counseling and behavioral interventions to promote sustained weight loss in obese adults and children and prevent morbidity and mortality associated with obesity, including:

- ↑ **risk of both cardiovascular and overall mortality.** In addition, there are clear associations between obesity and ↑ morbidity.
- ↑ risk of cardiovascular disease, hypertension, stroke, type 2 DM and insulin resistance, dyslipidemia, cancer (including cancers of the colon, kidney, and gallbladder), sleep apnea, gallbladder disease, GERD, and knee osteoarthritis.
- ↓ quality of life, including ↓ mobility and social stigmatization.

KEY FACT

A BMI ≥30 is associated with ↑ risk of both death from CVD and overall mortality. Intentional weight loss of 25 lb has been associated with a ↓ in CVD, cancer, and overall mortality.

Diagnosis

Overweight and obesity are diagnosed based on the **calculation of BMI (kg/m^2):**

$$BMI = weight\ (kg)\ /\ height^2\ (m^2)$$

See Table 2.6 for the categories of BMI.

Management

Consider the following modalities in the treatment of obesity:

- **Diet and exercise counseling with behavioral strategies** to help patients change eating patterns and become physically active. This may lead to small/moderate degrees of weight loss (1-6 kg) typically sustained for at least 1 year.

TABLE 2.6. BMI Categories for Overweight and Obesity

DEFINITION	BMI (kg/m^2)
Overweight	25-29
Obese	30-39
Morbidly obese	40-49
Super-obese	50-59

ANSWER 1

Calculate BMI, which for this patient is 35 kg/m², and offer referral for intensive, multicomponent behavioral interventions, as per USPSTF and AAFP recommendations for patients with BMI ≥30 kg/m². You explain that guar gum has not been shown to be effective for weight loss and recommend a diet and exercise regimen.

ANSWER 2

You check hematocrit, peripheral blood smear, and B_{12} and folate levels. Also consider checking an HbA_{1c}, as his loss of sensation could be caused by diabetic neuropathy. His alcohol use should be addressed as well including the risk of thiamine deficiency.

KEY FACT

Medications for the treatment of obesity allow for sustained weight loss only if they are used in combination with lifestyle changes.

■ **Medication (Table 2.7):** May be considered for patients with BMI >30 when diet and exercise attempts have failed and/or when the patient has comorbidities. Weight loss resulting from medication:
  ▪ Is modest (average 3-5 kg), and discontinuation of medications may lead to rapid weight gain.
  ▪ Will only be significant when combined with lifestyle changes.
  ▪ Is considered successful when a 5% to 10% reduction in initial weight. If that amount of weight loss is not achieved with a particular agent, the medication should be discontinued to avoid adverse effects.
■ **Surgery:**
  ▪ Consider patients for **gastric bypass and vertical banded gastroplasty** if they have a BMI >40 or BMI >35 with comorbidities, have failed to respond to previous nonsurgical weight loss attempts, and are well informed and motivated.
  ▪ Discuss with them postoperative complications, which may include a mortality rate of 0.2%, wound infection, re-operation, vitamin deficiency, diarrhea, and hemorrhage.
  ▪ Refer for **bariatric surgery** to high-volume centers with experienced surgeons.
  ▪ Prepare patients and offer appropriate support, including psychological screening and a diet and exercise program, for successful surgical weight loss.
  ▪ Patients who undergo Roux-en-Y gastric bypass will require lifelong vitamin supplementation (multivitamin, B_{12}, iron, zinc, magnesium) and yearly screening labs for nutritional deficiencies.

Nutrition

MALNUTRITION

Table 2.8 outlines the clinical manifestations and treatment of severe malnutrition.

TABLE 2.7. Medications Used to Treat Obesity

MEDICATION	MECHANISM	NOTES
Sympathomimetic drugs		
Phentermine and diethylpropion	Stimulates sympathetic nervous system	Can ↑ BP, contraindicated in CAD, HTN Use up to 12 weeks only (schedule IV drugs with abuse potential)
Drugs that alter fat digestion		
Orlistat	Inhibits pancreatic lipase	Can be used on a long-term basis, average loss of 8% initial weight Side effects include abdominal cramps, flatus, and oily spotting
Antidepressants		
Fluoxetine	Acts as an appetite suppressant	Not FDA approved for weight loss; must use ≥60 mg/day
Bupropion	Acts as a norepinephrine modulator	Not FDA approved for weight loss
Antiepileptic drugs		
Topiramate	Also approved for treatment of migraine	Not FDA approved for weight loss as a single agent; available in combination treatment with phentermine
Zonisamide	Has serotonergic and dopaminergic activity	Not FDA approved for weight loss

TABLE 2.8.   Presentation and Treatment of Severe Malnutrition

	MARASMUS	KWASHIORKOR
Definition	Total calorie malnutrition	Protein malnutrition
Etiologies (in developed countries)	COPD, HF, cancer, AIDS	Trauma, burns, sepsis
Symptoms/Exam	Weight loss/**wasting**	Normal weight; edema, ascites
Treatment	Correct fluid and electrolyte abnormalities; treat infections; give vitamins and minerals Start with 1 g protein/kg and 30 kcal/kg, preferably enterically	Treatment is the same as that for marasmus
Complications	Immunosuppression, poor wound healing, impaired growth and development, muscle atrophy leading to organ dysfunction	Same as those for marasmus

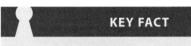

KEY FACT

Think about fat-soluble vitamin deficiencies in patients with any sort of intestinal malabsorption (IBD, CF).

KEY FACT

If neurologic deficits are present, think vitamin B_{12} deficiency. Immediate treatment is necessary to prevent irreversible peripheral neuropathy, balance problems, **dementia.**

VITAMIN DEFICIENCIES

Vitamin deficiencies may be more common in developed countries than is generally believed. Vitamins are needed for basic metabolism, but since most of them cannot be synthesized, they must be present in our diets. The presentation and treatment of fat- and water-soluble vitamin deficiencies are summarized in Tables 2.9 and 2.10.

TABLE 2.9.   Presentation and Treatment of Fat-Soluble Vitamin Deficiencies

VITAMIN	ETIOLOGY	SYMPTOMS/EXAM	TREATMENT
A (retinol)	Found in urban poor, elderly patients, and those with fat malabsorption syndrome	Night blindness, xerosis, Bitot spots (white patches on the conjunctivae) leading to keratomalacia, endophthalmitis, and blindness	High-dose vitamin A
D	Found in elderly patients, those with insufficient sun exposure or malnutrition/malabsorption, breastfeeding infants, and anticonvulsant users	**Children:** Rickets (restlessness, craniotabes, costochondral beading, bowlegs, kyphoscoliosis) **Adults:** Osteomalacia	High-dose oral vitamin D
E	Associated with severe malabsorption	Areflexia, peripheral neuropathy, gait abnormality, ophthalmoplegia, ↓ proprioception	Oral vitamin E
K	Poor diet, malabsorption, antibiotics	Clotting factor deficiencies (II, VII, IX, X)	Vitamin K SQ

TABLE 2.10. **Presentation and Treatment of Water-Soluble Vitamin Deficiencies**

VITAMIN	ETIOLOGY	SYMPTOMS/EXAM	TREATMENT
B$_1$ (thiamine)	The most common cause is alcoholism	Anorexia, muscle cramps, paresthesias. Dry beriberi leading to neuropathy and Wernicke-Korsakoff syndrome; wet beriberi leading to high-output heart failure	Oral thiamine
B$_2$ (riboflavin)	Usually occurs with other deficiencies	Nonspecific symptoms (eg, mouth soreness, glossitis, cheilosis, weakness, irritability) plus seborrheic dermatitis and anemia	Oral vitamin B$_2$
B$_3$ (niacin)	Associated with alcoholism	Nonspecific symptoms (see above); **pellagra** (Figure 2.2) (dermatitis, diarrhea, dementia)	Oral nicotinamide
B$_6$ (pyridoxine)	Associated with medication interactions (INH, OCPs) or with alcoholism; fat malabsorption syndromes may contribute	Nonspecific symptoms (see above); **peripheral neuropathy,** anemia, and seizures. Levels can be measured (normal >50 ng/mL)	Oral or intramuscular vitamin B$_6$
B$_{12}$ (cyanocobalamin)	Found in vegans, gastrectomy patients, gastric bypass patients, and those with pernicious anemia	Megaloblastic anemia, **glossitis,** anorexia, diarrhea. Peripheral neuropathy, balance problems, **dementia** (reversible if treated within 6 months)	Vitamin B$_{12}$ administered intramuscularly
C (ascorbic acid)	Found in urban poor, elderly, alcoholics, cancer patients, smokers, and those in renal failure	**Scurvy:** Poor wound healing, easy bruising, bleeding gums, subperiosteal hemorrhage, and anemia leading to edema, oliguria, neuropathy, and intracerebral hemorrhage	Oral vitamin C
Biotin	Caused by eating large quantities of raw eggs	Myalgias, dysesthesias, anorexia, and nausea leading to dermatitis and **alopecia**	Oral biotin
Folic acid	Caused by inadequate dietary intake	Megaloblastic anemia, neural tube defects	Oral folic acid

NUTRITIONAL AND HERBAL SUPPLEMENTS

Vitamin and Minerals in Disease Prevention

Current evidence is insufficient to assess the balance of benefits and harms of the use of the following:

- Multivitamins for the prevention of chronic disease such as cardiovascular disease and cancer.
- Vitamin D and calcium supplementation for prevention of fractures in premenopausal women or men and in postmenopausal women.

Be cautious in offering several vitamins, including A, C, and E, with antioxidant functions for protection against cancer, heart disease, and Alzheimer disease since studies report equivocal results for these effects, and several vitamins have been shown to be detrimental at high doses.

Herbal Supplements

More than 40% of the US population uses some type of complementary or alternative medicine. Effects of herbal supplements are difficult to evaluate due to problems in isolating the active component. Table 2.11 lists herbal supplements with demonstrated safety. Certain herbal remedies have been associated with deleterious effects and should be used with caution. Examples include:

- **Black licorice:** Causes hypertension.
- **Chromium:** ↓ blood sugar.
- **Garlic, ginger, gingko, ginseng, feverfew, CoQ10:** Prolong INR.

Domestic Violence

INTIMATE-PARTNER ABUSE

Defined as **intentional controlling by or violent behavior from** a person who was or is in an intimate relationship with the victim. This behavior may be **physical abuse, sexual assault, emotional abuse, economic control, and/or social isolation.**

- Women are more likely than men to be the victims of chronic physical abuse.
- Violence in gay and lesbian relationships appears to be as common as in heterosexual relationships.
- Most states do not currently require mandatory reporting of domestic violence against competent adults. Table 2.12 outlines risk factors for intimate-partner abuse.

TABLE 2.11. Effects of Selected Herbal Supplements

SUPPLEMENT	DISEASE/CONDITION	NOTES
Garlic powder	High cholesterol	Has modest effect; prolongs INR
Ginger root	Nausea, motion sickness	Studies are conflicting on whether ginger is effective for motion sickness; probably safe but may interact with many medications
Glucosamine	Osteoarthritis	Use with caution in the presence of seafood allergy
Horse chestnut	Venous insufficiency	β-escin, a mixture of triterpene saponins isolated from the horse chestnut seeds, has been shown in randomized controlled trials to have efficacy in chronic venous insufficiency; its mechanism of action remains unknown
Peppermint oil	IBS	Use supported by data from clinical trials
Saw palmetto	BPH	Give at a dose of 160 mg BID or 320 mg once per day
St John's wort	Depression	Comparable efficacy and safety when compared with SSRIs in patients with mild to moderate depression; caution with use is advised due to multiple drug interactions

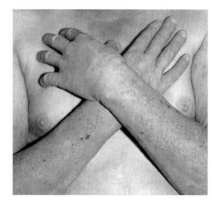

FIGURE 2.2. Pellagra. Characterized by an erythematous rash in sun-exposed skin. Findings range from obvious scaly erythema to subtle changes that are often mistaken for the photo-damage typically seen in elderly patients. (Reproduced from Oldham MA, et al. Pellagrous encephalopathy presenting as alcohol withdrawal delirium: A case series and literature review. *Addict Sci Clin Pract.* 2012;7(1):12; courtesy of Richard Johnson, MD, Department of Dermatology, Massachusetts General Hospital, Boston, MA USA, 2012.)

KEY FACT

Be aware of herbal remedies that interact with warfarin, including **g**arlic, **g**inger, **g**ingko, **g**inseng, feverfew, and CoQ10.

KEY FACT

Be alert for signs and symptoms of intimate-partner violence. Women abused by their intimate partners are more vulnerable to contracting HIV or other STIs due to forced intercourse or prolonged exposure to stress.

QUESTION

A 30-year-old businessman who is relocating to India in 5 weeks presents for a pre-travel check-up. He has no significant medical history and is generally in good health. He provides his immunization record. He is worried about contracting malaria and having bouts of diarrhea. How do you address his concerns?

TABLE 2.12. **Risk Factors for Intimate-Partner Abuse**

RISK FACTORS	WHEN TO SUSPECT
Female gender	Inconsistent explanation of injuries
Young age	Delay in seeking treatment
Low socioeconomic status	Multiple somatic complaints
Pregnancy	Gynecologic conditions such as premenstrual
Mental health problems	syndrome, STIs, unintended pregnancy, or
Substance abuse on the part of victims or	chronic pelvic pain
perpetrators	Lateness for prenatal care visits
Separated or divorced status	Frequent ED visits
History of childhood abuse	Patient noncompliance
	Central distribution of injuries (breasts,
	abdomen, genitals)

CHILD ABUSE

This important topic is addressed in the Child and Adolescent Medicine chapter.

Travel Medicine

Travel is associated with potential morbidity and even mortality from infectious sources, modes of transportation, environmental exposures, and adverse medical outcomes from illnesses independent of travel. In addition, always address safe sex strategies when a patient will be traveling. Offer the following guidelines and recommendations to those contemplating or planning travel to reduce the risk of adverse events. Please see the CDC Web site for up-to-date information regarding specific locations.

PRETRAVEL ASSESSMENT

 Determine the patient's **health status** (eg, infants, elderly persons, pregnant women, or those with chronic illnesses or underlying medical conditions).
 Identify potential **medical needs** (eg, allergy to vaccine components, medication use, immunosuppression).
 Evaluate the patient's **travel itinerary** (eg, planned destinations, climate and altitude, rural vs urban environment, duration of stay, accommodations, purpose of travel).

GENERAL GUIDELINES FOR SAFE TRAVEL

 Food: Advise patients that **fruits are safe only when peeled** and that **vegetables need to be fully cooked** to prevent contamination from fecally passed organisms in the soil. Unpasteurized dairy products and inadequately cooked fish or meat should be avoided.
 Water: Counsel patients to **avoid ice cubes** and that water is safe only after it has been boiled. Chlorination will kill most viral and bacterial pathogens, but protozoal pathogens such as *Giardia lamblia* can survive. Carbonated drinks, beer, wine, and drinks made from boiled water are safe.
 Insect repellents: Advise travelers to use at least **20% DEET** on clothing and exposed skin to prevent mosquito-borne infections such as malaria, yellow fever, dengue fever, and Zika virus. Protection with DEET lasts for several hours but is mitigated by swimming, washing, sweating, wiping, and rain. Travelers may also choose to

treat clothing and bed netting with **permethrin**, which can effectively repel mosquitoes for more than a week, even with washing.

- **Medications:** Advise travelers to bring adequate supplies of regularly used medications, since equivalent drugs may not be available at their destinations. Medications should be stored in carry-on luggage in the event that checked baggage is lost in transit.
- **Other advice:** Counsel patients to **avoid swimming in fresh water** in areas where schistosomiasis is prevalent. Swimming in chlorinated or salt water is safe. Give patients safe-sex counseling and advice regarding sun protection.

KEY FACT

Guidelines for travelers in regards to food and water: "Boil it, cook it, peel it, or forget it!"

RECOMMENDED VACCINATIONS BEFORE TRAVEL

Address three **categories of immunizations:**
- **Routine or standard:** Review childhood immunization programs and age-appropriate updates, regardless of travel (see Table 2.1).
- **Required:** Offer **yellow fever** vaccine for travel to certain parts of sub-Saharan Africa and tropical South America. Offer the **meningococcal** vaccine for travel to Saudi Arabia during the Hajj (required by the Saudi Arabian government).
- **Recommended:** Offer HAV, HBV, typhoid fever, meningococcal meningitis, Japanese encephalitis, rabies, and tick-borne encephalitis, depending on the trip-related risk and exposure to such diseases.

MALARIA PROPHYLAXIS

Address malaria prophylaxis with all patients planning travel to endemic regions. Malaria is transmitted by the female *Anopheles* mosquito and is most commonly caused by the organism *Plasmodium falciparum*; other species include *P vivax*, *P malariae*, and *P ovale*. Symptoms can begin from 8 days after initial infection to several months after departure from regions with high prevalence of malaria. The two most important components of malaria prevention are **avoidance of mosquitoes and chemoprophylaxis** (Table 2.13).

KEY FACT

Advise travelers to minimize exposure between dusk and dawn since mosquitoes that transmit malaria usually feed at night.

TRAVELER'S DIARRHEA

Approximately 40% to 60% of travelers to developing countries have diarrhea. Of these cases, 85% are caused by bacterial pathogens, the most common of which is **enterotoxigenic *E coli* (ETEC).** Parasites account for 10% and viruses for 5% of cases. Counsel patients traveling to developing countries on the following preventive measures:
- Advise travelers to pay attention to food and beverage selection (see the guidelines listed above).
- You may offer **bismuth subsalicylate,** the active ingredient in Pepto-Bismol, which has been shown to ↓ **the incidence of traveler's diarrhea** from 40% to 14%. Discuss side effects, which include blackening of the tongue and stool, nausea, constipation, and, rarely, tinnitus. **Avoid use in children** with viral infections because of the risk of Reye syndrome.
- Do not routinely offer prophylactic antibiotics to travelers.

KEY FACT

Avoid the use of bismuth subsalicylate in patients with aspirin allergy, renal insufficiency, and gout and in those taking anticoagulants, probenecid, or methotrexate.

Symptoms/Exam

- Patients may present with malaise, anorexia, nausea, vomiting, and abdominal cramps, followed by sudden onset of watery diarrhea 4 to 14 days after arrival, with symptoms lasting 1 to 5 days.
- Patients typically do not present with symptoms of colitis such as blood or pus in the stool ± low-grade fever.

TABLE 2.13. **Drugs Used for Malaria Prophylaxis**

DRUG NAME	INDICATION	ADMINISTRATION	SAFE FOR CHILDREN?	SAFE IN PREGNANCY?	SIDE EFFECTS
Atovaquone/ proguanil (Malarone)	Prophylaxis in areas with chloroquine-resistant or mefloquine-resistant *P falciparum*	Daily dosing Begin 1-2 days before travel and continue for 7 days after leaving the malarious area	Yes, if weight is >11 kg	No	Abdominal pain, nausea, vomiting, headache, rash
Chloroquine phosphate (Aralen and generic)	Prophylaxis only in areas with chloroquine-sensitive *P falciparum*	Weekly dosing Begin 1-2 weeks before travel and continue for 4 weeks after departure from the malarious area	Yes	Yes	GI disturbance, dizziness, blurred vision, headache, insomnia, pruritus
Doxycycline	Prophylaxis in areas with chloroquine-resistant or mefloquine-resistant *P falciparum*	Daily dosing Begin 1-2 days before travel and continue for 4 weeks after departure from the malarious area	Yes, if ≥8 years of age	No	Photosensitivity skin reactions
Mefloquine (Lariam and generic)	Prophylaxis in areas with chloroquine-resistant *P falciparum*	Weekly dosing Begin 1-2 weeks before travel and continue for 4 weeks after departure from the malarious area	Yes	Yes, in the second and third trimesters	Nausea, dizziness, vertigo Lightheadedness, bad dreams, paranoid ideation, seizures, psychosis in patients with significant psychopathology
Primaquine	Good choice for prophylaxis in areas where *P vivax* is the main species	Begin 1-2 days before travel and continue daily until 7 days after departure	Yes, if not G6PD deficient	No	In G6PD-normal persons, GI upset if taken on empty stomach is common In G6PD deficiency, primaquine can cause fatal hemolysis. Rule out **G6PD deficiency by appropriate lab test** before use

Management

- **Replace fluids:** The primary and most important treatment! Replete both fluid **volume** and **electrolytes.**
- Give **antibiotics** for those presenting with moderate to severe diarrhea characterized by more than four unformed stools daily; fever; or blood, pus, or mucus in the stool. Use **ciprofloxacin;** in areas of ↑ resistance to fluoroquinolones the recommended treatment is **azithromycin.**

- Do not use antimotility agents for mild to moderate cases; use only in severe cases in conjunction with antibiotics. Discontinue if abdominal pain worsens or if diarrhea persists after 2 days.
- You may use **bismuth subsalicylate,** which has antisecretory and antimicrobial properties, to ↓ stool frequency and shorten the duration of illness (15 mL or two tablets every 30 minutes for up to eight doses).
- Advise patients to seek medical care in the presence of high fever, severe abdominal pain, bloody diarrhea, or vomiting, and when antibiotics have not been helpful.

KEY FACT

Replace fluids in patients with diarrhea using a solution of ½ teaspoon of salt, ½ teaspoon of baking soda, and 4 tablespoons of sugar in 1 L of water.

Occupational Medicine

Work-related injuries and illnesses are prevalent and are associated with significant morbidity, mortality, and cost, both to the individual and to society.
- Pulmonary diseases predominate occupational illnesses. The etiologies and presentation of common occupational pulmonary illnesses are outlined in Table 2.14.
- Common nonpulmonary occupational illnesses include carpal tunnel syndrome, low back pain/injury, and contact dermatitis.

EVALUATION OF ILLNESS

Use the following guidelines to evaluate occupational illness:
- Take a **brief history** of possible work-related injuries or illnesses, including symptoms/review of systems; current and past jobs held; and the temporal relationship of the symptoms to jobs or work schedule.

KEY FACT

Occupational exposures that can present with fever include toxic organic dust syndrome, hypersensitivity pneumonitis, and metal fume fever (zinc exposure).

TABLE 2.14.   **Common Occupational Pulmonary Disorders**

ILLNESS	AGENTS/POTENTIAL EXPOSURE	CLINICAL PRESENTATION
Asthma	Isocyanates, flour, dyes, metals, wood dust, latex Rubber or plastic production, bakers	Rhinoconjunctivitis, wheezing
Silicosis	Crystalline silica mining, quarrying, sandblasting, masonry, foundry work, ceramics	May be asymptomatic, with an abnormal CXR (nodules or fibrosis), or may present with cough and dyspnea
Asbestosis	Textiles, shipbuilding, cement, insulation, plumbing, pipefitting, renovation of asbestos-containing buildings	After 20-30 years, presents with dyspnea on exertion; fine bibasilar crackles and clubbing may also be seen CXR shows interstitial fibrosis and pleural plaques **Can lead to mesothelioma**
Toxic organic dust syndrome	Moldy hay	Fever, cough, wheezing, dyspnea
Hypersensitivity pneumonitis (extrinsic allergic alveolitis)	Farmer's lung, hot tub lung, humidifiers, birds/poultry, grain processing, lumber milling/construction	**Acute:** Fever, malaise, cough, dyspnea, chest tightness (no wheeze!) 4-6 hours after exposure **Chronic:** Weight loss, fatigue, dyspnea, clubbing; consider in the presence of recurrent "pneumonias"

QUESTION

A 57-year-old male smoker presents with complaints of feeling out of breath when he takes walks with his wife. He denies any chest pain or other cardiac symptoms. He has worked in shipbuilding for >30 years. Pulmonary exam reveals some fine crackles. He also has fingernail clubbing. What are your next steps?

■ Include other components of the history such as **evaluation of products used** or manufactured at the workplace, examination of Material Safety Data Sheets (MSDSs), and assessment of the degree of protective measures taken (eg, protective clothing, appropriate ventilation).
■ **The physical exam** should include evaluation of the lungs, skin, and any painful musculoskeletal region as well as an examination of the extremities for clubbing.
■ **Diagnostic testing** will often begin with a CXR and PFTs.

The following groups may be of aid if on-site investigation is necessary:
■ **Occupational Safety and Health Administration (OSHA):** Within the Department of Labor. Creates and enforces workplace safety and health regulations.
■ **Environmental Protection Agency (EPA).**
■ **National Institute for Occupational Safety and Health (NIOSH):** Part of the Centers for Disease Control and Prevention (CDC) and within the Department of Health and Human Services (DHHS). Conducts research and makes recommendations for the prevention of work-related illnesses and injuries.
■ American College of Occupational and Environmental Medicine (ACOEM).
■ Association of Occupational and Environmental Clinics (AOEC).
■ **Private certified industrial hygienists.**
■ **Poison Control Centers.**

IMPAIRMENT VERSUS DISABILITY

In your assessment, you may state just the objective findings and degree to which the patient's functional capacity is limited. You do not need to and are not expected to make a disability determination.
■ **Impairment:** Defined as loss or abnormality of psychological, physiological, or anatomical structure or functioning of a body part or organ system, which can be shown by medically acceptable clinical and laboratory diagnostic techniques.
■ **Disability:** An impediment that prevents an individual from interacting with the environment at the specific level determined by the legal system. Defined by the Social Security Administration as "the inability to engage in any substantial gainful activity by reason of any medically determinable physical or mental impairment which can be expected to lead to death or which has lasted or can be expected to last for a continuous period of not less than 12 months."

Public Health

TUBERCULOSIS

Prevention of Active TB

■ Obtain **annual screen** with PPD or interferon gamma release assay test (in asymptomatic individuals) for:
  ■ People with an HIV infection.
  ■ Health care workers, prison guards, mycobacteriology laboratory personnel.
  ■ People with a medical condition that ↑ the risk of active TB (eg, diabetes, use of immunosuppressive medications, end-stage renal disease, alcoholism, conditions associated with rapid weight loss or chronic malnutrition).
  ■ Homeless individuals and people who inject drugs.
  ■ People who reside in a long-term care facility.
■ Obtain a **one-time screen** for:
  ■ Those with a single potential exposure to TB (repeat PPD in 6-12 weeks if the exposure is recent).

ANSWER

You suspect COPD as well as possible asbestosis and obtain a CXR and PFTs.

- Anyone with an incidentally discovered fibrotic lung lesion.
- Immigrants and refugees from countries with a high prevalence of TB.

Latent Tuberculosis Infection (LTBI)

LTBI represents a large subset of infections caused by *Mycobacterium tuberculosis*, which infects 19% to 43% of the world's population. The lifetime risk of acquiring reactivation TB with LTBI is roughly 10% to 20%, with 2% to 5% developing active TB in the first 2 years. If cases of LTBI are not detected and treated, new cases of TB will continually develop from this group.

Diagnosis

- Use **TST** via PPD to detect LTBI. A delayed-type hypersensitivity reaction mediated by T lymphocytes results in induration of the skin 48 to 72 hours after inoculation.
- False-negative skin tests may be seen in cases of:
  - Anergic states such as HIV and malignancy.
  - Newly diagnosed pulmonary TB or severe extrapulmonary TB.
  - Corticosteroids or immunosuppressive therapy.
  - Concurrent viral infection.
  - Poor nutrition.
- Because different types of exposures and varying baseline immune status result in a wide distribution of PPD reactions, criteria have been developed to minimize the number of false positives (Table 2.15).
- For persons who have received the BCG vaccine as children, interpret based on the criteria used for unvaccinated persons. Large PPD reactions in these individuals are still likely to represent TB infection.
- Obtain a CXR for all individuals with a ⊕ PPD to exclude active disease.

KEY FACT

Tuberculin skin test conversion occurs 2 to 12 weeks after 1° infection.

Management

- Offer INH therapy for 6 to 12 months (9 months ideally) to reduce the risk of reactivation TB in individuals with a ⊕ PPD. Its protective effect lasts at least 20 years and probably for life. Treat all individuals with a ⊕ PPD, regardless of age.
- Reserve rifampin for suspected INH-resistant strains in view of the ↑ incidence of rifampin-associated liver toxicity.
- Consider ordering initial and monthly liver panels in patients at ↑ risk for hepatitis (eg, alcoholics, those with chronic liver disease, HIV-positive patients, drug interaction).
- Warn patients of signs of hepatitis.
- Consider concurrent administration of pyridoxine (vitamin B_6, 25-50 mg/day) for patients at ↑ risk for peripheral neuropathy, paresthesias, and ataxia, such as the

KEY FACT

INH therapy ↓ the risk of reactivation TB in LTBI by roughly 70% if taken for 6 months and by >90% if taken for 12 months.

TABLE 2.15.   Criteria for a Positive PPD

≥5-mm INDURATION	10-mm INDURATION	15-mm INDURATION
Recent contact	Immigrants who have come	No risk factors
HIV infection	from a high-prevalence	
Chronic steroid use	country within the last 5	
Organ transplantation/	years	
immunosuppression	IV drug users	
Inactive TB on x-ray, untreated	Residents/employees of high-	
	risk facilities (hospitals, jails,	
	nursing homes, shelters)	
	Those <4 years of age	
	Those <18 years of age who	
	have been exposed to a	
	high-risk adult	

Q   QUESTION

A 43-year-old homeless man presents to your clinic to establish care. He has occasional wheezing but has had no fevers, night sweats, or cough. His medical problems include diabetes, hypertension, and tobacco use. He reports that some of the men who lived at his previous shelter were recently diagnosed with active TB infection. Should you screen for TB?

elderly, HIV-positive patients, children, people with diabetes, alcoholics, pregnant or breastfeeding women, those with chronic liver disease, and those in renal failure.

Epidemiology and Biostatistics

LEADING CAUSES OF DEATH

Table 2.16 outlines the principal causes of mortality, grouped by age.

TEST PARAMETERS

Common terms used in statistical methodology are as follows:
- **Incidence:** Defined as the **number of new cases** of a disease in a defined population over a specific period.
- **Prevalence:** Defined as the **number of existing cases** of disease in a given population over a specific period or a particular moment in time.
- **Sensitivity (Sn)—"PID" (Positive in Disease):** The probability that a test will be ⊕ in someone with the disease when compared with a gold standard; in other words, the test's **ability to correctly identify individuals who truly have the disease.**
- **Specificity (Sp)—"NIH" (Negative in Health):** The probability that a test will be ⊖ in someone who truly does not have the disease when compared with a gold standard; in other words, the test's **ability to correctly identify individuals who truly do not have the disease.**

In general, if a disease has a **low prevalence,** choose a **more specific test,** and if it has a **high prevalence,** choose a **more sensitive** test.
- **Positive predictive value (PPV):** The proportion of persons testing ⊕ who have the condition; in other words, **of all the people who test ⊕, the probability that they truly have the disease** (or the probability of disease in patient with a ⊕ test result).
- **Negative predictive value (NPV):** The proportion of persons testing ⊖ who do not have the disease; in other words, **of all the people who test ⊖, the probability that they truly do not have the disease** (or the probability of not having disease when test result is ⊖).
- **Likelihood ratio (LR):** Defined as the proportion of patients **with** a disease who have a certain test result over the proportion of patients **without** the disease who have the given test result (remember: "WOWO"—with over without).
  - Pretest odds of a disease × LR = posttest odds of a disease.
  - Positive LR = sensitivity / (1 − specificity) or true positives/false positives; for example, a high-probability V/Q scan has an LR of 14. This means that a ⊕ V/Q scan is 14 times more likely to be seen in patients **with** pulmonary embolism than in those **without** pulmonary embolism.
  - Negative LR = (1 − sensitivity)/specificity; it shows how much the odds of disease are ↓ if the test result is negative.

TABLE 2.16.   Leading Causes of Death by Age Group

1-24 YEARS	25-64 YEARS	65 YEARS AND OLDER
Unintentional injuries	Malignant neoplasms	Heart disease
Suicide and homicide	Heart disease	Malignant neoplasms
Malignant neoplasms	Unintentional injuries	Cerebrovascular disease
Heart disease	HIV	COPD
Congenital anomalies	Suicide and homicide	Alzheimer disease

- **Lead-time bias:** Lead time is the time by which a screening test advances the date of diagnosis from the usually symptomatic phase to an earlier presymptomatic phase. The time between diagnosis and death will always ↑ by the amount of lead time (Figure 2.3). To avoid lead-time bias, the lead time must be subtracted from the overall survival time of screened patients.
    - **Example:** A new screening test for pancreatic cancer is able to detect disease in a presymptomatic stage. Unfortunately, because the poor overall prognosis for the disease remains the same, screened patients know about their disease sooner and live with the disease longer but will still die of pancreatic cancer at the same rate.
- **Length-time bias:** Because cases vary in the length of their asymptomatic phase, screening will overdetect cases of slowly progressing disease (longer asymptomatic phases) and miss rapidly progressive cases (Figure 2.4).
- **Relative risk (risk ratio):** Used in cohort studies and randomized controlled trials. Defined as the incidence of a disease in exposed individuals divided by the incidence of disease in unexposed individuals.
    - **Example:** Individuals with a high dietary fiber intake and those with a low fiber intake are evaluated for colon cancer to determine if fiber intake is a risk factor for colon cancer. Results may be a statement such as "Individuals who do not have a high-fiber diet have been shown to have a relative risk of 1.7 of developing colon cancer."
- **Odds ratio:** Used in case-control studies. Defined as the odds that an individual with a specific condition has been exposed to a risk factor divided by the odds that a control has been exposed.
    - **Example:** Individuals with colon cancer are compared with matched controls without colon cancer in terms of fiber intake. Results may be a statement such as "Individuals with colon cancer were *x* times less likely to have had a high-fiber diet than those without colon cancer."
- **Absolute risk:** Calculated by subtracting the incidence of a disease in unexposed persons from the incidence of disease in exposed persons (usually in percentage points).
- **Number needed to treat (NNT):** The number of patients needed to treat to prevent one additional bad outcome. NNT is the inverse of absolute risk.

MAJOR STUDY TYPES

Table 2.17 outlines the types of studies conducted in epidemiologic and biostatistical analyses.

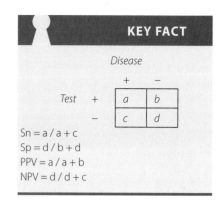

KEY FACT

Disease

		+	−
Test	+	a	b
	−	c	d

Sn = a / a + c
Sp = d / b + d
PPV = a / a + b
NPV = d / d + c

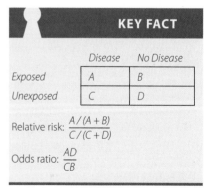

KEY FACT

Patients whose diseases are detected by screening will always live longer than patients whose diseases are detected clinically, even if early detection and treatment confer no benefit because of lead-time and length-time biases.

KEY FACT

	Disease	No Disease
Exposed	A	B
Unexposed	C	D

Relative risk: $\dfrac{A/(A+B)}{C/(C+D)}$

Odds ratio: $\dfrac{AD}{CB}$

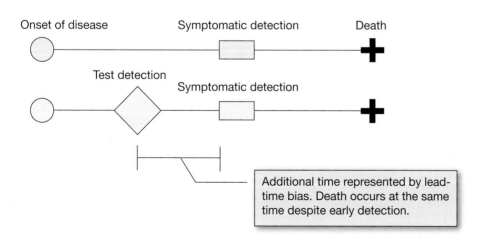

FIGURE 2.3. **Lead-time bias.**

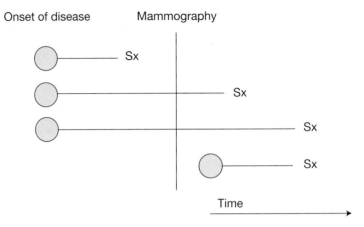

FIGURE 2.4.   **Length-time bias.** Two cases of breast cancer with brief time between disease onset and symptom appearance (top and bottom cases) are missed by routine mammography. Two other cases, with longer presymptomatic phases, are detected by mammography.

THREATS TO VALIDITY

- **Confounding factor** is a variable that is associated with both the predictor variable and the outcome variable but does not have a causal relationship with either.
- **Recall bias** is self-reporting by subjects that is often influenced by knowledge of the study hypothesis.
- **Misclassification bias** occurs when a person without disease is "misclassified" into the disease group or vice versa.
- **Random misclassification** occurs when subjects are randomly placed in the wrong group, biasing results to the null hypothesis.
- **Nonrandom misclassification** occurs when subjects are selectively placed in the wrong group, biasing results either toward or away from the null hypothesis. Also referred to as **systematic or differential misclassification.**
- **Selection bias** occurs when subjects are selected into or drop out of a study in a way that falsely changes the degree of association.

TABLE 2.17.   **Categories of Studies**

STUDY TYPE	DEFINITION	EXAMPLE	ADVANTAGES	DISADVANTAGES
Randomized controlled trial	Subjects are **assigned** to an exposure, and disease outcomes are observed	Assigning patients with hypertension to receive either a diuretic or an ACEI	Controls for unforeseen confounders	Expensive
Cohort study	Exposed subjects are identified and then **followed** for disease outcomes	Identifying obese children and then following them for the development of type 2 diabetes	The most robust observational study type; can evaluate multiple exposures	May take a long time to develop disease outcomes
Case-control study	Cases and noncases of the disease are identified **before** defining the exposure	Identifying children with certain birth defects and then looking for possible prenatal exposures	Inexpensive; fast; ideal for rare diseases	Prone to biases
Cross-sectional study	Exposures and disease outcomes are **identified at the same time** within a **specific population** of subjects	Checking for childhood diabetes while obtaining data on obesity in all children seen in specific community health clinics	Survey data	Cannot detect temporal relationship between exposure and outcome

HYPOTHESIS TESTING

- **Null hypothesis:** The theory that the exposure or intervention being studied is not associated with the outcome of interest.
- **P value:** Quantitative estimate of the probability that a study's outcome could occur by chance alone. A study with a $P < .05$ means that the probability of the results occurring by chance alone is <1 in 20 and is thus "statistically significant."
- **Type I error (α):** The probability of detecting a difference when none exists and thus rejecting the null hypothesis.
- **Type II error (β):** The probability of failing to detect a difference when one exists and thus failing to reject the null hypothesis.
- **Power:** The probability of avoiding a type II error in a study; in other words, the probability that a study will not accept the null hypothesis and conclude that there was no difference when there really was one.

CLINICAL TRIALS

Defined as studies in humans that answer specific health questions, including whether experimental treatments or new ways of using known treatments are safe and effective. Ideally conducted clinical trials provide one of the fastest and safest tools with which to change disease management and improve health in a population. Clinical trials must proceed through four phases (Table 2.18). Types of trials include the following:

- **Treatment trials:** Test experimental treatments, new combinations of drugs, or new approaches to surgery or radiation therapy.
- **Prevention trials:** Investigate better ways to prevent disease in a disease-free population or to prevent recurrent disease.
- **Diagnostic trials:** Investigate better tests or procedures for diagnosing a specific disease.
- **Screening trials:** Test the best way to detect disease and health conditions.
- **Quality-of-life trials:** Investigate for ways to improve comfort and quality of life for individuals with chronic diseases or illnesses.

EVIDENCE-BASED MEDICINE

Evidence-based medicine can provide you with the tools for finding, understanding, and using the most up-to-date data from clinical research and making sound recommendations for patient care. The criteria by which evidence is graded are listed in Tables 2.19 and 2.20.

TABLE 2.18. **Phases of Clinical Trials**

PHASE	DESCRIPTION
Phase I	The experimental drug or treatment is tested in a small group of people (20-80) for the first time to evaluate **safety,** to determine safe **dosage ranges,** and to identify **side effects**
Phase II	The experimental drug or treatment is tested in a larger group of people (100-300) to evaluate **efficacy** and further evaluate **safety**
Phase III	The experimental drug or treatment is given to large groups of people (1000-3000) to confirm **efficacy,** to monitor for **side effects,** and to **compare** it with treatments already in use
Phase IV	Postmarketing studies to determine additional information, including risks, benefits, and optimal use

TABLE 2.19.   **Levels of Evidence (Oxford Centre for Evidence-Based Medicine)**

LEVEL	DESCRIPTION
1a	Systematic review of randomized controlled trials
1b	Individual randomized controlled trial
1c	All-or-none[a]
2a	Systematic review of cohort studies
2b	Individual cohort study
2c	Outcomes research[b] and ecological studies
3a	Systematic review of case-control studies
3b	Individual case-control study
4	Case series
5	Expert opinion

[a]Met when all patients died before the treatment became available, but some now survive on it; or when some patients died before the treatment became available, but none now die on it.

[b]Looks at whether predicted outcomes (based on randomized controlled trials) are actually being observed in clinical practice.

Health Insurance Coverage

MEDICARE AND MEDICAID

The United States has two major publicly funded health insurance plans: Medicare and Medicaid. These plans are compared in detail in Table 2.21.

AFFORDABLE CARE ACT

In March 2010, President Obama signed into law the Affordable Care Act, which was then upheld by the Supreme Court in 2012. It went into effect in 2014. The overall goals of this bill were to improve quality and access to care while reducing costs.

- Insurance coverage was expanded and the uninsured percent of the population is now at the lowest rate since the presence of health insurance in the United States.
- Insurance companies have been limited in excluding coverage of a "preexisting condition."
- Young adults are able to stay on their parent's insurance coverage until the age of 26.
- Many routine preventive care services are now covered free of charge.

TABLE 2.20.   **Grades of Recommendation (Oxford Centre for Evidence-Based Medicine)**

GRADE	DESCRIPTION
A	Consistent level 1 studies
B	Consistent level 2 or 3 studies or extrapolations from level 1 studies
C	Level 4 studies or extrapolations from level 2 or 3 studies
D	Level 5 evidence or troublingly inconsistent or inconclusive studies of any level

TABLE 2.21.   **Comparison of Medicare and Medicaid**

FUNDING SOURCE	MEDICARE	MEDICAID
Eligibility	Federal government Those >65 years of age (who have worked and therefore have contributed to Medicare through payroll taxes) Those <65 years of age who are receiving Social Security disability Patients receiving dialysis	Federal and state governments (the federal government reimburses each state 50%-83% of costs) Pregnant women plus women and their children <6 years of age if their family income is <133% of poverty level Children 6-17 years of age if their family income is <100% of poverty level The elderly poor The disabled poor Other optional groups vary by state
Benefits	**Part A:** Inpatient services, skilled nursing facility, home health and hospice **Part B:** Outpatient care, x-rays, durable medical equipment, laboratory work **Part C (Medicare Advantage):** Allows enrollment in Medicare-eligible HMOs or PPOs; includes additional services such as dentures, eyeglasses, and drugs **Part D:** Prescription drug benefit **Medigap:** Private supplemental insurance	Physician services; laboratory, x-ray, inpatient hospital care, family planning, prenatal, and maternity services Nursing home care services **Optional benefits:** Rehabilitation services, dental care, physical therapy, eyeglasses, intermediate-care facilities, inpatient psychiatric care for individuals >65 or <21 years of age
Physician reimbursement	**Medicare-Approved Amount (MAA):** Government-determined payment for any given service The physician can bill only up to the MAA Medicare pays 80% of the MAA and the patient pays 20%	Providers receive reimbursement directly from Medicaid and must accept that amount as payment in full

DISABILITY PROGRAMS

The United States government publicly funds three major disability programs: Social Security Disability Insurance (SSDI), Supplemental Security Income (SSI), and workers' compensation.

- **SSDI:** Like Medicare, SSDI is funded through payroll taxes. Once an individual meets both the definition of disabled (see the section on Occupational Medicine) and the eligibility criteria based on length of time employed and wages earned, he/she and dependents qualify for benefits. After 2 years on SSDI, the individual becomes eligible for Medicare benefits.
- **SSI:** Funded through general taxes rather than payroll or Social Security taxes. To be eligible, an individual must be >65 years of age, blind, or disabled. In addition, only individuals with limited income and resources qualify.
- **Workers' compensation:** This program pays for medical expenses incurred from an injury or illnesses related to employment. A portion of the worker's wages is also paid out during the period of disability. Workers who are partially disabled can receive long-term payments of a portion of their salary.

HEALTH INSURANCE PORTABILITY AND ACCOUNTABILITY ACT

The first-ever federal privacy standards to protect patients' medical records and other health information, the Health Insurance Portability and Accountability Act (HIPAA), developed by the DHHS, set standards that apply to health plans, doctors, hospitals, and other health care providers. Under HIPAA, patients have the right to access their medical records and control how their personal health information is used and disclosed. Patient protections include the following:

- **Access to medical records:** Patients should be able to see and obtain copies of their medical records and request that corrections be made.
- **Notice of privacy practices:** Covered health plans, doctors, and other health care providers must notify patients of their rights and how their personal medical information may be used.
- Limits on use of personal medical information.
- **Prohibition of marketing:** Patient authorization must be obtained before specific information may be used for marketing purposes.
- Confidential communications.
- **Complaints:** Patients have the right to file formal complaints regarding the privacy practices of a health plan or provider.

CHAPTER 3

Cardiology

Marina Fomina-Nazarova, MD, MBA

Diagnostic Testing

PHYSICAL EXAM

Pulses

Table 3.1 addresses causes of ↑ and ↓ pulses.

Heart Murmurs

See the Child and Adolescent Medicine chapter for a discussion of heart murmurs. Sites for auscultation of the heart are shown in Figure 3.1.

Heart Sounds

- **S1:** Closure of the mitral and tricuspid valves. ↓ with LV systolic dysfunction and mitral regurgitation. See Figure 3.2 for the relation of heart sounds to other parts of the cardiac cycle.
- **S2:** Closure of the aortic and pulmonary valves. Normally, the aortic component (A2) precedes the pulmonic component (P2).
  - **Physiologic splitting:** ↑ time between A2 and P2 with inspiration. P2 is delayed during inspiration as negative intrathoracic pressure pulls more blood volume into right side of the heart. Normalizes when the breath is held.
  - **Wide splitting:** Early closing of A2 or delayed P2. Causes include right bundle branch block (RBBB), pulmonic stenosis, pulmonary embolism (PE), or pulmonary hypertension (HTN).
  - **Paradoxical splitting:** A2 comes after P2 so ↑ splitting with expiration. Causes include aortic stenosis (AS), left bundle branch block (LBBB), use of a pacemaker, and left ventricular (LV) systolic dysfunction.
  - **Fixed splitting:** Time between A2 and P2 does not vary with breath. Caused by atrial septal defect (ASD).
- **S3:** Low-pitched sound after S2 as ↑ blood volume flows into dilated ventricle. Best heard with the bell at the apex. Suggests ventricular enlargement and LV systolic dysfunction such as heart failure (HF) and dilated cardiomyopathy.
- **S4:** Low-pitched sound preceding S1 as atrial contraction forces blood into a stiff ventricle.

CARDIAC TESTING

Electrocardiography

The key elements of an ECG are shown in Figure 3.3.

TABLE 3.1.   Alterations in Normal Pulses

	INCREASED	DECREASED	NOTES
Peripheral	Aortic regurgitation, persistent ductus arteriosus, ↑ cardiac output (sepsis, hyperthyroid)	Peripheral vascular disease, low cardiac output	**Water-hammer:** Radial rapid rise/fall, seen in aortic regurgitation
Central		Delayed and weak in aortic stenosis	**Pulsus bisferien:** Two pulse peaks, seen in aortic regurgitation and large patent ductus arteriosus
Jugular venous	Distention with volume overload, tamponade		

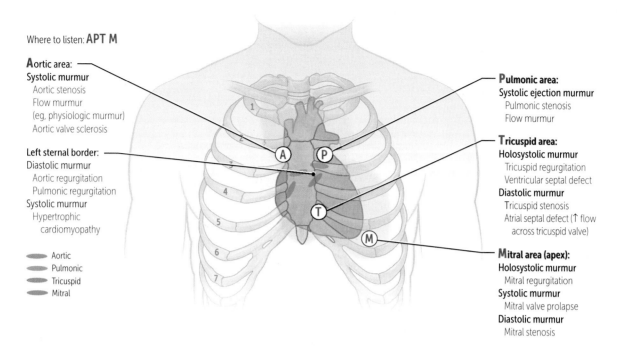

Where to listen: **APT M**

Aortic area:
Systolic murmur
  Aortic stenosis
  Flow murmur
  (eg, physiologic murmur)
  Aortic valve sclerosis

Left sternal border:
Diastolic murmur
  Aortic regurgitation
  Pulmonic regurgitation
Systolic murmur
  Hypertrophic
    cardiomyopathy

  Aortic
  Pulmonic
  Tricuspid
  Mitral

Pulmonic area:
Systolic ejection murmur
  Pulmonic stenosis
  Flow murmur

Tricuspid area:
Holosystolic murmur
  Tricuspid regurgitation
  Ventricular septal defect
Diastolic murmur
  Tricuspid stenosis
  Atrial septal defect (↑ flow
    across tricuspid valve)

Mitral area (apex):
Holosystolic murmur
  Mitral regurgitation
Systolic murmur
  Mitral valve prolapse
Diastolic murmur
  Mitral stenosis

FIGURE 3.1. **Common heart murmurs and where best to hear them.** (Reproduced with permission from USMLE-Rx.com.)

Definitions and guidelines pertinent to reading ECGs:
- **Dimensions:** One small box (1 mm) is 40 msec horizontally and 0.1 mV vertically.
- **Rate:** The normal rate is 60 to 100 bpm. For discussion of abnormal rates (bradycardia and tachycardia), see Dysrhythmias section.
- **Rhythm:** In sinus, there are P waves before every QRS complex. The P is upright in I, II, and avF. For discussion of abnormal rhythms such as atrial fibrillation (AFib), atrial flutter, and ventricular rhythms, see Dysrhythmias section.

QUESTION

Your patient requests help with pain management. Ultimately you decide to ↑ her current dose of methadone. What should you check after adjusting her dose?

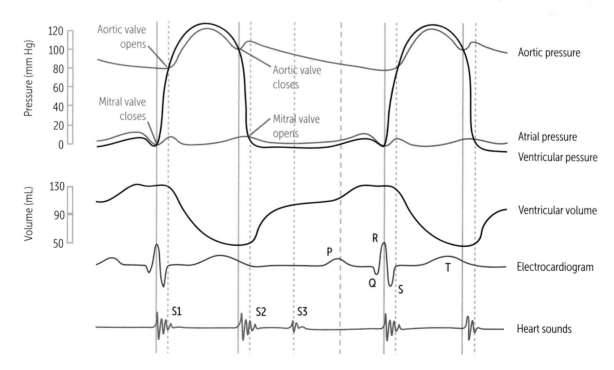

FIGURE 3.2. **Wiggers diagram.** Diagram shows the aortic, atrial, and ventricular pressures during the cardiac cycle and their relation to the ECG signal. (Reproduced with permission from USMLE-Rx.com.)

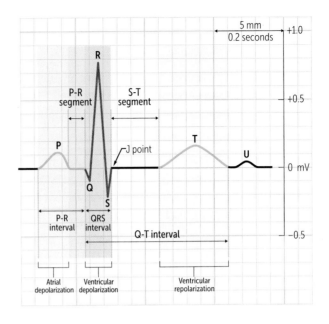

FIGURE 3.3. **Normal elements of an ECG.** (Reproduced with permission from USMLE-Rx.com.)

- **Axis:**
  - **Normal:** From −30 degrees to +90 degrees. **QRS** is net ⊕ in leads I and II.
  - **Left-deviated:** < −30 degrees. **QRS** is net ⊕ in I and net ⊖ in II. Associated with left anterior fascicular block (LAFB), left bundle branch block (LBBB), inferior MI, Wolff-Parkinson-White (WPW) syndrome with posteroseptal pathway, and COPD.
  - **Right-deviated:** >90 degrees. **QRS** is net ⊖ in lead I and net ⊕ in lead II. Associated with right ventricular hypertrophy (RVH), lateral or anterolateral MI, WPW syndrome with left-lateral pathway, and left posterior fascicular block (LPFB).
- **Intervals:**
  - **PR:** Normal 0.12-0.20 second. ↑ in AV blocks (see AV Blocks section).
  - **QRS:** Normal 0.12 second. Prolonged in bundle branch blocks, ventricularly paced rhythms (ventricular tachycardia or fibrillation, pacemakers), WPW, or aberrantly conducted supraventricular tachycardias (SVTs). See Dysrhythmias and Bundle Branch and Fascicular Blocks sections.
  - **QT:** Normal <50% of RR interval.
  - **QTc:** The corrected QT interval (QTc) estimates the QT interval at a heart rate of 60 bpm. This allows comparison of QT values at different heart rates and improves detection of patients at ↑ risk of arrhythmia. Abnormal defined as >0.44 second for men and >0.46 second for women.
  - Interval is **prolonged** in congenital conditions (long QT syndrome), metabolic abnormalities, drug use (antiarrhythmics, antibiotics, psychotropic drugs), MI, and mitral valve prolapse. Leads to ventricular arrhythmias such as torsades de pointes.
- **Hypertrophy:** ↑ LV mass associated with ↑ incidence of poor outcomes, including systolic dysfunction, HF, cerebrovascular accident, and death.
  - **LVH:** Many criteria—R in aVL is >11 mm (1.1 mV) **or** the sum of S in V_1 and R in V_5 or V_6 is >35 mm (3.5 mV).
  - **RVH:** Right-axis deviation. One criterion is R:S >1 in V_1. Another criterion is $RV_1 + SV_6$ >11 mm.

Noninvasive Cardiac Stress Testing

Used to diagnose CAD in patients in whom it is suspected and in the prognosis/management of patients with known CAD (Table 3.2).

TABLE 3.2.   **Stress-Testing Modalities**

MODE	STRESS METHOD	PLUSES/MINUSES	CONTRAINDICATIONS
Stress ECG	Exercise treadmill	+ **Widely available** – Less sensitive and specific than other modes, especially in women	Patient can't exercise to 85% of maximum heart rate Abnormal resting ECG (LBBB, WPW, ST-segment depressions, LVH) On digoxin or has pacemaker History of revascularization
Stress echocardiography	Exercise or pharmacologic (dobutamine)	+ Sensitivity and specificity are high (highest specificity) + Provides structural information + Lower cost than perfusion imaging – Interpretation is operator dependent	Symptomatic aortic aneurysm or high risk of ventricular arrhythmia Abnormal resting echo LBBB can lead to false ⊕ septal defect
Radionuclide myocardial perfusion imaging (sestamibi or thallium)	Exercise or pharmacologic (adenosine or dipyridamole)	+ Sensitivity and specificity are high (highest sensitivity mode) + **Can assess tissue viability with restriction study** (reversible vs fixed defects) – Involves radiation exposure	Hypotension, sick sinus syndrome, second/third-degree heart block, or severe reactive airway disease Use of caffeine within 24 hr or theophylline within 72 hr

Resting Echocardiography

Used to identify **anatomic abnormalities**; to assess the size, thickness, and function (ejection fraction, or EF) of chambers; and to evaluate valvular function. Wall motion abnormalities suggest CAD. Subtypes are as follows:
- **Transthoracic echocardiography (TTE):** Usually first modality tried due to ease of use.
  - **Doppler:** Characterizes blood flow and pressure gradients across valves. Useful for detecting stenotic or regurgitant blood flow.
  - **Bubble study:** Agitated normal saline injected intravenously to diagnose shunts.
- **Transesophageal echocardiography (TEE):** An ultrasound probe is placed in the esophagus to improve visualization of posterior cardiac structures.
  - **Indications:** Suspicion of left atrial thrombus, aortic dissection, or valvular vegetations.
  - **The sensitivity of TEE in endocarditis is 95% to 100%** (vs 40%-75% with TTE).

Cardiac Catheterization and Coronary Angiography

Indications:
- Stable angina with persistent symptoms despite medical management.
- **Acute coronary syndrome** (see section on Cardiac Ischemia/Acute Coronary Syndrome).
- Previous revascularization with recurrent symptoms to look for reocclusion.
- Aortic disease with concurrent angina to determine if coronary artery bypass grafting (CABG) might be performed at the time of valve replacement.
- Assessment of intracardiac pressures and oxygen saturations when pulmonary HTN or shunts are suspected.
- Assessment of severity of aortic stenosis.
- **Interventions include angioplasty and stenting.**

 QUESTION

A 34-year-old known IV drug user visits you because he has been feeling fatigued for the last several days and recently developed a painful rash on his hands. On physical exam, you notice a new pansystolic murmur over the fifth intercostal space at the left sternal border. You suspect endocarditis. What is the best imaging modality to confirm your diagnosis?

- **Coronary CT angiography:** Used in cases of atypical or low-risk cardiac chest pain to rapidly rule out obstructive CAD, where the expertise to obtain and interpret the study is available.
- **Cardiac MRI:** Assessment of myocardial viability for patients with ischemic cardiomyopathy and acute coronary syndrome, etiology and prognostic evaluation of nonischemic cardiomyopathies including myocarditis and arrythmogenic right ventricular cardiomyopathy, chronic pericarditis and cardiac masses, nonurgent aortic aneurysm and dissection, congenital cardiomyopathies, vascular malformations, and follow-up after curative or palliative surgery.

Dysrhythmias

BRADYCARDIA

Heart rate <55 to 60 bpm. Etiologies include:
- **Common:** Idiopathic degeneration, ischemic. Can be normal in highly conditioned athletes.
- **Rheumatologic:** SLE, RA, scleroderma.
- **Infectious:** Endocarditis, Chagas disease.
- **Infiltrative:** Sarcoidosis, amyloidosis, hemochromatosis, iatrogenic (due to SA or AV nodal blocking agents).
- **Autonomic:** ↑ vagal tone (carotid sinus hypersensitivity).
- **Iatrogenic:** Heart transplant, β-blockers, calcium channel blockers (CCBs), clonidine, digoxin, antiarrhythmics.
- **Metabolic:** Electrolyte abnormalities (hypo- and hyperkalemia), hypothyroidism, hypothermia.

Symptoms/Exam

- Dizziness, weakness, fatigue, and syncope. May be asymptomatic.
- Exam reveals ↓ pulse. Look for signs associated with the underlying cause of the bradycardia.

Diagnosis

- **ECG:** Heart rate <60 bpm. Look for dropped beats or AV dissociation.
- Metabolic workup, telemetry, event monitors, tilt-table testing, and electrophysiology studies can be helpful.

Management

- For unstable patients, follow the ACLS protocol.
- **Medications:** Atropine, glucagon (for β-blocker overdose), calcium (for CCB overdose).
- **Transcutaneous or transvenous pacing.**
- **Permanent pacemaker:** Consider for patients with documented symptomatic bradycardia, third-degree heart block, symptomatic 3-second or longer pause, 5-second or longer pause in atrial fibrillation (AF).

KEY FACT

Consider a permanent pacemaker for documented symptomatic bradycardia, third-degree heart block, symptomatic 3-second or longer pause, or 5-second pause in AF.

ANSWER

Transesophageal echocardiography.

NARROW QRS COMPLEX TACHYCARDIAS

Atrial Fibrillation

The **most common dysrhythmia in the general population** (0.5%-1.0%); prevalence ↑ with age. Of patients with diagnosis of stroke, 15% to 20% suffer from AF. The most common etiologies are **uncontrolled HTN and CAD.** Also common are valvular heart disease and HF. Less common etiologies include pulmonary disease (COPD,

PE), ischemia, rheumatic heart disease, hyperthyroidism, congenital heart disease, sepsis, alcoholism, WPW syndrome, and cardiac surgery.

Types of AF:
- **Paroxysmal:** Episodes last <7 days and usually <24 hours.
- **Persistent:** Lasts >7 days; responds to cardioversion but may recur afterward.
- **Permanent:** Present >1 year; failed cardioversion.
- **Lone:** One episode of AF in the absence of structural heart disease.

Symptoms/Exam

- Often asymptomatic. Palpitations, fatigue, dyspnea, dizziness, diaphoresis, HF, or ↓ exercise tolerance may be seen.
- Look for evidence of coexisting heart disease.

Diagnosis

- **ECG:** The most common cause of irregularly irregular rhythm is AF. The absence of P waves is diagnostic (Figure 3.4).
- **Echocardiogram:** Used to predict stroke risk with structural abnormalities such as left atrial enlargement, valvular disease, LVH, and ↓ EF. TEE is more effective for visualizing left atrial thrombi.
- Use the CHA_2DS_2-VASc score to evaluate the risk of ischemic stroke in patients with AF (Table 3.3).

Management

- **Rate control:** Preferred unless unstable. β-blockers and nondihydropyridone (DHP) CCBs (ie, verapamil, diltiazem) common. Administer digoxin in the presence of other comorbidities such as HF; administer amiodarone if hypotension is an issue.
- **Cardioversion:**
  - Indicated if the patient is unstable or if the duration of AF is <48 hours.
  - If >48 hours: First anticoagulate to prevent embolization of an atrial clot. Then perform TEE-guided cardioversion.
  - Anticoagulate for at least 4 weeks postcardioversion.
  - If AF recurs after cardioversion, treat with rate control and anticoagulation.
- **Anticoagulation:** To determine the need for anticoagulation, estimate stroke risk (see Table 3.3).

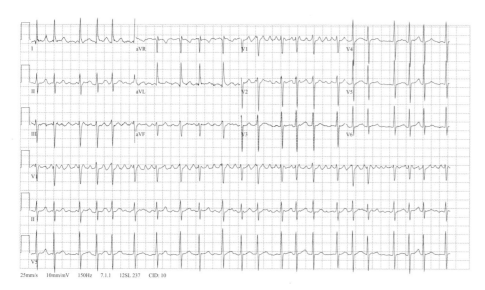

FIGURE 3.4. **Atrial fibrillation on ECG.** (Reproduced with permission from USMLE-Rx.com.)

25mm/s   10mm/mV   150Hz   7.1.1   12SL 237   CID: 10

QUESTION 1

An 85-year-old woman presents to the ED with intermittent palpitations and lightheadedness for the last month. Her medical conditions include HTN, diabetes, CAD with a previous stent, and hypothyroidism. Her BP is 145/80 mm Hg and pulse is 120 bpm. An ECG shows atrial fibrillation. Review of her records shows a previous ECG with this finding 3 years ago, with normal ECGs in the interim. In the ED, you determine that there is no urgent indication for cardioversion, and you lower her heart rate with β-blockers. She has no evidence of ischemia by biochemical markers and her TSH level is normal. An echocardiogram shows LVH but no other structural abnormalities or thrombus. How do you proceed?

QUESTION 2

A 62-year-old man is admitted to the ED with substernal chest pain radiating to his left jaw. The pain is not relieved with nitroglycerine. His BP is 85/50 mm Hg, pulse is 37 bpm, and respirations are 17/min. Physical exam is significant for fine crackles at lung bases bilateraly. ECG shows sinus bradycardia with 4-mm ST-segment elevations in leads II, III, and AVF. The patient reports feeling weak and dizzy. What is the next most appropriate step in management?

QUESTION 3

A 68-year-old man sees you in the office to discuss his anticoagulation treatment. He has been on warfarin for the last 4 years, but dislikes the medication because of the frequent INR checks and dose adjustments. He tells you that his neighbor also has AF but takes a medication that does not require blood tests. You review his history and notice that he has a prosthetic mitral valve. What is the best anticoagulation treatment for him?

TABLE 3.3. CHA$_2$DS$_2$-VASc Score

RISK FACTOR		POINTS[a]
C	Congestive heart failure	+1
H	Hypertension	+1
A$_2$	Age ≥75 yr	+2
D	Diabetes	+1
S$_2$	Stroke, TIA history, or thromboembolism	+2
V	Vascular disease	+1
A	Age 65-74 yr	+1
Sc	Sex category is female	+1

[a]In general, patients without clinical stroke risk factors do not need antithrombotic therapy, while patients with stroke risk factors (ie, CHA$_2$DS$_2$-VASc score of 1 or more for men, and 2 or more for women) are likely to benefit from oral anticoagulation.

Data from The Task Force for the management of atrial fibrillation of the European Society of Cardiology. *Eur Heart J.* 2016;37:2893-2962.

ANSWER 1

Control her heart rate with β-blockers and calculate her CHA$_2$DS$_2$-VASc score, which shows she has a high risk of embolism. You begin warfarin anticoagulation with a target INR of 2 to 3.

KEY FACT

Rhythm control and rate control have similar mortality benefit when combined with anticoagulation.

ANSWER 2

Administer IV atropine. Hypotension and bradycardia are common in acute inferior wall MI due to ↑ vagal tone after MI and sinus node ischemia caused by right coronary artery blockage. Bradycardia is usually transient and resolves in 24 hours, however symptomatic patients need to be treated.

ANSWER 3

A vitamin K antagonist is the only option for patients with valvular AF. New oral anticoagulation agents are used only for nonvalvular AF.

- **Rhythm control:** Not a mainstay of treatment; amiodarone, flecainide, propafenone, sotalol, dofetilide).
- Some patients, particularly young patients and patients who have failed pharmacologic rhythm control, may be candidates for radiofrequency catheter ablation to restore normal sinus rhythm. This technique can have significant risks and the success is operator dependent, but its use is becoming more common.

Atrial Flutter

Uncommon in a structurally normal heart. Can occur with LV dysfunction and rheumatic heart disease. Other etiologies, exam findings, and treatment are similar to those associated with AF; significant differences are listed below.

Diagnosis

ECG findings:
- **Typical isthmus-dependent flutter (counterclockwise):** Atrial rate of 250 to 350 bpm. Can present with or without typical flutter waves (Figure 3.5).
- **Clockwise flutter:** Presents with a sawtooth pattern in leads II, III, and aVF. Flutter rate should be around 300 bpm. Consider the diagnosis in patients with a ventricular rate of 150 bpm, as flutter usually presents with 2:1 conduction.

Management

- Approach to cardioversion, anticoagulation, and rate control similar to that of AF.
- Watchful waiting for reversion to normal sinus rhythm: Appropriate in stable patients with minimal atrial dilation and a known reversible cause such as hyperthyroidism or PE.
- **Radiofrequency ablation:** Highly effective and the preferred treatment.
- Alternatives: Antiarrhythmics or pacemakers, which require long-term anticoagulation.

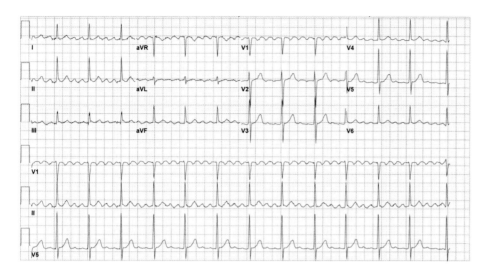

FIGURE 3.5. **Atrial flutter on ECG.** Typical sawtooth pattern on ECG. (Reproduced with permission from USMLE-Rx.com.)

Other Supraventricular Tachycardias

- **Reentrant SVT:** The point of reentry can be:
  - **AV node:** Also called AVNRT. Most common, accounting for 60% of cases of reentrant SVT.
  - The bypass tract or other site. Also called AVRT.
- Atrial: Sinus tachycardia, atrial tachycardia, multifocal atrial tachycardia.
- Arterioventricular: Junctional tachycardia.

Symptoms/Exam

Asymptomatic or may present with palpitations, pounding in the neck, lightheadedness, presyncope, syncope, or chest pain. Exam should focus on auscultation for evidence of valvular disease or cardiomyopathy.

Diagnosis

ECG shows regular rhythm. QRS is generally narrow, although it may be wide if aberrant conduction is present. Varying morphologies of P waves seen in **multifocal atrial tachycardia**. Retrograde P waves may be seen in AVNRT, AVRT, and junctional tachycardia.

Management

Valsalva; unilateral carotid sinus massage (if no prior TIA, prior serious cardiac arrhythmia, MI within last 6 months, or carotid bruit). Give adenosine if these maneuvers are unsuccessful. Cardioversion is indicated if the patient is unstable.

Ventricular Tachycardia and Ventricular Fibrillation

Causes include ischemia, infarction, cardiomyopathy, electrolyte abnormalities, and drug toxicities. Types of ventricular tachycardia (VT) are as follows (Figure 3.6):
- **Monomorphic:** Uniform QRS pattern (see Figure 3.6A). Usually associated with myocardial scar.
- **Polymorphic:** Bizarre and changing QRS. Often precipitated by ischemia.
- **Torsades de pointes** (in which the QRS complex oscillates around a baseline): Often associated with medications and electrolyte abnormalities that prolong the QT interval (see Figure 3.6B).

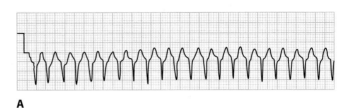

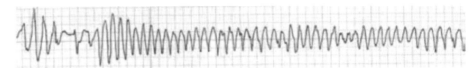

FIGURE 3.6.   **Monomorphic and polymorphic ventricular tachycardia.** (A) Rhythm strip shows wide-complex tachycardia with no clearly discernible P waves. (B) Rhythm strip shows torsades de pointes—a rapid polymorphic tachycardia with characteristic "twisting" of the QRS complexes around the baseline. (Image A reproduced with permission from Gomella LG, Haist SA. *Clinician's Pocket Reference,* 11th ed. http://www.accessmedicine.com. Copyright © The McGraw-Hill Companies, Inc. All rights reserved; image B source: Yates C, et al. Utility of the electrocardiogram in drug overdose and poisoning: theoretical considerations and clinical implications. *Curr Cardiol Rev.* 2012;8(2):137-151.)

Symptoms/Exam

Chest pain, dyspnea, syncope, **sudden cardiac death.**

Diagnosis

- Wide QRS complex. **Must be distinguished from SVT with aberrant conduction.** Baseline ECG may show bundle branch block or intraventricular conduction delay with a similar QRS morphology.
- **Unstable patients:** Assume VT.
- **Stable patients:** VT is evidenced by AV dissociation, complexes not typical of LBBB or RBBB, variation in QRS complexes, and fusion beats of simultaneously occurring ventricular and supraventricular beats.

Management

- **Unstable patients:** Cardioversion.
- **Stable VT:** First-line treatment is IV amiodarone.
- **Polymorphic VT** (including torsades de pointes): Can be treated with magnesium infusion and overdrive pacing.
- A defibrillator should be placed if the cause is not transient or reversible.

KEY FACT

VT must be distinguished from SVT with aberrant conduction; but in an unstable patient, treat as VT.

Conduction Abnormalities

BUNDLE BRANCH AND FASCICULAR BLOCKS

An impairment in the fast conduction of current through the septum/ventricles from the AV node (Table 3.4 and Figures 3.7 and 3.8). Can be due to age-related degeneration of the conduction system, CAD, cardiomyopathies, or acute ischemia. Pacemakers should be considered in some situations.

AV BLOCKS

Delayed conduction through the AV node → prolonged PR interval → eventual dissociation of atrial and ventricular rhythms if completely blocked. Increased with ↑ vagal tone, drugs (β-blockers, non-DHP CCBs), ischemic heart disease, cardiomyopathies, myocarditis, or congenital heart disease.

TABLE 3.4.   **ECG Changes in Intraventricular Blocks**

TYPE	AXIS	ECG	QRS	MISCELLANEOUS
LAFB	Left	Upright QRS in I; ⊖ QRS in aVF	Narrow	
LPFB	Right	⊖ QRS in I; ⊕ QRS in aVF	Narrow	
RBBB	Right or normal	rSR′ in V_1-V_2; **rabbit ears**	Wide	Can still read ischemia
LBBB	Left or normal	**Broad R wave in I; broad, deep S in V_1; RS in V_6** (see Figure 3.8)	Wide	Difficult to read ischemia
Bilateral block		Third-degree heart block	Wide and bizarre	

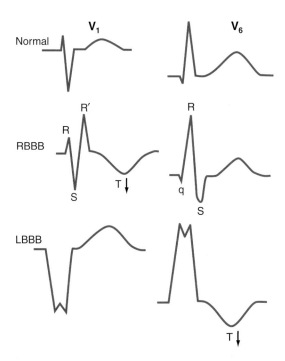

FIGURE 3.7.   **Changes in right and left bundle branch blocks on ECG.** (Reproduced with permission from Fauci AS, Kasper AL, Braunwald E, Hauser SL, Longo DL, Jameson JL, Loscalzo J. *Harrison's Principles of Internal Medicine,* 17th ed. http://www.accessmedicine.com. Copyright © The McGraw-Hill Companies, Inc. All rights reserved.)

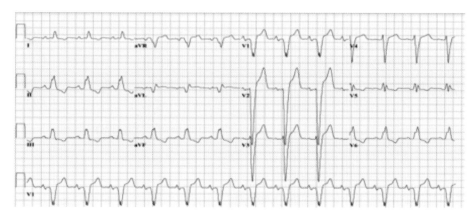

FIGURE 3.8.   **Left bundle branch block on ECG.** (Reproduced with permission from USMLE-Rx.com.)

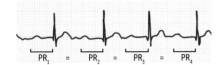

FIGURE 3.9.   **First-degree AV block on ECG.** Note the prolonged PR interval. (Reproduced with permission from USMLE-Rx.com.)

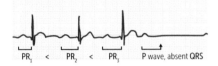

FIGURE 3.10.   **Mobitz type I second-degree AV block on ECG.** (Reproduced with permission from USMLE-Rx.com.)

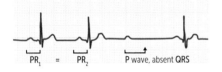

FIGURE 3.11.   **Mobitz type II second-degree AV block on ECG.** (Reproduced with permission from USMLE-Rx.com.)

MNEMONIC

Mobitz type **I:** PR interval gets longer and longer, then **ONE** drops ("longer, longer, **drop,** now you have a Wencke**bach**"). Mobitz type **II:** It's not **TWO** long until you need a pacemaker.

KEY FACT

Avoid all AV node blockers in patients with WPW. β-Blockers, CCBs, and digoxin can lead to dangerous tachycardia in these patients.

- **First-degree AV block:** Prolonged PR interval >200 msec (Figure 3.9). Try to treat underlying cause (lower medication dose) but can be observed untreated.
- **Second-degree AV block:** Some atrial impulses fail to reach ventricles.
  - **Mobitz type I (Wenckebach):** Progressively longer PR interval followed by a nonconducted P wave (Figure 3.10). Usually block is at AV node and is benign.
  - **Mobitz type II:** PR interval is stable but some P waves are not conducted (not followed by QRS), often in a regular patterns, 2:1, 3:2, etc (Figure 3.11). More serious condition; block is usually below AV node and can lead to complete heart block. Pacemaker often required.
- **Third-degree AV block:** No atrial impulses reach the ventricles. Complete dissociation of the atrial (P wave) and the ventricular (QRS) rhythm (Figure 3.12). "Escape rhythms" drive the ventricle from below the block. Escape rhythm is slower than a sinus rhythm and two-thirds of the time has a narrow QRS (focus for the escape rhythm is still within the conduction system). **Requires a pacemaker.**

WOLFF-PARKINSON-WHITE SYNDROME

A persistent accessory pathway between the atria and ventricles. May be found incidentally, but even asymptomatic patients are at risk for tachyarrhythmias. More common in those with first-degree relatives with WPW.

- **Antegrade accessory pathway conduction:** Impulses conduct from the atria to the accessory pathway to the ventricles. Characterized by ventricular preexcitation with **short PR and delta waves** (slurred upstroke of QRS; best seen in lead V_4). Delta waves with net-negative deflection can resemble Q waves (Figure 3.13).
- **Retrograde accessory pathway conduction:** Impulses conduct from the ventricles to the accessory pathway to the atria. Resting ECG is often normal; no delta wave is seen.
- Do an electrophysiologic study; ablate the bypass tracts.
- Serious complications usually happen in the setting of AF. Avoid AV nodal blockers in patients with a delta wave, as this can cause 1:1 conduction of AF → VF and cardiac arrest.

Electrolytes and ECGs

Some of the most common causes of abnormal ECGs are electrolyte abnormalities (Table 3.5).

Hypertension

High BP = systolic BP ≥140 mm Hg or a diastolic BP >90 mm Hg on more than two occasions. HTN is associated with MI, HF, stroke, and kidney disease and has a ↑ prevalence in ethnic minorities, women, and those with ↑ age.

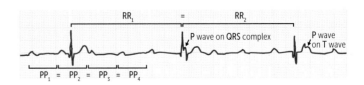

FIGURE 3.12.   **Third-degree AV block on ECG.** (Reproduced with permission from USMLE-Rx.com.)

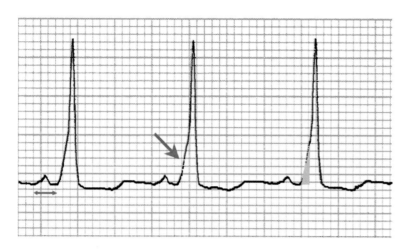

Table 3.6 describes the types of HTN and their causes. Table 3.7 defines the types of severe HTN.

Symptoms/Exam

- Headache, chest pain, SOB, vision changes.
- Exam should include a cardiopulmonary exam and an investigation for chronic changes associated with chronic HTN:
  - **Fundoscopic exam for retinopathy** to look for arteriolar narrowing or sclerosis, AV nicking (Figure 3.15), hemorrhages, and hard exudates.
  - PMI with left shift indicating LVH, signs of HF.
  - Signs of stroke with severe HTN.
- Look for signs of 2° HTN such as renal artery bruits, significant difference in right/left or upper/lower extremity BPs, ↓ or delayed femoral pulses, obesity, and physical findings of alcohol abuse or liver disease.

Diagnosis

- **Elevated BP on two separate occasions with correct cuff size.**
- **Labs:** Electrolytes, creatinine, hematocrit, UA, ECG, A_{1c}, urine albumin to creatinine ratio.
- Rule out 2° causes (see above) in those with severe or refractory HTN (on three meds, including a diuretic), proven age of onset before puberty, age <30 if nonobese

TABLE 3.5. ECG Findings in Electrolyte Abnormalities

ELECTROLYTE	ECG FINDING
Hyperkalemia	Tall peaked T waves, PR wide, QRS wide, bundle branch blocks, short QT, P waves disappear → Vfib (see Figure 3.14A)
Hypokalemia	ST and T wave depressions, **U wave** (at end of the T wave), pseudo-prolonged QT, large P waves (see Figure 3.14B)
Hypercalcemia	Short QTc
Hypocalcemia	Long QTc
Hypermagnesemia	Bradycardia
Hypomagnesemia	Long QT, prolonged PR, widened QRS

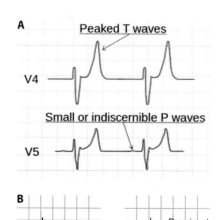

FIGURE 3.14. Effects of hyperkalemia and hypokalemia on the ECG. (A) Peaked T waves and indiscernible P waves characteristic of hyperkalemia. **(B)** Flattening of the T wave and progressive prominence of the U wave characteristic of worsening hypokalemia. (Image A reproduced from Wikimedia; courtesy of Mikael Häggström; image B reproduced with permission from USMLE-Rx.com.)

Counsel her about smoking cessation, exercise, and a low-cholesterol diet. Measure her BP on a different day before starting antihypertensive therapy. If 6 months later her BP is still elevated and her lipid profile has not changed significantly, start a statin.

KEY FACT

The goal of hypertension treatment is a BP <140/90 mm Hg, or <130/80 mm Hg in patients with diabetes, renal disease, or cardiovascular disease.

KEY FACT

Stages of HTN:
- Prehypertension: Systolic pressure of 120 to 139 mm Hg OR diastolic pressure of 80 to 89 mm Hg.
- Stage 1 HTN: Systolic pressure of 140 to 159 mm Hg OR diastolic pressure of 90 to 99 mm Hg.
- Stage 2 HTN: Higher than 160/90 mm Hg.

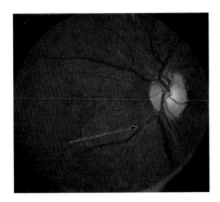

FIGURE 3.15. AV nicking. Arteriole crosses a venule and compresses the venule (arrow), which results in the compression of the vein with bulging on either side of the crossing. (Reproduced with permission from USMLE-Rx.com.)

TABLE 3.6. Types of Hypertension

TYPE	CAUSES
Essential	Idiopathic
Secondary	Common: Obesity, alcohol abuse, kidney disease, medications (steroids, OCPs, NSAIDs, antidepressants), recreational drug abuse including nicotine products, sleep apnea, hyper-/hypothyroidism
	Less common: Hyperaldosteronism, renovascular disease (renal artery stenosis), coarctation of the aorta, Cushing disease

and no family history of HTN, onset of stage 2 HTN after age 55, family history of early-onset HTN, or an acute ↑ in BP over a previously stable baseline.
- Additional labs to consider based on suspected causes of 2° HTN: TSH, renal ultrasound, plasma aldosterone-to-renin ratio.

Management
- The goal is <140/90 mm Hg, or <130/80 mm Hg in patients with **diabetes, renal disease,** or **cardiovascular disease.**
- Patients with prehypertension and stages 1 and 2 HTN should be counseled about lifestyle modifications, including weight loss, nicotine product use cessation, adherence to a low-sodium/DASH diet (rich in fruits, vegetables, and low-fat dairy), aerobic activity.
- Assess factors that may modify treatment choices (Table 3.8).

Hyperlipidemia

Coronary risk ↑ proportionally with total cholesterol. Accordingly, the control of hyperlipidemia is critical to ↓ the incidence of CAD, CVA, CKD, and PVD. Mortality benefits have been noted both in patients without known CAD and in patients with established CAD.

TABLE 3.7. Severe Hypertension

TYPE	DEFINITION
Hypertensive urgency	SBP >180-200 mm Hg or DBP >120 mm Hg without acute signs of end-organ damage
Hypertensive emergency	SBP >180 mm Hg or DBP >120 mm Hg with signs of acute end-organ effects: - Brain: confusion, lethargy indicate cerebral edema or hemorrhage - Eye: blurry vision, papilledema - Heart: chest pain or shortness of breath may indicate aortic dissection, acute coronary syndrome, or pulmonary edema - Kidney: oliguria, hematuria, or ↑ creatinine indicates acute renal failure
Hypertensive encephalopathy	Hypertension with signs of cerebral edema: altered sensorium, nausea, vomiting, headache
Malignant hypertension	Hypertension with retinal hemorrhages, exudates, or papilledema, usually with diastolic BP >120 mm Hg

TABLE 3.8.   Antihypertensive Medications

	THIAZIDES	β-BLOCKERS	ACE INHIBITORS	ANGIOTENSIN RECEPTOR BLOCKER	CALCIUM CHANNEL BLOCKERS
Drug examples	Hydrochlorothiazide, chlorthalidone	Atenolol, metoprolol	Captopril, enalapril, ramipril, lisinopril	Irbesartan, losartan, valsartan	Nondihydropyridines (non-DHPs): diltiazem, verapamil Dihydropyridines (DHPs): amlodipine, felodipine, nifedipine
Adverse effects	Hypokalemia, erectile dysfunction, ↑ insulin resistance, hyperuricemia, ↑ TG	Bronchospasm, depression, fatigue, erectile dysfunction, ↑ insulin resistance	Cough (10%), hyperkalemia, renal failure	Less cough, hyperkalemia, renal failure	Conduction defects (non-DHPs); lower extremity edema
Indications for use as first-line drug	**Most patients** as mono- or combination therapy (stage 1 or 2 HTN), **osteoporosis, kidney stones** Recurrent stroke prevention	**MI,** high CAD risk, rate control for AF/atrial flutter, HF	**Diabetes, MI,** HF, mild chronic renal failure	Diabetes, MI, HF, chronic renal failure, ACE inhibitor–related cough	Non-DHPs used for rate control for AF/ atrial flutter
Contraindications	Gout	Severe bronchospasm; high-degree (type II second- or third-degree) heart block, bradycardia	Pregnancy Moderate-severe renal failure; caution in renal artery stenosis	Pregnancy Moderate-severe renal failure; caution in renal artery stenosis	High-degree heart block

SCREENING GUIDELINES

The USPSTF recommends hyperlipidemia screening:
- In men age ≥35 years.
- In women age ≥45 years if they are at ↑ risk for CAD.
- In women age 20 to 45 years at ↑ risk for CHD.
  - Screening is generally **not** recommended for patients >75 years of age or children.
  - Measurement of fasting lipids is optimal, but nonfasting total cholesterol-to-HDL cholesterol ratio is an alternative.

RISK FACTORS

Patients with elevated blood cholesterol levels must have their atherosclerotic cardiovascular disease (ASCVD) risk calculated. Majority of calculators include categories of gender, age, race, total cholesterol, HDL cholesterol, SBP, treatment for ↑ SBP, history of diabetes, and smoking status.
- Patients with scores <7.5% are considered low risk and do not require statin therapy.
- In patients with scores ≥7.5%, consider moderate- to high-intensity statins, assuming no clinical ASCVD or diabetes, age 40 to 75 years, and LDL cholesterol 70 to 189 mg/dL.

QUESTION

A 65-year-old man with a history of MI and a three-vessel CABG 10 years ago comes to your office to establish care. He is a nonsmoker who is active and feels well, and he is currently on aspirin, a statin, and HCTZ. On exam, you note that he is obese, his BP is 160/80 mm Hg, and he has an S4. You check his lipids, and his LDL cholesterol is 125. What further interventions are necessary?

TABLE 3.9.   Types of Satin Therapy

TYPE	EXAMPLES
High intensity	Atorvastatin 40-80 mg
	Rosuvastatin 20-40 mg
Moderate intensity	Atorvastatin 10-20 mg
	Rosuvastatin 5-10 mg
	Simvastatin 20-40 mg
	Pravastatin 40-80 mg
	Lovastatin 40 mg
	Fluvastatin 80 mg
	Fluvastatin 40 mg (BID)
	Pitavastatin 2-4 mg

- Patients with ASCVD, 1° elevations of LDL ≥190 mg/dL, patients between 40 and 75 years old with diabetes and an LDL cholesterol 70 to 189 mg/dL without clinical ASCVD should be started on moderate- to high-intensity statin therapy.

MANAGEMENT

Table 3.9 outlines statins used to treat hyperlipidemia.

Coronary Artery Disease

CAD is the leading cause of mortality in women and men in the United States. It is associated with other forms of cardiovascular disease, including cerebrovascular disease, peripheral artery disease, and aortic atherosclerosis. Risk factors for CAD include the following:
- **Age:** Risk is ↑ in women >65 years of age or with premature menopause, and in men >55 years of age.
- **Family history:** Risk is ↑ with a family history of CAD in a first-degree female relative <55 years of age or a male relative <45 years of age.
- **Smoking.**
- **Hypertension** with a BP >140/90 mm Hg or use of an antihypertensive.
- **HDL cholesterol <40 mg/dL** on several occasions (an HDL cholesterol >60 mg/dL is a ⊖ risk factor).
- **Elevated LDL.**
- **Obesity** (BMI >30 kg/m²) and **physical inactivity.**
- **Chronic kidney disease.**
- **Diabetes:** Patients with diabetes are at a level of risk equivalent to those with established CAD.

More novel risk factors include elevated CRP, elevated homocysteine, coronary artery calcification on cardiac CT, and LVH.

PREVENTION

1° Prevention

Risk factor reduction includes the following:
- **Smoking cessation:** Yields an immediate ↓ in risk that reverts to a normal level after several years.
- **Diet:** Low in fat and high in whole grains, fruits, vegetables, and omega-3 fatty acids.
- **Hypertension:** The goal BP is based on the JNC8 guidelines. In the general population aged ≥60 years, initiate pharmacologic treatment to lower BP at an SBP ≥150 mm Hg or a DBP ≥90 mm Hg and treat to a goal SBP <150 mm Hg and goal DBP <90 mm Hg. (This is a grad A strong recommendation per the JNC8).
- **Hyperlipidemia:** Target LDL cholesterol levels should be based on the patient's 10-year risk for heart disease.
- **Diabetes:** Intensive control of type 2 diabetes has not been shown to lower cardiovascular events in most studies. Consider an A_{1c} target of <7.0 for most new-onset type 2 diabetics and 7.0-7.9 in frail diabetics and those with long-standing disease (8-12 years).
- **Other risk factors** that should be addressed include obesity and physical inactivity. Low to moderate alcohol intake (1-2 drinks a day) has been postulated to slightly ↓ the risk of CAD.
- **Pharmacologic therapy: Consider aspirin** therapy for 1° prevention in nondiabetics when 10-year CVD risk >20% and for diabetics when 10-year CVD risk >10%

KEY FACT

Diabetes is a CAD equivalent.

ANSWER

You add an ACEI and a β-blocker for BP control and for 2° prevention of CAD, and ↑ his statin dose to improve his LDL cholesterol toward his goal of 70 mg/dL. You also encourage him to continue to exercise and abstain from tobacco, and you discuss nutritional strategies to improve his cardiac health.

and no ↑ risk of bleeding. Use of 81 mg aspirin in patients with lower CVD risk is of uncertain benefit.

2° Prevention

Risk factor reduction measure are the same as those outlined above:
- **Pharmacologic therapy:**
    - **Aspirin:** ↓ mortality with daily use (81 mg). If contraindicated, clopidogrel may be used.
    - **Clopidogrel and ticagrelor:** ↓ mortality in patients with recent acute coronary syndrome (ACS) or in those with a stent. Dual antiplatelet therapy should be continued for at least 1 year if drug-eluting stent is placed.
    - **Statins:** ↓ mortality and the risk of acute cardiac events. Goal for those with CAD is an **LDL cholesterol <100 mg/dL,** although some groups recommend an LDL cholesterol goal of <70 mg/dL.
    - **β-blockers:** ↓ mortality. All patients with CAD should be on a β-blocker unless an absolute contraindication exists.
    - **ACE inhibitors (ACEIs):** ↓ mortality and risk of MI and stroke. If not tolerated, an angiotensin receptor blocker (ARB) may be used.

KEY FACT

β-blockers, ACEIs, statins, and aspirin ↓ CAD-related mortality.

STABLE ANGINA

Fixed artery stenosis limiting O_2 delivery in times of stress.

Symptoms/Exam

Classically presents with chronic, exercise-induced chest discomfort that is relieved by rest and nitroglycerin and does not change in severity or frequency. May be associated with dyspnea or nausea, and may radiate to the neck, jaw, or arms. Exam findings are nonspecific.

Diagnosis

Start with stress testing with either nuclear perfusion imaging or echocardiography. **Cardiac catheterization and now coronary CT angiography is the gold standard.**

Management

- The same as 2° prevention of CAD. Antianginal medical therapy includes nitrates, β-blockers, and CCBs.
- **Indications for revascularization with CABG:**
    - Chronic stable angina with three-vessel disease.
    - Two-vessel disease with prominent LAD involvement.
    - One- or two-vessel disease with high-risk features such as LV dysfunction.
    - Significant left main artery disease (>50% stenosis).
    - Refractory symptoms or chronic angina.

CARDIAC ISCHEMIA/ACUTE CORONARY SYNDROME

ACS encompasses three diagnoses: unstable angina (UA), non–ST-segment elevation MI (NSTEMI), and ST-segment elevation MI (STEMI), which reflect different levels of damage to the myocardium from ischemia.

Diagnosis

- ECG findings in ischemia (Figures 3.16 and 3.17):
    - Prolonged QTc, T-wave flattening, T-wave inversions (TWI), or normalization of previous TWI → ST depressions → ST elevations → Q waves.
    - New LBBB.

QUESTION

EMS brings to the ED a 47-year-old Hispanic woman with severe substernal chest pain and palpitations. Home medications include high-dose prednisone and hydroxychloroquine. Heart rate is in the 160s, respiratory rate is in the upper 30s, and she is afebrile. Despite the best efforts, she develops ventricular tachycardia and fails all resuscitative efforts. What is the most likely cause of her death?

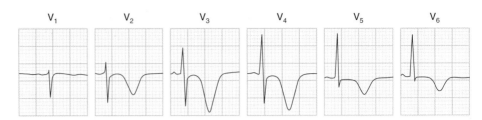

FIGURE 3.16. **Myocardial ischemia on ECG.** Note: T wave inversion in the precordial leads. (Reproduced with permission from Fauci AS, Kasper AL, Braunwald E, Hauser SL, Longo DL, Jameson JL, Loscalzo J. *Harrison's Principles of Internal Medicine,* 17th ed. http://www.accessmedicine.com. Copyright © The McGraw-Hill Companies, Inc. All rights reserved.)

- Heart block.
- Ventricular arrhythmias.
- Cardiac markers: Elevated troponin or CK-MB.
- Echo may show new wall motion abnormalities.

See Table 3.10 for summary of ECG changes characteristic of areas of the heart affected.

Diagnosis of ACS

See Table 3.11 for categorization of types of ACS based on serum markers and ECG findings.

Management

- Initial medical treatment of suspected MI in most cases: Morphine, oxygen, sublingual nitroglycerine, and ASA (MONA).
- If ACS:
  - Add high-dose statin, ACEI, and β-blockers in hemodynamically stable patients.
  - Anticoagulate with heparin drip or low-molecular-weight heparin.
  - Clopidogrel, ticagrelor.

MNEMONIC

For initial treatment of chest pain/ suspected MI:

MONA

Morphine
Oxygen
Nitroglycerin (sublingual)
Aspirin

ANSWER

CAD. SLE patients (based on her meds) are in ↑ risk for premature CAD, which predisposes them to MIs and consequently rhythm abnormalities.

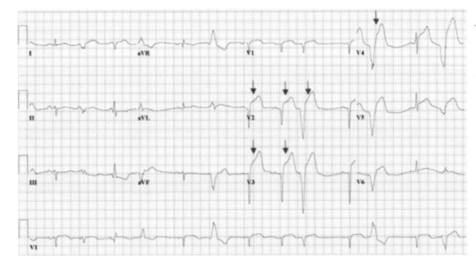

FIGURE 3.17. **ST-segment elevation myocardial infarction on ECG.** Anterior STEMI in V_2-V_4 precordial leads (arrows) with premature ventricular contractions (PVCs). (Reproduced with permission from USMLE-Rx.com.)

TABLE 3.10. **Localization of Transmural Infarction**

LEADS	LOCATION	ARTERY	MISCELLANEOUS
II, III, aVF	Inferior	Right coronary artery (80%) or left circumflex (20%)	Perform right-sided ECG (look for ST ↑ in $V_4R \rightarrow$ RV infarct)
I, aVL	Lateral	Left circumflex	
V_1-V_3	Anteroseptal	Left anterior descending (LAD)	
V_4-V_6	Apical/lateral	LAD or left circumflex	
V_4-V_6R	RV	Right coronary artery (+ branches of LAD)	Seen on right-sided ECG
V_1-V_2 depression V_7-V_9	Posterior	Left circumflex or right coronary artery	Check posterior ECG. If ST ↓ in V_1 or V_2, look for ST ↑ in V_7-V_9

- May also require GIIb/IIIa receptor antagonist or nitrate drip (contraindicated in RV infarction).
- Percutaneous coronary intervention (PCI)/percutaneous transluminal coronary angioplasty (PTCA), either emergently (STEMI) or urgently (UA/NSTEMI). Stents are usually placed, or if disease is extensive, CABG is performed.
  - Bare metal stents: Higher risk of restenosis, lower risk of thrombosis.
  - Drug-eluting stents: Lower risk of restenosis, higher risk of thrombosis.
- Thrombolytics such as tPA can be used to break up plaque if PCI/PTCA cannot be performed urgently.
- **Avoid β-blockers in RVMI:** Give IV fluids since patients are strongly dependent on RV function.

TABLE 3.11. **Diagnosis and Treatment of Acute Coronary Syndrome**

	POSSIBLE ACS	ACS		
		UNSTABLE ANGINA	NSTEMI	STEMI
History	Chest pain	Worsening of chest pain	Chest pain	Chest pain
ECG	Normal or nonspecific	Usually ischemic—contiguous TWI, ST depressions		ST ↑ >1 mm in 2 contiguous leads, or new LBBB, new Q waves
Serum markers	⊖	⊖	⊕	⊕
Medications	± β-blocker, nitrates, etc.	MONA; β-blocker; statin		
Anticoagulation	ASA	ASA + heparin + clopidogrel ± Gp IIb/IIIa inhibitors		

MONA, morphine, oxygen, nitroglycerine, and ASA.

KEY FACT

Most patients with HF have combined systolic and diastolic dysfunction.

Heart Failure

A condition in which the ability of the heart to maintain circulation is compromised. HF is most often chronic but may also be acute or subacute. Risk factors include ischemic heart disease, valvular disease, tobacco use, HTN, obesity, and diabetes. HF may be classified by symptom severity (Table 3.12), by stage of evolution, by type of dysfunction (systolic or diastolic), or by part of the heart primarily affected (right or left):

- **Stage A:** High risk for HF due to comorbidities (HTN, CAD, diabetes) without symptoms or structural disease.
- **Stage B:** Structural heart disease associated with the development of HF (LVH; enlarged, dilated ventricle; valvular disease; previous MI) without symptoms.
- **Stage C:** Structural heart disease with previous or current symptoms. This is the **largest group.**
- **Stage D:** Refractory HF despite medical therapy, requiring specialized interventions.
- **Systolic dysfunction:** Defined as ↓ EF seen on echocardiogram in the setting of signs or symptoms of HF.
  - **Left heart failure:** Most common. Etiologies include CAD (present in 70% of patients with systolic dysfunction), dilated cardiomyopathy, HTN, AF, and valvular disease.
  - **Right heart failure:** If in combination with left HF, usually due to ↑ pressures via pulmonary vasculature from LV systolic dysfunction. In isolated right HF, due to ↑ pulmonary pressures (from chronic lung disease such as severe COPD, bronchiectasis, PEs) or predominant RV infarction, there will be less lung involvement and more peripheral edema, causing a preload-dependent state.
- **Diastolic dysfunction: Abnormal LV filling** and normal systolic function. Etiologies are as follows:
  - ↓ myocardial relaxation due to ischemia, hypertrophy, cardiomyopathies, and aging.
  - Myocardial stiffness due to fibrosis, scarring, hypertrophy, and infiltration.
  - Endocardial fibrosis.
  - Constrictive pericarditis, tamponade.

Symptoms

- **Subacute or acute:** Usually related to excess fluid accumulation—dyspnea at rest or with exertion, orthopnea, paroxysmal nocturnal dyspnea, ascites.
- **Chronic:** Fatigue, edema, and anorexia may be more prominent.
- Diastolic dysfunction is often asymptomatic.

Exam

- **Systolic:** Signs of excess fluid accumulation related to ↓ EF of blood from the affected ventricle:
  - Left-sided: Lung crackles, S3, narrow pulse pressure.
  - Right-sided: Leg edema, ascites, elevated jugular venous pulse (JPV), hepatojugular reflex.
- **Diastolic:** The same as systolic except for the presence of an S4. An S3 should **not** be present in isolated diastolic dysfunction.

Differential

COPD, pneumonia, cirrhosis, nephrotic syndrome, PE.

TABLE 3.12.   NYHA Classification of HF by Symptom Severity

CLASS I	CLASS II	CLASS III	CLASS IV
Symptoms at levels identical to those of normal individuals	Symptoms with moderate exertion	Symptoms with mild exertion only	Symptoms at rest

Diagnosis

- **Labs:** CBC, electrolytes, and creatinine (for initiation of diuretics, assessment of renal failure from renal hypoperfusion), TSH, fasting glucose, LFTs, CXR, and ECG (to rule out ischemia, arrhythmias).
- **Brain natriuretic peptide:** Released with myocyte stretch. If ↑, helpful in distinguishing between HF and pulmonary causes of dyspnea. Not helpful in assessing severity. Tends to be ↓ in obese patients and ↑ in those with CKD or sepsis.
- **CXR:** May show cardiomegaly (cardiac-to-thoracic ratio >50%), Kerley B lines, pleural effusions (Figure 3.18).
- **Echocardiography:**
  - **Systolic dysfunction:** Demonstrates an **EF <40%** with an enlarged, dilated LV.
  - **Diastolic dysfunction:** EF is normal, but hypertrophy, RV enlargement, pericarditis, and infiltrative disease may be seen.

Management

- **Systolic dysfunction:**
  - Always start with lifestyle modifications: Smoking cessation, reduction of alcohol consumption, ↓ salt intake, weight loss, and monitoring.
  - **Stepwise medication approach** (see Table 3.13 for treatment targeted to area of dysfunction):
    - **Diuretics:** Used acutely to relieve symptoms of pulmonary edema. Confers **no mortality benefit.**
    - **ACEIs:** Mortality benefit in **all classes of HF.** If not tolerated, an ARB may be substituted.
    - **β-blockers:** Mortality benefits in **classes II, III, and IV** have been shown with carvedilol, metoprolol, and bisoprolol. Avoid starting in decompensated HF, but acceptable to continue during an exacerbation unless it is severe.
    - In patients with chronic symptomatic HF with reduced EF (HFrEF) NYHA class II or III who tolerate an ACEI or ARB, replacement by an angiotensin receptor-neprilysin inhibitor (ARNI) such as combination valsartan/sacubibiril) is recommended to further reduce morbidity and mortality.
    - **Digoxin:** May provide symptomatic relief, but confers **no mortality benefit.** Helpful for rate control in patients with concurrent AF. Symptoms of digoxin toxicity (seen more often in those with renal insufficiency, hypokalemia, hypomagnesemia, use of non-DHP CCBs) include fatigue, disturbed color perception, anorexia, vomiting, abdominal pain, confusion. **Bradycardia,** prolonged PR interval, hyperkalemia are also often seen.
    - **Hydralazine with nitrates:** Can be used as an alternative to other treat-

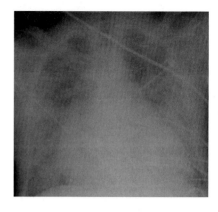

FIGURE 3.18. Heart failure. CXR shows enlarged cardiac silhouette in the setting of perihilar alveolar infiltrates, vascular congestion, and interstitial markings, compatible with pulmonary edema. (Reproduced with permission from USMLE-Rx.com.)

 QUESTION

An 81-year-old woman with a history of CAD, diabetes, HTN, and hyperlipidemia comes to your office complaining of progressive fatigue, chest pain, dyspnea, and lightheadedness over the previous several years. She has had several episodes of syncope over the last few weeks without accompanying palpitations but with chest pain and dyspnea. Her BP is 170/90 mm Hg. She has a late-peaking systolic murmur at the left upper sternal border radiating to the carotids. PMI is displaced and sustained. Her ECG is normal, and her echocardiogram shows severe aortic stenosis with a valve area of 0.75 cm². How do you proceed?

TABLE 3.13. Targeted Treatment of Heart Failure

	SYSTOLIC DYSFUNCTION	ISOLATED RIGHT-SIDED DYSFUNCTION	DIASTOLIC DYSFUNCTION
Acute treatment	Loop diuretics Oxygen, pain control, sodium/fluid restriction Vasodilators (nitrates)	Slow use of diuretics (high doses can cause hypotension since preload-dependent)	Rate control (β-blockers or non-DHP CCBs) Slow use of diuretics (preload-dependent) ACEIs
Chronic treatment (mortality benefit)	ACEIs or ARBs β-blockers Hydralazine/nitrates Spironolactone in class III/IV Exercise	Same as systolic	Rate control to ↑ filling time (β-blockers or non-DHP CCBs) ACEIs
Chronic treatment (symptom relief)	Diuretics Digoxin	Same as systolic	Diuretics

ments if contraindicated or as an addition for patients with moderate to severe symptoms on optimal therapy with ACEI, β-blocker, and diuretics.

- **Spironolactone:** Confers a mortality benefit in **class III–IV HF.** Creatinine should be <2.5 mg/dL in men or <2.0 mg/dL in women. For patients with EF <35% alternative is eplerenone, especially if patient develops gynecomastia on spironolactone.
- Advanced treatments:
  - **Mechanical therapy:** Consider a balloon pump for severe HF due to ischemia. Consider ventricular assist devices for very poor cardiac output as a bridge to transplantation.
  - **Implantable cardioverter-defibrillator (ICD):** For 2° prevention of sudden cardiac death (SCD) in those with a history of cardiac arrest, VF, or hemodynamically destabilizing VT. Consider for 1° prevention of SCD >40 days after an MI, LVEF ≤35, class II or III symptoms, and an expected survival >1 year.
  - **Cardiac resynchronization:** Pacers used with severe systolic HF (class III or IV), sinus rhythm, and wide QRS. More specifically, resynchronization is indicated for patients who have LVEF of ≤35%, sinus rhythm, LBBB with a QRS duration ≥150 ms, and NYHA class II, III, or ambulatory IV symptoms while receiving guideline-directed medical treatment.
  - **Cardiac transplantation:** Reserved for end-stage heart disease that either limits survival to <2 years or severely limits daily quality of life.
- **Isolated right-sided dysfunction:** Largely the same as left-sided systolic dysfunction management. Because of the risk of hypotension, avoid taking off too much fluid acutely with diuretics in preload-dependent state.
- **Diastolic dysfunction:**
  - Goals are to improve ventricular relaxation, ↓ heart rate, maintain sinus rhythm, and treat HTN to achieve LVH regression.
  - Usually β-blockers or non-DHP CCBs (verapamil, diltiazem). Other HF therapies are also used (see systolic dysfunction above).
  - Avoid using β-blockers with non-DHP CCBs together since combination may precipitate HF.

Valvular Heart Disease

See Table 3.14 for characteristic symptoms, exam findings, and treatment of different valvular pathologies. Table 3.15 lists disorders that are associated with congenital cardiac defects.

PROSTHETIC VALVES

- **Mechanical valves:** Last 20 to 30 years; require lifetime anticoagulation because of thrombosis risk but have ↓ risk of structural failure.
- **Bioprosthetic valves:** Last 10 to 15 years; do not have as great a risk of thrombosis but do have ↑ risk of structural failure. Can be porcine, bovine, human heterograft, or autograft.
- Major complication is thromboembolism:
  - Risk for mitral valves > aortic valves.
  - Risk for mechanical valves > bioprosthetic valves.
  - Risk ↑ if patient has other thrombosis risk factors such as AF.
  - Larger thrombi (>5 mm) require fibrinolysis or valve replacement. Heparin may be used with smaller thrombi.
  - See Table 3.16 for recommendations on when to use anticoagulation with prosthetic valves.

KEY FACT

ACEIs, β-blockers, hydralazine, and spironolactone provide mortality benefit in patients with HF; diuretics and digoxin are used for symptomatic relief.

ANSWER

Continue to work with her toward improved BP and lipid control, but also refer her to a cardiologist and a cardiothoracic surgeon for consideration of a valve replacement.

KEY FACT

Bioprosthetic valves are preferable to mechanical valves for older patients with a life expectancy of <10 years and for those who are unable to take long-term anticoagulants.

KEY FACT

Choose a prosthetic valve on the basis of life expectancy and suitability for long-term anticoagulation.

TABLE 3.14.   **Valvular Heart Disease**

	AORTIC STENOSIS	AORTIC INSUFFICIENCY	MITRAL STENOSIS	MITRAL VALVE PROLAPSE	MITRAL INSUFFICIENCY
Cause	Rheumatic (world), bicuspid valve, senile calcific stenosis	Valve leaflet destruction (endocarditis, rheumatic, aortic stenosis), acute aortic dissection (Marfan), or aortic dilatation (seen with bicuspid valve, Marfan syndrome, long-standing HTN)	Rheumatic (most), occasionally endocarditis, calcification of mitral annulus (elderly)	Idiopathic, familial, Marfan syndrome, Ehlers-Danlos syndrome, post-MI, $\downarrow$ LV size, flail leaflet	Endocarditis, MI, trauma to valve, MVP, rheumatic
Symptoms	**Angina, syncope, HF,** dyspnea, $\downarrow$ exercise tolerance	Often asymptomatic until HF develops. If acute, usually leads to HF and hemodynamic instability	Dyspnea, hemoptysis from bronchial vein rupture due to pulmonary edema, symptoms from pulmonary HTN, right HF, or PE	Often asymptomatic MVP syndrome = atypical chest pain, palpitations, dizziness **not** related to valve dysfunction	Acute: Cardiogenic shock. Chronic: $\downarrow$ exercise tolerance, fatigue, dyspnea
Murmur	Systolic crescendo-descrescendo, radiates to carotids (pulsus parvus et tardus)	Diastolic decrescendo blowing at base (ie, right upper sternal border) (in severe cases, apical diastolic rumble is heard, as in MS). **Austin Flint murmur** may be heard from regurgitant jet causing premature mitral valve closure by hitting the anterior mitral leaflet	Diastolic apical rumble after an opening snap	Midsystolic click and murmur at the apex	Holosystolic, high pitched, best heard at apex in left lateral decubitus position with diaphragm of stethoscope
Exam findings	Brachio-radial delay, sustained PMD, $\downarrow$ S2, systolic click if bicuspid	$\downarrow$ S1, wide pulse pressure, water-hammer pulses, pulsating retinal artery, pulsating uvula, pulsating nailbed, head bobbing	$\downarrow$ pulses, $\uparrow$ S1 (may be $\downarrow$ S1 if very severe), signs of right HF ($\uparrow$ JVP, edema)		$\downarrow$ S1, $\oplus$ S3, if acute signs of left HF
Diagnosis	Echo (asymptomatic until valve area <1 cm^3, mean pressure gradient >40 mm Hg)	Echo (if acute, may need TEE to r/o endocarditis) – however first test is usually TTE. Most sensitive test is TEE	Echo (evaluate valve area, pressure gradient, morphology)	Echo (assess if regurgitation or $\downarrow$ LV function)	Echo

(continues)

TABLE 3.14.   **Valvular Heart Disease** *(continued)*

	AORTIC STENOSIS	AORTIC INSUFFICIENCY	MITRAL STENOSIS	MITRAL VALVE PROLAPSE	MITRAL INSUFFICIENCY
Treatment	Valve replacement once symptomatic Survival is 2-5 years without treatment once symptoms develop High-risk patients benefit more from transcatheter aortic valve replacement more than from replacement	Afterload reduction (ACEI) Valve replacement if symptoms or worsening LV dilation/function	Percutaneous balloon valvotomy if no regurgitation or thrombus; valve repair or replacement	Usually not necessary, unless significant mitral regurgitation develops	Acute: Surgery Chronic: Valve repair/ replacement if new AF and ↓ LV systolic function
Complications	LVH, diastolic dysfunction LV systolic dysfunction may occur over time Left atrial enlargement, pulmonary HTN, right HF may occur as a result of long-standing LVH	Left atrial enlargement, pulmonary HTN, right HF, AF	AF is a very common complication of mitral stenosis, LA thrombus formation, pulmonary HTN, PE, right HF		HF, infectious endocarditis, AF

TABLE 3.15.   **Disorders Associated With Congenital Cardiac Defects**

DISORDER	FEATURE	CARDIAC DEFECT(S)
Alcohol syndrome	Facial and growth anomalies, intellectual disability	VSD, ASD
Down syndrome (trisomy 21)	Typical facies, intellectual disability, hypothyroidism, ALL	Atrioventricular septal defect (endocardial cushion defect) is most common, then VSD, ASD, PDA, tetralogy of Fallot
Edwards syndrome (trisomy 18)	Hypertonia, prominent occiput, micrognathia	VSD and PDA are most common
Patau syndrome (trisomy 13)	Holoprosencephaly, polydactyly, rocker-bottom feet	VSD and PDA are most common
Noonan syndrome	Short stature, downward eye slant, low-set ears, intellectual disability	Pulmonary stenosis, hypertrophic cardiomyopathy
Turner syndrome (chromosome XO)	Short stature, streak gonads, webbed neck, lymphedema	Coarctation of aorta, bicuspid aortic valve
DiGeorge syndrome (22q11.2 deletion)	Abnormal facies, thymic aplasia, cleft palate, hypocalcemia	Truncus arteriosus, tetralogy of Fallot
Williams syndrome (7q11.23 deletion)	"Elfin" facies, neurodevelopmental delay with preservation of language, hypervitamin D	Supravalvular aortic stenosis, pulmonic valvular stenosis, septal defects

(continues)

TABLE 3.15.   Disorders Associated With Congenital Cardiac Defects *(continued)*

DISORDER	FEATURE	CARDIAC DEFECT(S)
Marfan syndrome (*FBN1* gene mutation)	Wide arm span, arachnodactyly, scoliosis, pectus carinatum/excavatum	Aortic root dilatation, aortic insufficiency, mitral valve prolapse
Congenital rubella	Growth retardation, meningoencephalitis, hearing loss, cataracts, petechiae, hepatomegaly	Septal defects, PDA, pulmonary artery stenosis
Maternal diabetes	Macrosomia, spina bifida, caudal regression syndrome	Transposition of the great vessels, VSD, coarctation, PDA, ASD, single ventricle, hypoplastic LV, pulmonic stenosis, pulmonary valve atresia, double outlet right ventricle, truncus arteriosus

Reproduced with permission from USMLE-Rx.com.

TABLE 3.16.   Anticoagulation in Heart Disease

CONDITION	PRIMARY RECOMMENDATION	SECONDARY RECOMMENDATION
Cardiovascular disease		Clopidogrel if cannot take ASA
CAD	ASA	
Acute ACS	ASA + heparin + clopidogrel (or ticagrelor)	
After ACS	ASA, continue clopidogrel for at least 1 mo for patients managed medically without stent	
After bare-metal stent	ASA, clopidogrel for at least 1 mo	
After drug-eluting stent	ASA, clopidogrel for at least 1 y	
Arrhythmia		
AF/atrial flutter	Warfarin; see section on AF/atrial flutter for details	
Postcardioversion	Warfarin for 4 weeks if maintains normal sinus rhythm	
Heart failure	Routine anticoagulation for EF <30 is NOT indicated unless LV thrombus is present; presence of LV thrombus with any LVEF is an indication for anticoagulation	**Warfarin** if AF or history of systemic embolism also present
Valvular disease		
Mitral valve disease	**Not routine**	**Warfarin** if AF or history of systemic embolism also present, or if LA thrombus regardless of AF
Aortic valve disease	**Not routine**	**Warfarin + ASA** if repeated systemic embolism
Prosthetic heart valves		
Mechanical	**Warfarin** for lifetime	**Warfarin + ASA** if other thrombotic risk factors
Bioprosthetic	**Warfarin** for first 3 months, **ASA** for lifetime	**Warfarin + ASA** if other thrombotic risk factors
Cerebrovascular disease		If stroke while on ASA, give clopidogrel or GpIIb–IIIa antagonist
Ischemic embolic stroke	Depends on source of emboli (AF, carotid, endocarditis, etc)	
Ischemic thrombotic stroke	ASA	
Hemorrhagic stroke	Avoid	

ENDOCARDITIS

Endocarditis is usually caused by gram-positive cocci. Gram-negative and fungal organisms are less frequent and are associated with IV drug use and prosthetic heart valves. Clinical manifestations of endocarditis are shown in Figure 3.19.

Prophylaxis

Antibiotics to prevent endocarditis during procedures should be limited to patients with cardiac conditions with very high risk of adverse outcomes from endocarditis.

- The American Heart Association recommends prophylactic antibiotics for **prosthetic heart valves, prosthetic material** used in valve repair or repair of congenital heart disease, unrepaired **cyanotic congenital heart disease** (or partially repaired with residual defects), valve pathology in a **transplanted heart,** and **prior history** of endocarditis.
- Prophylactic antibiotics are no longer recommended for aortic stenosis, bicuspid aortic valve, aortic regurgitation, mitral stenosis, mitral valve prolapse, mitral regurgitation, and hypertrophic cardiomyopathy.
- Procedures that need prophylaxis include dental procedures and respiratory procedures **if** they involve biopsy or incision of mucosa (eg, tonsillectomy, bronchoscopy).
- Procedures that do not need prophylaxis include GI or GU procedures (unless patient has known active infection), C-section, or vaginal delivery.
- **Antibiotic regimen:** Amoxicillin. If patient is allergic, can use cephalexin, clindamycin, or azithromycin.

MNEMONIC

Prophylaxis for endocarditis in HEaRT:

Hole (unrepaired or partially repaired congenital lesion)
Endocarditis previously
Repair with prosthetic material (of valve or congenital lesion)
Transplanted heart with valve pathology

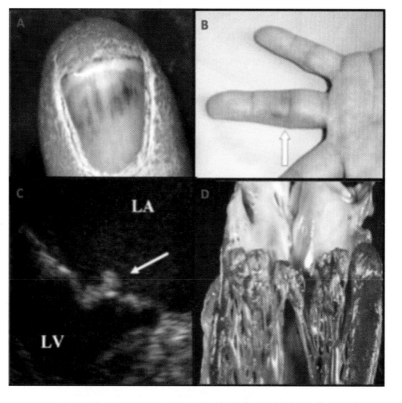

FIGURE 3.19.   **Clinical findings in endocarditis. (A)** Subungal splinter hemorrhages from infective endocarditis. **(B)** Painful, red, raised lesion of the fourth digit, compatible with an Osler node. **(C)** Vegetation on the mitral valve seen on echo. **(D)** Gross pathology demonstrating vegetations on the mitral valve. (Image A reproduced with permission from USMLE-Rx.com; image B reproduced from Yang M-L, et al. Case report: infective endocarditis caused by *Brevundimonas vesicularis. BMC Infect Dis.* 2006;6:179; image C reproduced from Norisada K, et al. Nonbacterial thrombotic endocarditis associated with cancer of unknown origin complicated with thrombus in the left auricular appendage: case report. *Cardiovasc Ultrasound.* 2011;9:8; image D reproduced from the CDC/Dr. Edwin P. Ewing, Jr.).

Anticoagulation in Heart Disease

Table 3.16 reviews the medications and indications for anticoagulation in various cardiovascular diseases.

Cardiomyopathies

Diseases of the heart muscle that have a variety of causes. Clinical presentation is variable and related to the underlying etiology.

- **Hypertrophic:** A genetic disorder with autosomal-dominant inheritance but variable penetrance. First-degree family members of affected individuals should be screened every year between ages 12 to 18, then every 5 years with an ECG, possibly an echocardiogram.
- **Restrictive:** Impaired diastolic filling with preserved systolic functioning.
  - Infiltrative (amyloid, sarcoid).
  - Noninfiltrative (familial, idiopathic).
  - Storage (hemochromatosis, Fabry disease).
  - Endomyocardial fibrosis (endemic in certain areas of the world, after radiation treatment).
- **Dilated:** Dilation and impaired contraction of one or both ventricles.
  - Ischemic.
  - Valvular.
  - Infectious (viral, Chagas disease, HIV, Lyme disease).
  - Toxic (alcohol, cocaine, methamphetamine, some chemotherapeutic agents).
  - Genetic.
  - Idiopathic.

Symptoms/Exam

- **Hypertrophic:** Often asymptomatic and found on routine family screening. Can present with symptoms of HF, SCD, syncope, or arrhythmias.
- **Restrictive:** Presents with symptoms of HF.
- **Dilated:** Can present with arrhythmias, HF, or SCD.

Diagnosis

- **Hypertrophic:**
  - Echo: LV thickening, may be asymmetric around the septum or apex → systolic pressure gradient.
  - ECG: LVH; prominent Q in II, III, aVF; P wave ↑ (LA enlargement).
  - Murmur: Systolic crescendo-decrescendo, radiating to axilla/base. ↑ with Valsava or standing (↓ blood return → less ventricular filling → ↑ obstruction). ↓ with squatting due to ↑ venous return into the LV. (Anything that makes the LV cavity smaller will worsen the obstruction and thus the murmur.)
- **Restrictive:** Ventricles have normal size and wall thickness but rigid walls on echocardiogram. Can have similar findings as constrictive pericarditis (see section on Constrictive pericarditis). Chest CT, cardiac MRI, or cardiac catheterization may assist in differentiating from constrictive pericarditis.
- **Dilated:** On echocardiogram: ↓ wall thickness, ↓ EF, ↑ LV volume.

Management

- **Hypertrophic:** Treatment with negative inotropes such as β-blockers or verapamil is directed toward improving diastolic filling in patients who are symptomatic. Avoid volume depletion, avoid vasodilators, and start activity restriction.

- **Restrictive:** Treatment aims to ↓ elevated filling pressures and treat symptoms of HF. Diuretics may relieve symptoms; CCBs may improve diastolic relaxation. Consider amiodarone or a defibrillator for high-risk patients with previous dysrhythmias, LVH, syncope, or specific genetic mutations.
- **Dilated:** Treatment is influenced by the development of HF.

Pericardial Disease

Pericardial disease often results from systemic disease. Often presents with both pericarditis and an effusion.

ACUTE PERICARDITIS

Etiologies of acute pericarditis are as follows:
- **Idiopathic:** The most common cause.
- **Infectious:** Usually viral (including HIV, coxsackie, Epstein-Barr virus, cytomegalovirus) but may also be caused by TB, other bacteria, or parasites.
- **Metabolic disorders:** Most commonly uremia, also hypothyroidism.
- **Other: Previous radiation, postinfarction** (Dressler syndrome), **inflammatory/autoimmune** (lupus, RA, scleroderma), **neoplastic** (often lung or breast cancer), **degenerative, traumatic, medications** (isoniazid, hydralazine).

Symptoms/Exam
- Presents with sudden onset, sharp, pleuritic chest pain that ↑ when the patient is supine and ↓ when the patient leans forward. Can be angina-like.
- **Pericardial friction rub.**
- **Diffuse ST-segment elevations** are found on ECG, as seen in Figure 3.20. PR depression. Sometimes cardiac markers are elevated, which may represent myopericarditis. Echocardiogram is often normal unless associated effusion is present.
- **High-risk features** include high fever, acute onset, evidence of tamponade or large effusion, acute trauma, leukocytosis, and failure to respond to medical therapy within 7 days.

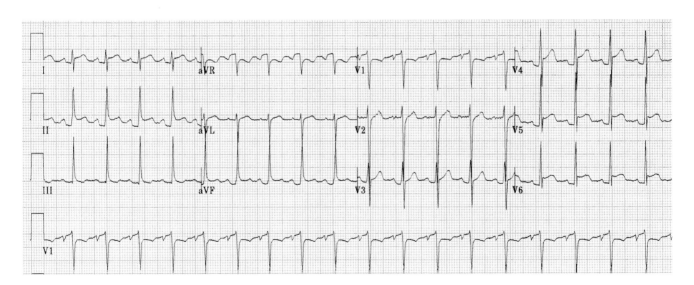

FIGURE 3.20. **Diffuse ST-segment elevations on ECG in pericarditis.** (Reproduced with permission from Knoop KJ, Stack LB, Storrow AB, Thurman RJ. *The Atlas of Emergency Medicine,* 3rd ed. http://www.accessmedicine.com. Copyright © The McGraw-Hill Companies, Inc. All rights reserved.)

Diagnosis

Diagnosed clinically based on the findings above. Usually benign course.

Management

NSAIDs in conjunction with colchicine. Steroids can also be used for refractory cases.

CONSTRICTIVE PERICARDITIS

Results from subacute or chronic scarring and loss of elasticity of the pericardial sac, so cardiac filling is impeded by external force. Because of less stretch, LV and RV are more interdependent. Many findings are similar to those in restrictive cardiomyopathy (Table 3.17 and Figure 3.21).

PERICARDIAL EFFUSION

Often accompanies acute pericarditis. Causes are similar to those of acute pericarditis, with the most common being idiopathic, infectious, malignancy, trauma, and post-MI.

- Symptoms and exam findings are similar to those of acute pericarditis; sometimes also persistent fever, L > R pleural effusion, cardiomegaly.
- **ECG** may show associated pericarditis; if large enough, effusion can look like tamponade (see tamponade information below—low-voltage, electrical alternans).
- **CXR** may show enlarged cardiac silhouette with a "water-bottle configuration" (Figure 3.22).
- **Echocardiography** can confirm the presence of effusion and determines the hemodynamic impact (impaired ventricular filling).
- **Pericardiocentesis** is most useful for cytology and cultures. Not always indicated, depending on cause/size of effusion. Acutely indicated if signs of tamponade are present (hemodynamic instability, pulsus paradoxus).
- Treatment is specific to the cause.

KEY FACT

Pericardial effusion may accompany acute pericarditis.

TABLE 3.17. Comparison of Restrictive Cardiomyopathy and Constrictive Pericarditis

	RESTRICTIVE CARDIOMYOPATHY	CONSTRICTIVE PERICARDITIS
Causes	Infiltrative (amyloid sarcoid), storage (hemochromatosis, Fabry disease), idiopathic, familial, hypereosinophillic syndromes	Scarring from previous pericardial disease (idiopathic, viral, radiation, postsurgical, connective tissue disease, TB)
Exam	↑ JVP, Kussmaul sign (lack of JVP decline during inspiration)	
ECG changes	Low voltage (more with constrictive pericarditis or amyloidosis), LVH, Q waves, impaired AV conduction, nonspecific ST-segment changes	
CXR/CT	Mild cardiomegaly	Mild cardiomegaly, occasional calcification of pericardium—seen as ↑ thickness on CT (see Figure 3.21)
Brain natriuretic peptide level	↑ (wall stretches)	Normal (wall can't stretch)

Chest pain better with sitting up, worse with laying down. Diffuse PR depressions and evidence of pericardial effusion on echo (not always present). A preceding viral illness or rheumatic disease should make you think of potential pericardial inflammation.

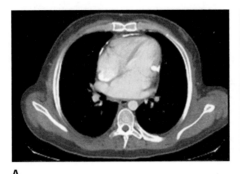

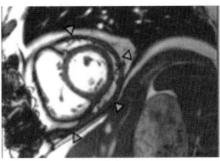

A   **B**

FIGURE 3.21. **Constrictive pericarditis.** (Image A reproduced with permission from Fuster V, O'Rourke RA, Walsh RA, Poole-Wilson P. *Hurst's The Heart,* 12th ed., Fig. 21-25. http://www.accessmedicine.com. Copyright © The McGraw-Hill Companies, Inc. All rights reserved; image B reproduced with permission from Fauci AS, Kasper DL, Braunwald E, et al. *Harrison's Principles of Internal Medicine,* 17th ed. New York: McGraw-Hill, 2008, Fig. 222-9.)

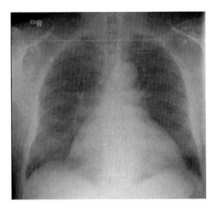

FIGURE 3.22. **Pericardial effusion.** CXR shows enlargement of the cardiac silhouette ("water-bottle heart") in a patient with pericardial effusion. (Reproduced with permission from USMLE-Rx.com.)

CARDIAC TAMPONADE

Caused by an effusion under pressure → impaired ventricular filling. May be acute or subacute. Etiologies are:
- **Acute:** Usually traumatic (penetrating trauma, aortic rupture, procedures such as pacemaker placement).
- **Subacute:** Neoplasm, pericarditis.

Symptoms/Exam
- **Acute:** Presents with chest pain and dyspnea. Classic exam findings include **elevated JVP, muted heart sounds, and hypotension.** Potentially life-threatening.
- **Subacute:** Presents with chest pain. Exam may reveal hypotension, tachycardia, and a narrowed pulse pressure.

Diagnosis
- **ECG:** Low-voltage, sinus tachycardia; "electrical alternans"—QRS shifts from beat to beat due to swinging of heart in large effusion (Figure 3.23).
- **Pulsus paradoxus:** An SBP ↓ of >10 mm Hg during inspiration. Occurs with tamponade, constrictive pericarditis, asthma, and COPD.
- **Echocardiography:** Shows right atrial collapse during diastole and equalization of RV and LV pressures (Figure 3.24).

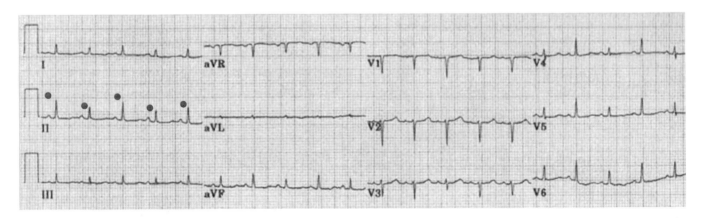

FIGURE 3.23. **Cardiac tamponade.** ECG shows low-voltage QRS complexes with electrical alternans (red dots). (Reproduced from Banham-Hall EJ, et al. Malignancy with unknown primary presenting as acute cardiac tamponade: a case report. *Cases J.* 2009;2:8176.)

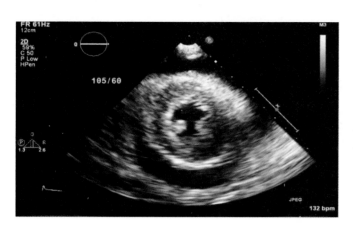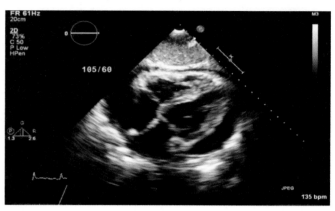

FIGURE 3.24. Pericardial tamponade. Transechocardiogram images show a large pericardial effusion with collapse of the right atrium and right ventricle in early diastole. (Reproduced with permission from USMLE-Rx.com.)

Management

Drainage via either pericardiocentesis or an open procedure is required. Pericardiectomy may also be necessary if frequently recurs.

> **KEY FACT**
>
> Cardiac tamponade is an effusion under pressure → impaired ventricular filling. Classic exam findings include ↑ JVP, distant heart sounds, hypotension, and pulsus paradoxus >12 mm Hg.

Peripheral Vascular Disease

Almost always due to peripheral atherosclerosis; therefore, risk factors are the same as those in coronary atherosclerosis (tobacco use, HTN, hyperlipidemia, diabetes).

Symptoms/Exam

- Often asymptomatic. **The classic symptom is claudication,** or pain in a muscle group that is reproduced with exercise and relieved by rest. Severity varies and symptoms do not always correlate with degree of vessel stenosis.
- The calf is the most frequently affected area, but the buttocks, thighs, and feet may also be affected.
- Poor wound healing.
- Rest pain is a late finding that often occurs at night.
- Exam findings include ↓ pulses, peripheral bruits, and cool, shiny extremities with ↓ hair.

Diagnosis

Ankle-brachial index (ABI) **<0.9** (indicates > 50% stenosis of one or more vessels). Higher systolic ankle pressure/systolic brachial pressure by Doppler. Performed at rest and after exercise. Calcified vessels can cause an abnormally high ABI (>1.3). ABI of <0.4 indicates ischemia.
- **Segmental limb pressures** are used to evaluate the extent of disease.
- Other modalities: Ultrasound with duplex, MRI, CT.

> **KEY FACT**
>
> Peripheral vascular disease is characterized by an ankle-brachial index <0.9.

Management

- **Risk factor reduction:** Tobacco cessation, treatment of hyperlipidemia, and control of glucose and BP. Rehabilitation and structured exercise programs.
- **Pharmacologic:**
  - **Aspirin:** Has only modest benefit. Ticlopidine and clopidogrel can also be used.
  - **Cilostazol:** Inhibits platelet aggregation and ↑ vasodilation.
  - **Pentoxifylline:** ↑ RBC deformity and ↓ serum viscosity.
  - **Ginkgo biloba:** Has been shown to be somewhat effective, although the mechanism is unclear.

- **Interventional procedures:**
  - Indicated for symptoms that limit activity as well as with rest pain or tissue loss (ischemic ulcers or gangrene).
  - Include percutaneous revascularization with percutaneous angioplasty or stents, generally for more focal lesions.
  - Surgical revascularization (endarterectomy or bypass grafting) if cannot be done percutaneously.

Endocrinology

Hannah Snyder, MD

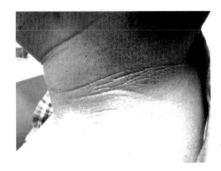

FIGURE 4.1. Acanthosis nigricans.
(Reproduced from Teelucksingh S, et al. Does insulin resistance co-exist with glucocorticoid resistance in the metabolic syndrome? Studies comparing skin sensitivity to glucocorticoids in individuals with and without acanthosis nigricans. *Cardiovasc Diabetol.* 2012;11:31.)

Diabetes Mellitus

Diabetes mellitus (DM) is an impairment in carbohydrate metabolism leading to hyperglycemia.

- **Type 1 (juvenile diabetes):** Due to absolute insulin insufficiency caused by destruction of pancreatic islet cells. Type 1 DM is typically autoimmune but can be idiopathic.
- **Type 2 (most common type of DM and becoming more common in children):** Due to insulin resistance and variable degrees of relative insulin deficiency.
- **Gestational diabetes:** A complication of pregnancy (see the Reproductive Health chapter).
- Other uncommon etiologies: Diabetes from pancreatic destruction (chronic pancreatitis, cystic fibrosis) and mature-onset diabetes of the young.

Symptoms/Exam

- **May be asymptomatic (common in type 2 DM).**
- Symptoms include polyuria, polydipsia, polyphagia, weight loss, blurry vision, acanthosis nigricans (a sign of insulin resistance; see Figure 4.1), dehydration, and neuropathy.
- **Diabetic ketoacidosis (DKA)** and **hyperosmolar hyperglycemic state** are acute complications and can be the initial presentation of diabetes (see below).

Diagnosis

The American Diabetes Association diagnostic criteria for DM are as follows:

- **Random plasma glucose concentration of ≥200 mg/dL combined with symptoms of diabetes.**
- Plasma glucose of ≥126 mg/dL after 8 hours of fasting.
- Plasma glucose of ≥200 mg/dL 2 hours after a 75-g glucose load during an oral glucose tolerance test.
- A_{1c} ≥6.5%.

For all but the first criterion, you must **repeat testing to confirm the diagnosis.**

Screening

- The USPSTF recommends screening overweight or obese adults 40 to 70 years old (see the Community and Preventive Medicine chapter).
- Symptomatic individuals should be tested.

Management

- **Glycemic control:** Nonpharmacologic modalities are typically the first approach to glycemic control but pharmacologic agents are often added early in the disease course.
- **Nonpharmacologic:** Diet, exercise, weight loss, and stress management can all help control glucose levels and ↓ the need for other medications in type 2 DM.
- **Pharmacologic:**
  - **First line:** Metformin is used in diabetics without contraindications because it is the only oral agent shown to reduce mortality.
  - If control is not achieved with metformin plus 1 to 2 additional agents despite good adherence, patients should be changed to insulin. There is no evidence that newer agents are more effective than insulin.
  - Table 4.1 outlines medications for the treatment of type 2 DM.
  - **Insulin** is appropriate for type 1 and type 2 DM. Options include a "basal–bolus" regimen (basal coverage with intermediate- to long-acting insulin plus

TABLE 4.1.   **Medications Used in Type 2 DM**

CLASS	DRUGS	MECHANISM	ADVERSE EFFECTS	CONTRAINDICATIONS	COMMENTS
Biguanides	Metformin	↑ insulin sensitivity, ↓ hepatic glucose production	GI side effects (nausea, diarrhea), lactic acidosis (↑ risk in renal disease)	Strict contraindication with GFR <30 mL/min, evaluate in patients with GFR 30-45 mL/min; hold prior to surgery or contrast, or in unstable HF	First-line treatment: Promote weight loss; hypoglycemia is rare; reduces mortality; often continued when on insulin
Sulfonylureas	Glipizide, glyburide, glimepiride	↑ insulin secretion	Hypoglycemia, weight gain	Dose adjust in renal insufficiency	Give with meals
Thiazolidinediones	Rosiglitazone, pioglitazone	↑ glucose uptake and ↓ glucose secretion from liver, ↑ insulin sensitivity	Rare hypoglycemia; weight gain/edema, liver disease	NYHA class III or IV HF, history of bladder cancer, osteoporosis	
Glucagon-like peptide-1 receptor agonists (GLP-1 RAs)	Exenatide, albiglutide, liraglutide	Delay gastric emptying, ↑ glucose uptake and ↓ glucose secretion from liver	Nausea, vomiting, diarrhea, pancreatitis	Gastroparesis, CrCl <30 mL/min, family/personal history of medullary thyroid cancer	Injectable; promote weight loss
Dipeptidyl peptidase 4 inhibitors	Sitagliptin, vildagliptin	↑ GLP-1 RA, ↑ insulin secretion	GI upset, rare hypoglycemia, pancreatitis		Weight neutral
Meglitinides	Repaglinide, nateglinide	↑ insulin secretion	Hypoglycemia		Short acting; use for postprandial hyperglycemia
Sodium-glucose cotransporter 2 inhibitors	Canagliflozin, dapagliflozin, empagliflozin	↓ renal glucose reabsorbtion	Yeast infections, UTIs, polyuria	Renal or liver failure	
α-glucosidase inhibitors	Miglitol, acarbose	Slow intestinal carbohydrate absorption	Gas, bloating, diarrhea	CrCl <25 mL/min	Start low and gradually ↑ dosage
Amylin replacement	Pramlintide	Slow gastric emptying, ↓ glucagon	Nausea, hypoglycemia	Gastroparesis	Injectable with meals in patients on bolus insulin, lower weight

a short-acting bolus insulin before meals), insulin in combination with other agents, or continuous insulin infusion via an insulin pump (Figure 4.2). Consider starting insulin as first-line treatment if A_{1c} is >10%.

- Generally metformin is continued if insulin is started, other oral antihyperglycemics are stopped. Metformin continues to help with weight and lower mortality.

QUESTION

A 70-year-old thin man presents for a diabetes test. He denies any diabetes symptoms. Lab results show a fasting blood glucose level of 150 mg/dL and creatinine level of 1.3 mg/dL. What further workup should you do before starting the patient on metformin?

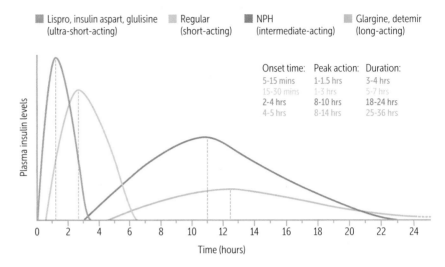

FIGURE 4.2. **Activity profiles of insulin types.** (Reproduced with permission from USMLE-Rx.com.)

ACUTE COMPLICATIONS

Hypoglycemia

A common occurrence in diabetic patients on insulin therapy. Can also occur with use of oral hypoglycemics, especially sulfonylureas.

- **Symptoms/Exam:** May present with **autonomic symptoms** of tachycardia, palpitations, sweating, tremulousness, nausea, hunger, or with **neuroglycopenic symptoms**—confusion, stupor, coma, focal neurologic findings—resulting from low glucose delivery to the brain.
- **Diagnosis:** Whipple's triad.
- **Management: Conscious patients:** Give glucose tablets, juice, and other high-glucose drinks or snacks. **Unconscious patients:** Administer 50% dextrose IV or IM glucagon.

Diabetic Ketoacidosis

Much more common in type 1 than in type 2 DM. Can be the initial manifestation of type 1 or may occur later in either type 1 or type 2. Look for a stressor (eg, infection, surgery, infarction, medical noncompliance) that may have precipitated DKA.

- **Symptoms/Exam:** Abdominal pain, vomiting, Kussmaul respirations (rapid deep breaths), a fruity breath odor (from acetone), and lethargy. Can progress to coma.
- **Diagnosis:** Lab findings include hyperglycemia, hyperosmolality, and a high anion-gap metabolic acidosis—serum HCO_3 <18 mEq/L; pH <7.3; serum ketones (Table 4.2).
- **Management:**
    - **Insulin drip:** To close the anion gap and ↓ plasma glucose. Switch to SQ insulin only when the anion gap has closed, regardless of the glucose level.
    - **Fluids:** Start with NS at 1 L/hour in adults. Add D5 when glucose is <200 mg/dL.
    - **Electrolytes: Potassium** is usually falsely elevated initially because of acidosis + hyperglycemia and will ↓ with treatment. Unless K is >5.3 mEq/L, it should be added to fluids. If K <3.3 mEq/L it should be given prior to starting insulin since insulin drives K into cells.

MNEMONIC

Symptoms of DKA:

Dehydration/**D**elerium
Ketones/**K**ussmaul breathing/**K** low
Acidosis/**A**bdominal pain

KEY FACT

In DKA, continue IV insulin until the anion gap closes, even after glucose has normalized (add dextrose to IV to prevent hypoglycemia if needed).

A   **ANSWER**

Glycated hemoglobin (A_{1c}) to confirm the diagnosis and monitor treatment; also calculate glomerular filtration rate (GFR), as serum creatinine can be misleading in elderly individuals with low muscle mass.

TABLE 4.2.   Diabetic Ketoacidosis Versus Hyperosmolar Hyperglycemic State

	DKA	HHS
Pathophysiology	Shortage of insulin → lack of intracellular fuel → ketosis → acidosis	Excess of glucose → hyperosmolality → polyuria → dehydration
Onset	Short (hours to days)	Insidious (days to weeks)
Blood glucose	>250 mg/dL	>600 mg/dL
pH	<7.3	>7.3
HCO_3	<18 mEq/L	>18 mEq/L
Osmolality	Variable	>320 mOsm/kg
Anion gap	>12	Variable
Total body water deficit	5-7 L	8-10 L

- ▪ **Bicarbonate: Not indicated** unless there is severe acidosis (pH <6.9).
- ▪ **Treat the underlying stressor.**

Hyperosmolar Hyperglycemic State

Defined as significant hyperglycemia, hyperosmolality, and dehydration without ketosis. Look for a precipitating stressor (eg, infection, infarction, intoxication, medical noncompliance).

- ▪ **Symptoms/Exam:** Presents with **polyuria, polydipsia, polyphagia,** weakness, lethargy, confusion, and coma.
- ▪ **Diagnosis:** Serum glucose is often >800 mg/dL, osmolality is elevated >320 mOsm/kg, pH is >7.3 (see Table 4.3). The name tells you everything you need: hyperosmolar and hyperglycemic (more than in DKA).
- ▪ **Management: Treat the underlying stressor;** give fluids, insulin drip, and electrolyte replacement. Similar to treatment for DKA but fluids are the cornerstone of treatment—more important than insulin. Often need 8 to 10 L of fluids in these patients (more than in DKA). Watch for pulmonary edema and volume overload in elderly patients.

CHRONIC COMPLICATIONS

Most of the **chronic complications** of DM begin about 5 years after disease onset. Screening for complications in patients with type 1 DM begins 5 years after diagnosis. However, for patients with type 2 DM, screening begins immediately after diagnosis, as these patients usually have had the disease for years before diagnosis.

- ▪ **Microvascular:**
  - ▪ **Retinopathy:** Schedule an annual eye exam by an ophthalmologist. Retinal neovascularization can be treated with photocoagulation therapy (Figure 4.3).
  - ▪ **Nephropathy:** Screen annually for microalbuminuria. ACEIs or ARBs can slow progression of renal disease in patients with microalbuminuria.
  - ▪ **Neuropathy:** Peripheral neuropathy starts in the distal feet and moves to the hands. Stress the importance of foot care and annual foot exams to prevent complications. Autonomic neuropathy may cause orthostatic hypotension, gastroparesis, neurogenic bladder, and impotence. Manage with improved glycemic control and pain management.

KEY FACT

For both DKA and HHS, always look for a precipitating stressor (eg, infection, infarction, intoxication, medical noncompliance).

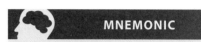

MNEMONIC

Chronic complications of diabetes:
KNIVES

Kidney
Neuropathy
Infection
Vascular
Eyes
Skin changes

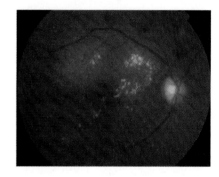

FIGURE 4.3.   Diabetic retinopathy.
Fundus photograph shows intraretinal hemorrhages, hard exudates, and microaneurysms in the posterior pole associated with diabetic macular edema. (Reproduced from Stefanini FR, et al. Anti-VEGF for the management of diabetic macular edema. *J Immunol Res.* 2014;2014:632307.)

QUESTION

A: A 10-year-old boy presents to the ED with lethargy, nausea, and vomiting. Exam reveals that he is tachypneic. UA shows 4+ glucose and ketones; glucose level is >500 mg/dL. What treatment would you start?
B: Additional lab results show a K^+ level of 4.0 mEq/L, a blood glucose level of 550 mg/dL, and a pH of 7.29. What can now be added to his fluids?
C: Subsequently his blood glucose level decreases to 210 mg/dL, K^+ level is 4.2 mEq/L, and he has a serum anion gap of 18 mEq/L. Should you switch to an SQ insulin regimen?

TABLE 4.3. **Routine Management of Diabetes**

Glucose control	Goal A_{1c} is <7% for most nonpregnant adults, <8% for those with short life expectancy, symptomatic hypoglycemia, multiple comorbidities or advanced vascular disease A_{1c} reflects glucose levels for the last 3 months; check at least twice a year in stable patients
BP control	Goal BP is <140/90 mm Hg regardless of age
Lipid control	All diabetics 40-75 years with LDL 70-189 should be on moderate-dose statin If 10 year ASCVD ≥7.5%, known ASCVD, or LDL ≥190 should be on high-dose statin
Aspirin therapy	Daily 81-mg aspirin therapy is recommended as followed: 1. 2° prevention in high-risk groups such as those with a history of MI, CAD, and PVD 2. 1° prevention in diabetic patients with ↑ cardiovascular risk (10-year risk >10%) and not at ↑ bleeding risk
Smoking cessation	Advise all patients to stop smoking
Nephropathy screening	Screen annually for microalbuminuria with urine albumin:creatinine and eGFR as follows: 1. Type 2 DM patients: screen immediately after diagnosis 2. Type 1 DM patients: screen 5 years after diagnosis Treat with ACEIs or ARBs; tolerate up to a 15%-20% ↑ in serum creatinine with the initiation of ACEIs/ARBs Tight BP and glucose control also delays development
Retinopathy screening	Schedule an annual ophthalmology exam as follows: 1. Type 2 DM patients: immediately after diagnosis 2. Type 1 DM patients: 5 years after diagnosis Maintain tight glucose and BP control for prevention Laser therapy can slow diabetic retinopathy and ↓ the risk of vision loss May space to every 2 years if prior exams normal
Foot care	Perform an annual complete foot exam with monofilament testing, pinprick/vibration/temperature sensation, visual inspection on each visit, and prophylactic foot care education for all diabetic patients
Immunizations	Vaccinate adults with the PPSV23 if <65, PCV 13 followed by PPSV23 if >65, and the annual influenza vaccine

ANSWER

A: NS and IV insulin.
B: K⁺.
C: Not yet; add 5% dextrose to his fluids and continue IV insulin until the anion gap closes.

- **Diabetic ulcers and osteomyelitis:** Neuropathy and trauma may result in bony deformations, including those of the foot, such as a Charcot joint. People with diabetes are also at higher risk for infections of the soft tissue (cellulitis) and bones (osteomyelitis; Figure 4.4).
- **Macrovascular complications:** Associated with an ↑ risk of MI and stroke. Control risk factors with the following measures (see Table 4.3):
  - Daily aspirin.
  - Smoking cessation.
  - **BP control:** Goal is <40/90 mm Hg.
  - **Lipids:** Start statin if LDL >70 mg/dL, do not treat to a goal.
  - Diet and exercise.

METABOLIC SYNDROME

Also known as insulin resistance syndrome or "syndrome X." Represents a combination of traits associated with insulin resistance and an ↑ risk of type 2 DM.
- **Diagnosis:** Based on any **three** of the following:
  - Abdominal obesity (waist circumference: men >40 in, women >35 in).
  - TG ≥150 mg/dL.
  - HDL <40 mg/dL in men and <50 mg/dL in women.
  - BP ≥130/85 mm Hg.
  - Fasting glucose ≥100 mg/dL.

- **Management:** Directed toward preventing the development of type 2 DM and coronary vascular disease. Focus on lifestyle modifications (diet, weight loss, exercise) and, if needed, metformin.

Pituitary Disorders

The pituitary gland releases eight hormones that regulate the body's endocrine functions. The hypothalamus produces oxytocin and antidiuretic hormone (ADH, vasopressin), which are then stored and released by the posterior pituitary. The anterior pituitary produces six hormones: Adrenocorticotropic hormone (ACTH), thyroid-stimulating hormone (TSH), follicle-stimulating hormone (FSH), luteinizing hormone (LH), growth hormone (GH), and prolactin (see Table 4.4 and Figure 4.5).

PITUITARY TUMORS

Pituitary tumors may arise from any cell. They are classified as **microadenomas** (<1 cm) and **macroadenomas** (>1 cm). They may ↑ or ↓ hormones produced by the cells of origin by mass effect. Subtypes include the following:
- **Functional pituitary adenomas (in order from most to least common):**
  - Prolactinomas (the most common pituitary microadenoma).
  - GH-secreting.
  - ACTH-secreting.
  - TSH-secreting (rare).
- Nonfunctioning (account for one-third of pituitary tumors; the most common macroadenoma).

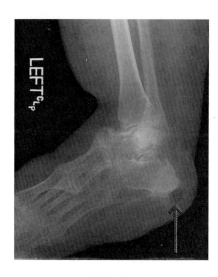

FIGURE 4.4. Diabetic foot.
Osteopenia and destruction of the ankle and tarsal joints (Charcot joints). Also, note the soft-tissue ulcer at the heel (arrow) with sclerosis of the underlying calcaneus that likely represents chronic osteomyelitis. (Reproduced with permission from USMLE-Rx.com.)

TABLE 4.4. Pituitary Hormones

HORMONE	EFFECT	INCREASED BY	DECREASED BY	EXCESS	DEFICIENCY
ADH/vasopressin	Vasoconstriction, ↑ free water retention in kidneys, thirst	Reduced plasma volume, high serum osmolality	Low serum osmolality	Syndrome of inappropriate secretion of ADH	Diabetes insipidus
ACTH	↑ cortisol release from adrenals	Corticotropin-releasing hormone (CRH), stress	High cortisol	Cushing syndrome	Adrenal insufficiency
TSH	↑ T_4 production in thyroid	Thyroid releasing hormone (TRH)	High T_4 and/or T_3	Hyperthyroidism	Hypothyroidism
LH/FSH	↑ sex hormone production	Gonadotropin-releasing hormone	Gonadal sex steroids		Hypogonadism
GH	Linear growth, protein synthesis	GHRH, hypoglycemia, testosterone	Somatostatin, glucocorticoids	**Childhood:** gigantism **Adulthood:** acromegaly	**Childhood:** short stature **Adulthood:** poor well-being
Prolactin	Lactation	Pregnancy, nursing, TRH, stress, medications	Dopamine is constantly secreted and inhibits prolactin	Galactorrhea, hypogonadism	Inability to lactate

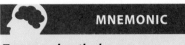

MNEMONIC

To remember the hormones released by the pituitary gland:
Anterior **P**ituitary **L**ets **F**olks **G**row **T**hyroid (**A**CTH, **p**rolactin, **L**SH, **F**SH, **G**H, **T**SH)
Posterior pituitary: **A**dds **O**xytocin (**A**DH, **o**xytocin)

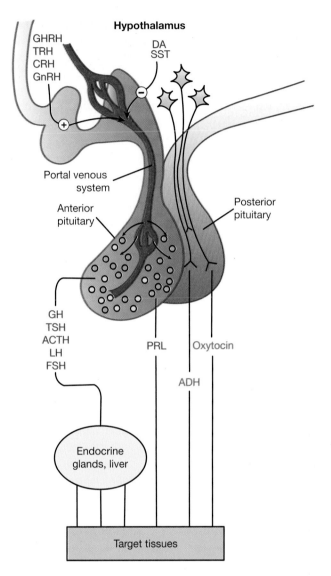

FIGURE 4.5. **The hypothalamic-pituitary endocrine system.** Except for prolactin, hormones released from the anterior pituitary stimulate the production of hormones by a peripheral endocrine gland or the liver. Prolactin and the hormones released from the posterior pituitary (ADH and oxytocin) act directly on target tissues. Hypothalamic factors regulate the release of anterior pituitary hormones. (Reproduced with permission from Katzung BG, et al. *Basic and Clinical Pharmacology*, 11th ed. New York: McGraw-Hill, 2009, Fig. 37-1.)

Symptoms/Exam

- Incidental discovery on MRI is very common; between 10% and 20% of pituitary adenomas may be unsuspected or found incidentally.
- Symptomatic cases may present as follows:
    - **Neurologic:** Headaches; visual field deficits (bitemporal hemianopia due to mass effect on the optic chiasm; Figure 4.6A).
    - **Hormonal excess/deficiency:** Hypothyroidism, hypogonadism, hyperprolactinemia (see specific sections for symptomatology).

Differential

The differential for intrasellar masses includes benign lesions (craniopharyngioma, meningioma), malignancies (1°—germ cell tumors and lymphomas; metastases—especially breast and lung cancer), cysts (Rathke cleft, arachnoid, and dermoid cysts can cause sellar enlargement), and infections (abscesses, TB).

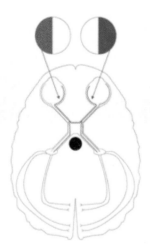

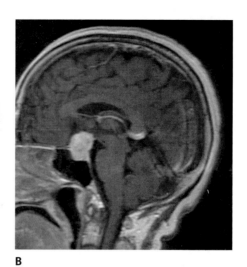

A   B

FIGURE 4.6.   **Pituitary adenoma.** (A) A pituitary adenoma represented by the black spot compresses the optic chiasm resulting in bitemporal hemianopia. (B) Gadolinium-enhanced sagittal MRI shows an expanding lesion inside the sella with suprasellar extension; histological examination of the resected mass confirmed the diagnosis of a prolactin-secreting adenoma. (Image A reproduced with permission from USMLE-Rx.com; image B reproduced from Wang CS, et al. Pituitary macroadenoma coexistent with supraclinoid internal carotid artery cerebral aneurysm: a case report and review of the literature. *Cases J.* 2009;2:6459.)

Diagnosis

- **Labs:** Check **prolactin** (most high yield) first. If normal, consider checking insulin-like growth factor-1 (IGF-1), 24-hour urine for cortisol, ACTH, TSH, LH, FSH, and testosterone levels.
- **Imaging:** MRI of the pituitary/sella (Figure 4.6B).

Management

- Observation with serial MRIs and labs may suffice if the tumor is nonfunctioning and is not causing visual field defects.
- Treatment for symptomatic disease is as follows:
    - **Medical:** Treat hormone deficiency or excess as appropriate (discussed in following sections).
    - **Surgical:** The transsphenoidal approach is successful in approximately 90% of microadenomas.
    - **Radiation:** Side effects include panhypopituitarism (seen in up to 90% of cases) requiring lifelong hormonal supplementation.

HYPOPITUITARISM

↓ secretion of one or more pituitary hormones. May be idiopathic or caused by:
- **Invasion:** Pituitary adenomas, craniopharyngiomas.
- **Infarction:**
    - **Sheehan syndrome:** Infarction of the pituitary occurring postpartum following substantial blood loss in childbirth. Presents with the inability to lactate, lethargy, and amenorrhea.
    - **Pituitary apoplexy:** Sudden hemorrhage, often into a pituitary adenoma. Presents with severe headache, visual field defects, and hypotension. May resolve spontaneously or require high-dose steroids ± decompression.
- **Injury:** Head trauma can cause anterior pituitary dysfunction and vasopressin deficiency.

- **Iatrogenic:** Postradiation therapy or after surgery.
- **Empty sella syndrome:** Enlarged sella turcica not entirely filled with pituitary. May be 1° or 2°.
    - 1°: A defect in the diaphragm sella leading to infiltration with CSF fluid.
    - 2°: Enlargement of the sella by a mass that is then removed by surgery, radiation, or infarction.
- **Other:** Infiltrative causes like sarcoidosis, immunologic causes, or infections like TB and fungi.

Symptoms/Exam

Screen patients after brain injury or high-risk surgery. May be asymptomatic or may present with symptoms 2° to mass effect and/or signs of hormone deficiency:

- **ACTH deficiency:** ↓ cortisol secretion (hypotension and shock, nausea, electrolyte disturbance).
- **TSH deficiency:** Hypothyroidism.
- **LH/FSH deficiency:** Hypogonadism. In women, presents with anovulation, infertility, and ↓ estrogen secretion. In men, infertility and ↓ testosterone are seen.
- **GH deficiency:** Presents as short stature in children. May cause a variety of subtle effects in adults, including ↓ muscle mass, ↓ bone mineral density (BMD), and ↓ energy.
- **Prolactin deficiency:** Inability to lactate postpartum.

Diagnosis

Diagnosed by testing basal hormone levels and by stimulation tests:

- **ACTH:** Abnormal ACTH and cortisol levels with failure of synthetic corticotropin stimulation test.
- **TSH:** Low free T_4 (TSH may be low or normal).
- **FSH/LH:** Low FSH/LH.
- **GH:** Low IGF-1.
- **Prolactin:** Low prolactin.

Management

Treat the underlying cause. Correct hormone deficiencies as follows:

- **ACTH:** Glucocorticoids.
- **TSH:** Levothyroxine.
- **FSH/LH:** In men, treat with testosterone replacement. In women, consider estrogen and progesterone therapy. Keep in mind ↑ cardiovascular risk and ↑ estrogen-dependent cancers with unopposed estrogen.
- **GH:** Human GH, although not usually used in adults.
- **Prolactin:** No treatment needed.

DIABETES INSIPIDUS

Low ADH activity causes diabetes insipidus (DI), which is characterized by polyuria and an inability to concentrate urine. There are two types of DI:

- **Central:** ↓ release of ADH. Causes include pituitary injury (neurosurgery, trauma, tumors, ischemia, autoimmune), genetic, or idiopathic.
- **Nephrogenic:** Resistance to ADH at the level of the kidneys. The most common cause is lithium toxicity. Other causes are electrolyte disturbances, malnutrition, and aging.

KEY FACT

ACTH deficiency differs from 1° adrenal insufficiency in that it does not cause hyperkalemia or hyperpigmentation. Hyperpigmentation happens when cortisol is low so ACTH synthesis is ↑—the precursor hormone is cleaved into ACTH and melanocyte stimulating hormone.

ANSWER

Diabetes insipidus. Confirm your diagnosis with water deprivation test, then do vasopressin challenge to see if it is central or peripheral.

Symptoms/Exam

- Inappropriately **dilute** urine (low urine osmolality) in the setting of ↑ **serum osmolality and hypernatremia.** ↓ ADH action means free water is not being retained; there is a relative excess of free water in the urine.
- **Polyuria,** nocturia, and polydipsia.
- There is no glucose dysregulation with DI.

Differential

Osmotic diuresis (eg, elevated serum and urine osmolality), **diabetes mellitus, psychogenic polydipsia** (low serum and urine osmolality).

Diagnosis

See Figure 4.7.

Management

- **Central DI:** Treat any underlying lesion if present. Administer intranasal desmopressin (DDAVP).
- **Nephrogenic DI:** Encourage fluids and restrict sodium; discontinue lithium. Thiazide diuretics and amiloride may help ↑ renal sodium excretion (paradoxically have antidiuretic effect).

Complications

Dehydration, hydronephrosis.

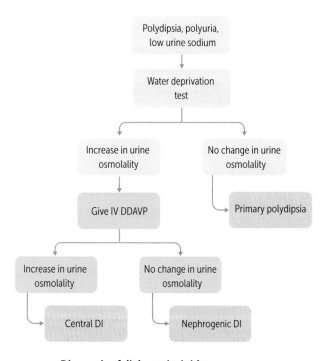

FIGURE 4.7. **Diagnosis of diabetes insipidus.** (Reproduced with permission from USMLE-Rx.com.)

SYNDROME OF INAPPROPRIATE SECRETION OF ADH

Syndrome of inappropriate secretion of ADH (SIADH) is defined as an excessive secretion of ADH that may be idiopathic or caused by the following factors:

- **CNS disturbances:** CNS pathology, including hemorrhage, stroke, or infection, can enhance ADH secretion.
- **Pulmonary disease:** pneumonia, cystic fibrosis, asthma.
- **Tumors:** Tumors (the most common being **small-cell lung carcinoma**) may cause ectopic production of ADH.
- **Drugs:** Many drugs can ↑ the release of ADH or enhance its effects. These include carbamazepine, SSRIs, vincristine, haloperidol, amitriptyline, and amiodarone.

Symptoms/Exam

Initially, mild SIADH may be asymptomatic. Later symptoms of **hyponatremia,** with nausea and malaise progressing to headaches, lethargy, and eventually seizures and coma, may develop.

Diagnosis

SIADH should be suspected in any euvolemic hypoosmolar patients with hyponatremia. See the Nephrology chapter, section on hyponatremia for evaluation.

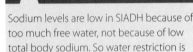

KEY FACT

Sodium levels are low in SIADH because of too much free water, not because of low total body sodium. So water restriction is the cornerstone of treatment.

Management

- **Water restriction and correction of underlying cause:** The mainstay of treatment. Avoid in subarachnoid hemorrhage, as it may precipitate cerebral vasospasm or infarction.
- **Salt administration:** IV hypertonic saline may be needed if hyponatremia is severe or symptomatic.
- **Loop diuretics:** Can enhance the effect of hypertonic saline.

GROWTH HORMONE EXCESS

Etiologies of GH excess are as follows:

- **Pituitary adenoma:** Accounts for >99% of cases. Insidious onset, causing the diagnosis to be delayed for >10 years. Accounts for approximately one-third of hormone-secreting tumors.
- **Iatrogenic:** Exogenous GH.
- **Ectopic GH or GHRH:** Very rare; can be seen with lung carcinoma, carcinoid, and pancreatic islet cell tumors.

Symptoms/Exam

- **Childhood: Gigantism** from delayed epiphyseal closure, leading to extremely tall stature.
- **Adulthood:**
  - Presents with **acromegaly, enlargement of the hands and feet,** glucose intolerance, hypertension, heat intolerance, weight gain, and fatigue.
  - May affect the heart by causing hypertrophic cardiomyopathy.

Diagnosis

- **Labs:** IGF-1 levels must be assessed (secreted by liver in response to GH). Random GH is not helpful.
- **Imaging: MRI** of the pituitary.

ANSWER

SIADH probably from pulmonary pathology. In this case, the most likely cause would be small cell lung carcinoma.

Management

- **Surgery: Usually surgery is first line.** Transsphenoidal resection is curative in 60% to 80% of cases but has risk of hypopituitarism or DI.
- **Medical:** First line is somatostatin analogs (octreotide). Also consider dopamine agonists (cabergoline), or GH receptor agonists (pegvisomant).

HYPERPROLACTINEMIA

Elevated serum prolactin can be caused by a variety of conditions:
- **Prolactinomas:** The most common type of pituitary tumor, also the most common cause of elevated prolactin. Most are microadenomas (<1 cm).
- **Drugs:** Medications associated with hyperprolactinemia include dopaminergic drugs (eg, antipsychotics, antihypertensives) as well as estrogen and SSRIs.
- **↓ dopamine:** Prolactin is elevated when dopamine no longer inhibits it. This can be due to hypothalamic/pituitary damage, or drugs such as antipsychotics.
- **Pregnancy:** Prolactin can reach 200 ng/mL in the second trimester.
- **Hypothalamic lesions:** May cause pituitary stalk compression or damage.
- **Hypothyroidism:** TRH stimulates prolactin secretion (Figure 4.8).

Symptoms/Exam

↑ prolactin inhibits GnRH, leading to ↓ FSH/LH, in turn leading to ↓ estrogen and testosterone, with the following clinical features:
- **Women: Galactorrhea;** anovulatory cycles with amenorrhea or oligomenorrhea.
- **Men:** Impotence, ↓ libido, galactorrhea (very rare).
- **Both:** Mass effect from large tumor (headache, visual field cuts, and hypopituitarism).

Diagnosis

- **Labs:** Show ↑ prolactin (typically >200 ng/mL) with normal TSH; ⊖ pregnancy test.
- **Imaging:** Obtain an MRI in anyone with hyperprolactinemia in the absence of pregnancy or drugs known to cause elevation.

Management

- **Pharmacologic:** Treat with a dopamine agonist such as **bromocriptine** or **cabergoline. Stop any medications that can elevate prolactin.**
- **Surgical:** Transsphenoidal resection is sometimes necessary if medical therapy is ineffective or if the tumor is causing a mass effect.

KEY FACT

The most common cause of amenorrhea and galactorrhea in a premenopausal woman is pregnancy! Prolactinomas are usually associated with a prolactin level >200 ng/dL.

KEY FACT

Dopamine agonists are first-line treatment of prolactinomas. In contrast, almost all other pituitary tumors are treated with surgical resection.

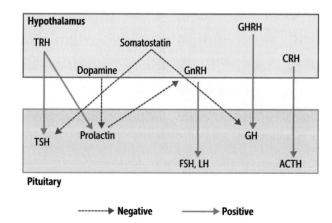

FIGURE 4.8. Hypothalamic-pituitary hormone regulation. (Reproduced with permission from USMLE-Rx.com.)

QUESTION

A 31-year-old woman who is on OCPs presents with bilateral galactorrhea and absent menses. Her serum prolactin level is >200 ng/dL. What is the most likely diagnosis and what treatment should you start?

MULTIPLE ENDOCRINE NEOPLASIA

Inherited in an autosomal-dominant pattern. There are three types of multiple endocrine neoplasia (MEN):

- Type 1: Pancreatic (insulinoma, gastrinoma), parathyroid, pituitary tumors.
- Type 2A: Medullary thyroid carcinoma (calcitonin secreting), pheochromocytoma (Figure 4.9), parathyroid hyperplasia.
- Type 2B: Medullary thyroid carcinoma, mucosal neuromas, pheochromocytoma.

Thyroid Disorders

HYPERTHYROIDISM

Etiologies, classified by nuclear imaging findings of radioactive iodine (RAI) uptake by the thyroid, are as follows (see also Table 4.5):

- ↑ **RAI uptake:**
    - **Graves disease:** An autoimmune disorder in which **TSH receptor antibodies**—also known as **thyroid-stimulating immunoglobulin (TSI)**—stimulate the receptor to produce excess thyroid hormone. The most common cause of hyperthyroidism (60%-90% of cases). Women are affected more often than men (5:1).
    - **Solitary toxic hyperactive nodule.**
    - **Toxic multinodular goiter.**
- ↓ **RAI uptake:** Thyroiditis (gland destruction releases preformed hormone); exogenous thyroid hormone.
- **Drug induced:** Amiodarone (can cause hypo- or hyperthyroidism), also lithium and antiretrovirals.

Symptoms/Exam

- Presents with anxiety, weakness, palpitations, heat intolerance, diaphoresis, weight loss, and oligo- or amenorrhea.
- Exam reveals tachycardia, hyperreflexia, thin hair, lid lag, exophthalmos, and pretibial myxedema. Goiter may be present.

KEY FACT

Exophthalmos and pretibial myxedema are pathognomonic for Graves disease, not present in other forms of hyperthyroidism.

KEY FACT

First-line test for hypothyroidism or hyperthyroidism should always be TSH alone. If abnormal, can follow up with free T$_4$, total T$_3$. Imaging of choice is RAI, not ultrasound (only indicated if there is a palpable nodule).

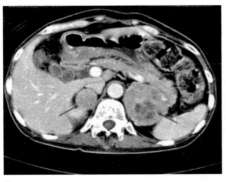

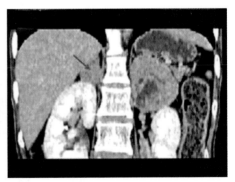

A   B

FIGURE 4.9. Pheochromcytoma. Contrast-enhanced coronal (**A**) and sagittal (**B**) CT images of a patient with MEN 2A shows bilateral adrenal masses (arrows). (Reproduced from Cui Q, et al. Integrated DNA-based/biochemical screening for early diagnosis of multiple endocrine neoplasia type 2A (MEN2A). *J Biomed Res.* 2013;27(2):145150.)

A   **ANSWER**

With a prolactin level of >200 ng/dL, prolactinoma is the most likely etiology. If a prolactinoma is found, start a dopamine agonist such as bromocriptine or cabergoline.

TABLE 4.5.   **Causes and Treatment of Hyperthyroidism**

DISORDER	CLINICAL FINDINGS	UNIQUE FINDINGS	RAI UPTAKE AND SCAN	TREATMENT
Graves disease	Diffusely enlarged thyroid; possibly bruit	**Exophthalmos,** periorbital edema, **pretibial myxedema; TSI $\pm$ TPO antibodies**	Diffusely $\uparrow$ uptake	MMI and PTU; β-blockers; RAI; **surgery for very large, obstructing goiters**
Solitary toxic nodule	Single palpable nodule	Autoantibodies are usually absent; may have predominantly **T$_3$ toxicosis**	Single-focus $\uparrow$ uptake	**Definitive therapy is RAI or surgery**
Multinodular goiter	"Lumpy-bumpy," enlarged thyroid	Autoantibodies are usually absent; may have predominantly T$_3$ toxicosis	Multiple hot and/or cold nodules	**Definitive therapy is RAI or surgery**
Thyroiditis (transient destruction of thyroid tissue)	Tender, enlarged thyroid	Subacute thyroiditis occurs following a viral infection; can also be postpartum or silent ("painless"); thought to have an autoimmune etiology $\downarrow$ **TSH, classically followed by a hypothyroid phase and then by euthyroidism Can be caused by medications (eg, amiodarone)**	Diffusely $\downarrow$ uptake	β-**blockers, NSAIDs, corticosteroids if indicated**
Exogenous hyperthyroidism	Normal or nonpalpable	The patient may be taking weight loss medications or have psychiatric illness **Distinguish from thyroiditis by $\downarrow$ TSH levels**	Diffusely $\downarrow$ uptake	Discontinuation of thyroid hormone

Diagnosis

- TSH: First line if suspected hyperthyroidism. If low, follow with free T$_4$ and total T$_3$.
- If presentation consistent with Graves disease (ophthalmopathy, Figure 4.10; symmetric goiter), no additional workup is needed.
- If diagnosis is unclear, consider the following:
  - Thyrotropin receptor antibodies (TRAb, TSI).
  - RAI uptake scan in nonpregnant patients (see Table 4.5).
- Rarely TSH is elevated when T$_3$/T$_4$ are high, this suggests TSH-secreting parathyroid adenoma.
- No thyroid ultrasound is indicated unless there is a palpable nodule.

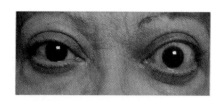

FIGURE 4.10.   Graves ophthalmopathy. Proptosis of the left eye. (Reproduced from Lee S, et al. Thiazolidinedione induced thyroid associated orbitopathy. *BMC Ophthalmol.* 2007;7:8.)

Management

- **Medications:**
  - **Antithyroid medications—methimazole (MMI) and propylthiouracil (PTU):** Block thyroid hormone production; can induce remission in 50% of patients with Graves disease. Check periodic leukocyte counts as they can cause agranulocytosis. MMI is first line except in first trimester of pregnancy.
  - **β-blockers:** For symptomatic treatment.
- **RAI:** Works by destroying thyroid follicular cells. Highly effective in toxic nodules and multinodular goiters; 90% effective in Graves disease, most common treatment in the United States. May result in hypothyroidism requiring lifelong levothyroxine supplementation. Contraindicated in pregnancy/nursing.
- **Surgery:** Subtotal thyroidectomy is used only in rare cases (eg, for uncontrolled disease in pregnancy, very large goiters, goiters obstructing the airway, or patient preference). Side effects include hypothyroidism, hypoparathyroidism, or recurrent laryngeal nerve damage.

Complications

- **Cardiac:** HF, arrhythmias (atrial fibrillation is most common).
- **Graves ophthalmopathy:** Occurs in approximately 20% of patients. More common in **smokers.** Can be worsened by RAI therapy. Treatment includes corticosteroids. Treatment of hyperthyroidism does not cure exophthalmos, only stops progression.
- **Thyroid storm:** Presents with fever, tachycardia, delirium, diarrhea, vomiting, and HF. Treat with high-dose propranolol, PTU, corticosteroids, and iodide. This is a **life-threatening** medical emergency. Look for an underlying stressor that may have triggered the storm.

KEY FACT

All patients with new atrial fibrillation should be screened with TSH for hyperthyroidism.

HYPOTHYROIDISM

May be caused by a variety of conditions, including the following:

- **Hashimoto thyroiditis:** An autoimmune thyroiditis that commonly leads to hypothyroidism but may initially present as hyperthyroidism. The most common cause of hypothyroidism in the United States.
- **Iodine deficiency:** Rare in developed countries, but the most common cause of hypothyroidism worldwide.
- **Drugs:** Amiodarone and lithium are most common drugs to cause hypothyroidism, but can also cause hyperthyroidism.
- **Iatrogenic:** Neck irradiation, thyroidectomy, RAI, antithyroid medications.
- **Subacute thyroiditis:** Typically transient.
- **Other:** 2° hypothyroidism (hypopituitarism); 3° hypothyroidism (hypothalamic dysfunction); peripheral resistance to thyroid hormone.

KEY FACT

Screening asymptomatic adults for thyroid disease is not evidence-based.

Symptoms/Exam

- Causes a generalized slowing of metabolic processes, leading to a vague, nonspecific constellation of symptoms that includes **fatigue, weight gain, cold intolerance, dry skin, constipation, menstrual irregularities,** and **depression.**
- During exam, look for bradycardia and delayed relaxation of deep tendon reflexes. Accumulation of matrix glycosaminoglycans in many tissues can also cause symptoms of coarse hair, enlargement of the tongue, hoarseness, and periorbital edema.

KEY FACT

Hypothyroidism may cause galactorrhea and amenorrhea because TSH stimulates prolactin secretion.

Diagnosis

Always start with TSH. If elevated, follow with free T_4.

- **1° hypothyroidism,** if TSH is elevated and free T_4 is low: Consider checking for TPO, although often unnecessary and can just presumptively treat for Hashimoto with levothyroxine.

- **Subclinical hypothyroidism**, if TSH is elevated and free T_4 is normal: Treatment generally is not indicated, although may vary based on age.
- **2° (pituitary) or 3° (hypothalamic) hypothyroidism**, if TSH is low and free T_4 is low.

Management

- Thyroid hormone replacement: Levothyroxine (T_4). Titrate to normalize TSH.
- Pregnancy as well as some drugs (eg, OCPs and other hormones) can affect the amount of thyroid-binding globulin and may therefore ↑ the need for T_4. In pregnancy, treat elevated TSH even if free T_4 is normal.

KEY FACT

Excess thyroid hormone replacement can cause ↓ bone density.

Complications

- Hypothyroidism may precipitate depression and hyperlipidemia and may cause modest weight gain. Consider checking TSH in patients presenting with these symptoms.
- **Myxedema coma:** Severe hypothyroidism constituting a medical emergency. Characterized by ↓ mental status and hypothermia. Can progress to shock and death. Treatment is IV glucocorticoids and T_3 and/or T_4 along with supportive therapy, especially rewarming.

THYROID NODULES AND CANCER

Etiologies of thyroid nodules and cancer include the following:
- **Benign lesions:** Cysts, benign multinodular goiter, thyroiditis.
- **1° thyroid cancer:**
  - **Papillary:** The **most common type.** Excellent prognosis. Many tumors secrete thyroglobulin, a precursor to thyroid hormone.
  - **Follicular:** A more aggressive form associated with metastasis to bone, lungs, and brain. Often retains the ability to form thyroglobulin and occasionally thyroid hormone (ie, "functioning thyroid cancer").
  - **Medullary:** May secrete **calcitonin** and can be associated with MEN 2A and 2B.
  - **Anaplastic:** Undifferentiated thyroid gland tumors. Very aggressive.
- **Other:** Lymphoma, metastasis to thyroid (breast, kidney, melanoma, lung).

MNEMONIC

Thyroid nodules:
90% of nodules are benign
90% are cold on RAI uptake scan
90% of cold nodules are benign
90% of thyroid malignancies present as a thyroid nodule or lump

Symptoms/Exam

- Typically presents with a single, firm, palpable nodule. Otherwise, often asymptomatic unless associated with thyroid hormone abnormalities or advanced carcinoma.
- Risk factors for thyroid carcinoma are female gender; age <14 or >70 years; a ⊕ history of head/neck irradiation; a ⊕ family history of thyroid cancer; a hard, fixed nodule >4 cm; rapid growth of the nodule; and symptoms related to local invasion (dysphagia, hoarseness).

MNEMONIC

Thyroid cancers from most to least common and least to most aggressive:
Please **F**eed **M**y **A**lligator
Papillary
Follicular
Medullary
Anaplastic

Diagnosis

- Start with TSH and thyroid ultrasound in all patients with a thyroid nodule (Figure 4.11).
- If TSH is low, follow with RAI scan:
  - If a hot nodule (↑ iodine uptake), low likelihood malignancy. Do not do FNA! Evaluate and treat for hyperthyroidism.
  - If a cold nodule (↓ iodine uptake), FNA is indicated to rule out malignancy.
- If ultrasound is concerning for malignancy, FNA is indicated.

QUESTION

A 62-year-old woman presents for a routine visit. Physical examination reveals a 2-cm thyroid nodule but is otherwise normal. What tests do you order?

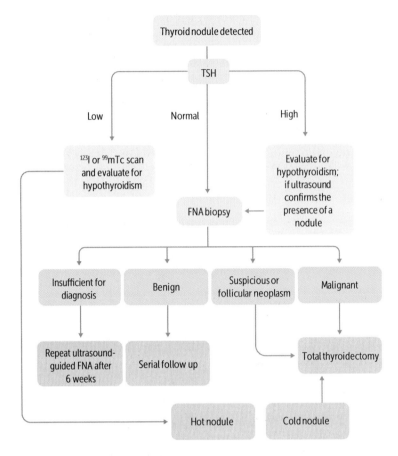

FIGURE 4.11.   Thyroid nodule workup. (Reproduced with permission from USMLE-Rx.com.)

Management

- **Benign nodules:** Observe with serial ultrasound if asymptomatic and confirmed to be benign. T_4 suppression therapy is only 50% effective. Surgical excision can be considered.
- **Malignancies:** Total thyroidectomy or lobectomy. Most will need thyroid hormone therapy; some may need additional **RAI ablation.**

Calcium and Bone Disorders

CALCIUM METABOLISM

Figure 4.12 illustrates the hormonal control loop that governs vitamin D and calcium metabolism and function.

HYPERCALCEMIA

High levels of calcium in the blood can stem from a variety of causes, but **1° hyperparathyroidism** and **malignancy** account for 90% of cases. Pathophysiologic mechanisms are as follows:

- **Malignancy-associated hypercalcemia:** Occurs in 10% to 30% of cancer patients via several mechanisms:
  - **Tumor release of PTH-related peptide (PTHrP):** Most common. PTHrP is

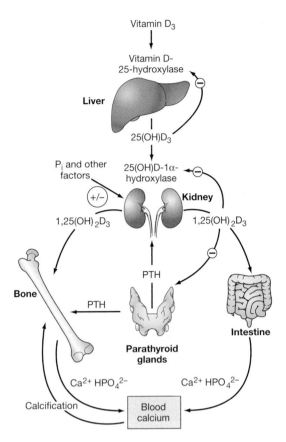

FIGURE 4.12. **Hormonal control loop for vitamin D metabolism and function.** Low serum calcium levels prompt a proportional ↑ in PTH concentration, which mobilizes calcium from the bone. PTH also increases the synthesis of $1,25(OH)_2$ vitamin D in the kidney, which in turn stimulates the mobilization of calcium from bone, increases absorption of calcium in the intestine, and downregulates PTH synthesis. (Reproduced with permission from Kasper DL, et al. *Harrison's Principles of Internal Medicine*, 16th ed. New York: McGraw Hill, 2005:2246.)

homologous to PTH but is not detected as PTH by serum assays and does not ↑ 1,25-dihydroxycholecalciferol (DHD) production (Table 4.6).

- **Tumor release of 1,25-DHD.**
- **Local osteolysis:** From metastases, adjacent tumor mass, or multiple myeloma.
- **Hyperparathyroidism:** See section below.
- **Granulomatous disorders: Sarcoidosis,** especially, can ↑ vitamin D production.
- **Endocrine disorders:**
  - Thyrotoxicosis can be associated with mild hypercalcemia due to ↑ bone resorption.
  - Adrenal insufficiency.
  - Familial hypocalciuric hypercalcemia.
- **Drug induced:** Thiazides, lithium, vitamin A, vitamin D, estrogens, androgens.
  - Milk alkali syndrome: Overconsumption of calcium-based antacids causing hypercalcemia, renal insufficiency, and metabolic alkalosis.

Symptoms/Exam

- Renal stones.
- Bone pain.
- Abdominal pain, often with constipation, nausea, vomiting, and anorexia.
- Psychiatric symptoms: Anxiety, depression, cognitive dysfunction.

KEY FACT

Elevated calcium with low PTH is strongly suggestive of malignancy. PTHrP causes hypercalcemia without showing up on PTH assays.

MNEMONIC

Hallmarks of hypercalcemia:

Stones, bones, groans, and psychiatric overtones.

QUESTION

A 52-year-old man presents with nausea, constipation, lethargy, and impaired concentration and memory. His physical exam is essentially normal. Lab results show elevated calcium and low PTH. What is the likely cause of this patient's hypercalcemia?

TABLE 4.6. **Laboratory Findings Associated With Hypercalcemia**

	CALCIUM	PHOSPHORUS	PTH	PTHRP	OTHER
PTH mediated	↑	↓	↑	↓	
PTHrP mediated	↑	↓	↓	↑	
Sarcoidosis, non-Hodgkin	↑	↑	↓	↓	↑ 1,25-DHD
Vitamin D intoxication	↑	↑	↓	↓	↑ 25-HD

Diagnosis

- Figure 4.13 provides a stepwise algorithm for the evaluation of hypercalcemia. See Table 4.6 for pertinent laboratory findings.
- **Imaging:** In a patient with normal PTH, perform CXR to look for sarcoidosis or malignancy.

Management

Hypercalcemia should be treated if severe (>14 mg/dL) or symptomatic.
- **Fluids:** Key to acute treatment. Start with IV isotonic saline to expand volume and ↑ urinary excretion.
- **Bisphosphonates (IV):** Toxic to osteoclasts; first line, if treatment beyond fluids is needed.
- **Calcitonin (SQ):** A thyroid produced hormone. ↓ bony reabsorption by interfering with osteoclast function; also ↑ renal excretion.
- **Glucocorticoids:** ↓ calcitriol (1,25-vitamin D) therefore ↓ GI absorption of calcium.

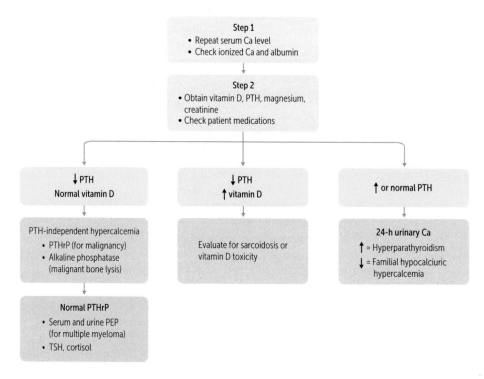

FIGURE 4.13. **Diagnostic workup for hypercalcemia.** (Reproduced with permission from USMLE-Rx.com.)

Complications

Long-standing or very high levels of hypercalcemia can cause deposition of calcium in heart valves, coronary arteries, and myocardial fibers and can also cause severe renal disease and neurologic deficits.

HYPERPARATHYROIDISM

Hyperparathyroidism has three different etiologies:
- 1° hyperparathyroidism: Autologous elevated PTH causing elevated calcium (Table 4.7).
- 2° hyperparathyroidism: Due to vitamin D deficiency, usually in the setting of chronic kidney disease. PTH is being appropriately secreted in this state. Marked by low or normal calcium despite elevated PTH.
- 3° hyperparathyroidism: In patients with long-standing vitamin D deficiency, PTH secretion becomes autologous, and even when 2° hyperparathyroidism is treated the PTH secretion continues.

Diagnosis
- Preoperative imaging with sestamibi scanning can help determine the surgical technique (ie, minimally invasive vs bilateral neck exploration) for a parathyroidectomy.
- Consider dual-energy x-ray absorptiometry (DEXA) in patients with 1° hyperparathyroidism.

Management
- 1° hyperparathyroidism:
  - **Parathyroidectomy** is the only curative treatment. The cure rate is 95%, and the complication rate is low.
  - **Indications for surgery** include symptomatic patients, age <50 years, serum calcium >1 mg/dL above normal, osteoporosis, renal insufficiency. Also treat osteopenia.
- 2° hyperparathyroidism:
  - Treat underlying cause, usually CKD.
  - Vitamin D and phosphate binders lower PTH.
  - Parathyroidectomy is rarely indicated.
- 3° hyperparathyroidism:
  - Parathyroidectomy is mainstay of treatment.

Complications

Nephrolithiasis, nephrocalcinosis with renal insufficiency, osteopenia, osteoporosis.

HYPOCALCEMIA

Low serum calcium concentrations are most often caused by disorders of vitamin D or PTH. These include the following, see also Table 4.8:
- Renal failure due to phosphate retention, changes in vitamin D metabolism and resistance of bones to PTH.
- Vitamin D deficiency:
  - Caused by malabsorptive states (eg, IBD, celiac sprue), lack of sun exposure, and dark skin.
  - In children: Rickets (bony deformities with rachitic rosary, bowing of the lower extremities, and frontal bossing).
  - In adults: Osteomalacia with myopathy and poor bone mineralization.
  - Diagnose with a low 25-HD level (<20 ng/mL), hypocalcemia, hypophosphatemia, and 2° hyperparathyroidism.
  - Treatment is high-dose oral vitamin D replacement and calcium.

TABLE 4.7. Laboratory Findings Associated With Hyperparathyroidism

	CALCIUM	PTH
Primary	↑	↑
Secondary	↑↑	Normal or ↓
Tertiary	↑	↑

KEY FACT

Approximately 80% of cases of 1° hyperparathyroidism are due to a single parathyroid adenoma; the remainder are due to gland hyperplasia and cancer.

KEY FACT

In 1° and 3° disease, mainstay of treatment is parathyroidectomy. In 2°, treat the underlying cause and give vitamin D.

KEY FACT

Renal failure is the most common cause of hypocalcemia.

QUESTION

A 50-year-old man comes to your office for a routine screening. Lab studies indicate that he has elevated serum calcium. In addition to rechecking serum calcium with albumin and ionized calcium, you check PTH, which is elevated. What are the indications for parathyroidectomy?

TABLE 4.8.   **Laboratory Findings Associated With Hypocalcemia**

	CALCIUM	PHOSPHORUS	PTH	OTHER
Hypoparathyroidism	↓	↑	↓	
Chronic kidney disease	↓	↑	↑	
Vitamin D deficiency	↓	↓	↑	↓ 25-HD
1,25-DHD resistance	↓	↓	↑	↑ 1,25-DHD
Hypomagnesemia	↓	↓	↓	

KEY FACT

If you suspect vitamin D deficiency, 25-hydroxy vitamin D should be the first-line test, not 1,25-hydroxy vitamin D.

- Hypoparathyroidism: Most often follows thyroid or parathyroid surgery. Can also be autoimmune, familial, infiltrative, or idiopathic. Treat with chronic oral calcitriol (1,25-DHD) and calcium.
- Hypomagnesemia: Inhibits PTH release.

Symptoms/Exam

- Neuromuscular manifestations:
  - Tetany: Neuromuscular irritability, leading to muscular and sensory nerve dysfunctions. Test with Chvostek sign (contraction of the facial muscles in response to tapping of the facial nerve) and Trousseau sign (induction of carpal spasm by inflation of a BP cuff to 20 mm Hg above SBP for 3 minutes).
  - Paresthesias, especially of the fingertips and perioral area.
  - Seizures, psychiatric symptoms.
- Cardiac: Prolonged QT (Figure 4.14), arrhythmia.
- Other: Cataracts, skeletal abnormalities.

Diagnosis

- Check ECG to determine need for emergent treatment.
- Lab studies reveal a ↓ calcium level when corrected for albumin. If PTH is ↑ or normal, check 25-HD and renal function (see Table 4.8).

Management

- **Acute:** If symptomatic or calcium <7.6 mg/dL, give IV calcium gluconate. Monitor with ECG and give PO calcium and calcitriol (1,25-vitamin D) if due to PTH deficiency.
- **Chronic:** Oral calcium and calcitriol, if needed.

KEY FACT

The most common fractures in Paget disease are vertebral crush fractures.

PAGET DISEASE

A skeletal disease with **accelerated bone turnover** due to ↑ osteoclast activity. Most often occurs in those >55 years, whites. Quite common, prevalence is 1% to 2% of US population.

A   ANSWER

Symptomatic patients. Consider parathyroidectomy for asymptomatic patients aged <50 years, renal insufficiency, serum calcium >1 mg/dL above normal, osteoporosis.

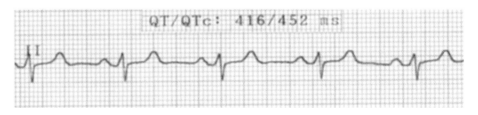

FIGURE 4.14.   **Prolonged QTc in hypocalcemia.** Note: normal QTc interval in men is <430 ms. (Reproduced from Rosa RG, et al. Mood disorder as a manifestation of primary hypoparathyroidism: a case report. *J Med Case Rep.* 2014;8:326.)

Symptoms/Exam

- Two-thirds of patients are asymptomatic, incidentally found on imaging or with elevated alkaline phosphatase.
- Symptoms can include **pain** (worsens with weight-bearing and often occurs at night), **fractures**, hearing loss (if the skull is affected), and bony **deformity**.

Diagnosis

- **Labs:** ↑ **alkaline phosphatase**, but normal GGT and other markers of liver function. Ca⁺⁺ and phosphorus are usually normal.
- **Imaging:** Plain films of involved bones show ↑ density and size (Figure 4.15); erosions can be seen in the skull. Bone scintigraphy shows ↑ uptake in affected areas.

Management

Bisphosphonates: Treatment of choice, often leads to remission.

Complications

↑ risk of bone tumors. Immobilizing a patient with active Paget disease can cause hypercalcemia. If large volumes of total bone are involved, can cause high-output HF.

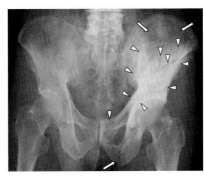

FIGURE 4.15. Paget disease.
X-ray of the pelvis shows ↑ osteoclast activity (arrows) and sclerotic lesions (arrowheads) in the left acetabulum, half the ilium, and the pubic bone.
(Reproduced from Iba K, et al. Five-year follow-up of Japanese patients with Paget's disease of the bone after treatment with low-dose oral alendronate: a case series. *J Med Case Reports.* 2010;4:166.)

OSTEOPOROSIS

Age-related decline in bone mass, leading to bone fragility and ↑ fracture risk. Although osteoporosis affects >10 million individuals in the United States, only a small proportion are properly diagnosed and treated. See the Community and Preventive Medicine chapter for recommendations on osteoporosis screening.

Symptoms/Exam

- Typically asymptomatic until fractures occur; often presents with pathologic fractures, particularly of the vertebrae, hip, or wrist.
- Hip, neck, and back pain.
- Sudden acute back pain while performing routine activities such as lifting or bending may indicate a vertebral compression fracture.
- Classic findings include thoracic kyphosis and loss of height in **thin older women**; however, men may be affected as well.

Differential

Osteomalacia, osteopenia, multiple myeloma. 2° osteoporosis may be caused by medications, hyperthyroidism, hyperparathyroidism, and hypogonadism.

Diagnosis

- CBC, chem 7, TSH, and PTH.
- **DEXA scan** (Figure 4.16). T-score is the number of standard deviations BMD is above or below the average BMD of a young, healthy control of the same sex.
  - T-score < −2.5 establishes osteoporosis.
  - T-score between −1 and −2.5 establishes osteopenia.
- Commonly diagnosed clinically after a fragility fracture.

Management

- **Nonpharmacologic therapy** (first line): Lifestyle changes, including ↑ weight-bearing exercise, modification of risk factors (smoking cessation, avoidance of excessive alcohol intake), and ↑ dietary intake of calcium and vitamin D.

KEY FACT

Risk factors for osteoporosis: Low body weight, smoker, alcoholic, white or Asian race, personal or first-degree family history of fragility fracture, chronic corticosteroid use, anti-androgen therapy, rheumatoid arthritis, postmenopausal status (in women).

Q QUESTION

An 83-year-old, overweight woman with a history of hypertension presents with sudden onset of severe left-sided back pain that radiates to her left buttock. Her symptoms occurred when she bent over to pick up a laundry basket. She denies a loss of urine, but reports numbness in her left leg. On exam, she is in obvious pain, especially when sitting. You are unable to perform a straight-leg test because of her discomfort. What is the diagnosis?

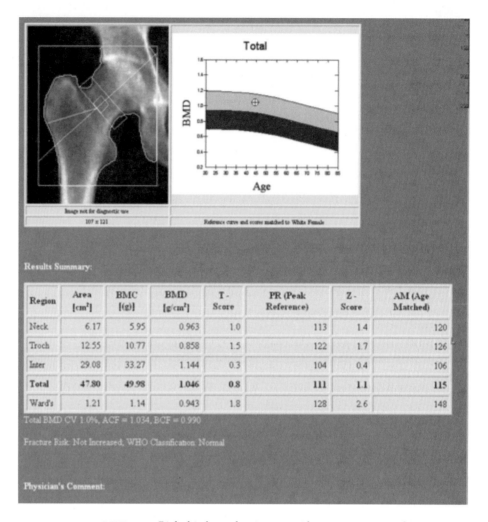

Region	Area [cm²]	BMC [(g)]	BMD [g/cm²]	T-Score	PR (Peak Reference)	Z-Score	AM (Age Matched)
Neck	6.17	5.95	0.963	1.0	113	1.4	120
Troch	12.55	10.77	0.858	1.5	122	1.7	126
Inter	29.08	33.27	1.144	0.3	104	0.4	106
Total	47.80	49.98	1.046	0.8	111	1.1	115
Ward's	1.21	1.14	0.943	1.8	128	2.6	148

Total BMD CV 1.0%, ACF = 1.034, BCF = 0.990

Fracture Risk: Not Increased; WHO Classification: Normal

Physician's Comment:

FIGURE 4.16. DEXA scan. Right hip bone density scan with measurements and scoring to investigate osteoporosis in an elderly woman with right hip pain. (Reproduced with permission from USMLE-Rx.com.)

- **Pharmacologic therapies:**
  - Bisphosphonates (eg, alendronate and risedronate) are the first-line agents. May be dosed weekly, ↓ fracture risk by as much as 50% in the first year. Side effects include erosive esophagitis and jaw necrosis, therefore stop after 5 years.
  - **Selective estrogen receptor modulators (SERMs):** Raloxifene ↑ BMD and ↓ total LDL cholesterol concentrations while ↓ the incidence of vertebral fractures. Less effective than bisphosphonates.
  - **PTH:** Teriparatide is a recombinant human PTH that stimulates bone formation. It is a good choice for high-risk patients who have failed previous treatment. Drawbacks include high cost, daily injection, and ↑ risk of osteosarcoma. Contraindicated in patients with Paget disease.
  - **Calcitonin:** Second-line therapy for osteoporosis, but can be used for its analgesic effect in patients who have substantial pain from an acute osteoporotic fracture.

 ANSWER

Vertebral fracture secondary to osteoporosis. Her age and sudden onset of back pain are core features of symptomatic disease.

Adrenal Disorders

The adrenal gland is controlled by the hypothalamus and the pituitary. The hypothalamus secretes CRH, which acts on the pituitary to produce ACTH. ACTH then acts on the adrenal gland to produce cortisol. The adrenal gland consists of the medulla and the cortex.

- **Medulla:** Produces catecholamines (epinephrine, norepinephrine, and dopamine).
- **Cortex:** Made up of three layers:
    - **Glomerulosa:** Produces mineralocorticoids (aldosterone).
    - **Fasciculata:** 1° producer of cortisol, also produces some androgens.
    - **Reticularis:** Produces androgens, also produces some cortisol.

MNEMONIC

Layers of the cortex in order of depth:

GFR

Glomerulosa
Fasiculata
Reticularis
(Think "the deeper you go, the sweeter it gets." Hormones produced by each in order of depth in the adrenal gland act on salt, then sugar, then sex.)

ADRENAL INSUFFICIENCY

1° adrenal insufficiency is known as **Addison disease.** 2° adrenal insufficiency is much more common. Hallmark is cortisol deficiency. Etiologies are as follows:

- 1° adrenal insufficiency (Addison disease):
    - **Autoimmune** destruction of the adrenal gland: **Most common** etiology in the United States.
    - **Infiltration:** Metastasis, sarcoidosis, amyloidosis.
    - **Hemorrhage:** Can occur in critical illness, pregnancy, coagulopathic patients, and Waterhouse-Friderichsen syndrome from meningococcemia.
    - **Infection:** Associated with HIV, TB, fungi, and CMV. Most common cause in the developing world.
    - **Congenital adrenal hyperplasia:** Most commonly due to 21-hydroxylase deficiency. Without this enzyme cortisol cannot be produced. Low levels of cortisol cause ACTH production, which leads to androgen production instead of cortisol production. Presents with ambiguous genitalia, virilization, precocious puberty, and adrenal insufficiency.
- 2° adrenal insufficiency:
    - **Iatrogenic:** Due to glucocorticoid and anabolic steroid administration. Often leads to relative lack of cortisol during acute illness.
    - Pituitary or hypothalamic dysfunction.

KEY FACT

The most common cause of 2° adrenal insufficiency is exogenous glucocorticoid use, while the most common cause of 1° adrenal insufficiency is autoimmune destruction of the adrenal gland.

Symptoms/Exam

- Presents with weakness, fatigue, anorexia, weight loss, vitiligo, alopecia, nausea, vomiting, diarrhea, abdominal pain, and orthostatic hypotension, coma, and death.
- Hyperpigmentation of the oral mucosa and palmar creases is found in 1° disease, not in 2°. ACTH precursor is cleaved to make ACTH and melanocyte-stimulating hormone, causing hyperpigmentation.

Diagnosis

- **Early-morning serum cortisol:** <3 µg/dL strongly suggests adrenal insufficiency.
- **Cosyntropin stimulation test:**
    - Obtain baseline ACTH and cortisol levels.
    - Inject cosyntropin (synthetic ACTH) 250 µg IM or IV.
    - Check cortisol level 45 to 60 minutes later.
    - A peak ≥18 µg/dL excludes adrenal insufficiency. Can be falsely ⊖ in acute 2° adrenal insufficiency.
- **ACTH:** An ↑ ACTH level in a patient with adrenal insufficiency is consistent with 1° adrenal insufficiency. In 2° disease, ACTH is low because pituitary doesn't make it—either due to a intrinsic issue or high levels of exogenous steroids.
- Evaluate the cause: Exclude exogenous or iatrogenic steroids. In 1° adrenal insufficiency, obtain a CT of the adrenal gland. In 2° disease, obtain a brain MRI.

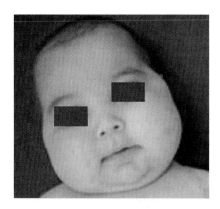

FIGURE 4.17. **Cushing syndrome.**
Moon facies in a child after 2 months of topical steroid application. (Reproduced from Katar, S, et al. Infantile iatrogenic Cushing's syndrome. *Indian J Dermatol.* 2008;53(4):190-191.)

Management

- **Hydrocortisone** or **prednisone** daily. In 1° adrenal insufficiency, use fludrocortisone (a mineralocorticoid) as well as a glucocorticoid.
- Administer "stress-dose" steroids IV as well as IV fluids during illness or surgery.

Complications

Adrenal crisis, an acute deficiency of cortisol, usually occurs due to abrupt discontinuation of exogenous steroids or major stress in the setting of adrenal insufficiency. Presents with headache, nausea, vomiting, confusion, fever, hypotension, and coma. Treat immediately with IV steroids as complications include death.

CUSHING SYNDROME

Due to excess exogenous or endogenous cortisol.
- **Exogenous corticosteroids:** The **most common** cause.
- **Ectopic ACTH:** ACTH secretion from a nonpituitary neoplasm (**small-cell lung carcinoma**).
- **Cushing disease:** Caused by ACTH hypersecretion from a **pituitary** microadenoma. More common in women.
- **Adrenal disease:** Adenoma, carcinoma, or nodular adrenal hyperplasia.

Symptoms/Exam

Presents with central obesity, with moon facies (Figure 4.17) and buffalo hump, menstrual irregularities, hypertension, emotional lability, dermatologic manifestations (eg, plethora, hirsutism, purple striae), and glucose intolerance. Excess ACTH may also cause hyperpigmentation.

Diagnosis

Do not test during an acute illness as levels will not be reflective. Check the following:
- Overnight dexamethasone suppression test, midnight cortisol, or 24-hour urine cortisol to establish diagnosis of Cushing syndrome.
- Plasma ACTH:
  - If ↓ or normal, the etiology is adrenal. Do CT/MRI of adrenals.
  - If ↑, order MRI the pituitary for Cushing disease. If MRI is ⊖, order CT chest/abdomen and octreotide scan for ACTH-secreting malignancy.

Management

- **Adrenal tumors:** Adrenalectomy.
- **Cushing disease:** Transsphenoidal pituitary adenoma resection.
- **Ectopic ACTH:** Treat underlying neoplasm.
- Mainstay of treatment is surgical, but if unsuccessful or not possible, medications include ketoconazole, cabergoline, and mitotane.

Complications

Complications may arise from long-term excess glucocorticoids (diabetes, hypertension, CVD, obesity, osteoporosis). May also ↑ susceptibility to infections.

HYPERALDOSTERONISM

Excess aldosterone can stem from a variety of sources and can be a cause of 2° hypertension and hypokalemia (hormone function in normal kidneys is shown in Figure 4.18). The two most common etiologies are:

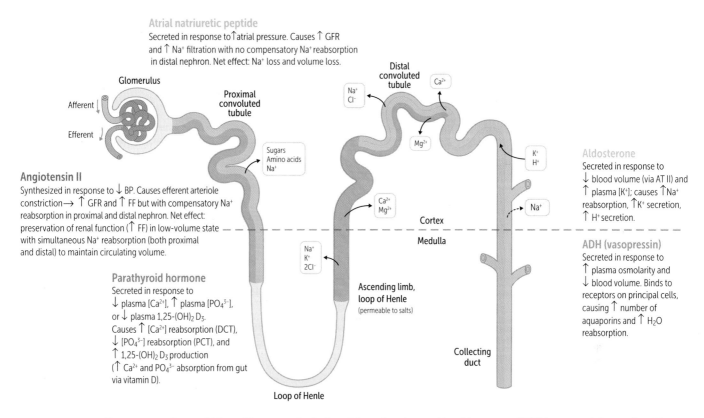

FIGURE 4.18. **Hormones acting on kidney.** Hormones include atrial natriuretic peptide, aldosterone, ADH (vasopressin), parathyroid hormone, and angiotensin II. (Reproduced with permission from USMLE-Rx.com.)

- **Aldosterone-producing adenoma (Conn disease):** More common in women than in men. Accounts for more than half 1° aldosteronism.
- **Idiopathic hyperaldosteronism:** Bilateral adrenal hyperplasia accounts for approximately one-third of cases.

Symptoms/Exam

- **Most patients are asymptomatic. Hypertension** and **hypokalemia** are classic, but potassium can be normal.
- Consider workup in patients with hypertension refractory to three agents or BP above 160/100 mm Hg, or hypertension in the setting of hypokalemia or adrenal mass.

Diagnosis

- Check morning ratio of **plasma aldosterone concentration:plasma renin activity.**
- In patients with hyperaldosteronism, CT should be performed to search for an adrenal adenoma.

Management

- **Spironolactone:** Give high-dose **spironolactone** or **eplerenone** mineralocorticoid receptor to normalize potassium levels. Side effects include gynecomastia in men, rash, impotence, and epigastric discomfort.
- **Unilateral adrenalectomy** in patients with unilateral disease.

PHEOCHROMOCYTOMAS AND PARAGANGLIOMAS

Rare tumors that produce **epinephrine and/or norepinephrine.**
- Ninety percent are pheochromocytomas that arise in the adrenal gland itself.
- Ten percent are paragangliomas that arise extra-adrenally in sympathetic ganglia.

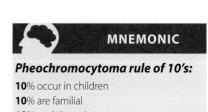

MNEMONIC

Pheochromocytoma rule of 10's:

10% occur in children
10% are familial
10% are bilateral
10% are malignant
10% are extra-adrenal (paragangliomas)
10% recur after resection

Symptoms/Exam

Patients most commonly present with episodic attacks of hypertension, throbbing headaches, diaphoresis, and palpitations.

Diagnosis

Pheochromocytoma is usually suggested by the history of a symptomatic patient, particularly those with a history of familial disease. Diagnose as follows:

- Establish biochemistry: The finding of markedly elevated urinary metanephrines in a 24-hour urine collection or plasma metanephrines confirms a biochemical diagnosis.
- Next, localize the lesion with MRI/CT imaging of the abdomen and pelvis.

Management

- **Surgical resection:** Treatment of choice. Has a 90% cure rate. It is important to hydrate patients and control symptoms before surgery.
- **Adrenergic blockade:** Phenoxybenzamine is the key first step.
- **β-blockers:** Used to control heart rate, but only after adrenergic blockade.

Complications

Hypertensive crises, MI, CVAs, arrhythmias, renal failure, dissecting aortic aneurysm.

ADRENAL INCIDENTALOMAS

Adrenal lesions are found incidentally in approximately 2% of patients undergoing abdominal CT scans for unrelated reasons. Autopsies indicate a prevalence of approximately 10%. Subtypes are as follows:

- **Functioning:**
  - Cushing syndrome (central obesity, striae, hypertension).
  - Pheochromocytoma (hypertension, palpitations, sweating).
  - Hyperaldosteronism (hypertension, hypokalemia).
- **Nonfunctioning:** Carcinoma, benign adenoma, metastatic lesion.

Diagnosis

- **Rule out functioning tumor:**
  - Plasma metanephrines or 24-hour urine metanephrines to rule out pheochromocytoma.
  - Dexamethasone suppression test to rule out Cushing disease.
  - If the patient is hypertensive, check plasma renin activity and aldosterone level.
- **Imaging:** Characteristics of a CT with contrast can help define whether a lesion is likely benign or malignant (Figure 4.19).

KEY FACT

Do not use β-blockers in patients with pheochromocytoma before adequate adrenergic blockade is achieved as this can lead to unopposed α-adrenergic stimulation, which can cause a hypertensive crisis.

KEY FACT

All patients with adrenal incidentaloma should be tested for Cushing syndrome.

KEY FACT

Before any adrenal biopsy or surgery, you must rule out pheochromocytoma! Biopsy of a pheochromocytoma can cause hypertensive crisis.

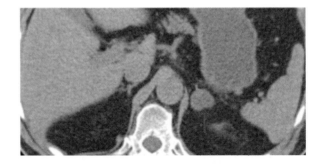

FIGURE 4.19. **Adrenal adenoma.** Cropped transaxial image from a noncontrast CT scan showing a small, low-density mass in the left adrenal gland (arrow). (Reproduced with permission from USMLE-Rx.com.)

Management

Treat based on the size and functional status of the lesion:

- **Lesions <4 cm and nonfunctioning:** Repeat imaging in 3 to 6 months, then annually for 1 to 2 years; hormone testing annually.
- **Lesions >4 cm:** Resect.
- **Functioning lesions:** Treat as appropriate for the disorder (see previous sections).

NOTES

Gastroenterology

Nicole Person-Rennell, MD, MPH

Esophageal Disorders

ESOPHAGEAL DYSPHAGIA

A sensation of **difficulty swallowing.** Patients typically complain of symptoms **seconds after swallowing** and identify the **suprasternal notch** or **retrosternal area** as the source of their discomfort. Not to be confused with:

- **Odynophagia:** Pain with swallowing.
- **Globus sensation:** Persistent or intermittent sensation of a lump or foreign body in the throat for >12 weeks that is present **even when the patient is not swallowing.** Unclear pathogenesis—not due to pathology of esophageal structure, motility, or GERD.
- **Oropharyngeal dysphagia: Difficulty initiating swallowing.** Patients complain of food getting stuck **immediately upon swallowing, frequently followed by coughing and choking.** Commonly caused by a variety of neurologic disorders (eg, CVA, Parkinson disease).

Etiologies of dysphagia include (identify most likely based on history):

- **Gastroesophageal reflux.**
- **Anatomic abnormalities of the esophagus:** Zenker diverticulum, cricopharyngeal bars, peptic strictures, radiation injury, esophageal webs/rings, and esophageal carcinoma.
- **Esophageal motility disorders:**
  - **Achalasia:** Inflammatory idiopathic degeneration of neurons in esophageal wall → failure of lower esophageal sphincter (LES) relaxation and distal peristalsis. 2° achalasia or pseudoachalasia is due to Chagas disease, malignancy, or other motor disease. Symptoms are progressive, worsen at night, and usually occur without heartburn (Figure 5.1).
  - **1° motility disorders:** A group of disorders with an unclear pathologic or pathophysiologic basis, each characterized by specific manometric findings. Features include diffuse esophageal spasm, nutcracker esophagus, and hypertensive LES. Chest pain is common.
- **Autoimmune disorders:** Scleroderma, Sjögren syndrome (dysphagia is independent of xerostomia but is worsened by it).
- **Cardiovascular abnormalities:** Can lead to dysphagia via compression of the esophagus (eg, vascular rings, aneurysms, left atrial enlargement).
- **Xerostomia** (eg, anticholinergics).
- **Functional dysphagia:** Dysphagia for >12 weeks for 1 year with no identifiable cause.
- **Esophageal cancer:** Progressive dysphagia, weight loss, anemia/heme-positive stools.

Diagnosis

Dysphagia warrants immediate workup:

- **Esophagogastroduodenoscopy (EGD):** Most commonly used for the diagnosis of esophageal dysphagia.
- **Barium swallow:** Less diagnostic but safer than EGD; the initial test of choice for suspected achalasia, revealing classic "bird's beak" narrowing (see Figure 5.1).
- **Esophageal manometry:** Usually performed if the aforementioned studies are ⊖ to evaluate for a 1° esophageal dysmotility disorder. Also, confirmatory for achalasia.
- **Video fluoroscopic swallow study:** Useful in the evaluation of oropharyngeal dysphagia.
- **Laryngoscopy:** Consider in patients with globus sensation to rule out malignancy.

Management

Directed at the underlying cause.

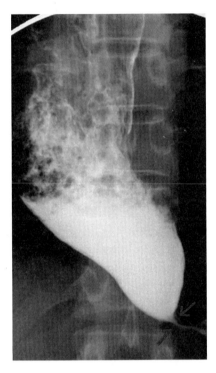

FIGURE 5.1. Achalasia. Note the dilated esophagus tapering to a "bird's-beak" narrowing at the LES. (Reproduced with permission from Doherty GM. *Current Diagnosis & Treatment: Surgery,* 13th ed. New York: McGraw-Hill, 2010, Fig. 20-5.)

KEY FACT

Dysphagia for only solids suggests a mechanical obstruction (but severe obstruction often progresses to include liquids). Dysphagia equally for solids and liquids suggests a motility disorder.

KEY FACT

Rule out cardiac chest pain in a patient suspected of having a 1° esophageal dysmotility disorder.

ESOPHAGITIS

Inflammation of the esophagus with variable etiologies (Table 5.1). Can be asymptomatic or can present with odynophagia, dysphagia, heartburn, retrosternal chest pain, or GI bleeding.

Diagnosis

- Use presentation to guide diagnostic choices; first line is usually EGD but can be a clinical diagnosis.
- Candida esophagitis may present with oral thrush (Figure 5.2), but **the absence of thrush does not preclude diagnosis.**
- Drug history is important to rule out pill esophagitis. Commonly implicated drugs include antibiotics (tetracycline, doxycycline, clindamycin), vitamin C, $FeSO_4$, KCl, NSAIDs/ASA, and bisphosphonates.

Management

Depends on etiology.

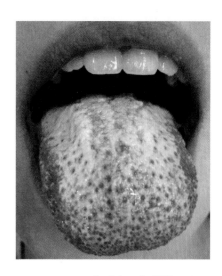

FIGURE 5.2.   **Oral thrush.** Diffuse *Candida albicans* infection on a child's tongue after taking antibiotics. (Reproduced from Wikimedia; courtesy of Dr. James Heilman.)

TABLE 5.1.   **Etiologies and Presentation of Esophagitis**

SUBTYPE	CHARACTERISTICS	DIAGNOSIS	TREATMENT
Reflux	See section on GERD		
HSV	Often immunocompromised patient Acute onset; exam may reveal concomitant oral or perioral vesicles	EGD, biopsy, culture	Acyclovir
CMV	Often immunocompromised patient Presents with odynophagia, chest pain, hematemesis, nausea, and vomiting	EGD, biopsy, culture	Ganciclovir
HIV	May present in 1° infection	HIV testing	Usually self-limited
Candida	Often immunocompromised patient Exam may reveal thrush (see Figure 5.2)	EGD, biopsy; alternatively, therapeutic trial	Fluconazole

Radiation for head and neck tumors	May present as acute (2-3 weeks after
	    radiation) or chronic (3 months after
	    therapy, due to inflammation, fibrosis)
		Usually clinical, EGD, barium swallow if stricture symptoms	Acutely, viscous lidocaine, supportive care; manage complications such as stricture, perforation

Corrosive	Caustic ingestion	Usually clinical, EGD if stable	Acutely, prednisone (**no** emetics or neutralizing agents); strictures formed later require balloon dilation

Pill	Relatively sudden onset; classically caused
	    by taking an offending medication
	    without water before sleep
		Usually clinical	Prevention: Hold meds if possible or give
			    liquid form
			Consider PPI short term, although data
			    are mixed

Eosinophilic	Idiopathic or allergic; usually leads to
	    refractory GERD, dysphagia, and food
	    impaction due to stricture/ring formation
		EGD, biopsy	Esophageal dilation, swallowed aerosolized fluticasone, systemic steroids, elimination diet trial, PPI trial

GASTROESOPHAGEAL REFLUX DISEASE

Etiology is LES dysfunction. High prevalence: 14% of US adults have symptoms.

Symptoms/Exam

- Think GERD when patients present with regurgitation of food or sour material in the mouth or heartburn (usually postprandial). Can also present with dysphagia, sore throat, chest pain, and/or water brash (hypersalivation).
- Severe cases: Laryngitis, chronic coughing, morning hoarseness, dysphonia, and pulmonary aspiration.
- Exam is usually normal.

Differential

Esophagitis of other etiology, esophageal motility disorders, gastritis, functional dyspepsia, peptic ulcer disease (PUD), biliary tract disease, CAD, laryngopharyngeal reflux, or malignancy.

Diagnosis

- First line:
    - For mild, low-risk cases (ie, those with no dysphagia, epigastric mass, anemia, bleeding, or weight loss) usually **diagnosed clinically** and supported by patient's response to empiric treatment.
    - For higher risk or those unresponsive to treatment, obtain **EGD.** Can be used to evaluate for Barrett esophagus, erosions, strictures, or ulcers.
- **Barium swallow** is used less because of its lower sensitivity in milder cases of GERD. Still, should be ordered when complaint is prominently dysphagia and there is concern for achalasia.
- **Wireless capsule endoscopy:** Approved by the FDA for evaluation of the esophagus in patients with heartburn. Sensitivities are nearly equal to those of EGD.
- **24-hour pH probe monitoring:** Use to confirm disease in patients with persistent symptoms despite treatment and ⊖ EGD. Manometry is usually only for preoperative evaluation.
- There is no indication for *Helicobacter pylori* screening in GERD; use only if concern for PUD or dyspepsia.

Management

- First line and concurrent with medications: **Lifestyle modifications:**
    - Weight loss.
    - **Elevation of the head of the bed:** Especially beneficial for nocturnal or laryngeal symptoms. Elevation should be approximately 6 inches.
    - **Dietary modifications:** Minimal evidence for benefit unless specific trigger. Avoidance **reflux-inducing foods** (chocolate, peppermint, alcohol, fatty foods); avoidance of **acidic foods** (orange juice, coffee, colas, red wine); consumption of **smaller, more frequent meals;** and use of lozenges or chewing gum (to promote salivation, which neutralizes gastric contents).
    - **Other:** Avoidance of recumbence after meals; smoking and alcohol cessation.
- Antacids (Figure 5.3).
    - **PPIs:** More effective than H$_2$ blockers in healing and providing symptomatic relief. However, have a considerable side effect profile.
    - Use a trial of daily therapy with 8 weeks of any PPI. Can ↑ to BID if refractory.
    - Use maintenance therapy for recurrence after stopping PPI, erosive esophagitis, or Barrett esophagus. Avoid long-term use if possible due to side effects.
    - **H$_2$ blockers:** More effective than placebo. Frequently used first in step-up approach or after PPI in step-down approach.

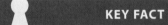

KEY FACT

Indications for EGD in patients with GERD include failure to respond to PPI trial (at least 4-8 weeks), bleeding, anemia, dysphagia, or weight loss.

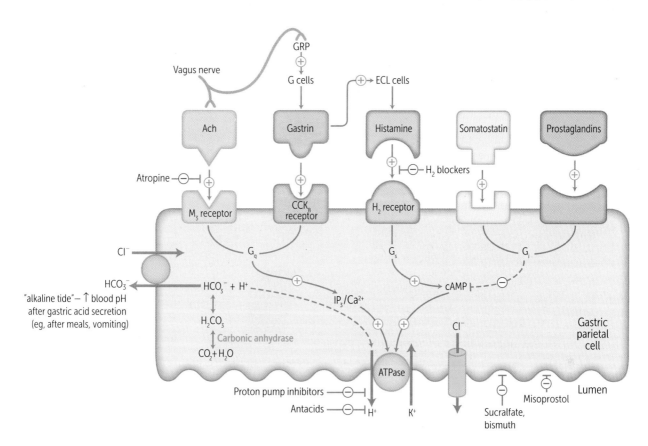

FIGURE 5.3. **Acid suppression therapy. Sites of action.** (Reproduced with permission from USMLE-Rx.com.)

- **Prokinetic:** Can be useful adjunct after formal evaluation, but not appropriate as monotherapy or first line.
- **Surgery:**
  - Generally reserved for patients whose symptoms persist despite optimal medical therapy, those who are unable to tolerate or comply with medical management, or those preferring surgery over long-term medical treatments.
  - No consensus on preferred surgical technique.

Complications

- **Complications of prolonged PPI use:** Osteoporosis, pneumonia, ↑ CV risk, ↑ risk of enteric infections (due to easier colonization of pathogens in the upper GI tract) as well as malabsorption, including vitamin B_{12}, magnesium, and iron. An association between PPI use and dementia is also under investigation.
- **Barrett esophagus:**
  - Metaplastic process in which stratified squamous epithelium is replaced by **intestinal-type (columnar) epithelium** during the healing phases of esophagitis (Figure 5.4). Occurs in 4% to 10% of patients with significant heartburn.
  - The presence of Barrett esophagus ↑ the risk of esophageal adenocarcinoma, with an annual cancer incidence of 0.2% to 2.0%. Treatment includes aggressive antireflux therapy.
  - There is no well-established guideline or evidence for cancer surveillance; however, the American Gastroenterological Association recommends consideration for EGD and biopsy with multiple risk factors (age >50, male, white, chronic GERD, abdominal obesity, hiatal hernia).
- **Peptic stricture:** Suggested by progressive dysphagia and episodic obstruction. Barium swallows are helpful in diagnosis. Treatment of choice is endoscopic balloon dilation along with high-dose acid suppression.

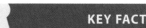

KEY FACT

There is no clear relationship between H pylori and GERD and no evidence that H pylori eradication relieves GERD symptoms.

QUESTION

Your patient is a 45-year-old woman with a history of 2 years of a sour taste in her mouth after large meals, epigastric pain, and chronic cough that is worse at night. She denies dysphagia or weight loss. What is your first step?

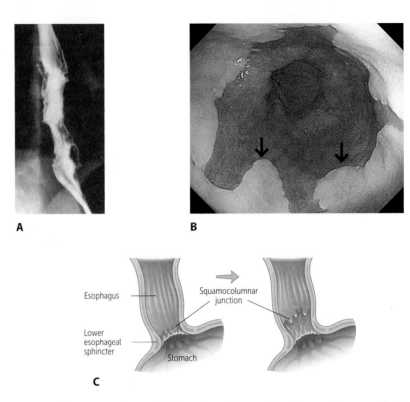

A   B

C

FIGURE 5.4. **Barrett esophagus.** (A) Barrett esophagus with adenocarcinoma on barium esophagram. Note the nodular mucosa (arrow) and the raised filling defect (arrowhead), representing adenocarcinoma. (B) Endoscopic image showing the pink tongues of Barrett esophagus (arrows indicate normal esophagus). (C) Location of Barrett esophagus, with ↑ gastric mucosa within the lower esophagus as a result of reflux of gastric contents. (Image A reproduced with permission from Chen MY, et al. *Basic Radiology.* New York: McGraw-Hill, 2004, Fig. 10-19; image B reproduced with permission from Fauci AS, et al. *Harrison's Principles of Internal Medicine,* 17th ed. New York: McGraw-Hill, 2008, Fig. 285-3A; image C reproduced with permission from USMLE-Rx.com.)

Diagram labels: Esophagus; Lower esophageal sphincter; Stomach; Squamocolumnar junction

- **Asthma:** Caused by microaspiration and ↑ vagal tone from acid stimulation of the esophagus. Consider in asthmatic patients who fail to respond to conventional asthma therapy.
- **Others: Chronic cough,** periodontal disease, chronic sinusitis, recurrent pneumonitis, nocturnal choking, chronic hoarseness, pharyngitis, subglottic stenosis, laryngeal/tracheal stenosis.

Disorders of the Stomach

GASTRITIS/GASTROPATHY

Gastritis: Injury to the mucosa of the stomach, with epithelial cell damage and regeneration, 2° to inflammatory response.
- **Acute gastritis:** Typically caused by an acute *H pylori* infection, although etiologic agents such as CMV have been implicated in immunocompromised and iatrogenic cases. Can progress to chronic gastritis if not treated.
- **Chronic (metaplastic) gastritis:**
  - Includes **achlorhydria** and **autoimmune gastritis,** in which antibodies against parietal cells and intrinsic factor (IF) lead to **pernicious anemia** (cobalamin deficiency, megaloblastic anemia, subacute combined degeneration).

KEY FACT

Asthma unresponsive to conventional therapy is highly suspicious for GERD.

ANSWER

Based on your patient's lack of red flags, she can be treated empirically with a PPI for 4 to 8 weeks followed by symptom reassessment.

- Includes **chronic infection, such as *H pylori*.** Can lead to multifocal atrophic gastritis, gastric atrophy, and metaplasia, ↑ the risk of developing gastric adenocarcinoma. If chronic gastritis persists, consider empiric *H pylori* treatment.
- **Gastropathy:** Injury to the mucosa of the stomach, with epithelial cell damage and regeneration, **unrelated to inflammation.** Etiologies include drugs (**NSAIDs**), alcohol, bile reflux, severe illness, and portal hypertension.

Symptoms/Exam

- There is a **poor correlation** between symptoms (eg, pain and dyspepsia) and endoscopic findings. However, acute *H pylori* gastritis can cause **sudden onset of epigastric pain, nausea, and vomiting,** while gastropathy caused by NSAID use, alcohol, or portal hypertension can present with GI bleeding.
- Exam is usually unremarkable, but abdominal tenderness may be seen.
- Signs of vitamin B_{12} deficiency (anemia, neurologic signs) may also be noted.

Differential

Functional dyspepsia, gastric cancer, sarcoidosis, Crohn's disease, infections (TB, strongyloidiasis, giardiasis), GERD, biliary tract disease, gastroparesis, pancreatitis, malabsorption, and Ménétriere disease (characterized by giant thickened folds of mucosa).

Diagnosis

- Diagnosis is largely clinical. Include ***H pylori*** testing (Table 5.2) based on availability, history, or need for endoscopy. Evaluate for suspected autoimmune gastritis via antiparietal cell and IF antibodies.
- Consider testing for eradication if ulcer or persistent symptoms despite treatment.
- **EGD** with biopsy can provide a pathologic diagnosis. Obtain if alarming symptoms.

Management

- Treatment generally consists of avoidance of causative factors (eg, NSAIDs, alcohol) along with **prophylaxis** (acid suppression; nonselective β-blockers for varices).
- *H pylori* eradication: Treatment regimen includes PPI BID, clarithromycin 500 mg BID, amoxicillin 1 g BID for 14 days. Metronidazole may be substituted for amoxicillin if patient is penicillin-allergic, but resistance is common. Add bismuth subsalicylate 525 mg QID and a tetracycline if retreating or resistance to clarithromycin >15%; parenteral vitamin B_{12} for pernicious anemia.

PEPTIC ULCER DISEASE

The principal cause of PUD is ***H pylori* infection,** which causes 70% to 80% of duodenal and 60% to 70% of gastric ulcers. Second most likely etiology is **NSAID** use. Other causes include Zollinger-Ellison syndrome, tobacco use, medications (ie, aspirin, KCl, mycophenolate), physiologic stress (ie, ICU), and, less often, CMV, HSV-1, and chemoradiation.

Psychological stress is not a cause and corticosteroids are not a contributing factor unless they are used in association with NSAIDs.

Symptoms/Exam

- May be asymptomatic ("silent disease"; more common in the elderly and in NSAID users), or may present with dyspepsia or with severe, hunger-like epigastric pain accompanied by burning and gnawing. Can radiate to upper quadrants or back.

KEY FACT

Indications for prophylactic PPI use in hospitalized patients:

- Coagulopathy (platelets <50,000 µL, INR >1.5)
- Intubated >48 hours
- History of GI bleed or ulcer in the last year
- Two or more of the following criteria:
  - Sepsis
  - ICU admission >1 week
  - Occult GI bleed >6 days
  - Glucocorticoid treatment (>250 mg hydrocortisone or equivalent)

KEY FACT

Alarm findings for dyspepsia requiring further workup include: age >55, bleeding, anemia, unexplained weight loss, progressive dysphagia, odynophagia, vomiting, family history of GI cancer, and history of esophagogastric malignancy.

QUESTION

A 50-year-old man presents for follow-up after EGD significant for a duodenal ulcer and ⊕ biopsy urease test for *H pylori*. What are your next steps?

TABLE 5.2.   Testing Methods for *H pylori*

TYPE	ADVANTAGES	DISADVANTAGES
Invasive		
Biopsy urease test	The test of choice if using endoscopy; sensitivity is 90%-95% and specificity 95%-100%	False negatives occur with use of PPIs and H_2-blockers as well as with GI bleeding, antibiotics, and bismuth
Histology	Useful in excluding gastritis, intestinal metaplasia, and MALT lymphoma	Prone to sampling error and interobserver variability; has ↓ sensitivity if the patient is on antisecretory therapy
Brush cytology	Sensitivity and specificity are similar to those of the biopsy urease test	Not commonly done unless the patient has a bleeding disorder
Culture for *H pylori*		Not done routinely; mostly for suspected antibiotic resistance if sensitivities are needed
Noninvasive		
Urea breath test	Uses urea with radiolabeled carbon, allowing liberated CO_2 to be detected; has 88%-95% sensitivity and 95%-100% specificity, as good as the urea breath test	The same factors causing false negatives with the biopsy urease test are less accurate if the patient is on PPI or bismuth
Stool antigen testing	Recently developed rapid stool antigen developed for office use	Specificity is 76%-96%; reliable if high population prevalence (high PPV)
H pylori serology (IgG, IgA)	Inexpensive and has good sensitivity (90%-100%)	Cannot differentiate from old infection

KEY FACT

Many tests for *H pylori* (except serology testing) will be falsely ⊖ if a patient is on acid suppression therapy.

ANSWER

You prescribe triple therapy. Two months later, the patient reports some improvement but continues to have symptoms and remains on his PPI. Before discussing eradication testing (ideally performed while patient is off PPI), you find that he never filled his prescription for his antibiotics due to medication costs. You connect the patient with a prescription support program and his symptoms resolve after therapy.

- Symptoms can be further distinguished as follows, but can't be reliably used to differentiate:
  - **Gastric ulcers:** Classically present with **severe pain soon after meals. Relief with antacid intake or food consumption is less frequent than with duodenal ulcers.**
  - **Duodenal ulcers:** Classically present as **pain 2 to 5 hours after meals** along with night symptoms occurring from 11 PM to 2 AM. **Food and antacids tend to relieve symptoms.**
- Exam may reveal epigastric tenderness.

Differential

See differential above for gastritis.

Diagnosis

- **EGD:** The diagnostic **gold standard,** allowing for the **differentiation of benign ulcers from cancer** (Figure 5.5). Indicated to rule out malignancy if any **alarm signs** are present.
- **Upper GI series:** Common distractor answer. Less favored because of its variable sensitivity (50%-90%).
- *H pylori* testing (see Table 5.2).

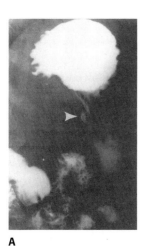
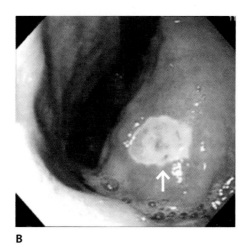

A   **B**

FIGURE 5.5.   Gastric ulcer. (A) Barium upper GI study shows a benign gastric ulcer as pooling of contrast (arrowhead) extending beyond the adjacent gastric wall. **(B)** Benign gastric ulcer (arrow) at endoscopy. (Image A reproduced with permission from Chen MY, et al. *Basic Radiology.* New York: McGraw-Hill, 2004, Fig. 10-21; image B reproduced from Moriya M, et al. Stress-induced hemorrhagic gastric ulcer after successful *Helicobacter pylori* eradication: two case reports. *J Med Case Rep.* 2011;5:252.)

Management

- **Lifestyle modifications:** Smoking cessation; alcohol and caffeine avoidance; and avoidance of NSAIDs or aspirin.
- **Acid suppressors:** Include H_2-blockers, PPIs, and sucralfate. Maintenance acid suppression may be required to prevent recurrence or to treat complications.
- ***H pylori* infection:** Eradicate *H pylori* if indicated. Continued acid suppression is necessary to allow the ulcer to heal. In complex cases, *H pylori* testing should be repeated approximately 4 weeks after healing to confirm disease resolution. See Gastritis section for treatment regimens.
- **Surgical intervention:** Indications include failure of medical management; suspicion of cancer (ie, a gastric ulcer that fails to heal after 12 weeks); perforation; outlet obstruction (failing to resolve after >72 hours); and failure to arrest bleeding.

> **KEY FACT**
>
> The prevalence of peptic ulcers in patients with dyspepsia who test ⊕ for *H pylori* is 15% to 30%. Therefore, if a patient has no alarm symptoms, *H pylori* treatment without endoscopic evaluation is recommended.

Complications

- **Lack of response:** Causes of treatment failure include *H pylori* resistance, noncompliance with medical therapy/supportive measures, giant ulcers (ulcers >2 cm have a lesser chance of healing), H_2-blocker/PPI resistance or tolerance, cancer, Crohn's disease, infection, and **Zollinger-Ellison syndrome** (pancreatic gastrinoma; ↑ **fasting serum gastrin**).
- Penetrating ulcers (more localized and intense pain radiating to the back): perforation (sudden diffuse abdominal pain and peritonitis), gastric outlet obstruction (early satiety, vomiting, nausea, weight loss, pain, and bloating), and hemorrhage.

GASTROPARESIS

Obstructive symptoms in the stomach/bowel in the **absence of an anatomic lesion.** Most commonly due to diabetes, postsurgical changes, or idiopathic, but can also be caused by hypothyroidism, neurologic disorders, rheumatologic disease (scleroderma), amyloidosis, paraneoplastic disease, or drugs (ie, anticholinergics, calcium channel blockers, α_2-adrenergic agonists).

Symptoms/Exam

- Presents with early satiety, nausea, bloating/distention, abdominal pain, and vomiting soon after meals.
- Exam may reveal abdominal distention, tenderness, and/or succussion splash (heard when shaking the abdomen by holding the pelvis, indicating free fluid).

Diagnosis

- **Upper GI series with small bowel follow-through:** Used to rule out mechanical obstruction. Also consider EGD or CT/MRI for structural evaluation.
- **Gastric scintigraphy:** Establishes delayed gastric emptying. Necessary for diagnosis.

Management

- **Acute episodes:** Treat with NPO, NG suction, and IV fluids.
- **Nutritional support:** Small, frequent meals with fewer fatty, bulky, or gas-forming foods. Parenteral nutrition if necessary.
- **Prokinetics: Metoclopramide** (first line), macrolide antibiotics (**erythromycin** more standard, but also azithromycin) for 4 weeks at a time 2/2 tachyphylaxis.
- Antiemetics for symptom control; avoid QTC prolongation if combining agents.
- **Strict glycemic control** in diabetic gastroparesis is recommended.
- Discontinue drugs that slow intestinal motility (ie, anticholinergics, opioids).

Disorders of the Bowel

ACUTE DIARRHEA

KEY FACT

Etiologies of bloody diarrhea include most commonly *E coli* O157:H7, then *Shigella*, *Campylobacter,* and *Salmonella*.

Defined as diarrhea lasting ≤2 **weeks.** One of five leading causes of death worldwide. **Ninety percent** of cases are caused by **infectious agents.** Most are viral, but severe cases are more frequently caused by bacteria (1.5%-5.6% of mild cases are due to bacterial infection, vs 87% of severe cases). The remaining 10% are from **medications, toxin ingestion,** and **ischemia.** Some chronic cases present acutely, as in **IBD** or **diverticulitis.** Risk factors for acute infection are as follows:

- **Travel:** Approximately 40% of travelers to Asia, Latin America, or Africa get "traveler's diarrhea." The most common infectious agents are enterotoxigenic *Escherichia coli*, enteroaggregative *E coli* (EAEC), *Campylobacter*, *Shigella*, and *Salmonella*. Norovirus, rotavirus, and parasites including *Giardia*, cryptospora, and microsporidia also commonly cause traveler's diarrhea, though less likely than *E coli*.
- **Contaminated food ingestion:** Usually associated with food consumption at picnics, banquets, or restaurants. Commonly implicated foods include chicken, hamburger (enterohemorrhagic *E coli*), fried rice (*B cereus*), mayonnaise (staph), eggs (*Salmonella*), and raw seafood (*Vibrio*).
- **High-risk populations:** Include immunocompromised patients, day care workers and their contacts, and health care workers.
- **Recent antibiotic use:** Risk factor for *Clostridium difficile* infection.
- **Viral gastroenteritis:** Etiology includes rotavirus, norovirus, enteric adenovirus, and astrovirus. Usually has rapid onset (24 to 48-hour incubation period) and is short-lasting (12-60 hours). Symptoms often include vomiting. Most adult outbreaks (cruise ships, nursing homes, military environments, etc) are caused by norovirus. Rotavirus is leading cause of childhood diarrhea.

KEY FACT

Do not give antibiotics to patients with suspected enterohemorrhagic *E coli* infection (bloody stools, abdominal pain/tenderness, little or no fever), as there is no evidence that antibiotics are of benefit, and there is a theoretical risk of causing hemolytic-uremic syndrome.

Diagnosis

First-line choice is guided by history. Most acute diarrhea not evaluated with lab studies and treated supportively. Indications for evaluation include: profuse diarrhea with dehydration, grossly bloody stools, fever ≤38.5°C (101.3°F), illness lasting >7 days, age >65, severe abdominal pain, community outbreaks, more than six stools in 24 hours for >48 hours, recent use of antibiotics, and hospitalization.

- **Fecal leukocytes:** Sensitivity and specificity for inflammatory diarrhea vary (70%-90%). Useful to support evaluation for inflammatory diarrhea along with cultures. Fecal lactoferrin has greater sensitivity and specificity but is not widely available.
- **Bacterial stool culture:** Controversial because acute infectious diarrhea is often viral, and bacterial cases are usually self-limited. However, stool cultures should be obtained for the above indications and in immunocompromised patients, those with significant comorbidities, and those with IBD (to differentiate flare from infection).
- Routine cultures will identify *Salmonella*, *Shigella*, and *Campylobacter* but not *Yersinia* or *Aeromonas*. The **false-negative rate is low** (ie, repeat testing is not necessary).
- **Viral stool culture and antigens: only if history directs or in setting of outbreak.**
- **Stool ova and parasites (O&P):** Usually obtained if diarrhea is persistent (>2 weeks) or for patients who have traveled to developing countries, men who have sex with men (MSM), immunocompromised patients, those involved in waterborne outbreaks, and those with bloody diarrhea with few or no fecal leukocytes (suggestive of amebiasis). Send O&P on 3 consecutive days, each spaced >24 hours apart.
- **Endoscopy/colonoscopy:** Appropriate if IBD or pseudomembranous/ischemic colitis is suspected.
- **Other:** Toxin assays (ie, *C difficile*); stool *Giardia* antigen; *Entamoeba histolytica* antigen if concern based on history.

Management

- **Fluid and electrolyte replacement:** Consists of ½ teaspoon of salt, ½ teaspoon of baking soda, and 4 tablespoons of sugar in 1 L of water for oral rehydration. IV fluids may be needed if oral rehydration fails.
- **Loperamide and diphenoxylate:** Consider for the alleviation of symptoms in afebrile and nonbloody cases. Avoid in suspected *C difficile* infection, as this can lead to toxic megacolon.
- **Bismuth subsalicylate:** Another option for symptomatic relief, but slower acting compared with loperamide.
- **Antibiotics** if indicated.
  - Consider empiric antibiotics if high clinical suspicion for inflammatory diarrhea:
    - Severe symptoms: Fever, bloody stools, more than eight stools/day, symptoms >1 week, consider hospitalization, immunocompromise.
    - Traveler's diarrhea with moderate to severe symptoms.
    - Avoid antibiotics if concern for EHEC.
    - Direct antibiotic therapy to culture results when possible.
  - **Fluoroquinolones:** For suspected bacterial infection: give for 3 to 5 days.
  - **Macrolides:** If resistance is suspected, especially with concern for *Campylobacter* infection.
  - **Metronidazole:** For cases suspected to be related to *Giardia* or *C difficile*.
  - **Vancomycin (PO):** May need as second-line agent for recurrent or resistant cases of *C difficile*.
- **Probiotics:** Proven to aid recolonization in pediatric patients and in traveler's diarrhea, but their efficacy less well established in adults. Examples include *Saccharomyces*, *Lactobacillus*, *Bifidobacterium*.

Q   QUESTION

A 48-year-old woman presents with 3 days of five watery stools each day; she has no fever, travel history, hypovolemia, or a significant medical history. How would you evaluate and treat?

CHRONIC DIARRHEA

Defined as diarrhea **lasting >4 weeks.** In developing countries, it is most often due to chronic infections, whereas in developed countries it is primarily caused by IBS, IBD, and malabsorption syndromes. Subtypes are as follows:

- **Secretory:** Deranged transport of fluid and electrolytes across the mucosa. Usually presents with frequent, watery, large-volume diarrhea that persists with fasting, occurring night and day. Causes include medications, laxatives, chronic alcohol consumption (enterocyte injury), toxins, cholorrheic diarrhea, partial obstruction/strictures/fecal impaction (leading to paradoxical hypersecretion), carcinoid, gastrinoma, and VIPoma.
- **Osmotic:** Due to a poorly absorbed osmotically active substance. Diarrhea is usually watery and worsens with ↑ solute load. Characterized by ↑ **stool osmotic gap, calculated as 290 − [2 (Na + K)].** Causes include carbohydrate malabsorption (leading to watery diarrhea) and fat malabsorption (leading to greasy diarrhea).
- **Inflammatory:** Due to mucosal inflammation. Diarrhea is generally bloody and accompanied by fever and abdominal pain. Causes include infections, IBD, radiation enterocolitis, and eosinophilic gastroenteritis.
- **Dysmotile:** Associated with hyperthyroidism, diabetes, carcinoid, drugs, and IBS.

Diagnosis

Figure 5.6 shows an algorithm to guide the diagnosis of chronic diarrhea.

Management

- Treat the underlying cause.
- **Pharmacotherapy for symptom management:**
  - **Loperamide and diphenoxylate:** Can be used for mild or moderate watery diarrhea.
  - Fluid, electrolyte, and vitamin replacement as needed.

KEY FACT

Nocturnal diarrhea is not characteristic of IBS and must be evaluated for another cause.

ANSWER

Given the lack of severe symptoms, no laboratory evaluation is indicated. You treat supportively with oral rehydration solution and loperamide. If she had presented with recent travel, you could treat with fluoroquinolone.

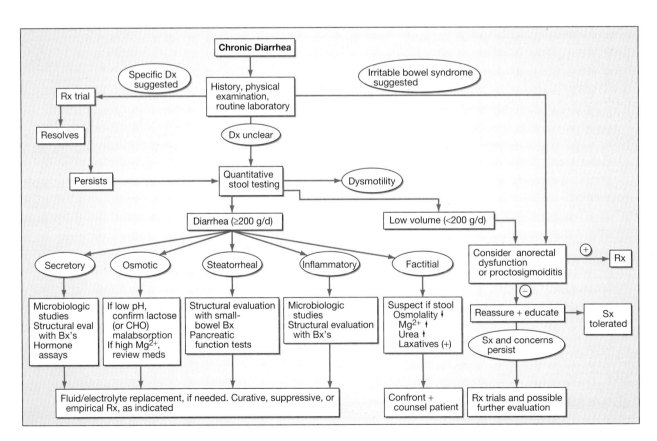

FIGURE 5.6. Diagnosis of chronic diarrhea. (Reproduced with permission from Kasper DL, et al. *Harrison's Principles of Internal Medicine,* 16th ed. New York: McGraw-Hill, 2005:230.)

FAT MALABSORPTION

Results from failure to digest, absorb, or transport fat or from a deficiency of bile with failed compensatory hepatic synthesis.

Symptoms/Exam

- Classically presents with diarrhea, steatorrhea, and weight loss; however, can also have more subtle symptoms (anorexia and flatulence).
- Symptoms of fat-soluble vitamin deficiencies (A, D, E, K) may be seen (associated blindness, osteopenia, and bleeding).

Differential

Most likely cause driven by history: commonly mucosal dysfunction (ie, celiac disease), lipolysis defects (ie, chronic pancreatitis), ↓ bile acid synthesis (liver disease) or secretion (biliary disease), bile acid deconjugation (ie, bacterial overgrowth) or loss (ie, Crohn's disease, ileal resection), or postabsorption defects (ie, abetalipoproteinemia).

Diagnosis

- **Best initial test: Fecal fat collection** (72-hour stool collection): The gold standard. Fat malabsorption is defined as stool fat excretion >6 g/day; however, patients with steatorrhea excrete >20 g/day. The inconvenience of the test limits its use.
- **Sudan III stain for fecal fat: Can detect >90% of patients with steatorrhea** if performed properly, but consistency is a shortcoming.
- **Stool acid steatocrit:** Sensitivity and specificity >95% compared with fecal fat collection. Alternate test if unable to perform fecal fat test.

Management

- Address the underlying disorder.
- Restrict long-chain fatty acids to 40 g/day, with supplementation of medium-chain fatty acids to maintain nutritional balance.
- Treat fat-soluble vitamin deficiencies by supplementing **5 to 10 times** the recommended daily value. **Water-soluble preparations** are necessary.
- Calcium and magnesium bind fatty acids in severe fat malabsorption, requiring supplementation.

CARBOHYDRATE MALABSORPTION

Most common malabsorption disorder is **lactose intolerance,** with a high prevalence in East Asians and Native Americans and a moderate prevalence in African Americans. Least common in whites (but still has up to 20% prevalence).

Symptoms/Exam

- Presents with diarrhea, cramps, abdominal pain, and/or flatus following the ingestion of carbohydrate. Symptom severity depends on the amount ingested and the fat content of the product (eg, skim milk empties from the stomach faster, causing more symptoms).
- Exam may reveal abdominal distention and hyperactive bowel sounds.

Differential

See the differential for chronic diarrhea above.

KEY FACT

Steatorrhea is not synonymous with cholorrhea ("bile acid diarrhea"). In the latter, excessive bile enters the colon and causes a secretory diarrhea, as seen in patients with ileal disease/resection.

KEY FACT

Vitamin deficiencies may result from fat malabsorption. Fat-soluble vitamins: A, D, E, K.
- ↓ vitamin A → night blindness, keratomalacia, xerophthalmia
- ↓ vitamin D → bone disease, hypocalcemia
- ↓ vitamin E → ataxia, hyporreflexia, and myopathy
- ↓ vitamin K → bleeding disorders

KEY FACT

Although lactose intolerance is commonly a 1° disorder, it may also be caused by a number of conditions (ie, celiac disease, bacterial overgrowth, gastroenteritis) because of the susceptible location of lactase on the distal villi.

QUESTION 1

A 12-year-old African American boy is brought in by his mother because of 4 weeks of diarrhea and abdominal cramping, worse after breakfast. What is the most likely diagnosis and how do you test?

QUESTION 2

You are working up a 25-year-old female German-American patient with diarrhea and weight loss, and are concerned for celiac disease. What test do you order first?

Diagnosis

Usually clinical, with trial of empiric restriction of carbohydrate (usually lactose) intake. Best initial test empiric trial of avoidance or:

- **Lactose tolerance test:** Measures serum glucose in blood 0, 60, and 120 minutes after the ingestion of 50 g of lactose. An ↑ in glucose of <20 mg/dL in conjunction with symptoms is diagnostic.
- **Breath test:** Measures hydrogen or $(13)CO_2$ in the breath at 30-minute intervals following an oral challenge. An ↑ in breath hydrogen of >20 ppm is diagnostic (the ↑ is due to bacterial fermentation of nonabsorbed sugars).
- **D-xylose:** Tests absorption of small intestinal epithelium with urine and blood levels of D-xylose after load. False-positive tests with antibiotic use, bacterial overgrowth, or impaired gastric emptying.
- **Other:** Nonspecific tests such as stool pH, stool-reducing substances, and stool osmotic gap (osmotic diarrhea) can aid in diagnosis.

Management

- Carbohydrate restriction (eg, milk and ice cream have more lactose than cheese).
- For lactose intolerance:
  - Lactase preparations can ↓ symptoms.
  - Calcium and vitamin D supplementation needed because of ↓ intake of milk products.

CELIAC DISEASE

An immune disorder triggered by the **gliadin component of gluten;** can affect any part of the intestine. Presents usually between 10 to 40 years of age. **Spontaneous remissions and exacerbations** are common. Associated with autoimmune disorders (type 1 diabetes, autoimmune thyroiditis, autoimmune hepatitis) as well as with dermatitis herpetiformis and IgA deficiency. More common among patients from Northern European backgrounds.

Symptoms/Exam

- Can range from symptoms of a single nutrient deficiency to diarrhea, steatorrhea, and weight loss.
- Exam may reveal no abnormalities or only those due to a particular nutrient deficiency.

Diagnosis

- **Best initial test: Anti–tissue transglutaminase (anti-TTG) IgA and anti-endomysial IgA:**
  - Excellent screening tests, with sensitivities >95%. Can also be used to follow titers to gauge clinical improvement; can be ⊖ after treatment and falsely ⊖ in patients on a gluten-free diet during testing.
  - Screenings should be followed by endoscopy with biopsy.
  - Antigliadin IgA is no longer favored because of its lower sensitivity and specificity.
- **Gold standard test: Small intestinal biopsy.** Reveals suggestive (not diagnostic) changes of villous atrophy that are confirmed by reversion to normal histology following initiation of a gluten-free diet.
  - If disagreement between biopsy findings and serologic results, can perform genetic testing and measure IgA levels.

Management

- **Dietary modifications:**
    - Institute a **gluten-free diet** (avoidance of wheat, rye, and barley products), supplemented by nutritional counseling.
    - Avoid lactose, as 2° intolerance is common.
    - Specific dietary deficiencies, such as deficiencies of iron, folic acid, calcium, vitamin D, and, rarely, vitamin B_{12}, should be corrected.
- Educate patients about the relapsing and remitting nature of the disease.
- Obtain a DEXA scan for osteopenia/osteoporosis screening due to vitamin D deficiency.
- Consider pneumococcal vaccination, as celiac disease is associated with hyposplenism.

Complications

Refractory sprue. Associated with ↑ risk of progressive malabsorption, risk of T-cell lymphoma, and death. Treatment consists largely of immunosuppression (steroids).

SHORT GUT SYNDROME

A malabsorptive state following massive small bowel resection, usually for Crohn's disease, malignancy, mesenteric ischemia, or radiation.

Symptoms/Exam

Presents with diarrhea and symptoms or signs of specific nutrient or vitamin deficiencies, depending on the nature of the resection. Common examples include resection of >60 cm of terminal ileum → malabsorption of IF-bound vitamin B_{12}; resection of >100 cm of ileum → bile salt wasting and subsequent fat malabsorption; loss of ileocecal valve → bacterial overgrowth and ↓ intestinal transit time.

Diagnosis

Usually clinical and suggested by the surgical history.

Management

- **Best initial:** Enteric feeding to promote intestinal adaptation. Fiber can help absorb water and also ↑ bacterial production of short-chain fatty acids to provide additional calories.
- **Cholestyramine** for choleraic diarrhea.
- Monitor and replace vitamins and minerals (eg, monthly vitamin B_{12} IM).
- TPN may be necessary if alimentary feeds are insufficient.

BACTERIAL OVERGROWTH

↑ in bacteria in the more proximal GI tract. This can result from abnormal stasis (eg, stricture, blind loops), ↓ motility, or abnormal communications between the proximal and distal GI tract (eg, fistula, ileocecal valve resection). Bacterial overgrowth can lead to **carbohydrate malabsorption** (due to bacterial consumption), **fat malabsorption** (through deconjugation of bile, which also has a direct toxic effect on the mucosa, aggravating carbohydrate malabsorption), and **vitamin B_{12} deficiency** (as bacteria compete with the host for vitamin B_{12}). Altered intestinal motility is also seen.

KEY FACT

Bacterial overgrowth should be suspected in any patient with a predisposing condition who presents with malabsorptive symptoms.

Symptoms/Exam

- Presents with diarrhea, steatorrhea, bloating, flatulence, anemia, subacute combined degeneration, weight loss, and associated calcium and fat-soluble vitamin deficiencies.
- Exam may reveal a succussion splash or distention.

Diagnosis

- Best initial test: Carbohydrate breath testing (lactulose or glucose).
- Alternatively, an empiric trial of antibiotics can be attempted.
- The gold standard is a **jejunal aspirate** showing a bacterial count of >**1000**; perform this if symptoms persist and diagnosis is still in question.

Management

- First: Treat the disorder predisposing to overgrowth.
- Next: **Antibiotics** to alter (not eliminate) flora include rifaximin (expensive), amoxicillin-clavulanate, cephalexin plus metronidazole, or TMP-SMX plus metronidazole. Usually given for 7 to 10 days, but it may be necessary to prolong treatment, offer repeat courses, and rotate antibiotics to prevent resistance.
- ↓ drugs that slow motility or gastric acidity (including PPIs).
- A high-fat, low-carbohydrate diet is of benefit, as bacteria rely more on carbohydrates. Avoid lactose if 2° lactose deficiency develops.

INFLAMMATORY BOWEL DISEASE

Chronic inflammatory disease of the GI tract. The two main subtypes are **Crohn's disease** (Figure 5.7) and **ulcerative colitis** (Figure 5.8). Table 5.3 outlines symptoms and disease characteristics of these two subtypes.

Suspect IBD with diarrhea >4 weeks, especially if bloody, however the diagnosis requires endoscopy/sigmoidoscopy and excluding other sources with stool studies, history and exam. Serologic tests are not useful to diagnose IBD or differentiate between Crohn's disease and UC.

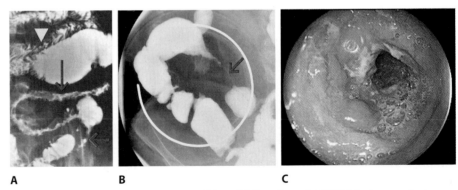

A   **B**   **C**

FIGURE 5.7.   **Crohn's disease. (A)** Small bowel follow-through (SBFT) barium study shows skip areas of narrowed small bowel with nodular mucosa (arrows) and ulceration. Compare with normal bowel (arrowhead). **(B)** Spot compression image from SBFT shows "string sign" narrowing (arrow) due to stricture. **(C)** Cobblestone appearance and surrounding erythema of the colon seen in Crohn's disease. (Image A reproduced with permission from Chen MY, et al. *Basic Radiology*. New York: McGraw-Hill, 2004, Fig. 10-30; image B reproduced with permission from USMLE-Rx.com; image C reproduced from Bataduwaarachchi VR, et al. The concurrent association of inflammatory polymyositis and Crohn's ileo-colitis in a Sri Lankan man: a case report of a rare association and literature review. *BMC Gastroenterol*. 2014;14:35.)

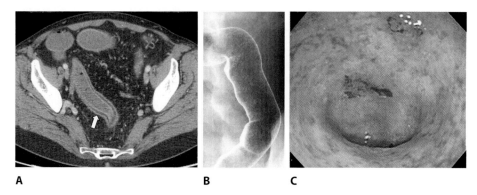

A   **B**   **C**

FIGURE 5.8. **Ulcerative colitis.** (**A**) CT scan shows wall thickening and enhancement of the colon with a featureless ("lead pipe") colon (arrow). (**B**) Double contrast barium enema shows granular mucosa in a patient with active ulcerative colitis. (**C**) Endoscopic image of ulcerative colitis shows loss of vascular pattern of the sigmoid colon, granularity, and some friability of the mucosa. (Images A and B reproduced from Deepak P, et al. Radiographical evaluation of ulcerative colitis. *Gastroenterol Rep (Oxf)*. 2014;2(3):169-177; image C reproduced from Wikimedia Commons.)

TABLE 5.3. **Crohn's Disease Versus Ulcerative Colitis**

	CROHN'S DISEASE	ULCERATIVE COLITIS
Symptoms	Chronic diarrhea, crampy abdominal pain, fever, weight loss, and fatigue Strictures leading to obstructive symptoms Fistulization causing recurrent UTIs/pneumaturia, gas/feces from vagina, psoas abscesses, and ureteral obstruction	Chronic bloody diarrhea, abdominal pain, cramps, tenesmus, and fecal urgency
GI tract involvement	**Transmucosal inflammation** leading to ulceration, strictures, fistulas, and abscesses May affect any part of the GI tract, from the mouth to the anus, but typically affects the **small bowel and colon;** 30% of cases involve the ileum; 20% involve the colon; and in 50% of cases both ileum and colon are involved	**Mucosal inflammation** leading to friability, erosions, and bleeding The **rectum** is invariably involved Extends **proximally** in a **continuous** fashion to involve the colon; 50% of cases involve the rectosigmoid colon; 30% extend to the splenic flexure; and 20% extend proximal to the splenic flexure
GI bleeding manifestations	Guaiac-positive stools are common; **grossly bloody stools are uncommon**	**Bloody stools are common**
Exam	Exam may reveal pallor, weight loss, a palpable mass (in some cases of perforation and localized peritonitis), **aphthous ulcers, anal fissures, perirectal abscesses,** and **anorectal fistulas**	Exam reveals abdominal tenderness and **gross blood on DRE**
Extraintestinal manifestations	Aphthous ulcers, anal fissures; less common, but those seen in ulcerative colitis may also be seen in Crohn's disease	Uveitis, episcleritis, erythema nodosum, pyoderma gangrenosum (see Figure 5.9), arthritis, ankylosing spondylitis, venous/arterial thromboembolism, sclerosing cholangitis
Differential	Ulcerative colitis, acute infectious diarrhea (*Shigella, Salmonella, Campylobacter, E coli* O157:H7), acute ileitis (*Yersinia* spp), TB of the bowel, amebiasis pseudomembranous colitis, CMV colitis (in the immunosuppressed), appendicitis, diverticulitis, ischemic colitis, lymphoma, carcinoma	Crohn's disease, radiation proctitis, ischemic/pseudomembranous/infectious colitis, infectious proctitis (gonorrhea, chlamydia, herpes, syphilis), amebiasis, CMV or Kaposi sarcoma in the immunosuppressed

(continues)

TABLE 5.3.   Crohn's Disease Versus Ulcerative Colitis (continued)

	CROHN'S DISEASE	ULCERATIVE COLITIS
Endoscopic evaluation	**Colonoscopy** with intubation of the terminal ileum (reveals skip lesions, linear ulcers, and cobblestone mucosa) with biopsy An upper GI series with small bowel follow-through or barium enema may also be needed to identify disease in the small bowel	**Flexible sigmoidoscopy** is usually adequate (shows pseudopolyps, bleeding, petechiae, ulcers, and exudates) with biopsy Colonoscopy may cause perforation in severe disease but may be used to evaluate the extent of disease
Autoantibodies (sent if diagnosis after endoscopy remains uncertain)	**ASCA** is present in 60%-70% of cases; **p-ANCA** is present in 5%-10% **ASCA-positive/p-ANCA-negative** findings are 90% specific for Crohn's disease	**p-ANCA** is present in 50%-70% of cases; ASCA is present in 10%-15% **p-ANCA-⊕/ASCA-⊖** findings are 98% specific for ulcerative colitis
Labs	Micro- or macrocytic anemia, leukocytosis, hypoalbuminemia Stool studies are ⊖ for an infectious cause	Same (but macrocytic anemia is less likely)
Suggested diet	High-fiber diet with colonic involvement; conversely, ↓ roughage if obstructive symptoms are present A trial of lactose elimination may benefit those with 2° intolerance	High-fiber diet; limit caffeine and gas-producing foods A trial of lactose elimination may be beneficial
Medical therapy	Ileitis: 5-ASA agents: mesalamine (sulfasalazine is activated in the colon, so it should not be used) Ileocolitis/colitis: first-line: mesalamine or sulfasalazine Next: Steroids or antibiotics (ciprofloxacin or metronidazole) Refractory cases require immunemodulators or biologics Surgery is not curative	Proctitis: 5-ASA suppositories (or steroid suppositories/foams); 5-ASA enemas (or steroid enemas) for left-sided colitis Extensive/pancolitis: Combined oral/rectal ASA agents and/or steroid enemas/suppositories, with oral corticosteroids for refractory cases Treat severe/fulminant cases with bowel rest, IV steroids, and antibiotics if the patient appears septic Colectomy is curative
Complications	Localized perforation/peritonitis, abscess, fistulas, bowel obstruction, massive hemorrhage, toxic megacolon, short gut syndrome (after resection)	Massive hemorrhage, fulminant colitis, toxic megacolon, perforation, stricture, colon cancer

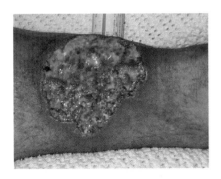

FIGURE 5.9. Pyoderma gangrenosum. A medical condition in which the body attacks itself in painful ulcers seen in patients with Crohn's disease. This is a picture of the lower half of the left leg. Inflammatory bowel disease. (Reproduced from Wikimedia Commons.)

IRRITABLE BOWEL SYNDROME

A functional disorder characterized by **abdominal pain and discomfort,** with associated **disturbed defecation.** Its etiology is believed to be multifactorial, involving altered gut motility/secretion, visceral hypersensitivity, and brain-gut axis dysregulation. IBS is the most commonly diagnosed GI condition and the second most common cause of work absenteeism, exceeded only by the common cold. It is more prevalent in women and generally presents at 30 to 50 years of age.

Symptoms/Exam

- **1° symptoms:** Abdominal discomfort, relief of discomfort with defecation, a change in frequency and/or form of stool (may be diarrhea- or constipation-predominant).
- **Other symptoms:** Straining, urgency, or a feeling of incomplete evacuation; passage of mucus; bloating.
- Exam typically yields no physical findings, but mild lower abdominal tenderness may be seen.

Differential

IBD, colon cancer, hyperthyroidism, hypothyroidism, chronic diarrhea (infectious, malabsorption), chronic constipation, celiac sprue.

Diagnosis

- Presumes the absence of a structural or biochemical explanation for the symptoms.
- The absence of alarm signs (ie, fever, weight loss, blood in the stool, anemia, a family history of IBD, celiac disease, or colon cancer, progressive symptoms, pain preventing sleeping or awakening the patient from sleep) is essential to diagnosis.
- Best first tests after history: stool hemoccult, CBC, ESR (especially in younger patients), serum chemistry, albumin, stool O&P × 3, TSH, and anti-endomysial/anti-TTG antibodies.

Management

- Best first choice: **Dietary modification:** Trial of limiting gas-producing foods (eg, beans, onions) and fermentable oligo-, di-, and mono-saccharides and polyols (FODMAPs; includes certain fruits, dairy, and grains), or limited trial of lactose or gluten if no improvement with first two modifications. A symptom diary to identify possible triggers may be useful.
- **Pain medications:**
  - **Antispasmodics:** Dicyclomine or hyoscyamine.
  - **Antidepressants: If no relief from dietary changes,** use low-dose TCAs or occasionally SSRIs, especially with comorbid depression.
  - For **constipation:** First use ↑ **dietary fiber or psyllium.** If bloating is a major factor, use polyethylene glycol, then lubiprostone.
  - For **diarrhea:** Best first is loperamide; next best, cholestyramine. If refractory, alosetron (serotonin antagonists) or dicyclomine (antispasmodic).

CONSTIPATION

Defined as **<3 stools per week,** however, many patients with daily bowel movements report "constipation" with feelings of incomplete defecation or difficulty stooling. Chronic constipation is more common in women, nonwhites, and those >60 years of age. Causes of constipation in adults are described in Table 5.4.

Constipation can also be idiopathic, characterized by patterns seen on bowel function studies. In **slow-transit constipation,** there is normal resting colonic motility but little or no ↑ after meals or with stimulants. In **dyssynergic defecation,** the pelvic floor muscles and external anal sphincter fail to relax during defecation, making evacuation difficult.

Diagnosis

- Largely clinical. Best initial step: Exclude IBS and review medication list.
- If alarm signs for obstruction 2° to malignancy (weight loss, a family history of colon cancer or IBD, anemia, hematochezia, a ⊕ FOBT, or acute onset of symptoms) are present, pursue further work-up starting with lab tests and imaging, then endoscopy.
- Laboratory tests include serum calcium for hypercalcemia and TSH for hypothyroidism.
- Barium enemas can detect structural changes, megacolon, and megarectum.
- If no improvement with treatment trial and negative imaging, consider idiopathic constipation. Workup with anorectal manometry, marker studies for assessing colonic transit, and defecography.

Management

- Best initial treatment: **Patient education:** Recommend that patients ↑ fluid and fiber intake, take advantage of ↑ colonic transit after meals (go to the bathroom

KEY FACT

Pursue further workup for IBS in the absence of alarm signs, including fever, weight loss, melena/hematochezia, iron-deficiency anemia, family history of IBD, celiac disease, or colon cancer, worsening symptoms, and nocturnal symptoms.

KEY FACT

An anorectal exam is essential in evaluating neurologic causes of constipation. ↓ rectal tone and sensation suggests sacral nerve or cauda equina lesions, which can lead to hypomobility, dilation, ↓ tone/sensation, stasis, and impaired defecation.

Q QUESTION

A 35-year-old woman complains of 6 months of intermittent lower abdominal discomfort, bloating, and diarrhea. She has no fever, weight loss, nocturnal symptoms, or bloody stools. Initial tests, including a complete metabolic panel, CBC, TSH, fecal occult blood test (FOBT), and stool O&P, have all been ⊖, and 2 weeks of a food journal have revealed no dietary triggers. What is the most likely diagnosis and how would you treat?

TABLE 5.4.   **Causes of Constipation in Adults**

TYPE OF CONSTIPATION	EXAMPLES
Recent onset	
Colonic obstruction	Neoplasm, stricture (ischemic, diverticular, inflammatory)
Anal sphincter spasm	Anal fissure, painful hemorrhoids
Medications	Narcotics
Chronic	
IBS	Constipation-predominant, alternating
Medications	Narcotics, calcium channel blockers, antidepressants
Colonic pseudo-obstruction	Slow-transit constipation, megacolon (rarely, Hirschsprung and Chagas disease)
Disorders of rectal evacuation	Pelvic floor dysfunction, anismus, descending perineum syndrome, rectal mucosal prolapse, rectocele
Endocrinopathies	Hypothyroidism, hypercalcemia, pregnancy
Psychiatric disorders	Depression, eating disorders, drugs
Neurologic disease	Parkinsonism, multiple sclerosis, spinal cord injury
Generalized muscle disease	Progressive systemic sclerosis

Reproduced with permission from Fauci AS, et al. *Harrison's Principles of Internal Medicine,* 17th ed. New York: McGraw-Hill, 2008, Table 40-5.

after eating), and participate in regular physical activity (immobility worsens the condition).

- **Pharmacotherapy: First line:** Fiber (psyllium). Next: stimulant laxatives (eg, bisacodyl, senna) or osmotic laxatives (eg, lactulose, polyethylene glycol). Stool surfactants (eg, docusate) are least efficacious.
  - If severe constipation with no improvement with treatment, use enemas, biofeedback, digital rectal stimulation/disimpaction. Use suppositories for defecatory dysfunction.
  - Slow-transit constipation requires aggressive medical treatment. Treatment failure or the presence of a megarectum or megacolon may suggest the need for surgery.

FECAL INCONTINENCE

Affects men and women equally (about 0.5%-2.0% of the US population), but tends to be more severe in women and elderly patients. Usually multifactorial, but generally due to sphincter dysfunction, abnormal rectal compliance, ↓ rectal sensation, or abnormal puborectalis muscle function. Specific etiologies include anal sphincter tears or pudendal nerve trauma during vaginal childbirth, surgical trauma (during fistula or hemorrhoid repairs), ulcerative/radiation proctitis, impaired rectal sensation (eg, neurologic disease, dementia), fecal impaction, or a cancer/obstructing mass.

Symptoms/Exam

- Anal wink reflex should be elicited bilaterally; its absence suggests nerve damage.
- DRE may show a mass or fecal impaction or reveal weakened anal tone.

Differential

Incontinence must be distinguished from bowel urgency and frequency **without loss of bowel contents,** which suggests etiologies such as IBD or IBS.

Diagnosis

- Mostly **clinical,** based on the history and physical exam.
- Next: **Sigmoidoscopy** to evaluate for inflammatory causes or a mass.

KEY FACT

There is little evidence to support using docusate in chronic constipation, despite its widespread use.

KEY FACT

Diarrhea should be excluded in patients who complain of fecal incontinence.

A   ANSWER

Irritable bowel syndrome. Treat with diet and lifestyle modifications.

- Anorectal manometry, pudendal nerve terminal latency, endorectal ultrasound, defecography, and EMG of the anal sphincter can be done if further evaluation is required.

Management

- Treat underlying cause.
- **Stool disimpaction and bowel regimen:** If fecal impaction is the cause.
- **Regular defecation program:** Appropriate if the disorder is related to mental dysfunction or physical disability.
- **Biofeedback programs.**
- **Pharmacotherapy:**
  - **Bulk-forming laxatives:** Indicated with low-volume, loose stools.
  - **Loperamide:** ↓ stool frequency and ↑ internal anal sphincter tone.
  - **Anticholinergics** (hyoscyamine, atropine) may be helpful.
  - **Surgical repair:** Usually successful in patients with single anal sphincter tears following vaginal delivery or fistula surgery.

Liver Disease

Table 5.5 outlines the differential diagnosis and treatment of common liver diseases. Viral hepatitis (HAV, HBV, and HCV) is not included in this table, as it is covered in

TABLE 5.5.   **Common Liver Diseases**

DISEASE	CLINICAL CAVEATS	SYMPTOMS/EXAM	LFT PATTERN	OTHER FINDINGS	TREATMENT
Drug/toxin-induced liver disease (always review meds in patients with liver disease)	Common offenders include **acetaminophen, isoniazid, tetracyclines,** and some antiepileptics	Variable	Variable		**Stop the offending medication** For acetaminophen toxicity, give **N-acetylcysteine** if **toxicity is likely** based on nomogram (>200 µg/mL at 4 hr)
Alcoholic liver disease	Includes alcoholic fatty liver (develops in 90% of patients), alcoholic hepatitis (develops in 10%-20%), and alcoholic cirrhosis. Women are affected more than men; concomitant HCV is a risk factor	**Fatty liver:** May be asymptomatic or present with hepatomegaly. **Alcoholic hepatitis:** Begins after a recent period of heavy drinking and presents with anorexia, nausea, hepatomegaly, and jaundice	**Fatty liver:** Modest elevation of aminotransferases (100-200 U/L). **Alcoholic hepatitis: AST usually** <300-400 U/L and 2 × ALT, ALP, and bilirubin are generally ↑	Fatty liver on ultrasound, CT, or MRI; biopsy shows **macrovesicular** fatty change; PMNs and Mallory bodies are seen	**Abstinence;** alcohol rehabilitation (AA, family therapy); aggressive nutritional support **(thiamine, folate); prednisolone if encephalopathic** or **discriminant function >32** (PT – control × 4.6 + total bilirubin). **Liver transplantation** can be considered with abstinence **>6 months**

(continues)

TABLE 5.5.   Common Liver Diseases *(continued)*

DISEASE	CLINICAL CAVEATS	SYMPTOMS/EXAM	LFT PATTERN	OTHER FINDINGS	TREATMENT
Nonalcoholic steatohepatitis	A condition in which **biopsy findings are indistinguishable from alcoholic hepatitis** in patients without significant alcohol consumption Most commonly found in patients 40-60 years of age; affects women more than men Metabolic syndrome is a risk factor	Usually asymptomatic, but may present with fatigue, malaise, RUQ discomfort, and hepatomegaly	↑ ALT and AST are seen in 90% of patients; unlike alcoholic hepatitis, the **ALT-to-AST ratio is** >1	Indistinguishable from that in alcoholic hepatitis	**Gradual weight loss** (rapid loss can exacerbate condition), dietary **fat restriction, exercise** Can recur following liver transplantation
Ischemic hepatopathy (shock liver)	Liver disease due to an acute ↓ in cardiac output (eg, MI, arrhythmia)	Variable; signs of fulminant failure may be present (eg, encephalopathy, jaundice, coagulopathy)	A **striking ↑ of transaminases** (often >**5000 U/L**); corrects quickly if cause reversed, ↑ prothrombin time may occur		Restore perfusion; aminotransferases usually correct quickly **(within 1 week)**
Hemochromatosis	**Most common genetic disorder in whites** Characterized by inappropriately ↑ absorption of dietary iron, causing deposition in the liver, heart, pancreas, and pituitary (leading to end-stage liver disease, hepatocellular carcinoma, dilated cardiomyopathy, diabetes, and hypogonadism) Associated with mutations of the *HFE* **gene on chromosome 6**	Presents with weakness, fatigue, malaise, hepatomegaly, RUQ pain, arthralgias, impotence, amenorrhea, and slate-gray pigmentation of the skin (due to iron and melanin deposition; also known as "bronze diabetes")	Variable (usually mild) elevation of AST and ALP is seen, depending on the stage of the disease	Fasting **transferrin saturation >45%; ↑ ferritin; genotype testing** (performed if iron studies are ⊕ or there is a history of the disease in first-degree relatives) Liver biopsy should be offered to document the degree of fibrosis in homozygotes >40 years of age with ↑ AST and ferritin >1000 ng/mL **Hepatic iron index** has **fallen out of favor** for diagnosis with genetic testing	**Phlebotomy therapy** (remove 1 unit of blood 1-2 times per week) **Deferoxamine** is **rarely needed** A normal diet is acceptable, but avoid iron supplements, vitamin C, **shellfish** (↑ susceptibility to *Vibrio vulnificus* and others) Liver transplant has relatively low survival because of concurrent cardiac disease and ↑ infection risk

(continues)

TABLE 5.5.   **Common Liver Diseases** *(continued)*

DISEASE	CLINICAL CAVEATS	SYMPTOMS/EXAM	LFT PATTERN	OTHER FINDINGS	TREATMENT
Wilson disease	An **autosomal-recessive** disease (involving the **ATP7B gene**) causing ↓ transmembrane transport (excretion) of copper in hepatocytes, leading to copper accumulation in organs (liver, brain, kidneys, cornea)	Presents with symptoms of liver failure ⊖ Coombs, hemolytic anemia, ARF, **Kayser-Fleischer rings,** behavior change, cognitive decline, tremor, lack of motor coordination, drooling, dysarthria, dysphonia, spasticity, oropharyngeal dysphagia, depression, anxiety, and psychosis	↑ **aminotransferases** are seen ALP is usually low	**Low copper** and serum **ceruloplasmin** (<5 mg/dL is strongly suggestive; low because of ↓ incorporation causing ↓ half-life); ↑ **24-hour urinary copper excretion** (>40 μg is suggestive); **slit-lamp exam** for Kayser-Fleischer rings (diagnostic with ceruloplasmin <20 mg/dL) Confirm with **hepatic copper content on biopsy** (>250 μg/g is the best biochemical evidence of disease; <40-50 μg/g excludes the diagnosis); brain MRI to evaluate for neurologic complications	D-**penicillamine** (binds copper and enhances urinary excretion); trientene is an alternative for patients who cannot tolerate D-penicillamine or with 1° neurologic symptoms **Oral zinc** interferes with the absorption of copper in the GI tract; reduction of copper-containing foods (shellfish, organs, legumes) is essential Liver transplant for end-stage liver disease and fulminant failure
Autoimmune hepatitis	Heterogeneous group of liver disorders characterized by **autoantibodies** and **high serum globulins** Can be seen with other autoimmune diseases (hemolytic anemia, ITP, diabetes, ulcerative colitis, celiac disease, thyroiditis) Female predominance	May be asymptomatic or fulminant (20%-25%, with jaundice and coagulopathy) A subset of patients are **young, otherwise healthy women** with fatigue, malaise, spider nevi, anorexia, amenorrhea, acne, arthralgias, and jaundice	**Aminotransferases are ↑ (100-1000 U/L)**	↑ **gamma globulin** (SPEP) Autoantibodies include **ANA, AMA, ASMA (type 1), and in kids, ALKM1.** Exclude other chronic liver diseases Liver biopsy may be nonspecific but aids in diagnosis, prognosis, and monitoring response to therapy	Treat if aminotransferases are elevated 10-fold or with significant changes of lab or biopsy studies based on guidelines Treat with **prednisone with azathioprine** or **6-MP** Disease can recur after liver transplantation (especially as immunosuppression is ↓)

(continues)

TABLE 5.5.   Common Liver Diseases *(continued)*

DISEASE	CLINICAL CAVEATS	SYMPTOMS/EXAM	LFT PATTERN	OTHER FINDINGS	TREATMENT
1° biliary cirrhosis	An **autoimmune disorder** causing granulomatous destruction of the intrahepatic bile ducts and cholestasis, T-cell mediated 95% of patients are women; onset at 40-60 years of age Osteopenia/osteoporosis develops in 25% of patients because of osteoblast dysfunction Frequently associated with other autoimmune disorders such as Sjögren and CREST	**Usually asymptomatic** (60% are asymptomatic at the time of diagnosis), but fatigue and pruritus are common presenting symptoms Jaundice, skin hyperpigmentation, xanthomas, hepatosplenomegaly, and other findings of end-stage liver disease may be present **Osteoporosis** is seen	Usually diagnosed in the presymptomatic phase, with **ALP** often more than **twice normal** (with elevations of GGT and 5-NT) **Bilirubin** ↑ with disease progression. AST and ALT may be normal	**Antimitochondrial antibodies** are 95% sensitive and 98% specific for the disease **Liver biopsy** is confirmatory Other causes of cholestasis should be excluded (eg, by ultrasound or cholangiography) **DEXA scans** to evaluate for concurrent osteoporosis	**Ursodeoxycholic acid** delays progression, enhances survival **Cholestyramine** improves pruritus (rifampin is second line) **Liver transplantation** is appropriate for treatment failure or severe osteoporosis
1° sclerosing cholangitis	Characterized by diffuse inflammation, fibrosis, and stricturing of the biliary tract as well as an ↑ risk of cholangiocarcinoma (associated with a 10%-15% lifetime risk), unknown etiology **90%** of patients have **ulcerative colitis** (but only 5% of ulcerative colitis patients have 1° sclerosing cholangitis) Affects males more than females	Presents with **progressive jaundice,** with associated malaise, pruritus, anorexia, and indigestion May have occasional bouts of acute cholangitis Steatorrhea, fat-soluble vitamin deficiency, and osteopenia develop	Usually diagnosed in the presymptomatic phase with ↑ **ALP;** aminotransferases may be ↑ to 300 U/L	Diagnosis is established by **ERCP** (or MRCP) unless the disease is **confined to small intrahepatic ducts,** in which case a **liver biopsy** is needed to establish the diagnosis and staging ANCA, ANA, anticardiolipin antibodies, anti-TPO antibodies, and RF may be ⊕ Rule out 2° causes of cholangitis	Medical therapy has failed to show consistent benefit in survival **Ursodeoxycholic acid** use is controversial Dominant biliary strictures should be **biopsied to rule out carcinoma, with balloon dilation or stent placement** to relieve obstruction **Liver transplantation** significantly improves survival

detail in the Infectious Diseases chapter. The subtopics that follow discuss cirrhosis and related complications.

CIRRHOSIS

Progressive scarring of the liver, with fibrosis and nodular regeneration. In the United States, cirrhosis is usually caused by chronic HCV infection, alcoholic liver disease, and nonalcoholic liver disease, although can also be caused by rarer etiologies such as medications or the liver diseases listed in Table 5.5.

The fibrosis and resulting distorted vasculature in cirrhosis lead to numerous physiologic changes (Figure 5.10).

Symptoms/Exam

- Fatigue, anorexia, nausea/vomiting, disturbed sleep, muscle cramps, or weight loss.
- If decompenstated disease, may have abdominal distention, jaundice, pruritis, or GI bleeding.
- Men may develop impotence, loss of libido, sterility, and gynecomastia; women may develop amenorrhea.
- The liver can be enlarged, normal, or shrunken, and usually is firm. Splenomegaly, spider nevi, palmar erythema, Dupuytren contractures, clubbing, gynecomastia, caput medusa, weight loss, and wasting may be seen.
- Late signs include jaundice, ascites, pleural effusions, ecchymoses, encephalopathy, asterixis, tremor, fetor hepaticus, and GI bleeding.

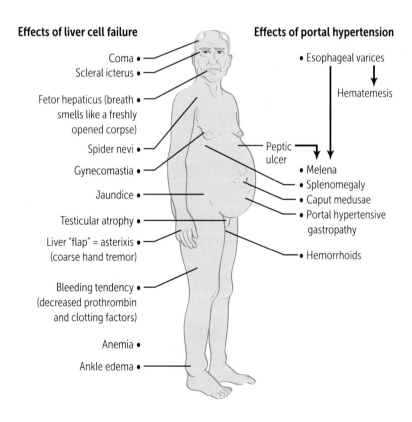

FIGURE 5.10.   **Clinical effects of cirrhosis.** (Reproduced with permission from USMLE-Rx.com.)

QUESTION

A 50-year-old woman presents with fatigue, pruritus, and mild jaundice. A liver panel reveals an alkaline phosphatase level 2× normal with mildly elevated bilirubin and normal AST/ALT. What is your next step and what is your differential?

Diagnosis

- Best initial test: **Ultrasound** to assess the extent of disease and to detect nodules (which can be further evaluated by CT/MRI if suspicious for HCC); include Doppler studies (to assess flow patterns in vasculature). Figure 5.11 shows a CT scan in a cirrhotic patient, with subsequent portal hypertension.
- **Labs:** Anemia, leukopenia, and thrombocytopenia may be seen. AST and alkaline phosphatase may be mildly ↑, and albumin is low. Rising total bilirubin, INR, and creatinine indicate worsening liver function. **Liver biopsy:** The gold standard, but diagnosis is usually made with clinical, lab, and radiologic findings.

Management

Treat reversible causes (eg, autoimmune hepatitis); discontinue alcohol use; treat HBV and HCV if possible. Immunize against HAV and HBV; limit hepatotoxic drugs (eg, acetaminophen <2 g/day), manage complications (see next sections), and consider transplantation referral.

END-STAGE LIVER DISEASE

Most common causes are alcohol and chronic viral hepatitis. Other etiologies include autoimmune, metabolic (hemochromatosis, Wilson disease, α_1-antitrypsin antibodies), biliary (1° biliary cirrhosis, 1° sclerosing cholangitis), and vascular disorders (Budd-Chiari, nonalcoholic fatty liver disease).

Symptoms/Exam

Jaundice, spider angiomata, icterus, palmar erythema, asterixis, ascites, splenomegaly, peripheral edema (see Figure 5.10).

Diagnosis

- Clinical history of liver injury.
- Best initial test is **ultrasound of liver.** Also obtain liver studies, coagulation studies, metabolic panel, GGT.

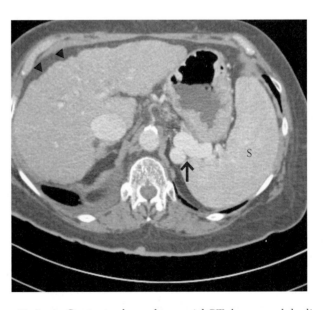

FIGURE 5.11. **Cirrhosis.** Contrast-enhanced transaxial CT shows a nodular liver contour (arrowheads) and the stigmata of portal hypertension, including splenomegaly (S) and perisplenic varices (arrow). (Reproduced with permission from USMLE-Rx.com.)

A   **ANSWER**

Order RUQ ultrasound and antimitochondrial antibodies to evaluate for 1° biliary cirrhosis versus 1° sclerosing cholangitis. Your patient has a normal ultrasound with ⊕ antimitochondrial antibody, suggesting biliary cirrhosis, confirmed by liver biopsy. You order a DEXA and start ursodeoxycholic acid and cholestyramine.

Prognosis

- MELD score: A scoring system reflecting total bilirubin, INR, and creatinine. Directly correlates with mortality. Calculators can be used to determine 90-day mortality risk. MELDNa incorporates serum sodium and is used for assigning rank for patients listed for liver transplant.
- Child-Pugh classification system helps rank severity of cirrhosis and predict survival. Used by surgeons for preoperative risk stratification (Table 5.6).

ASCITES

Intra-abdominal fluid accumulation caused by transudative movement of fluid into the abdominal cavity as a result of portal hypertension and ↓ serum oncotic pressure. Table 5.7 lists causes of ascites.

Symptoms/Exam

Presents with abdominal distention; exam may reveal flank dullness (eg, shifting dullness), indicating at least 1500 mL of ascitic fluid.

Diagnosis

- Usually clinical but can be difficult in obese patients. Best initial test after clinical diagnosis is ultrasound.
- Usually occurs in the presence of portal hypertension (**SAAG >1.1 g/dL**).

Management

- Best initial choice: **Sodium restriction:** Restrict patients to 2 g (88 mmol) per day. Fluid restriction should be reserved for patients with sodium level <120 mEq/L.
- Next best: **Spironolactone and furosemide:** If sodium restriction is inadequate, 90% of patients will respond to sodium restriction and spironolactone/furosemide starting at 100 mg/40 mg, respectively (ratio ensures normokalemia with normal renal function).
- **Repeated large-volume paracentesis:** Albumin replacement should be considered if >4 to 5 L of fluid is removed.
- **Transjugular intrahepatic portosystemic shunt (TIPS):** Controversial. Improves ascites (and is a last resort for variceal hemorrhage), but can ↑ encephalopathy and has a high occlusion rate.
- **Liver transplantation:** For refractory cases.
- With ascites due to cirrhosis: Discontinue alcohol use (regardless of underlying cause of liver disease), avoid renal-toxic medications, and with refractory ascites, consider discontinuing β-blockers.

KEY FACT

Use **diagnostic paracentesis** for new-onset clinically apparent ascites; send fluid for albumin, total protein, cell count, Gram stain, and culture.

TABLE 5.6. Child-Pugh Scoring System

	1 POINT	2 POINTS	3 POINTS
Encephalopathy grade	None	Mild confusion/lethargy	Marked confusion/coma
Bilirubin (mg/dL)	<2	2-3	>3
Ascites	None	Mild-moderate	Severe or refractory
Albumin (mg/dL)	>3.5	2.8-3.5	<2.8
INR	<1.7	1.7-2.3	>2.3

Total Points	Classification	1-Year Survival	2-Year Survival
5-6	Class A	100%	85%
7-9	Class B	80%	60%
10-15	Class C	45%	35%

QUESTION

A 57-year-old woman with a history of IV drug use is admitted with fever of 39.0°C (102.2°F) and a fluid wave noted on exam. What are your next diagnostic and treatment steps?

TABLE 5.7.   **Causes of Ascites**

HIGH ALBUMIN GRADIENT (SAAG >1.1 G/DL)	LOW ALBUMIN GRADIENT (SAAG <1.1 G/DL)
Cirrhosis	Peritoneal carcinomatosis
Portal hypertension	Peritoneal tuberculosis
Alcoholic hepatitis	Pancreatitis
Nonalcoholic steatohepatitis	Serositis
Chronic hepatitis C	Nephrotic syndrome
Heart failure	Dialysis
Massive hepatic metastases	Chlamydial peritonitis
Hypothyroidism	
Budd-Chiari syndrome	

SAAG (serum ascites albumin gradient) = serum albumin − ascites albumin.

SPONTANEOUS BACTERIAL PERITONITIS

Defined as infection of ascitic fluid caused by translocation of enteric bacteria across the gut wall or mesenteric lymphatics. Most common organisms are *E coli*, *Klebsiella*, or *Streptococcus* species.

Symptoms/Exam

Patients present with fever, ascites, abdominal pain, or altered mental status.

Diagnosis

Established by a PMN count >250 cells/mm³, a ⊕ **culture** of ascitic fluid, and exclusion of a surgical infection.

Differential

- **Culture-negative neutrocytic ascites:** PMN >250 cells/mm³; ⊖ culture. Treat as spontaneous bacterial peritonitis (SBP).
- **Alcoholic hepatitis:** If PMN >250 cells/mm³, treat as SBP. If <250 cells/mm³, treat as SBP for 48 hours and discontinue treatment if all cultures are ⊖.
- **Perforated viscus:** PMN >250 cells/mm³; multiple organisms found on culture. The presence of two of the following suggests SBP: Total protein >1 g, LDH > normal for serum, or glucose <50 mg/dL.

Management

- **Cefotaxime (or other third-generation cephalosporin):** Administer IV × 5 days, narrow as culture results become available.
- Consider **albumin** infusion if creatinine >1 mg/dL, BUN >30 mg/dL, or total bilirubin >4 mg/dL (to ↓ the incidence of hepatorenal syndrome).
- Discontinue nonselective β-blocker (ie, propranolol) permanently due to mortality benefit.
- **Prophylaxis:** (note: **norfloxacin not available in the United States**)
  - **Prior SBP:** TMP-SMX DS tablet daily, or ciprofloxacin 500 mg daily.
  - **GI bleeding in the setting of cirrhosis: Ceftriaxone 1 g daily, then** TMP-SMX or ciprofloxacin × 7 days total (there is an ↑ risk of SBP in these patients).
  - Ascitic protein <1.5 g/dL with renal dysfunction (creatinine >1.2 mg/dL, BUN >25 mg/dL, sodium <130 mEq/L) or liver failure (bilirubin >3 mg/dL): Daily TMP-SMX or ciprofloxacin.
  - **Ascitic protein <1 g/dL and hospitalized for condition other than SBP:** TMP-SMX once per day or ciprofloxacin 500 mg daily during hospitalization.

KEY FACT

Indications for prophylaxis for SBP include history of SBP, GI bleeding with history of cirrhosis, history of ascitic fluid protein <1.5 g/dL with renal dysfunction (creatinine >1.2 mg/dL) or liver failure, or ascitic fluid <1 g/dL (prophylaxis during hospitalization).

ANSWER

Perform a diagnostic paracentesis with cell count, culture, albumin, total protein, glucose, and LDH. Measure serum LDH and albumin and calculate SAAG. Start cefotaxime and give albumin if creatinine is >1 mg/dL to reduce risk of renal failure.

HEPATORENAL SYNDROME

Characterized by **progressive renal failure, low urine sodium,** and **<500 mg/dL of proteinuria** in the presence of **advanced liver failure** and **portal hypertension** without other 2° cause. Also characterized by lack of response to albumin and cessation of diuretics.

Believed to be caused by splanchnic arterial vasodilation with ↓ renal perfusion despite intense renal vasoconstriction. Can be rapidly progressive (type 1, creatinine >2.5 mg/dL in <2 weeks, often as consequence of SBP or GI bleed) or insidious (type 2).

Survival is essentially zero without liver transplantation. Management involves the following:

- **Supportive care until liver transplantation:** IV albumin, with octreotide, midodrine, and norepinephrine or vasopressin to ↑ mean arterial pressure.
- Reverse underlying cause of liver failure if possible.
- Hemodialysis alone does not improve patient outcomes and is used only for patients awaiting transplantation.

HEPATIC ENCEPHALOPATHY

Causes are multifactorial, but the **ammonia hypothesis** is still the predominant etiology. **Usually has a precipitating cause,** including GI bleeding, metabolic changes (hypokalemia or hypoglycemia), alkalosis (favors $NH_4 \rightarrow NH_3$, which crosses the blood-brain barrier), infection, renal failure, hypoxia, TIPS placement, sedative/tranquilizer use, or constipation (↓ GI clearance of ammonia).

Symptoms/Exam

Progressive psychiatric and neuromuscular changes: Sleep changes, disorientation and confusion, with asterixis, bradykinesia, and other neurologic signs.

Diagnosis

Usually clinical.
- Common distractor: ↑ **ammonia** is common, but level is not diagnostic and does not correlate with severity of disease.
- Rule out other etiologies of mental status changes and evaluate for precipitating cause.

Management

- **Correct the precipitating event**—eg, replace potassium, IV fluids, antibiotics targeted to infection.
- Supportive care: No protein restriction needed.
- **Pharmacotherapy:**
  - First choice: **Lactulose;** a retention enema can be used if oral lactulose is not well tolerated.
  - If no improvement after lactulose, nonabsorbable antibiotic such as **rifaxamin.**

HEPATOPULMONARY SYNDROME

Characterized by intrapulmonary vascular dilatations → to ventilation-perfusion mismatch with underlying liver disease and usually with portal hypertension. Thought to be caused by failure of the liver to clear pulmonary vasodilators.

Symptoms/Exam

Usually characterized by dyspnea; **platypnea** (shortness of breath received when lying down) and **orthodeoxia** (shortness of breath and deoxygenation in the upright position) are suggestive. There is a correlation between hepatopulmonary syndrome and the presence of **spider angiomata.**

Diagnosis

- Clinical diagnosis in a patient with liver disease, impaired oxygenation, and ruling out other causes.
- Best first choice: Alveolar-arterial gradient >15 mm Hg or arterial oxygen tension <80 mm Hg on room air.
- Next best choice: Contrast-enhanced echocardiography is useful for screening pulmonary vascular dilatations.

Management

Supplemental oxygen and ultimately liver transplantation with disease progression.

ESOPHAGEAL VARICES

Dilated submucosal veins due to portal hypertension. The mortality rate associated with variceal bleed is 20%; risk factors include size, the presence of "red signs" markings, high Child-Pugh class, location (eg, gastric fundal varices have ↑ risk of bleeding), and active alcohol use. Gastric and rectal varices are also common. Approximately 70% of patients have a repeat episode of variceal bleeding.

Symptoms/Exam/Diagnosis

Asymptomatic unless there is acute hemorrhage (see the discussion of Upper GI bleeding below). Patients with cirrhosis should be screened with endoscopy for risk stratification.

Management

- First line: **Endoscopic variceal ligation (EVL) or sclerotherapy:** Acute therapy for bleeding varices. EVL preferred over sclerotherapy due to fewer complications.
- Supportive cares: Fluid resuscitation avoiding hypervolemia, monitor for alcohol withdrawal.
- **Prophylaxis against SBP** or other serious infection (see section on SBP above).
- **Somatostatin, vasopression, or octreotide drips:** ↓ splanchnic flow and portal pressures.
- **Balloon tube tamponade:** Has a high complication rate (esophageal ulceration, aspiration, perforation); used when bleeding cannot be controlled medically or endoscopically while awaiting TIPS/portosystemic shunt.
- Second line if failed endoscopy and medical management: **TIPS/portosystemic shunt** creates a decompressive shunt between the portal and hepatic veins. Associated with high complication and mortality rates.
- 1° prophylaxis for variceal hemorrhage: First choice: prophylaxis with nonselective β-blockers (propranolol, nadolol) for all varices except large ones. For large varices, first choice is esophageal variceal ligation (EVL), which offers a slightly better reduction in the risk of bleeding, but is more invasive. The goal for medical prophylaxis is generally to ↓ resting heart rate to 50 to 60 bpm.
- Nitrates are **not** recommended.

See the section on upper GI bleeding below for further discussion.

KEY FACT

Approximately 25% to 40% of patients with cirrhosis with experience variceal hemorrhage; the mortality rate associated with variceal bleeding is 20%.

 ANSWER

Nonselective β-blocker such as propranolol or nadolol, titrated gradually to ↓ his heart rate to 50 to 60 bpm.

Biliary Disease

CHOLELITHIASIS AND ACUTE CHOLECYSTITIS

Caused by **aberrations in the solubilization of cholesterol**. In the United States, cholelithiasis is found in 6% of men and 9% of women. Risk factors include obesity, insulin resistance, rapid weight loss, and pregnancy. Most patients with cholelithiasis are asymptomatic; 15% have symptomatic disease. Cholecystitis is usually caused by an impaction of a gallstone (90% of cases).

Symptoms/Exam

- **Cholelithiasis:** Majority are asymptomatic; may cause variable amounts of **RUQ or epigastric pain,** often after eating (biliary colic).
- **Acute cholecystitis:** Presents with **fever** and **severe RUQ or epigastric pain** that may radiate to the infrascapular area. Symptoms are usually precipitated by a large or fatty meal. Vomiting and malaise are common.
- Exam is usually normal or may reveal mild RUQ tenderness in cholelithiasis.
- In acute cholecystitis, exam reveals RUQ tenderness, a ⊕ **Murphy sign,** guarding, and rebound pain. The gallbladder may be palpable.

Differential

- **Biliary dyskinesia:** Biliary colic in the setting of ⊖ initial radiographic studies. Usually caused by undetected stenosis, adhesions, or kinking in the cystic duct. Diagnosed by ↓ gallbladder emptying on scintigraphy following cholecystokinin injection. Cholecystectomy is curative.
- **Acalculous cholecystitis:** 10% of cholecystitis. Found in patients who are critically ill.
- **Infectious cholecystitis:** Found in HIV-positive patients, those with CMV, or those with crypto- or microsporidiosis.
- **Cholangitis:** Highly suspicious if **jaundice** is present (a component of the Charcot triad, along with **fever** and **RUQ pain**). See next section for further discussion.

Diagnosis

- **Labs:** Labs are usually normal in cholelithiasis. In acute cholecystitis, there may be leukocytosis.
- **Imaging:**
  - First choice: **RUQ** ultrasound will reveal the presence of stones in cholelithiasis (Figure 5.12). In cholecystitis, ultrasound can demonstrate cholelithiasis, gallbladder wall thickening, pericholecystic fluid, and a sonographic Murphy sign.
  - Second line: **HIDA scan:** Can demonstrate obstruction in the cystic duct using injected contrast, taken up by hepatocytes and excreted into bile.
- **Cholangiography:** Usually performed intraoperatively to rule out choledocholithiasis or preoperatively by ERCP or MRCP.

Management

- **Asymptomatic gallstones:** Cholecystectomy usually not indicated. Indicated if the gallbladder wall appears calcified (porcelain gallbladder) or other risk factors for gallbladder cancer, or in young patients with sickle cell disease.
- **Symptomatic gallstones: Laparoscopic cholecystectomy** is indicated.

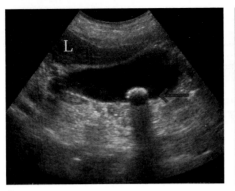 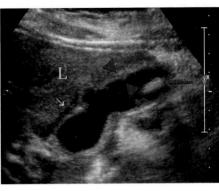

A   B

FIGURE 5.12.   **Gallstone disease.** (A) Cholelithiasis. Ultrasound image of the gallbladder shows a gallstone (arrow) with posterior shadowing. (B) Acute cholecystitis. Ultrasound image shows a gallstone (red arrow), a thickened gallbladder wall (arrowheads), and pericholecystic fluid (white arrow). L = liver. (Reproduced with permission from USMLE-Rx.com.)

KEY FACT

Acute cholecystitis is characterized by the triad of fever, RUQ pain, and leukocytosis; recurrence risk and risk of complications are high without definitive stone management.

- Chenodeoxycholic acid and ursodeoxycholic acids can dissolve some cholesterol stones in patients who refuse cholecystectomy or are poor surgical candidates.
- **Acute cholecystitis:**
  - First line: NPO, IV fluids, pain control.
  - Antibiotics: Provide coverage for gram-negative rods and anaerobes to address potential for 2° infection.
- Laparoscopic cholecystectomy is indicated during hospitalization; emergently if suspicion for perforation, progressive symptoms, or hemodynamic instability. Percutaneous cholecystostomy/ultrasound-guided aspiration may be considered in patients with a high operative risk.

Complications

- **Gangrene: 20% of cases without treatment.** Suggested by progression of symptoms, including severe abdominal pain, fever, vomiting, and hypotension. Cholecystectomy is mandatory.
- **Perforation:** May progress to abscess versus generalized peritonitis, although pain usually remains anatomically localized. Cholecystectomy is mandatory.
- **Gallstone ileus:** Mechanical obstruction by a stone in the bowel (usually the ileocecal valve) caused by passage of a gallstone through a cholecystenteric fistula.
- **Emphysematous cholecystitis:** 2° infection of gallbladder with gas-forming bacteria; frequently leads to gangrene, perforation, or other complications.
- **Repeated episodes** can cause chronic inflammation, leading to choledocholithiasis, fistulization to the bowel, pancreatitis, and, rarely, carcinoma of the gallbladder.

CHOLEDOCHOLITHIASIS AND CHOLANGITIS

Choledocholithiasis is the presence of gallstone in the common bile duct (occurs in 15% of patients with gallstones). **Cholangitis** is an infection within the common bile duct, usually (85% of the time) resulting from a common bile duct stone.

Symptoms/Exam

- Symptoms develop if **obstruction occurs** and causes biliary colic and jaundice.
- RUQ or epigastric **pain, jaundice, and fever (Charcot triad)** are classic findings in cholangitis.
- In acute suppurative cholangitis, patients may also present with **confusion and hypotension (Reynolds pentad).**
- Exam reveals RUQ tenderness, jaundice, scleral icterus, and hepatomegaly.

Differential

Most likely: obstruction due to choledocholithiasis. Also can be due to carcinoma, Mirizzi syndrome (gallbladder neck stone compressing the common bile duct), benign biliary stricture, cholestatic liver disease (1° sclerosing cholangitis, 1° biliary sclerosis, drug-induced cholestasis), external obstruction, congenital disease (biliary atresia, choledochal cysts), parasites (*Ascaris lumbricoides, Echinococcus* spp).

Diagnosis

- First choice: RUQ **ultrasound:** Evaluate for bile duct dilation and underlying cause (stone, stent, stricture).
- Second choice: **Labs, used to stratify need for intervention:** ↑ bilirubin, alkaline phosphatase, GGT, and PT/INR. Elevation of aminotransferases in the 1000s may be seen if acute necrosis of hepatocytes occurs.
- **ERCP:** Determines the cause, location, and extent of biliary obstruction; also preferred for interventions. **MRCP** for patients who cannot undergo ERCP.

Management

- **Choledocholithiasis: ERCP with** stone extraction followed by cholecystectomy.
- **Choledocholithasis with cholangitis:** Broad-spectrum antibiotics plus:
  - First choice: ERCP with sphincterotomy and stone extraction on an urgent or emergent basis.
  - Second choice: If first choice unavailable or unsuccessful, percutaneous drainage.

KEY FACT

ERCP should be performed within 24 to 48 hours of diagnosis of acute cholangitis and emergently for acute suppurative cholangitis (fever >39°C [102°F], hypotension, confusion).

Pancreatic Disease

ACUTE PANCREATITIS

Disease ranges from Atlanta classification of edematous versus necrotizing categories with severity of mild to severe, which determines presentation and prognosis. The most common etiologies are **biliary disease** and **alcohol.** Other etiologies include drugs (2%-5%), postoperative or post-ERCP, trauma, hypertriglyceridemia, viral infection (eg, mumps), vasculitis, pancreas divisum, sphincter of Oddi dysfunction, and hypercalcemia. May also be idiopathic.

KEY FACT

Gallstones are the most common cause of pancreatitis, but only about 5% of patients with gallstones develop pancreatitis.

Symptoms/Exam

- Presents with a steady, usually epigastric or diffuse upper abdominal pain, with radiation to the back, chest, and lower abdomen.
- Pain worsens in a supine position and improves in a fetal position or leaning forward.
- Nausea, vomiting, and distention due to GI hypomobility are common.
- Patients may appear distressed, with fever, tachycardia, hypotension, and shock as well as with variable degrees of abdominal tenderness and rigidity.
- Bowel sounds may be diminished.
- **Cullen sign** (ecchymosis at the umbilicus) and **Grey Turner sign** (ecchymosis of the flanks) point to severe necrotizing pancreatitis (Table 5.8 lists other signs of severity).

Differential

Perforated viscus (peptic ulcer), acute cholecystitis or cholangitis, biliary colic, acute intestinal obstruction, mesenteric ischemia, renal colic, ACS, dissecting aortic aneurysm or hepatitis.

MNEMONIC

Causes of acute pancreatitis:
I GET SMASHED
Idiopathic
Gallstones
Ethanol
Trauma
Steroids
Mumps
Autoimmune (PAN)
Scorpion stings
Hyperlipidemia/**H**ypercalcemia
ERCP
Drugs (including azathioprine and diuretics)

TABLE 5.8.   Apache II Score

Temperature >38.5°C or <35.9°C
MAP or HR outside of 70-109 bpm
RR outside of 12-24/min
Pao$_2$ <70 mm Hg
pH outside of 7.33-7.49
Na outside of 130-149 mEq/L
K outside of 3.5-5.4 mEq/L
Creatinine outside of 0.6-1.4 mg/dL
Hematocrit outside of 30%-45.9%
WBC outside of 3-14.9 cells/mm³
GCS <15
Age >44 years
Presence of chronic diagnoses

↑ points given for values further from normal. Use most abnormal values in previous 24 hours.

Diagnosis

- **Labs:**
  - First choice: **serum lipase:** Specificity is 85% to 100%.
  - Next, additional studies to evaluate for other causes: CBC may show leukocytosis and anemia (due to hemorrhage); chemistry may show hyperglycemia and hypocalcemia. LFTs may reveal transient elevation of transaminases, ALP, and bilirubin. An **ALT >150** is 96% sensitive for gallstone-related pancreatitis.
- **Imaging:**
  - First line: **Ultrasound:** Often used for initial investigation if pancreatitis is suspected and for etiology work-up. Efficacy is limited by obesity and intestinal gas.
  - **CT scan** (IV contrast preferred): The best imaging study. Can confirm the diagnosis when amylase levels are normal; also indicates severity. Not as sensitive or specific as serum lipase level. CT scan is not indicated unless pancreatic necrosis or other developing complication is suspected or the diagnosis of pancreatitis is in doubt (Figure 5.13).
  - **MRI/MRCP:** More sensitive than CT for early disease and used when patients cannot tolerate contrast. Advantages include absence of ionizing radiation, excellent assessment for fluid collections, and detection of choledocholithiasis rivaling ERCP. Cons include cost and availability.

Prognosis

- Multiple scoring systems for severity and prognosis; less helpful for severity due to limited accuracy, but frequently used to triage to ICU care. Average mortality risk from pancreatitis is 2%, but can be much higher with severe disease.
  - Apache II: Not a direct scoring system for pancreatitis, but is a general acuity score that can be used daily to trend severity and prognosticate (see Table 5.8).
  - **Ranson criteria:** Uses data at admission and at 48 hours to predict severity; however, poor predictor.
  - **CT Severity scale: Uses data from imaging to prognosticate mortality.**
  - SIRS: Persistent SIRS criteria at 48 hours poor prognostic sign.

Management

- **NPO** and **IV fluids; NG tube** if needed.
- **Analgesics: Parenteral.** Typically patient-controlled morphine or fentanyl.
- **Early refeeding** (with fat restriction): As soon as there is improvement.
- **Early enteral nutrition (jejunum)** if unable to restart PO within 5 to 7 days. Anticipate use in severe pancreatitis. Patient may also need parenteral feeding if unable to tolerate enteral.

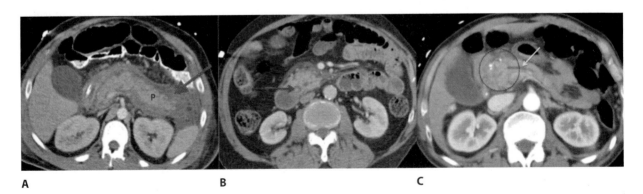

FIGURE 5.13.   Acute and chronic pancreatitis. (A) Uncomplicated acute pancreatitis. Peripancreatic fluid and fat stranding can be seen (arrows) surrounding the pancreas (P). **(B) Gallstone pancreatitis.** Gallstone (arrow) lodged within the proximal pancreatic duct, which caused acute pancreatitis with dilated pancreatic duct and peripancreatic fluid. **(C) Chronic pancreatitis.** Dilated pancreatic duct (arrow) with enlarged pancreatic head with associated pancreatic calcifications (circle). (Reproduced with permission from USMLE-Rx.com.)

- **Antibiotics:** Broad-spectrum antibiotics only if extrapancreatic infection identified.
- For gallstone pancreatitis with cholangitis, urgent ERCP with papillotomy; planned cholecystectomy. No indication for ERCP without common bile duct obstruction, even if pancreatitis is severe.

Complications

- **Pancreatic necrosis:** Frequently acute, but over >4 weeks, can become walled off.
- **Pancreatic abscess** 4 to 6 weeks after onset.
- **Pseudocysts** usually develop after 4 weeks, diagnosed by sonography or CT; resolves in 25% to 40% of patients; drainage considered if complicated (ie, infection) or if >5 cm and persists for >6 weeks.

CHRONIC PANCREATITIS

The causes of chronic pancreatitis are outlined in the mnemonic **TIGAR-O.** The majority of cases are associated with alcohol use.

Symptoms/Exam

- May present with symptoms identical to those of acute pancreatitis; however, the pain pattern may be variable and located in the upper quadrants of the back or upper abdomen.
- Late symptoms and signs include signs of malabsorption such as weight loss, steatorrhea, and diabetes.

Differential

First concern: pancreatic cancer. Also consider acute pancreatitis, endocrine tumors, autoimmune pancreatitis, or lymphoma.

Diagnosis

- **Classic triad: Pancreatic calcifications, steatorrhea,** and **diabetes are pathognomonic.**
- First choice: **Imaging: Abdominal x-ray,** sonography, or contrast CT to evaluate for calcifications.
- **MRCP** first line, if available, due to visualization without radiation.
- **ERCP:** Consider if calcifications are not present or the diagnosis is uncertain, to delineate anatomy and to find a possible source amenable to intervention.
- **Labs:**
  - **Amylase and lipase: not recommended for chronic pancreatitis work-up.**
  - ↑ ALP or bilirubin is seen if inflammation leading to ductal obstruction is present.
  - ↑ fasting glucose, ↑ fecal fat or ⊕ fecal elastase, and coalbumin malabsorption are seen in later stages.
  - **Secretion stimulation test:** Perform if the classic triad is not present (⊕ when 60% of exocrine function is lost).
  - Genetic testing not recommended.

Management

- **Treat pain:** Avoid alcohol, tobacco, and large fatty meals; narcotics may be needed for pain management.
- Pancreatic enzyme replacement with acid suppression; treat diabetes.
- Ductal decompression or pancreatic resection in selected cases.

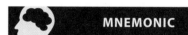

MNEMONIC

Causes of chronic pancreatitis:
TIGAR-O
Toxic/metabolic (alcohol, hypercalcemia, severe protein-calorie malnutrition)
Idiopathic
Genetic
Autoimmune
Recurrent severe/acute
Obstructive

KEY FACT

Evidence of malabsorption due to exocrine pancreatic failure occurs after >90% of pancreatic function is lost.

KEY FACT

Approximately 70% to 80% of chronic pancreatitis cases are associated with alcohol use.

Complications

Associated with ↑ risk of pancreatic carcinoma. Also monitor for complications similar to acute pancreatitis (see above).

GI Malignancies

ESOPHAGEAL CANCER

Most often affects patients 50 to 70 years of age, with a male-to-female ratio of 3:1. **Squamous cell carcinoma** is strongly associated with chronic alcohol use and smoking. In the majority of cases, **adenocarcinoma** develops from Barrett esophagus. A diet low in fruits and vegetables is a risk factor, as is obesity.

Symptoms/Exam

- Presents with solid food dysphagia that progresses over weeks to months. Weight loss is common.
- Cough on swallowing, chest or back pain, and voice hoarseness are seen with invasive disease.

Diagnosis

- First choice: **Endoscopy with biopsy:** Disease is usually incurable at the time of diagnosis (Figure 5.14).
- Next best: **CT of the chest and liver:** For disease staging. Perform positron emission tomography (PET) scans if CT ⊖.
- If CT is ⊖, **endoscopic ultrasound** should be performed to evaluate wall involvement as well as local mediastinal and lymph node involvement (in conjunction with FNA).
- Bronchoscopy to evaluate airways for invasive disease in locally advanced disease without metastases.

Management

- **Early-stage disease:** May be cured by **surgery alone** (transhiatal esophagectomy with anastomosis of the stomach with cervical esophagus). Comprehensive treatment plan with radiation and systemic chemotherapy most effective, but ideal agents controversial.
- **Advanced local spread or distant metastases:** Surgery is not warranted. Palliative treatment should be directed toward dysphagia and pain relief. Radiation and chemotherapy have significant side effects and may be considered in otherwise healthy patients with good functional status and minimal medical problems.
- Prognosis is poor, with a 5-year survival rate of 15%.

KEY FACT

Fifty percent to 60% of patients with esophageal cancer present with incurable disease. Even in patients with resectable disease treated trimodally (surgery, radiation, chemotherapy), recurrence occurs in >50% of patients.

GASTRIC CANCER

Adenocarcinoma is the most common form of gastric cancer. Mean age at diagnosis is 63 years; uncommon in patients <40 years of age. The male-to-female ratio is 2:1. It is more common among patients of Hispanic, African American, and Asian descent. Additional risk factors include chronic *H pylori* gastritis, diets high in salt and nitrous compounds, alcohol use, tobacco use, chronic atrophic gastritis, pernicious anemia, and a history of partial gastric resection.

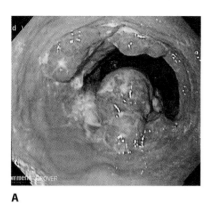 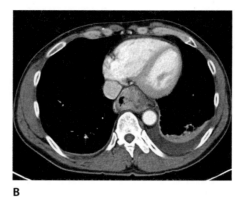

A   **B**

FIGURE 5.14. **Esophageal cancer.** (A) EGD with fungating nodular intraluminal mass consistent with esophageal adenocarcinoma. (B) Contrast-enhanced CT of the chest shows enhancing irregular circumferential mass (red outline) arising from the esophagus that is suspicious for esophageal cancer. (Reproduced from Wikimedia Commons; image A courtesy of Samir and image B courtesy of Tdvorak.)

Symptoms/Exam

- Presents with dyspepsia, epigastric pain, anorexia, early satiety or vomiting, weight loss, occult fecal blood (and iron deficiency anemia), hematemesis, dysphagia, or melena. A gastric mass is palpable in 20% of cases.
- Metastatic spread may reveal palpable **left supraclavicular or umbilical nodes** (Virchow and Sister Mary Joseph nodes, respectively), a **rigid rectal shelf** (Blumer shelf), or **ovarian metastases** (Krukenberg tumor).

Diagnosis

- First line: **Endoscopy with brush cytology and biopsy** should be performed on any patient >50 years of age with dyspepsia who does not respond to a short course of acid suppression (Figure 5.15).
- **Staging:** Performed with abdominal CT and endoscopic ultrasound. If ⊖, then PET scan to assess for metastases.
- Barium swallow not first line due to low sensitivity in early disease.

Management

- **Localized disease: Surgical resection** (depending on the location and extent of disease) can be curative.
- Adjuvant chemotherapy and radiation are also being used for ↑ survival in multi-modal therapy for localized and potentially resectable disease.
- **Advanced disease:** Patients may have palliative tumor resection or, for unresectable tumors, a gastrojejunostomy (to prevent bleeding and obstruction by tumor). Chemotherapy may be used for palliation.

Prognosis

The 5-year survival rate is 15%. However, long-term survival rate is >45% in patients who undergo curative resection.

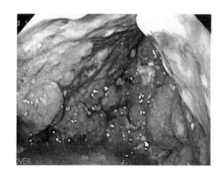

FIGURE 5.15. **Gastric cancer.** EGD of irregular and nodular stomach rugae compatible with diffuse infiltrative cancer of the stomach seen in linitis plastica. (Reproduced from Wikimedia Commons.)

KEY FACT

Two-thirds of patients present with stage III or IV disease and only 10% have stage I disease. Mortality is high due to late-stage presentation and aggressive disease biology.

COLORECTAL CANCER

The **third leading cause of death due to cancer** in the United States. Almost all cases are **adenocarcinomas,** and slightly <50% are distal to the splenic flexure. Colorectal cancer is believed to arise from transformation of adenomatous polyps. Risk factors include age, IBD, diet high in fats and red meat, male sex, African American race, tobacco use, diabetes, history of abdominal irradiation, and a ⊕ family history. **Specific risk factors** include the following:

- **Adenomatous polyps:** Present in 35% of patients >50 years of age. The risk of progression to cancer ranges from <4% to >10%, depending on size and histologic features (larger size and villous features carry an ↑ risk). Commonly removed by colonoscopic polypectomy.
- **Familial adenomatous polyposis (FAP):** An autosomal-dominant syndrome characterized by **>100 colonic adenomatous polyps.** Polyps appear by 15 years of age, adenomatous polyps by 35 years of age, and **colorectal cancer by 50 years of age.** Colectomy or proctocolectomy is indicated before 20 years of age.
- **Lynch syndrome:** An autosomal-dominant syndrome; also ↑ risk for endometrial and other cancers. Associated with a **70% to 80% lifetime risk of colorectal cancer.** Typically, only a **few adenomas** develop, but these tend to be villous, with high-grade dysplasia. If cancer is found, treatment is subtotal colectomy.

Symptoms/Exam

- Presents most commonly with rectal bleeding, unexplained iron deficiency anemia, colicky abdominal pain, or altered bowel habits due to obstruction in the left colon.
- Rectal cancers may present with tenesmus, urgency, and hematochezia. Weight loss is uncommon.
- DRE may reveal a mass or fixation. Abdominal masses may be palpable, and the liver edge may be enlarged in the presence of metastases.

Diagnosis

- First choice: **Colonoscopy:** permits biopsy. If the cecum cannot be reached, CT colonography or barium enema may be considered (Figure 5.16).
- **CEA:** Not reliable for diagnosis; sensitivity 46%. However, can be obtained for prognosis; a level of >5 ng/mL is predictive of a poorer prognosis.
- **Staging:**
  - **Colon cancer:** CT of the abdomen and pelvis ± CXR or chest CT. PET scan gives limited additional information.

> **KEY FACT**
>
> One-fifth of patients with colon cancer have metastatic disease at presentation, with metastases most common in the regional lymph nodes, peritoneum, liver, and lungs.

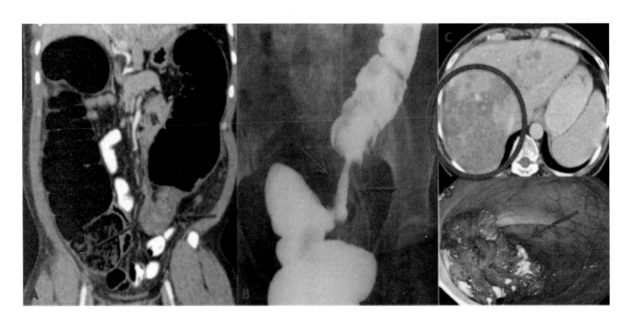

FIGURE 5.16.   Colon cancer. (**A**) Contrast-enhanced CT demonstrating proximal sigmoid colon circumferential mass (arrows) creating an "apple core lesion" with proximal large bowel dilation. (**B**) Barium enema showing the "apple core lesion" seen on the CT. (**C**) Axial CT demonstrating multiple hypoenhancing masses within the liver, largest within the right hepatic lobe (circle), consistent with hepatic metastases from colon cancer. (**D**) Colonoscopy reveals an adenocarcinoma growing into the lumen of the colon. (Images A, B, and C reproduced with permission from USMLE-Rx.com; image D reproduced with permission from Fauci AS, et al. *Harrison's Principles of Internal Medicine,* 17th ed. New York: McGraw-Hill, 2008, Fig. 285-6.)

- **Rectal cancer:** Above plus pelvic MRI or endorectal ultrasound for regional staging.

Management

- First line: **Resection and regional lymph node dissection,** which is recommended for local disease or in selected cases with resectable metastases (liver, lung). Consider palliative resection to ↓ the likelihood of complications such as obstruction or bleeding, although majority of patients with stage IV disease treated with chemotherapy do not need palliative resection. Transanal resections may be performed for some rectal cancers.
- **Adjuvant chemotherapy and radiation:**
    - **Colon cancer:** Chemotherapy recommended for node-positive disease. Radiation may be considered with locally advanced disease, but is not usual.
    - **Rectal cancer:** Treatment is more aggressive, involving **combination chemotherapy** and **radiation** with locally advanced disease due to difficulty with anatomy and resection.
- Surveillance in survivors:
    - **Colon cancer:** Differs by stage; for all, HP for 3 to 6 months initially. For stage II or III disease, evaluate with yearly colonoscopy, CT, and CEA.
    - **Rectal cancer:** As with colon cancer, but sigmoidoscopy every 6 to 12 months for 3 years (frequency varies by guideline).

Prevention

Measures of **2° prevention** include the following:
- Screening frequency determined by level of risk:
    - **Average risk:** No family history or one second- or third-degree relative with cancer. Begin screening at 50 years of age.
    - **Elevated risk:** Describes patients with a first-degree relative diagnosed with cancer/advanced adenoma at <60 years of age or two first-degree relatives with cancer/advanced adenoma. Begin screening at 40 years of age or when the patient is 10 years younger than the family member's age at diagnosis; repeat every 5 years.
- Screening methods:
    - Annual gFOBT/fecal immunochemical test (FIT).
    - FIT-DNA every 3 years.
    - Flexible sigmoidoscopy every 10 years with FIT annually or every 5 years if stool testing is not available.
    - Colonoscopy every 10 years.
    - CT colonography every 5 years is now an option; weigh risks of radiation and extracolonic findings.
- Special cases for screening:
    - **Adenomatous polyp on screening colonoscopy:** Repeat colonoscopy in 5 years, unless polyp was >9 mm in size or there were three or more adenomatous polyps found, in which case repeat in 3 years. If villous adenoma, repeat in 3 years.
    - **FAP:** Genetic testing offered to first-degree family members after 10 years of age; flexible sigmoidoscopy annually with colonoscopy if polyps found and annually while awaiting colectomy.
    - **Lynch syndrome:** Offer genetic counseling and testing if the family history is suggestive. If testing is ⊕, screen with colonoscopy every 1 to 2 years starting at 25 years of age or when the patient is 5 years younger than the age of the family member at diagnosis (whichever earliest). Also, screen annually for endometrial cancer among patients 25 to 35 years of age with pelvic exam, endometrial biopsy or transvaginal ultrasound (or consider prophylactic total abdominal hysterectomy and bilateral salpingo-oophorectomy in women after reproductive age).

QUESTION

A 44-year-old male construction worker complains of intermittently seeing blood on the toilet paper following a bowel movement. His father was diagnosed with colorectal cancer at age 52. Anoscopy reveals internal hemorrhoids. What is the next appropriate step?

Prognosis

The 5-year survival rate is 75% with early-stage cancer but is 5% with metastatic disease. The prognosis for rectal cancer worsens with each stage.

HEPATOCELLULAR CARCINOMA

Strongest risk factors include cirrhosis and HBV/HCV. Other risk factors include alcohol use, tobacco use, aflatoxin exposure, hemochromatosis, α_1-antitrypsin deficiency, nonalcoholic fatty liver disease, and diabetes.

Symptoms/Exam

- Patients typically present without symptoms other than chronic symptoms of end-stage liver disease.
- Symptoms of decompensation of previously compensated cirrhosis; ascites, variceal bleeding, or jaundice.
- Exam may show hepatomegaly or a palpable mass. A bruit may be audible over the tumor.

Diagnosis

- First choice: **Triple- or quad-phase liver CT scan:** Preferred initial imaging studies (Figure 5.17). If follow-up imaging needed, use MRI to better characterize lesions >1 cm.
- Next best: **α-fetoprotein (AFP):** ↑ in 70% of cases but is **nonspecific.**
- **Liver biopsy:** Diagnostic and used if previous studies are equivocal, but characteristic imaging with ↑ AFP can be sufficient. Biopsy may be deferred if surgical resection is planned because of possible seeding of the needle tract, although risk is low.

Management

- **Surgical resection:** May result in cure, but not possible in advanced cirrhosis or when the tumor is multifocal.

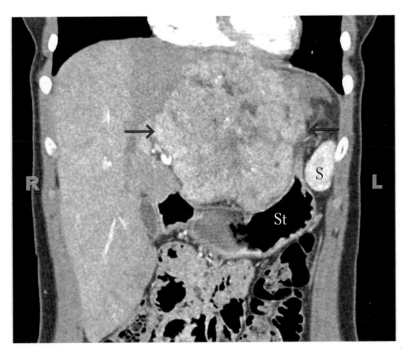

FIGURE 5.17.   Hepatocellular carcinoma. Coronal reformation from a contrast-enhanced CT shows a large HCC in the left hepatic lobe (arrows). St = stomach; S = spleen. (Reproduced with permission from USMLE-Rx.com.)

- Chemotherapy: Used for metastatic disease, although modest benefit only. Chemotherapy with **sorafenib** (a tyrosine kinase inhibitor) may help to prolong survival.
- **Liver transplantation:** Associated with 5-year survival in up to 75% of cases.
- **Palliative measures:** Include chemoembolization via the hepatic artery; small tumors may be amenable to ethanol injection, radiofrequency ablation, or cryotherapy.

Prevention

- Screening for liver cancer is controversial. Screening recommended for those with chronic HBV and ↑ risk for HCC as well as patients with cirrhosis who would be candidates for treatment for HCC.
- First line: **Ultrasound:** Noninvasive and widely available, but sensitivity range is 40% to 78%. Consider every 6 to 12 months.
- Second line: **AFP:** Often ↑ in HCC, but levels do not correlate with size or stage. Also ↑ in pregnancy, gonadal tumors, and chronic liver disease (especially HCV). At low cutoff values, the test is nonspecific; at high cutoffs, the test loses sensitivity despite high specificity (>500 μg/L in high-risk patients is virtually diagnostic).

Prognosis

No consensus on best staging system for prognosis. Median survival from diagnosis is 6 to 20 months. For locally resectable disease, 5-year survival is 55%. For unresectable disease, 5-year survival is virtually zero.

PANCREATIC CANCER

Ninety-five percent of pancreatic cancer is adenocarcinoma from the exocrine pancreas. Risk factors include age, obesity, tobacco use, chronic pancreatitis, pancreatic cysts, prior abdominal radiation, and a ⊕ family history of pancreatic cancer.

Symptoms/Exam

- Presents with vague, diffuse pain in the epigastrium or LUQ (if the tail is involved) with occasional radiation to the back. Pain that is relieved by sitting or leaning forward suggests inoperable spread of disease. However, may also be painless. Weight loss is common and diarrhea may be an early symptom.
- May also present with pancreatitis, and jaundice (sometimes painless) may be present with obstruction. A palpable gallbladder (**Courvoisier sign**) may be present. A hard, fixed epigastric mass may be palpable.

Diagnosis

- First choice: RUQ ultrasound if primary complaint jaundice or obstructive symptoms. If jaundice is not present, use **multiphase thin-cut spiral CT,** which detects most tumors, demonstrates vessel invasion, delineates the extent of disease, and allows for FNA (Figure 5.18).
- **ERCP or MRCP** can aid in diagnosis if CT is ambiguous, but is mainly used for treatment of obstructive symptoms.
- **Endoscopic ultrasonography:** Also aids in diagnosis by demonstrating venous or gastric invasion if diagnosis unclear on RUQ U/S or CT.
- Biopsy: Gold standard, but not always required if imaging is conclusive.
- **CA 19-9** has not proved sensitive enough (70%) for early detection. Specificity is 87%; ↑ values are also found in acute and chronic pancreatitis and cholangitis.
- **Other:** Mild anemia, impaired glucose intolerance, and ↑ amylase/lipase may be seen. LFTs may suggest obstructive jaundice.

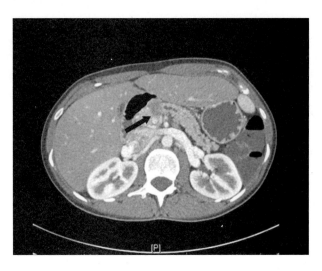

FIGURE 5.18.   **Pancreatic cancer.** Contrast-enhanced CT scan of the abdomen demonstrates hypoenhancing pancreatic head mass (arrow) with distal pancreatic duct dilation. (Reproduced from Bass LM, et al. Pancreatic adenocarcinoma in type 2 progressive familial intrahepatic cholestasis. *BMC Gastroenterol.* 2010;10:30.)

Prevention

In patients with a ⊕ family history, consider screening with **spiral CT or endoscopic ultrasound** beginning 10 years earlier than the age of the family member at diagnosis or at age 45 (whichever is earliest) if patient is a surgical candidate.

Management

- Lesions limited to the head, periampullary zone, and duodenum: Resection by a **Whipple procedure** (pancreaticoduodenectomy) is associated with a 10% 5-year survival rate, ↑ to 20% to 30% in the presence of ⊖ margins and lymph nodes. Adjuvant chemotherapy is beneficial.
- **Unresectable lesions:** Treatment is usually palliative. Treat jaundice with endoscopic stenting of the bile duct or cholecystojejunostomy; duodenal obstruction can be treated or prevented by gastrojejunostomy or endoscopic placement of a self-expandable duodenal stent. Combined irradiation and chemotherapy may be used for palliation of unresectable cancer confined to the pancreas.
- **Metastatic disease:** Chemotherapy has shown limited efficacy in metastatic pancreatic cancer, but gemcitabine is standard agent.
- Celiac plexus nerve block or thoracoscopic splanchnicectomy may improve pain control.

KEY FACT

Only 10% to 20% of patients with pancreatic cancer are candidates for surgery at time of diagnosis due to metastatic disease.

KEY FACT

The etiology of upper GI bleeding is unable to be identified in 10% to 15% of cases due to healing by the time of endoscopy or difficulty with visualization/identification.

GI Bleeding

ACUTE UPPER GI BLEEDING

More common in patients >60 years of age and in men. Associated with a mortality rate of 10%, but mortality is usually due to complications of underlying disease, not exsanguination. Etiologies include most commonly peptic or duodenal ulcers, varices, Mallory-Weiss tears; erosive esophagitis; gastritis (eg, NSAIDs, alcohol) and duodenitis, malignancy, vascular anomalies (ectasias, Dieulafoy lesion, angiodysplasia), portal hypertensive gastropathy, aortoenteric fistula, and hemobilia (Figure 5.19).

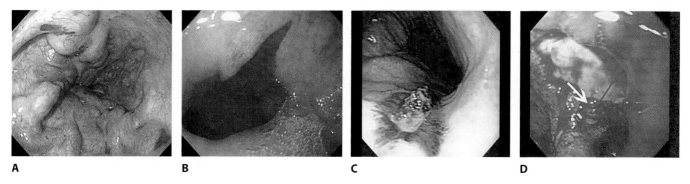

FIGURE 5.19. **Causes of upper GI bleed at endoscopy.** (A) Esophageal varices. (B) Mallory-Weiss tear. (C) Gastric ulcer with protuberant vessel. (D) Duodenal ulcer with active bleeding (arrow). (Reproduced with permission from Fauci AS, et al. *Harrison's Principles of Internal Medicine,* 17th ed. New York: McGraw-Hill, 2008, Figs. 285-16, 285-18, and 285-15D and E.)

Symptoms/Exam

- Commonly presents as **melena** or **hematemesis** (bright red or coffee-ground emesis). Melena develops with as little as 50 to 100 mL of bleeding.
- About 10% of cases present with hematochezia, but this requires massive bleeding.
- Symptoms and signs of predisposing diseases may be present (eg, a history of vomiting; stigmata of liver disease).

Diagnosis/Management

- **Initial resuscitation and stabilization:**
  - Patients should be **NPO; discontinue aspirin, NSAIDs,** and any **anticoagulants.**
  - Place two 18-gauge IVs and initiate **aggressive fluid resuscitation** if there is hemodynamic compromise.
  - Place an **NG tube** for lavage if contents (blood, particulates) need to be removed prior to endoscopy. Aspiration of red blood or coffee-ground emesis confirms an upper GI source, but clear aspirate does not exclude it (eg, duodenal bleed).
- **Type and cross RBCs.**
- The decision to transfuse should be based on the following criteria:
  - **Hemoglobin:** Consider transfusion if hemoglobin <7 g/dL or if continued bleeding and hemodynamic instability, transfuse at normal hemoglobin levels. Do not overtransfuse (>10 g/dL) in variceal bleeding.
  - **Platelets:** Transfuse if the platelet count is <50,000 cells/mm³ or if bleeding is due to platelet dysfunction.
  - **INR:** Transfuse with fresh frozen plasma for values >1.5. One unit of FFP is required for every 5 units of packed RBCs transfused.
  - Send laboratory studies based on suspicion for disease etiology (eg, *H pylori*, LFTs, INR, BUN, creatinine).
- **Triage:**
  - **Discharge:** Healthy patients with normal hemodynamics and normal labs may be discharged. Endoscopy should be scheduled as an outpatient procedure. The risk of rebleeding is low if the patient presents <48 hours after the event.
  - **Admit to the hospital:** All other patients must be admitted for observation and/or endoscopy.
  - **ICU admission:** Those with active bleeding, hemodynamic instability, or advanced liver disease or serious comorbidities.
- First line for diagnosis and treatment: **Endoscopy: diagnostic, prognostic,** and **therapeutic** (cautery, injection, or endoclips; injection of a sclerosant or application of a rubber band to the bleeding varix). Surgical intervention may be necessary if endoscopic interventions fail.

KEY FACT

- HR >100 bpm suggests mild to moderate hemorrhage.
- Orthostatic hypotension suggests moderate to severe acute hemorrhage with 15% blood volume loss.
- Hypotension suggests severe acute hemorrhage with 40% blood volume loss.

- Other medical therapy:
  - **IV PPIs:** ↓ the risk of rebleeding in peptic ulcers with high-risk features following endoscopic treatment. High doses of oral PPIs may also be effective.
  - **Octreotide infusion:** ↓ splanchnic blood flow and portal BP; effective in the initial control of variceal bleeding.
  - **Antibiotics** for patients with suspected variceal bleed.
  - **Refractory bleeding: Surgical intervention;** intra-arterial embolizations/vasopressin; **TIPS** for acute variceal hemorrhage.

ACUTE LOWER GI BLEEDING

Bleeding occurring below the ligament of Treitz. Approximately 95% of cases arise from the colon. Lower GI bleeds tend to have a **more benign course** than upper GI bleeds, largely because there is less likelihood of hemodynamic compromise (see Table 5.9 for other factors that distinguish upper from lower GI bleeding). Etiologies correlate with age:
- **Patients <50 years of age:** Associated with infectious colitis, hemorrhoids, fissures, and IBD.
- **Patients >50 years of age:** Associated with diverticulosis, vascular ectasias, neoplasm/malignancy, ischemia, and recent polypectomy (generally 2 weeks post procedure).

Symptoms/Exam

- Black stools (melena) generally indicate bleeding proximal to the ligament of Treitz; maroon stools point to the right colon or small intestine. Brown stools mixed or streaked with blood indicate a source in the rectosigmoid or anus.
- Examine for source with DRE and consider anoscopy.

Diagnosis/Management

- **Initial resuscitation and stabilization:** Measures are the same as those for upper GI bleeding. An upper tract source should be excluded by EGD, especially if the patient is hemodynamically unstable. If moderate suspicion, can perform NG lavage and also give bowel prep.

KEY FACT

About 10% of cases of hematochezia are due to a brisk upper GI bleed and usually have concomitant hypotension and shock.

TABLE 5.9.   **Upper Versus Lower GI Bleed**

	CAUSES	SYMPTOMS/SIGNS
Upper GI bleed	Peptic ulcer disease	Epigastric pain
	Mallory-Weiss tear	Hematemesis (fresh blood or coffee-
	Varices	ground emesis)
	Gastritis	Melena
	Esophagitis	
	Angiodysplasia	
	Cancer	
Lower GI bleed	Diverticulosis	Hematochezia
	Bowel ischemia	Abdominal pain
	Anorectal disease	Tenesmus
	Colon cancer	Maroon-colored stools (rarely,
	Angiodysplasia	melena)
	IBD	Physical exam may reveal
	Infectious diarrhea	hemorrhoids, fissures, mass

- Diagnostic and treatment options:
  - First choice: **Colonoscopy.** Diagnostic, prognostic, and therapeutic (epinephrine injection, cautery, or application of metallic endoclips). Diagnostic accuracy is ↓ with inadequate prep (eg, with severe, active bleeding).
  - **Nuclear bleeding scan** (technetium-labeled RBC scan) or **angiography:** Can identify the bleeding site for arterial embolization or bowel resection, but has poor diagnostic accuracy unless bleeding is brisk.
  - **Small intestine push enteroscopy** (a small-diameter endoscope that can reach the distal jejunum)/**wireless capsule imaging:** May help identify a source of persistent recurrent bleeding.
  - **Surgery:** Indicated with ongoing bleeding that requires >4 to 6 units of blood within 24 hours or >10 units in total. May also be indicated in patients with two or more hospitalizations for diverticular hemorrhage.

DIVERTICULOSIS AND DIVERTICULITIS

- **Diverticulosis: Protrusions of the colonic mucosa in the wall of the colon** (see Figure 5.20B). Most commonly in the sigmoid colon. Risk factors include low-fiber/high-fat diet, ↑ age, constipation, and connective tissue disorders (eg, Marfan syndrome). Often asymptomatic. No specific treatment necessary, but a high-fiber diet may help.
- **Diverticulitis: Infection within the diverticula** (see Figure 5.20C). Colonoscopy and barium enema are contraindicated because of the ↑ risk of perforation. Clinical features include fever, LLQ pain, and leukocytosis with left shift. Treatment includes antibiotics against colonic flora (oral or IV, depending on severity) and slowly advancing diet. Surgery with resection or diverting colostomy is indicated if patient has not responded to medical therapies or has experienced complications including abscess or fistula formation, obstruction, or peritonitis.

Diagnosis

- First choice: CT scan for acute diverticulitis. Perform colonoscopy as outpatient after acute flare to evaluate for colon cancer.
- For diverticulosis: Usually seen on colonoscopy, barium enema, CT, or MRI.

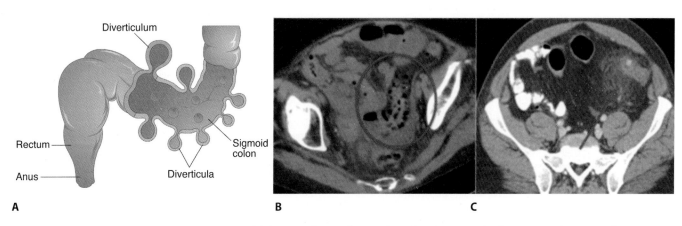

A   **B**   **C**

FIGURE 5.20. **Diverticulosis and diverticulitis. (A)** Drawing depicts diverticula within the sigmoid colon. **(B)** Axial CT scan shows multiple air-filled sigmoid diverticula. **(C)** Axial CT demonstrates pericolonic stranding and inflammatory changes in the setting of sigmoid diverticulosis, consistent with diverticulitis. (Reproduced with permission from USMLE-Rx.com.)

INTESTINAL ISCHEMIA

Can present with acute or chronic disease and affecting small bowel (mesenteric) versus colon (colonic). Acute mesenteric ischemia is 60% to 70% of disease. The four main causes are arterial embolism (often the SMA), arterial thrombosis (from preexisting vascular disease), nonocclusive etiology (low cardiac output with mesenteric vasoconstriction), and venous thrombosis.

Diagnosis

- Clinical history (chronic ischemia presents with postprandial abdominal pain and "food fear"). For acute mesenteric ischemia, look for history of vascular disease, recent low-volume state, cardiac disease, history of aortic surgery/instrumentation, or vasoconstriction.
- Signs include abdominal pain out of proportion to physical exam findings.
- **Labs:** Leukocytosis, hemoconcentration, ↑ amylase, ↑ LDH.
- **Imaging:** First choice: **CT** may show thickened bowel wall, bowel wall hemorrhage, and/or nonenhancing bowel wall and may show arterial or venous occlusion. May need **CT angiography** or angiography if diagnosis equivocal after initial CT.
  - KUB uncommonly used, but may show "thumbprinting" of the bowel wall.
  - Colonoscopy: Used for diagnosis of colonic ischemia.

Management

- Fluid resuscitation, restore blood flow.
- General surgery and interventional radiology consultation.
- Treat underlying condition as indicated (embolectomy, bypass, stenting, thrombolysis).
- Consider anticoagulation if there are no contraindications and if patient is not going to surgery.
- Prognosis: 60% mortality rate in acute mesenteric ischemia.

CHAPTER 6

Infectious Diseases

Sky Lee, MD

Common Antibiotics

These classes of antibiotics are most commonly used to treat infectious diseases:

- **β-lactams** include high-dose amoxicillin ± clavulanate, ampicillin ± sulbactam, and piperacillin + tazobactam (antipseudomonal); and cephalosporins such as ceftriaxone, cefotaxime, cefuroxime, and cefepime (antipseudomonal).
- **Fluorquinolones** include ciprofloxacin, levofloxacin (antipseudomonal), gemifloxacin, and moxifloxacin.
- **Macrolides** include azithromycin and clarithromycin (an erythromycin used less commonly and usually not as monotherapy for pneumonia).
- **Carbapenems** include ertapenem, meropenem (antipseudomonal), imipenem ± cilastatin (antipseudomonal), and doripenem (antipseudomonal).

Central Nervous System Infections

ACUTE BACTERIAL MENINGITIS

Meningeal infections are associated with profound inflammatory responses. Without treatment, mortality can be >50%. Survivors usually have severe morbidity. Typical bacterial pathogens include *Streptococcus pneumoniae*, *Neisseria meningitidis*, group B streptococci, and *Listeria monocytogenes* (Table 6.1).

Symptoms/Exam

- Symptoms include headache, photophobia, and nausea/vomiting. Neonates may present with fever or hypothermia and subtle signs, including lethargy, poor feeding, and/or bulging fontanelles.
- Less common presentations are rash (Figure 6.1); cranial nerve palsies; cerebral involvement in the form of seizures, aphasia, or focal neurologic deficits (eg, **syphilitic meningitis**); and coma.

KEY FACT

The classic triad of bacterial meningitis consists of fever, altered mental status, and nuchal rigidity. Virtually all patients have at least one of these symptoms.

MNEMONIC

Meningeal signs:
K is for **K**ernig and **K**nee.

TABLE 6.1.   Causes and Treatment of Bacterial Meningitis

AGE/TREATMENT GROUP	COMMON MICROORGANISMS	EMPIRIC ANTIBIOTICS—FIRST CHOICE	SEVERE PENICILLIN ALLERGY
<1 month of age	Group B strep, *E coli*, *Listeria*	Ampicillin and cefotaxime/gentamicin	N/A
1 month to 50 years of age	*S pneumoniae*, *N meningitidis*, *H influenzae*[a]	Ceftriaxone/cefotaxime + vancomycin	Aztreonam or carbapenem[b] + vancomycin
>50 years of age	*S pneumoniae*, *Listeria*, gram-negative bacilli	Ceftriaxone/cefotaxime + ampicillin + vancomycin	Fluoroquinolone or aztreonam or carbapenem[b] (*N meningitidis*) + TMP-SMX (*Listeria*) + vancomycin
Impaired cellular immunity (or alcohol use disorder)	*S pneumoniae*, *L monocytogenes*, gram-negative bacilli	Ceftazidime or cefepime + ampicillin + vancomycin	TMP-SMX + vancomycin
Postneurosurgery or post–head trauma	*S pneumoniae*, *S aureus*, gram-negative bacilli (incl. *Pseudomonas*)	Meropenem, cefepime, or ceftazidime + vancomycin	Aztreonam or ciprofloxacin + vancomycin

Adapted with permission from Tierney LM, et al. *Current Medical Diagnosis & Treatment*, 44th ed. New York: McGraw-Hill, 2005:1251.

[a]*H influenzae* type B has greatly ↓ in pediatrics as a result of vaccination.

[b]Agent choice depends on patient age and clinical situation.

- Traditional signs thought to correlate with meningeal irritation include **Kernig sign** (with the thigh and knee flexed, passive leg extension leads to pain) and **Brudzinski sign** (passive flexion of the neck leads to spontaneous flexion of the hip and knees). However, these signs are not sensitive for the diagnosis of bacterial meningitis.
- Atypical presentations are common in neonates, infants, the elderly, and immuno-compromised patients.

Differential

- Other forms of meningitis, such as viral, fungal (*Cryptococcus neoformans*), tuberculous, and aseptic (eg, medication-induced, autoimmune).
- Viral or bacterial encephalitis (eg, Rocky Mountain spotted fever, Lyme disease).
- A parameningeal focus such as epidural, subdural, or intraparenchymal abscess. **Epidural abscess** may present as headache, back pain, and neurologic deficits 2° to cord compression. Consider in patients with a history of IV drug use.
- Noninfectious causes of meningitis include subarachnoid hemorrhage, vasculitis, and connective tissue disease.

Diagnosis

- History and physical examination.
- **Labs:**
  - Best initial lab: CBC. Leukocytosis with PMN predominance or leukopenia (associated with severe infection).
  - Most accurate lab: **CSF analysis:** Opening pressure is typically ↑. Send CSF for cell count and differential, total glucose, protein, Gram stain, and bacterial culture (Table 6.2).
    - In the appropriate setting, test CSF for viral PCR (HSV), viral culture, cryptococcal antigen, AFB culture, or VDRL (syphilis).

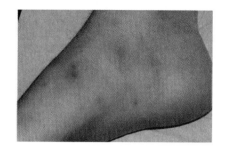

FIGURE 6.1. **Vasculitic skin eruption in meningococcal meningitis.** (Reproduced from Kernéis S, et al. Chronic meningococcemia in a 16-year-old boy: a case report. *Cases J.* 2009;2:7103.)

Q   QUESTION

A 45-year-old woman presents to the ED after 5 days of fever, cough, pleuritic chest pain, and purulent sputum. Her family brought her to the hospital today because she began complaining of a headache and neck pain. The family also notes that she has been acting strangely and seems confused. On exam, you note a temperature of 40.4°C (104.7°F) and nuchal rigidity. The patient is oriented only to self. What would you do first?

TABLE 6.2.   CSF Profiles in Common CNS Diseases

DIAGNOSIS	RBC (PER ML)	WBC (PER ML)	GLUCOSE (MG/DL)	PROTEIN (MG/DL)	OPENING PRESSURE (CM H$_2$O)	APPEARANCE
Normal[a]	<10	<5	About 2/3 of serum level	1-45	10-20	Clear
Bacterial meningitis	Normal	↑ (PMNs)	↓	↑	↑	Cloudy
Aseptic/viral meningitis, encephalitis	Normal (may be ↑ in encephalitis)	↑ (lymphs)[b]	Normal	Normal or ↑	Normal or ↑	Usually clear
Chronic meningitis (TB, fungal)	Normal	↑ (lymphs)[b]	↓	↑	↑	Clear or cloudy
Spirochetal meningitis (syphilis, Lyme disease)	Normal	↑ (lymphs)[b]	Normal	↑	Normal or ↑	Clear or cloudy
Neighborhood reaction[c]	Normal	Variable	Normal	Normal or ↑	Normal or ↑	Usually clear
SAH, cerebral contusion	↑↑	↑	Normal	↑↑	Normal or ↑	Yellow or red

[a] With traumatic tap, usually have 1 WBC/800 RBCs and 1 mg protein/1000 RBCs.

[b] May have PMN predominance in early stages.

[c] May be seen with brain abscess, epidural abscess, vertebral osteomyelitis, sinusitis/mastoiditis, septic thrombus, and brain tumor.

A   ANSWER

Perform a noncontrast head CT, perform an LP, and start empiric antibiotics (ceftriaxone and vancomycin)—all within the first 60 minutes of presentation. In cases such as this where there is moderate to high suspicion for pneumococcal meningitis, give steroids before or with the first dose of antibiotics. If the CT scan or LP is delayed, **do not delay antibiotics,** as CSF cultures usually remain ⊕ for the first few hours after antibiotics are given. The CSF Gram stain, cell counts, and chemistries will still be useful, even if the cultures have been rendered ⊖.

■ **Blood cultures:** Bacteremia is seen in 40% to 90% of patients with community-acquired bacterial meningitis.

Management

■ Untreated bacterial meningitis causes severe morbidity, and mortality exceeds 50%. Begin antimicrobial therapy ASAP: within 60 minutes of presentation. Choose empiric therapy based on patient factors (see Table 6.1) and tailor to results of CSF culture.

■ Unless allergic, all patients should receive a third-generation cephalosporin. For patients >1 month of age, add vancomycin to cover penicillin-resistant *S pneumoniae* infection. Ampicillin should be added in very young, elderly, or immunocompromised patients to cover *L monocytogenes*.

■ Consider giving corticosteroids (dexamethasone) in the 30 minutes before antibiotics. Steroids ↓ mortality and morbidity in adults with pneumococcal meningitis and ↓ hearing loss in children with *H influenzae* meningitis. Steroids may also ↓ other adverse outcomes in children with bacterial meningitis. Consider adding rifampin if giving corticosteroids due to ↓ vancomycin uptake into the CSF when steroids are given.

■ Patients with features of rickettsial meningitis (Lyme disease, Rocky Mountain spotted fever) may benefit from early antibiotics (ceftriaxone for Lyme disease and doxycycline for Rocky Mountain spotted fever). Patients suspected of TB meningitis should be isolated, and early antimycobacterial therapy and steroids initiated in consultation with an infectious disease specialist and a neurologist.

■ **Do not delay antibiotics** while waiting for imaging or LP.

Complications

■ Systemic complications result primarily from bacteremia and include septic shock, disseminated intravascular coagulation (eg, from meningococcal meningitis), ARDS, and septic or reactive arthritis.

■ Neurologic complications include cerebral edema and ↑ ICP, hydrocephalus, seizures, cognitive impairment, hearing loss and other cranial neuropathies, subdural effusion, empyema, epidural abscess, and SIADH. Permanent neurologic morbidity may occur.

VIRAL MENINGITIS AND ENCEPHALITIS

Viruses infiltrate the CNS in various ways, including hematogenous and axonal spread, causing a range of disease processes, including meningitis (Table 6.3) and encephalitis as well as postinfectious autoimmune demyelination.

Symptoms/Exam

■ Presents with headache, altered mental status, motor/sensory deficits, and speech/movement abnormalities.

■ Symptoms of meningitis and encephalitis can overlap. Both can have rash (meningococcus, Rocky Mountain spotted fever, Lyme disease, VZV), fever, headache, nausea/vomiting, seizures, or focal neurologic deficits (flaccid paralysis in West Nile virus). However, photophobia and stiff neck are less common findings in pure encephalitis.

■ HSV encephalitis can cause bizarre behavior, olfactory hallucinations and aphasia. This is due to the predilection for involvement of the **medial temporal lobes** (Figure 6.2).

TABLE 6.3.   **Etiologic Agents in Viral Meningitis**

VIRUS	INCIDENCE	SOURCE	SUSCEPTIBLE POPULATION	SEASONALITY, ASSOCIATED SYMPTOMS, LABORATORY FINDINGS
Echoviridae	30%	Fecal-oral	Children, family contacts	Summer/fall; rash, gastroenteritis common
Coxsackievirus A/B	A: 10%; B: 50%	Fecal-oral	Children, family contacts	Summer/fall; rash, gastroenteritis, herpangina (in A) serositis, myocarditis, orchitis (in B)
Mumps virus	15%	Inhalation	Children, male more than female	Winter/spring; parotitis, orchitis, oophoritis, pancreatitis; CSF glucose may be ↑ or ↓
HSV type 2	Uncommon	Genital infection	Neonates with affected mothers	Vesicular genital lesions
Adenovirus	Uncommon	Inhalation	Infants, children	Pharyngitis, pneumonia
Lymphocytic choriomeningitis virus	Uncommon	Mouse	Laboratory workers	Late fall/winter; pharyngitis and pneumonia; marked CSF pleocytosis
Hepatitis viruses	Uncommon	Fecal-oral, venereal, transfusion	IV drug users, high-risk sexual activity, transfusion recipients	Jaundice, arthritis; LFT abnormalities
EBV (infectious mononucleosis)	Uncommon	Oral contact	Teenagers, young adults	Atypical lymphocytes, ⊕ heterophil, LFT abnormalities; lymphadenopathy, pharyngitis, splenomegaly, skin/palatal rash
Flaviviruses (West Nile, Japanese B, St Louis, yellow fever)	Uncommon	Mosquitoes	Rural, near standing water	Variable geographic distribution; rash, myocarditis, hepatitis, pancreatitis
Alphaviruses (Eastern/Western/Venezuelan equine)	Uncommon	Mosquitoes	Rural, near standing water	Neurologic sequelae common in EEE, uncommon in WEE and VEE
Orbivirus (Colorado tick fever)	Uncommon	Ticks	Western and Rocky Mountain states	Rash
Rabies	Rare	Rodent, bat, canine, feline vectors	Worldwide; individuals bitten/scratched by animal vectors (dogs in most of world; bats in the United States)	Invariably fatal unless treated promptly with vaccine and antiserum before symptoms

Adapted with permission from Aminoff MJ, et al. *Clinical Neurology*, 6th ed. New York: McGraw-Hill, 2005:27.

Differential

- See the differential for bacterial meningitis above.
- Other common causes of altered mental status.

Diagnosis

- The 1° goal is to **distinguish HSV from other causes.**
- A thorough history is essential and should include season, sexual activity, travel, and insect or animal bites.
- **MRI is the best imaging study** to visualize brain parenchyma. CT scan is an acceptable alternative, if MRI is unavailable or contraindicated.

KEY FACT

With rare exceptions, HSV is currently the only treatable type of viral encephalitis. IV acyclovir is the drug of choice.

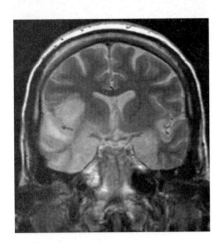

FIGURE 6.2.   HSV encephalitis. T2-weighted MRI shows high signal in the temporal lobes including hippocampal formations and parahippocampal gyrae, insulae, and right inferior frontal gyrus. (Reproduced from Wikipedia; courtesy of Dr. Laughlin Dawes.)

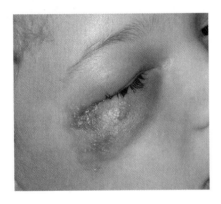

FIGURE 6.3.   Periorbital cellulitis in a 7-year-old boy with recent URI and 3-day history of progressive eye swelling and pain. (Reproduced with permission from USMLE-Rx.com.)

Management

- Untreated HSV encephalitis is associated with high morbidity and mortality. Therefore, in suspected cases of encephalitis without an obvious source, **empiric IV acyclovir** should be used until HSV is ruled out. Young children and the immunocompromised are at greatest risk for HSV disease.
- Supportive measures are the mainstay of treatment for all other types of viral encephalitis.
- If rabies exposure is possible by history, consult infectious disease clinicians and consider administration of antiserum and rabies vaccine.
- Failure to improve within **48 hours** should prompt reevaluation of the diagnosis.

Head and Neck Infections

ORBITAL AND PERIORBITAL CELLULITIS

Bacterial infection of the soft tissues surrounding the eye following a URI, sinusitis, dental infection, or trauma. Common causative agents include *Staphylococcus* spp, *Streptococcus* spp, and, until recently, *H influenzae* (now a less common cause due to routine vaccination). An important clinical distinction is made between **periorbital cellulitis** (ie, preseptal) and **orbital cellulitis** (around and posterior to the globe).

Symptoms/Exam

- **Periorbital (preseptal) cellulitis:** Presents with swelling and erythema of the eyelids, minimal pain, and fever. Conjunctivitis, proptosis, restricted eye movements, and visual deficits are **NOT** generally present (Figure 6.3).
- **Orbital cellulitis:** Presents with very painful erythematous swelling of the eyelid, **conjunctivitis,** proptosis with **ophthalmoplegia,** and fever. Patients may also have ↓ visual acuity, pain with eye movement, and an afferent pupillary defect.

Diagnosis

- Most accurate test: CT scan of the orbit to evaluate for postseptal extension or **abscess** is imperative in the presence of symptoms or signs of orbital cellulitis. Patients with low clinical suspicion of orbital extension do not require a CT scan (Figure 6.4).
- If there is concern for associated cavernous sinus thrombosis, obtain an MRI with venous phase.
- Consider blood cultures, although these are generally ⊖.

Management

- Usually requires hospital admission and IV antibiotics for approximately 10 to 21 days (broad-spectrum antistaphylococcal and antistreptococcal coverage). Typically, vancomycin, ceftriaxone, and metronidazole OR vancomycin and piperacillin-tazobactam. Most patients recover with antibiotics alone.
- Promptly drain an abscess or the paranasal sinuses if there is a large abscess, vision deteriorates, or the patient fails to improve despite antibiotics.

Complications

Abscess, blindness, or extension into the CNS, causing meningitis or septic cavernous sinus thrombosis.

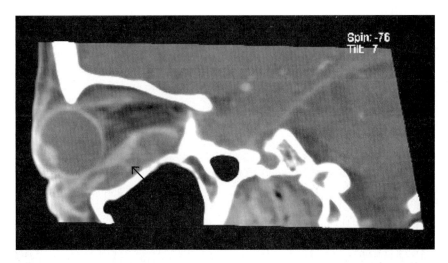

FIGURE 6.4. **Orbital cellulitis.** Sagittal contrast-enhanced CT demonstrating enhancing fluid collection extending into the inferior extraconal fat (arrow), compatible with postseptal (orbital) cellulitis. (Reproduced from Henney SE, et al. Dacryocystitis presenting as post-septal cellulitis: a case report. *J Med Case Rep.* 2007;1:77.)

CONJUNCTIVITIS

The most common cause of a red eye. Can be caused by viruses or bacteria. Although usually a self-limited infection, conjunctivitis occasionally requires treatment (Table 6.4).

NOSE AND SINUS INFECTIONS

Common Cold

- Usually caused by **rhinoviruses.** Other viruses include coronavirus, parainfluenza virus, respiratory syncytial virus (RSV), influenza virus, and adenoviruses.

QUESTION

A 15-year-old boy is being seen in urgent care for a 1-day history of right eye pain and swelling. On exam, you note significant erythema and periorbital swelling, and the patient reports pain when asked to look to his left. What is your next step in this patient's management?

TABLE 6.4. **Manifestations and Treatment of Infectious Conjunctivitis**

	VIRAL	BACTERIAL
Etiologies	Adenovirus, HSV	*Staphylococcus* spp, *Streptococcus* spp, *H influenzae*, *Neisseria gonorrhoeae*, *Chlamydia trachomatis*
Symptoms/Exam	Erythema, watery discharge, photophobia Frequently bilateral Concomitant URI "Pink eye"	Erythema, mucopurulent discharge, "morning crustiness" Usually unilateral
Treatment	Symptomatic; cold compresses	Topical erythromycin, bacitracin-polymyxin, trimethoprim, fluoroquinolone For *N gonorrhoeae*, ceftriaxone IM/IV × 1 For *C trachomatis*, erythromycin syrup PO
Prevention	Frequent hand washing (highly contagious)	Frequent hand washing
Complications	Corneal abrasion 2° to rubbing	Untreated *C trachomatis* conjunctivitis is a common cause of **blindness** worldwide

- **Management:** Generally, treat with supportive measures, including fluids, rest, and contact precautions. The FDA recommends against OTC cold preparations in children <2 years of age and cautious use in children 2 to 11 years of age. A 2014 Cochrane review suggests that honey may provide symptomatic relief; however, honey cannot be used for children <1 years old due to concern for botulism.

Bacterial Sinusitis

Infection of the sinus resulting from impaired mucociliary clearance and obstruction of the osteomeatal complex; viral or allergic rhinitis is a predisposing factor. The majority of cases are viral, with about **20% due to bacteria.** Infections lasting >1 week are more likely to have a bacterial etiology, commonly *S pneumoniae*, *H influenzae*, and occasionally *S aureus* and *Moraxella catarrhalis*. *Pseudomonas aeruginosa* and anaerobes are implicated in cases of **chronic sinusitis.**

Symptoms/Exam

- Frequently presents with unilateral or bilateral pain over the maxillary sinuses or teeth as well as with fever and nasal discharge (at times purulent).
- Acute sinusitis can last 1 to 4 weeks; sinusitis >4 weeks is considered chronic.

Differential

- **Zygomycosis:** A rare but dangerous fungal infection that occurs in immunocompromised patients.
  - Presents as **facial pain** with a necrotic eschar of the nasal mucosa and subsequently with cranial nerve palsies.
  - Early diagnosis is paramount because the infection can spread rapidly. Treat emergently with antifungal therapy (traditionally amphotericin B; possibly posaconazole) and surgical debridement.
- **Other:** In chronic or resistant sinusitis, consider anatomic obstruction, common variable immunodeficiency, a variant of cystic fibrosis, granulomatosis with polyangiitis (Wegener), or periodontal or dental infection.

Diagnosis

- Usually made by the history and physical exam.
- **Routine imaging is not indicated** in uncomplicated acute sinusitis. However, in chronic, resistant, or complicated sinusitis, CT scan is much more sensitive than x-rays. Imaging may identify air-fluid levels, bony abnormalities, and extension outside of the paranasal sinuses.

Management

- **General:** Intranasal saline irrigation or intranasal corticosteroids. Oral and/or nasal decongestants (eg, oral pseudoephedrine, intranasal oxymetazoline) may be useful in viral infections, especially if eustachian tube dysfunction is present.
- **Acute bacterial sinusitis:** Recommendations on starting antibiotics vary from immediately after diagnosis to only for persistent symptoms or if there are severe symptoms. If needed, 5 to 10 days of amoxicillin or a macrolide are standard therapy. Consider amoxicillin/clavulanate if risk factors for anaerobes or β-lactamase-producing organisms (eg, *H influenzae* [30% produce β-lactamase] and *M catarrhalis*) are present. Risk factors include diabetes, other immunocompromised states, and recent antibiotic use. There is insufficient evidence to support the use of decongestants for acute bacterial sinusitis.
- **Chronic sinusitis:** Amoxicillin/clavulanate for at least 3 to 4 weeks along with intranasal glucocorticoids.

Complications

Rare; extension into the CNS and orbital or periorbital cellulitis.

ANSWER

Perform a CT scan of the orbits, obtain blood cultures, and admit to the hospital for IV antibiotics.

OROPHARYNGEAL INFECTIONS

Pharyngitis

An infection or irritation of the pharynx and/or tonsils. Etiologies include:

- **Bacterial:** The most important bacterial etiology is group A streptococci (GAS, or *Streptococcus pyogenes*), causing "strep throat" (see below). Other bacterial agents include groups C and G streptococcus, *N gonorrhoeae*, *M pneumoniae*, *C pneumoniae*, and, rarely, *Corynebacterium diphtheriae*.
- **Viral:** Viruses are the **most common** etiology of pharyngitis (see below). These include rhinovirus, coronavirus, adenovirus, and many others. Pharyngitis may also occur secondary to systemic viral infections such as mononucleosis (EBV), herpangina (coxsackievirus), and acute retroviral syndrome (HIV).
- **Other:** Allergy, gastroesophageal reflux, trauma, toxins, malignancy.

Bacterial Pharyngitis, Including Group A Streptococci (Strep Throat)

Symptoms/Exam

- Prominent sore throat and odynophagia. Patients with acute bacterial pharyngitis typically have purulent **tonsillar exudates.**
- In cases of **gonococcal** or **chlamydial** pharyngitis, patients may have associated **GU symptoms** (dysuria, discharge) or **joint complaints.**
- Testing and treatment for GAS, the major cause of bacterial pharyngitis, are based on the Modified **Centor criteria/McIssac score.**
- When to test for GAS: Test if the McIssac score indicates a reasonable clinical suspicion it is bacterial pharyngitis:
  - McIssac score = 2: Optional testing.
  - McIssac score ≥ 3: Consider testing.
- Do not test for GAS when there is high suspicion for viral etiology. Testing not recommended in children <3 years unless they have risk factors, such as an older sibling with known GAS.

Diagnosis

- If needed, the **most accurate and initial test of choice** for GAS is the **rapid antigen test,** which has >90% specificity but slightly lower sensitivity (70%-90% depending on the manufacturer). Cultures are not necessary if the rapid test is positive. If rapid test is ⊖ but clinical suspicion continues, send a GAS culture for children only. Culture is not recommended for adults as bacterial pharyngitis is less common. Pharyngitis due to GAS is more common in children than adults, which is reflected in the McIssac score.
- A routine bacterial culture is not indicated unless there is high suspicion of a bacterial infection other than GAS (eg, gonococcal pharyngitis.)

Management

- Treat for GAS **only** if it is confirmed with a rapid test or culture. Also consider for recurrent GAS infections, the patient may be colonized with GAS with recurrent viral pharyngitis.
- For GAS, give one dose IM benzathine penicillin or a 10-day course of oral penicillin VK. For penicillin-allergic patients, a first-generation cephalosporin, azithromycin, or clindamycin can be used. Other antistreptococcal antibiotics (eg, cefuroxime or amoxicillin) may be used, but their efficacy in preventing rheumatic fever has not been adequately studied.
- Patients may return to work or school 24 hours after initiation of therapy.
- Tonsillectomy is not recommended to ↓ the recurrence of GAS pharyngitis.
- For uncomplicated **gonococcal** pharyngitis, treat with both ceftriaxone and azithromycin due to resistance patterns of gonorrhea; if patient is allergic to ceftriaxone, use gentamicin and azithromycin. If complicated by pelvic or joint infection, treat-

KEY FACT

Prompt antibiotic treatment for group A streptococcus is the number one intervention to prevent acute rheumatic fever.

KEY FACT

Modified Centor criteria and McIssac Score
- Age: 3 to 14 years (+1), 15 to 44 years (0), ≥45 years (–1).
- Temperature >38.0°C (100.4°F) (+1).
- Tender or swollen anterior cervical lymphadenopathy (+1).
- Absence of cough (+1).
- Presence of pharyngotonsillar exudates or tonsillar swelling (+1).

QUESTION

An otherwise healthy 25-year-old woman presents to the urgent care clinic with a very sore throat, subjective fever, and swollen glands in her neck. She has a temperature of 38.5°C (101.3°F). On exam, you note palatal petechiae, purulent tonsillar exudates, and tender cervical lymphadenopathy. What is your treatment plan?

ment may require IV antibiotics and hospitalization. For **chlamydia,** doxycycline or azithromycin can be used as first-line therapy.

Complications

- Peritonsillar abscess and, rarely, pharyngeal abscesses.
- In GAS, postinfectious phenomena can occur, including **acute rheumatic fever** (see Special Topics: Acute Rheumatic Fever, at the end of this chapter) and glomerulonephritis.

Viral Pharyngitis

Suggested by upper respiratory symptoms and the absence of tonsillar exudates. Usually due to common viral causes of URIs including adeno-, corona-, and rhinoviruses. Pharyngitis secondary to other systemic viral infections presents as follows:

- **Mononucleosis:** Characterized by the triad of **lymphadenopathy, fever,** and **tonsillitis.** Symptoms also include severe fatigue, headache, and malaise. More common in young adults. Transmitted in saliva and may persist for up to 18 months after 1° infection (Figure 6.5).
- **Herpangina:** Presents with fever, sore throat, myalgias, and a vesicular exanthem on the soft palate. Commonly caused by coxsackievirus A16 (Figure 6.6) and may be associated with vesicular rash on the palms and soles in hand-foot-mouth disease.
- **Acute retroviral syndrome:** Nonexudative pharyngitis and fever are common symptoms of acute HIV infection.

Diagnosis

- **Mononucleosis:** Diagnosed with a ⊕ heterophil antibody (Monospot) test or a high anti-EBV antibody titer.
- Consider HIV or other viral testing.

Management

- **Supportive care,** including acetaminophen or NSAIDs and saltwater gargling for symptomatic relief. Oral steroids may occasionally be needed for severe pharyngitis.
- Patients may return to work or school when fever resolves and they are well enough to participate in normal activities.

Complications

- **Mononucleosis:** Complications include hepatitis, a morbilliform rash following antibiotic administration (especially ampicillin/amoxicillin), and splenomegaly occurring within the first 3 weeks. To ↓ the risk of **splenic rupture,** noncontact sports must be avoided for 3 to 4 weeks and contact sports for 4 to 6 weeks after the onset of symptoms.
- For **HIV** disease, see section on HIV.

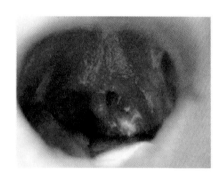

FIGURE 6.5.   Exudative tonsilitis in mononucleosis pharyngitis. (Reproduced from Balfour HH Jr, et al. Infectious mononucleosis. *Clin Transl Immunol.* 2015;4(2):e33.)

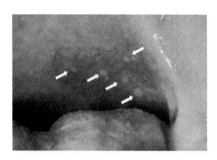

FIGURE 6.6.   Herpangina. Acute, multiple papulovesicular lesions progress to form shallow ulcerations (arrows), with brisk marginal erythema. (Reproduced with permission from Wolff K, et al. *Fitzpatrick's Dermatology in General Medicine,* 7th ed. New York: McGraw-Hill, 2008, Fig. 192-18.)

ANSWER

She meets the modified Centor criteria/ McIssac score for testing. Treat with a 10-day course of penicillin for group A streptococci (*S pyogenes*) if her rapid strep or culture is positive.

DENTAL AND PERIODONTAL INFECTIONS

Dental Caries

The most common chronic childhood disease. For a patient to develop caries, three factors must be present: a **host,** a **substrate (sucrose),** and **bacteria.** The most common bacterial agent is *Streptococcus mutans.*

Differential

Isolated gingival infections, sinus disease, trigeminal neuralgia, TMJ.

Treatment

- Antibiotics that cover oral flora include penicillins (Penicillin VK, amoxicillin), clindamycin, and erythromycin for penicillin-allergic patients.
- Refer to a dentist or oral surgeon for dental extraction or incision and drainages as appropriate.

Complications

- Acute pulpitis, periapical abscess, granuloma, or cyst. Abscesses may track and lead to serious infections.
- **Ludwig angina:** A life-threatening infection of the sublingual and submandibular spaces that causes nonpitting sublingual edema, potentially leading to airway obstruction. Requires hospitalization and IV antibiotics, ampicillin/sulbactam, clindamycin, or high-dose penicillin plus metronidazole.
- **Lemierre syndrome:** A suppurative thrombophlebitis of the internal jugular vein located in the posterior compartment of the lateral pharyngeal space caused by *Fusobacterium necrophorum*. Can lead to bacteremia, septic pulmonary emboli, and other septic embolic complications.

Prevention

Fluoridated water, good oral hygiene, and regular dental care are effective in reducing dental caries. Fluoride varnish can be applied in primary care settings for children who do not have adequate dental care.

Oral Lesions

Table 6.5 outlines the differential diagnosis of common mouth ulcers.

Cardiovascular Infections

ENDOCARDITIS

An infection of the endothelium of the heart that most frequently involves the valves. A vegetation consists of bacteria, platelets, fibrin, and inflammatory cells. Endocarditis is classified as acute versus subacute and **native valve endocarditis (NVE)** (Figure 6.7) versus **prosthetic valve endocarditis (PVE)**. People who use IV drugs are at particularly high risk for tricuspid valve endocarditis (Table 6.6).

QUESTION

A 33-year-old man is brought to the ED complaining of fever and shortness of breath of 3 days' duration. On exam, the only pertinent findings are warm skin and some track marks in the left antecubital fossa. The nurse tells you that his current temperature is 39.5°C (103.1°F). You order a CXR, UA, and blood cultures. Six hours later, the patient's blood cultures reveal gram-negative cocci. On reexamination, you note a II/VI systolic ejection murmur. Which antibiotic would be the most appropriate empiric choice?

TABLE 6.5. Differential of Common Mouth Ulcers

	APHTHOUS ULCER (CANKER SORE)	HERPES STOMATITIS
Cause	Common; unknown cause (possible association with HHV-6)	Common; HSV
Symptoms	Pain up to 1 week; heals within a few weeks	Initial burning, followed by small vesicles and then scabs
Exam	Small ulcerations, with yellow centers surrounded by red halos on **nonkeratinized** mucosa (buccal and lip mucosa, tongue)	Vesicles → ulcers → scabs on **keratinized** tissue (lips, hard palate)
Treatment	Anti-inflammatory: topical steroids	No need for treatment, but oral **acyclovir** × 7-14 days may shorten the course and postherpetic pain
Prognosis	Recurrent	Resolves quickly; may recur; frequent reactivation in immunocompromised patients
Differential diagnosis	If large or persistent, consider erythema multiforme, HSV, pemphigus, Behçet disease, IBD, or squamous cell carcinoma	Aphthous ulcer, erythema multiforme, syphilis, cancer

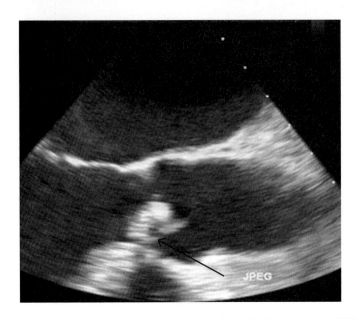

FIGURE 6.7.   Tricuspid valve endocarditis. Transesophageal echocardiogram (TEE) demonstrating degenerated aortic valve with associated valvular vegetation (arrow). (Reproduced from Alozie A, et al. Arthralgia and blood culture-negative endocarditis in middle age men suggest tropheryma whipplei infection: report of two cases and review of the literature. *BMC Infect Dis.* 2015;15:339.)

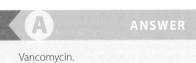

Vancomycin.

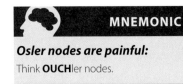

Osler nodes are painful:
Think **OUCH**ler nodes.

Symptoms

- **Acute bacterial endocarditis:** Presents with high fever (80%) and chills and can cause symptoms related to embolic phenomena (<50%) and HF.
- **Subacute endocarditis:** Presents with fever, weight loss, and poor appetite; has an indolent course. May also have signs or symptoms of HF.

TABLE 6.6.   Etiologies of Endocarditis

TYPE	ETIOLOGY (INCIDENCE)
NVE	*S aureus* (32%), viridans group streptococci (18%), *Enterococcus* (11%), coagulase-negative staphylococci (10%), *S gallolyticus* (formerly *S bovis;* 6.5%), HACEK group (1.7%), culture negative (8.1%)
PVE	*S aureus* and coagulase-negative staphylococci, gram-negatives, and fungi (in valves <2 months old), agents similar to NVE in valves >2 months old, except more coagulase-negative staphylococci
IV drug use	*S aureus* (60%), unusual gram-negatives, and fungi
Notes	**HACEK** organisms (*Haemophilus, Actinobacillus, Cardiobacterium, Eikenella, Kingella*) previously required special media or longer incubation time Consider *Candida* and *Aspergillus* in people who inject drugs and patients with long-term indwelling catheters or immunosuppression Causes of culture-negative infective endocarditis: *Chlamydia psittaci*, the "ellas" (*Bartonella, Legionella, Brucella, Coxiella*), and recent antibiotic use

Exam

- Fever and a heart murmur are most commonly seen; 85% have heart murmurs, but only 5% to 10% have a new murmur.
- Other symptoms and signs are as follows:
    - **Osler nodes:** Tender nodules on the finger and toe pads.
    - **Janeway lesions:** Nontender hemorrhagic macules on the palms and soles.
    - **Splinter hemorrhages:** Reddish-brown streaks in the proximal nail beds (Figure 6.8).
    - **Roth spots:** Retinal hemorrhages seen with an ophthalmoscope.
    - Petechiae, especially conjunctival and mucosal.
    - Signs of right or left heart failure or CVA may also be seen.

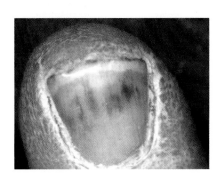

FIGURE 6.8.   Splinter hemorrhage of infective endocarditis. Patient was a 60-year-old man who presented 3 months after aortic valve replacement. (Reproduced with permission from USMLE-Rx.com.)

Differential

Atrial myxoma, marantic endocarditis (nonbacterial thrombotic endocarditis, seen in cancer and chronic wasting diseases), Libman-Sacks endocarditis (autoantibodies to heart valve, seen in SLE), acute rheumatic fever, suppurative thrombophlebitis, catheter-related sepsis, renal cell carcinoma, carcinoid syndrome.

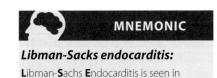

MNEMONIC

Libman-Sacks endocarditis:
Libman-**S**achs **E**ndocarditis is seen in **S**ystemic **L**upus **E**rythematosus.

Diagnosis

- Duke criteria:
    - Diagnosis of definite endocarditis must meet two major, one major plus three minor, or five minor criteria (Table 6.7). Duke criteria sensitivity is 95%.

TABLE 6.7.   Duke Criteria for the Clinical Diagnosis of Infective Endocarditis

MAJOR CRITERIA

1. A ⊕ blood culture:
    - A typical microorganism consistent with infective endocarditis from 2 separate blood cultures, as follows:
        - Viridans streptococci, *S gallolyticus* (formerly *S bovis*), HACEK group, *S aureus* **OR**
        - Community-acquired enterococci in the absence of a 1° focus **OR**
    - A persistently ⊕ blood culture, defined as recovery of a microorganism consistent with infective endocarditis from:
        - Two or more blood cultures drawn >12 hours apart **OR**
        - All of 3 or a majority of 4 or more separate blood cultures, with the first and last drawn at least 1 hour apart **OR**
        - A single ⊕ blood culture for *Coxiella burnetii* or anti–phase 1 IgG antibody titer of >1:800
2. Evidence of endocardial involvement:
    - A ⊕ echocardiogram, defined as follows:
        - An oscillating intracardiac mass on the valve or supporting structures, in the path of regurgitant jets, or in implanted material in the absence of an alternative anatomic explanation **OR**
        - Abscess **OR**
        - New partial dehiscence of a prosthetic valve **OR**
        - New valvular regurgitation (an ↑ or change in a preexisting murmur is not sufficient)

MINOR CRITERIA

1. **Predisposition:** A predisposing heart condition or IV drug use
2. **Fever:** ≥38.0°C (≥100.4°F)
3. **Vascular phenomena:** Major arterial emboli, septic pulmonary infarcts, mycotic aneurysm, intracranial hemorrhage, conjunctival hemorrhages, Janeway lesions
4. **Immunologic phenomena:** Glomerulonephritis, Osler nodes, Roth spots, RF
5. **Microbiologic evidence:** A ⊕ blood culture but not meeting major criteria as noted previously,[a] or serologic evidence of active infection with an organism consistent with infective endocarditis

[a]Excluding single ⊕ cultures for coagulase-negative staphylococci and diphtheroids, which are common culture contaminants, and organisms that do not cause endocarditis frequently, such as gram-negative bacilli.

- Diagnosis of possible endocarditis includes one major plus one minor or three minor criteria.
- To reject a diagnosis of endocarditis, there must be an alternate diagnosis, resolution of clinical manifestations after 4 days of antibiotic therapy, failure to meet the clinical criteria for possible or definite infective endocarditis, or $\ominus$ pathology.
- **Labs:** Leukocytosis with left shift, mild anemia, and ↑ ESR.
  - Initial test: **Blood cultures.** Critical in establishing the diagnosis; $\oplus$ in 85% to 95% of cases. It is recommended that **three sets** of blood cultures be taken at least **1 hour apart** before antibiotics if subacute endocarditis is suspected.
  - Most accurate test: **Echocardiogram.** In NVE, transthoracic echo (TTE) is 60% to 75% sensitive, whereas transesophageal echo (TEE) is 95% sensitive. Both are 95% specific. TTE is insensitive (15%-30%) with prosthetic valves—use TEE. An echocardiogram should be done as soon as possible and ideally within 12 hours of initial evaluation.
- **ECG:** May show varying degrees of **heart block** if the conduction system is involved. Consider perivalvular abscess if PR is prolonged.
- **CXR:** May show multiple peripheral infiltrates with cavitation or effusions from septic emboli in patients with right-sided heart valve involvement.

Management

- In general, therapy must be intravenous and administered for prolonged periods. The choice of antibiotic should be guided by clinical and epidemiologic clues in the absence of culture data or before culture data are available. Consult an infectious disease specialist to help tailor antibiotics.
- **NVE (empiric therapy):** Starting with vancomycin plus ceftriaxone is reasonable before blood culture results are available. Adjust antibiotics on the basis of culture results and treat for 4 to 6 weeks. Uncomplicated right-sided and left-sided methicillin-sensitive staphylococcal endocarditis (with no systemic embolic disease and with intact pulmonary function) can be treated with nafcillin. If methicillin-resistant *Staphylococcus aureus* is the organism responsible, treat for minimum of 6 weeks with vancomycin, or daptomycin if there is a vancomycin allergy.
- **PVE (empiric therapy):** Vancomycin plus rifampin for a minimum of 6 weeks. Additionally, gentamicin should be given for the first 2 weeks for *S aureus* and coagulase-negative staphylococci. Adjust antibiotics in accordance with culture results and treat for 6 weeks.
- **Persistent fever** after 1 week suggests a septic embolic focus or inadequate antibiotic coverage.
- Reappearance of fever **after initial defervescence** suggests septic emboli, drug fever, or, less commonly, the emergence of antimicrobial resistance.
- **Indications for surgery** are individualized. Common indications include refractory HF, valvular obstruction, myocardial abscess, perivalvular extension (new conduction abnormalities), persistent bacteremia, fungal endocarditis, recurrent emboli, and valvular dysfunction.

Complications

- **HF:** Caused by valvular destruction or myocarditis. The **most common cause of death** due to endocarditis.
- **Embolic phenomena:** Mycotic aneurysms, infarction, or abscesses in the CNS, kidney, coronary arteries, or spleen. Right-sided disease can lead to pulmonary emboli, but if a patent foramen ovale is present, it can also lead to systemic emboli ("paradoxic embolus").
- **Conduction abnormalities:** Arrhythmia and heart block.
- **Myocardial or perivalvular abscess:** May extend to cause pericarditis and tamponade. Most common with *S aureus*.

Prevention

- **Antibiotic prophylaxis** is largely theoretical. Recommended only for patients at the highest risk with prosthetic valve, patch, or devices; surgical systemic pulmonary shunts; unrepaired cyanotic congenital heart defects, including palliative shunts; or prior endocarditis; and also for patients <6 months of age postcardiac surgery with prosthetic material, or cardiac transplantation with valvulopathy.
- Daily oral and dental hygiene with consistent brushing and flossing should be stressed to prevent gingivitis and periodontal disease, which can cause recurrent infective endocarditis.
- **Procedures requiring prophylaxis:** Dental procedures involving manipulation of gingiva, oral mucosa, or periapical regions of teeth; respiratory tract procedures with incision or biopsy of the respiratory tract mucosa; procedures on infected skin or soft tissues. Prophylaxis no longer required for GI or GU procedures.
- **Antibiotic choice for prophylaxis:** PO amoxicillin or clindamycin 1 hour before procedure. If giving parenterally, IV vancomycin 120 minutes before procedure.

MYOCARDITIS

Inflammation of the myocardium (Figure 6.9); postulated to be a common cause of "idiopathic" dilated cardiomyopathy. The typical patient is young and healthy and may have had a recent viral URI. Can be a cause of sudden cardiac death. Etiologies include the following:

- **Infectious:** Usually **viral** (eg, coxsackievirus, HIV, influenza) but may also be caused by other pathogens, including bacteria such as *Borrelia burgdorferi* in Lyme disease (most commonly on the East Coast and in the Rocky Mountain regions of the United States) and parasites such as *Trypanosoma cruzi* in Chagas disease (almost exclusively found in Central and South America).

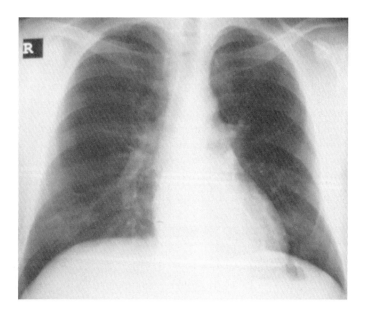

FIGURE 6.9. X-ray findings in viral myocarditis. A 27-year-old man who had influenza infection 1 week before admission was initially diagnosed as having asthma with acute viral bronchitis and pericarditis. Lack of response to treatment led to further evaluation with echocardiography, which showed global hypokinesia in the left ventricle and a ↓ ejection fraction of 40%. Viral myocarditis was diagnosed. (Reproduced from Sertogullarindan B, et al. A case of viral myocarditis presenting with acute asthma attack. *J Clin Med Res.* 2012;4(3):224-226.)

- **Immune mediated:** Medication allergy, sarcoidosis, scleroderma, SLE, and other autoimmune conditions.
- **Toxin related:** Medications (anthracyclines), EtOH, heavy metals, and others.
- **Postpartum.**

Symptoms/Exam

- Nonspecific. Flulike symptoms, fever, arthralgias, and malaise may be seen. In severe cases, patients may present with chest pain, dyspnea, and symptoms of HF.
- Physical exam may be normal or may reveal findings consistent with HF.

Differential

CAD/MI, aortic dissection, pericarditis, pulmonary embolism, other pulmonary and GI processes.

Diagnosis

- Diagnosis of myositis relies more on clinical suspicion (ie, unclear reasons for HF) and exclusion of other causes than on a single test.
- Most accurate test: **Endomyocardial biopsy.** The **gold standard.** However, the test is insensitive because of the patchy involvement of the myocardium and it is not indicated in most cases. Consider for patients where there is a concern for fulminant lymphocytic myocarditis and giant cell myocarditis as they may respond to immunosuppressive therapy.
- Cardiac magnetic resonance (CMR): Helps distinguish ischemic versus nonischemic cardiomyopathy. Indicated in patients with persistent symptoms, evidence of significant myocardial injury, or suspected viral etiology.
- **ECG:** Can be abnormal, but is neither sensitive nor specific.
- **Cardiac enzymes:** May be ↑ in the acute phase.
- **Echocardiogram:** May reveal focal wall motion abnormalities and ↓ ejection fraction, but findings are nonspecific.
- Cardiac catheterization: To exclude CAD.

Management

- Can be focused if there is a known cause (eg, a parasite).
- Treat HF.
- Steroids have not been shown to be of use, except in small studies of autoimmune disease–mediated myocarditis (eg, sarcoidosis or giant cell myocarditis).
- Refer for evaluation of cardiac transplantation in severe cases.

Complications

Dilated cardiomyopathy, HF, arrhythmias, death.

PERICARDITIS

Inflammation of the pericardium that leads to chest pain, pericardial friction rub, and diffuse ST elevations on ECG. It is often accompanied by a pericardial effusion, which can lead to tamponade. Most cases are idiopathic.

Infectious etiologies include:
- **Viral:** Coxsackievirus A and B, echovirus, mumps, adenovirus, hepatitis, HIV, EBV, VZV, HSV.
- **Bacterial:** *S pneumoniae* and other streptococci, *S aureus*, *Neisseria* spp, *Legionella* spp, *Mycobacterium tuberculosis*, *Treponema pallidum*.
- **Fungal:** Histoplasmosis, coccidioidomycosis, *Candida* spp, blastomycosis.

Noninfectious etiologies of pericarditis include:

- **Autoimmune:** Most commonly rheumatoid arthritis and lupus (SLE).
- **Malignant:** Most commonly lung, breast, or metastatic disease.
- **Posttraumatic** (aka Dressler syndrome): After surgery, an MI, or radiation therapy.
- **Metabolic:** Dialysis-related or from uremia or hypothyroidism.

Symptoms/Exam

- Classically described as sharp, **pleuritic** chest discomfort that worsens when patients are supine and **eases when they lean forward.**
- On exam, a pericardial **friction rub** is the hallmark. The rub is classically described as having three components: atrial contraction, ventricular contraction, and ventricular filling.

Differential

Same differential as for myocarditis **plus:**

- Pneumothorax.
- Costochondritis.
- Aortic aneurysm and dissection.

Diagnosis

Diagnosis requires two or more of the following criteria:

- History of chest pain that is typical of acute pericarditis.
- Auscultation of friction rub.
- New or worsening pericardial effusion.
- Typical ECG changes: Diffuse ST-segment elevation, PR-segment depression (Figure 6.10).

KEY FACT

In patients with sharp chest pain while supine and diffuse PR-segment depression or ST-segment elevations on ECG, think pericarditis.

Management

- Usually supportive, although treatment should be directed to the likely etiology.
- Monitor for signs of enlarging pericardial effusion and/or tamponade (pulsus paradoxus, a >10 mm Hg ↓ in SBP during inspiration, hypotension, elevated JVP)—a medical emergency requiring pericardiocentesis and/or a surgical pericardial window.

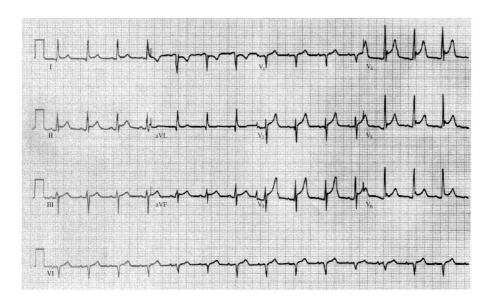

FIGURE 6.10. **ECG in acute pericarditis.** Note PR depression in I, II, V3, V4, V5, and V6 as well as diffuse ST elevations. (Reproduced with permission from Crawford MH, et al. *Current Diagnosis & Treatment in Cardiology*, 3rd ed. New York: McGraw-Hill, 2009, Fig. 17-2.)

- NSAIDs are first line. May use colchicine as adjunctive treatment (especially for patients with recurrent episodes).
- Low-dose steroids are often used as a last resort when patients do not respond to other therapies.
- Consider exercise restriction, at least 3 months for athletes.

Pulmonary Infections

ACUTE BRONCHITIS

A nonspecific term used to describe an acute productive cough without evidence of pneumonia in patients with or without underlying lung disease. By definition, the inflammation is limited to the trachea and to large and medium-sized bronchi. The most common causative organisms are respiratory viruses (RSV; rhino-, corona-, and adenoviruses; influenza and parainfluenza viruses) and, to a lesser extent, atypical bacteria (M pneumoniae, C pneumoniae, Bordetella pertussis).

Symptoms/Exam

- Cough (productive or not) may persist for 1 to 4 weeks, often with initial URI symptoms (rhinorrhea or sore throat).
- Lung exam findings range from clear to wheezes (from bronchospasm) or rhonchi.

Differential

- Community-acquired pneumonia (CAP).
- B pertussis in children with a "whooping" cough and in adults with a severe paroxysmal cough. Recent studies show that adolescents and young adults with waning immunity are a reservoir to infect unvaccinated or inadequately vaccinated children with pertussis. It is therefore recommended that all adults 19 to 64 years of age receive one Tdap booster vaccine in lieu of a Td vaccine.
- Conditions that may lead to chronic cough include GERD, asthma, postnasal drip, foreign body, malignancy, HF, and tuberculosis.

Diagnosis

Diagnosis is made clinically. CXR is not routinely indicated unless used to rule out pneumonia.

Management

- Because the most common etiologies are viral, antibiotics are **not generally indicated** except in the setting of a COPD exacerbation.
- Expectorants can be used for symptomatic treatment.
- Bronchodilators may be used if there is a reactive airway component.

INFLUENZA

An acute viral respiratory infection caused by influenza A and B, members of the Orthomyxoviridae family. Infection and mortality are most common in winter. Transmission via aerosolized droplets is highly contagious. Influenza is responsible for many **local epidemics as well as historical pandemics.**

Influenza infectivity and virulence vary yearly, related to the surface proteins hemagglutinin (H) and neuraminidase (N). Different combinations of H + N create a given influenza A serotype (eg, H1N1, or "swine flu").

Influenza A strains are harbored by animal reservoirs—pigs and birds—which can be asymptomatic carriers. New combinations of H + N are due to **antigenic shift**: the reassortment of H + N when virus serotypes exchange genetic material in a host animal or person.

Symptoms/Exam

- Presentation usually includes **abrupt onset** of fever (up to 5 days), chills, headache, myalgias, fatigue, anorexia, dry cough, sore throat, and/or clear rhinorrhea. Abdominal pain and diarrhea may be seen as well.
- Physical findings are nonspecific and may include hyperemic pharyngeal mucosa without exudates, lymphadenopathy, and scattered rhonchi or rales on lung exam.

Differential

Other respiratory viruses, atypical bacteria (*M pneumoniae*, *C pneumoniae*), bacterial pneumonia or pharyngitis, exacerbation of underlying comorbidities such as COPD.

Diagnosis

- Initial and most accurate test: **Rapid antigen immunoassay.** Rapid tests collected from the nasopharynx can detect viral particles within 30 minutes. In general, these tests are more specific than sensitive. Viral cultures and PCR for identification are usually available, but results can take up to 3 to 5 days.
- **Blood tests:** WBC counts vary from mild leukopenia to mild leukocytosis. Significant leukocytosis should prompt consideration of a bacterial etiology.

Management

- **Symptomatic treatment:** Treat fever, headache, and myalgias with acetaminophen. Avoid salicylates in patients <18 years of age because of the risk of **Reye syndrome.** Antitussives can be used sparingly. Encourage rest and hydration.
- **Antiviral therapy:** Most effective when administered within the first 6 hours of symptom onset. When used within the first 48 hours of illness, antivirals may ↓ the duration of illness by 1 to 2 days and in some studies ↓ the subjective symptom severity. Consider treatment for patients with severe illness or the immunocompromised even >48 hours after symptom onset.
- Since 2005, widespread resistance to the antivirals amantadine and rimantadine has developed, but influenza A and B remain mostly sensitive to **oseltamivir** and zanamivir (neuraminidase inhibitors).
- Consider hospitalization if there is concern about hydration and oxygenation or if the patient has significant comorbidities. Whereas zanamivir is used for postexposure prophylaxis, oseltamivir is generally used for hospitalized patients.
- Consider treatment for those who are hospitalized or at high risk for complications such as children <5 years of age (particularly <2 years of age), adults ≥65 years of age, pregnant women, the immunocompromised, patients with pulmonary conditions or chronic medical conditions, and residents of nursing home or chronic care facilities.

Prevention

- **Universal yearly vaccination** is recommended for all patients >6 months of age (Table 6.8). The vaccine is produced in eggs and thus is **contraindicated in serious egg allergy unless it is the recombinant influenza vaccine (RIV), which is egg free.**
- Chemoprophylaxis with antiviral medication may be considered in very-high-risk patients during an influenza epidemic but is not an evidence-based approach except in certain settings, such as skilled nursing facilities.

TABLE 6.8.   Recommendations for Influenza Vaccination

The CDC recommends **universal vaccination** for all patients >6 months of age.

Type of vaccine for administration:

- Three types of influenza vaccine are currently available: live attenuated influenza vaccine **(LAIV),** trivalent influenza vaccine **(TIV), and recombinant influenza vaccine (RIV).**
- LAIV contains weakened live virus, which can cause mild symptoms such as malaise, rhinorrhea, and cough; it is administered by nasal spray.
- TIV contains killed virus and cannot cause infection; it is administered by injection.
- RIV is egg free and can be given to those with egg allergies who are >18 years old.

Vaccination of specific populations:

- LAIV should only be administered to healthy, nonpregnant patients 2-49 years of age.
- TIV should be administered to all other patients, including pregnant women, any person with chronic illness >6 months of age, and adults >50 years of age.
- Because of the theoretical risk of transmission of live influenza virus, LAIV should not be administered to the contacts or caregivers of the severely immunocompromised, such as recipients of hematopoietic stem cell transplant while they require care in a protective environment (eg, positive pressure room).
- LAIV may be administered to contacts of pregnant women and moderate-risk patients (eg, those with chronic illness, including cancer and AIDS); there have not been any documented cases of severe influenza via transmission from an LAIV recipient.

Notes on children: Children 6 months to 8 years of age who have not been previously vaccinated should receive two sequential vaccine doses in their first year of vaccination.

Notes on H1N1: H1N1 has been incorporated into the seasonal influenza vaccine since the 2010-2011 season.

Complications

With most influenza strains, complications are common in very young patients, in patients >65 years of age with comorbid conditions, and during the second or third trimester of pregnancy.

- **Pulmonary:** ARDS, leading to hypoxemic respiratory failure, 2° bacterial pneumonia (including a higher relative risk of *S pneumoniae* and *S aureus* pneumonia).
- **Musculoskeletal:** Myositis, rhabdomyolysis, and myoglobinuria are rare.
- **Cardiopulmonary:** Myocarditis (especially in younger patients), pericarditis, and exacerbations of COPD, asthma, or HF.
- **Neurologic:** Encephalitis, transverse myelitis, Guillain-Barré syndrome.
- **Reye syndrome:** Children present with nausea and vomiting, followed by CNS changes several days after a viral illness. Currently, Reye syndrome is uncommon due to ↓ aspirin use in children.

ACUTE BACTERIAL PNEUMONIA

An infection of the lung parenchyma and airspaces. Caused by a diverse array of pathogens. The most common infectious cause of disease and death in the United States, responsible for 50,000 to 60,000 deaths yearly. Treatment is based on severity of symptoms, presumed pathogen, and the risk of multidrug resistance (MDR) in a given patient. Incidence increases with age. Risk factors include chronic comorbidities, smoking, and alcohol use. Common pathogens include *S pneumoniae, H influenzae, Staphylococcus aureus, Klebsiella* species, *Mycoplasma pneumoniae, Chlamydophila pneumoniae,* and *Legionella pneumophila.*

Symptoms/Exam

- Shortness of breath, productive cough, pleuritic chest pain, fever and chills, or rigors.
- Hyperthermia or hypothermia, tachypnea, tachycardia, and hypoxia are common. Severe cases may present with cyanosis and altered mental status and can advance to sepsis and multiorgan failure.

ANSWER

The differential diagnoses include CAP and influenza, among other etiologies. Obtain a CXR and a rapid test for influenza, discuss the treatment options and precautions with the patient, and consider early initiation of the antiviral medication oseltamivir if ⊕ for influenza.

- In addition to altered air movement and rhonchi or rales on lung exam, special findings due to lung consolidation may include egophony, whispered pectoriloquy, and tactile fremitus.

Differential

- **Infectious causes:** Viral or fungal pneumonia (including *Pneumocystis jiroveci*), TB, postobstructive pneumonia, and septic emboli from right-sided endocarditis.
- **Noninfectious causes:** Malignancy, foreign body, pulmonary infarct from emboli, collagen vascular disease with vasculitis leading to hemorrhage and hypersensitivity, radiation, chemical pneumonitis, aspiration pneumonitis, and asthma exacerbation.

Diagnosis

- Initial test: **CXR** is recommended to assist in diagnosis and treatment; may characterize pneumonia severity, extent, and whether the pneumonia is complicated (Figure 6.11). CT scan of the chest can provide more detailed information, but is recommended only in complicated cases or if the diagnosis is unclear.
- **Blood cultures:** Collect in hospitalized patients before antibiotic therapy. Cultures provide reliable data and may allow for the tailoring of antimicrobial therapy. However, cultures are ⊕ in only 10% of cases. Results may change the duration of antibiotic therapy.
- **Sputum Gram stain and culture:** Often not helpful due to low sensitivity and specificity. Must have <10 squamous cells to be considered an adequate sample. It is, however, recommended for ICU patients, those with outpatient treatment failure, pulmonary effusion, severe obstructive or structural lung disease, cavitary infiltrates, alcohol use, or a ⊕ US for *S pneumoniae* or *Legionella*.
- **Urine antigen testing for *S pneumoniae* and *Legionella*:** Recommended for those with severe pneumonia. Benefits include fast results and ability to detect antigen even after antibiotic initiation. However, there can be false positives for *S pneumoniae* for those with recent CAP, recent immunization, or children with chronic respiratory illness or colonization. *Legionella* can also remain positive in the urine after a recent illness.
- **Tests for specific etiologies:** If there is a high clinical suspicion for a specific etiologic organism, seek appropriate available testing (Table 6.9).

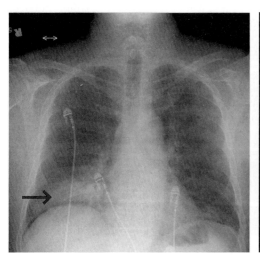
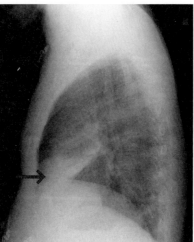

A   B

FIGURE 6.11. Community-acquired pneumonia. Frontal (**A**) and lateral (**B**) radiographs show airspace consolidation in the right middle lobe (arrows) in a patient with CAP. (Reproduced with permission from USMLE-Rx.com.)

TABLE 6.9. **Causative Organisms and Historical Features of Community-Acquired Pneumonia**

ORGANISM	CAUSE (%)	SUGGESTIVE HISTORICAL FEATURES
Streptococcus pneumoniae	20-60	Acute onset; often follows URI or influenza; underlying COPD
Haemophilus influenzae	3-10	Often follows URI; COPD
S aureus	3-5	May follow influenza infection; cavitary disease. May be methicillin resistant (MRSA), especially in HAP or VAP
Legionella spp	2-8	Exposure to humidifier, hot tub, or air-conditioning cooling towers; pleuritic chest pain and pleural effusion are common; diarrhea; hyponatremia
Klebsiella, other gram-negative rods	3-10	Ethanol abuse, diabetes, patients in long-term care, aspiration, VAP; some may display broad multidrug resistance
Mycoplasma pneumoniae	1-6	Young adults in summer and fall; associated rash and bullous myringitis
Chlamydia pneumoniae	4-10	Young adults; often follows prolonged sore throat
Pseudomonas aeruginosa	Rare	Important cause of VAP, high rate of morbidity from chronic lung disease and mortality
Stenotrophomonas and *Acinetobacter*	Rare	Additional causes of VAP; can display broad resistance patterns; usually require 14+ days of antibiotics
Q fever (*Coxiella burnetii*)	Rare	Exposure to livestock (cattle, goats, sheep); elevated LFTs
Chlamydia psittaci	Rare	Exposure to birds, including parrots, pigeons, and chickens; headache; temperature-pulse dissociation

■ In ventilated patients, attempt noninvasive sampling prior to invasive sampling such as bronchoalveolar lavage before administering antibiotics. Quantitative culture can provide more specific information if a pathogenic organism is present. Ten percent to 20% of patients who are mechanically ventilated will develop VAP.

Management

■ Outpatient therapy is appropriate in low-risk patients. By assigning risk categories, indices such as the pneumonia PORT severity index (PSI) and CURB-65 can help determine which patients are appropriate for outpatient care and which should be hospitalized (Tables 6.10 and 6.11).

■ Per Infectious Diseases Society of America (IDSA) and American Thoracic Society (ATS) guidelines, acute bacterial pneumonia treatment is divided into settings by risk category for multidrug-resistant pathogens and by level of care needed (Table 6.12). MDR risk factors include use of antibiotics in the last 90 days, current hospitalization for >5 days, prevalence of MDR in the community, and immunosuppression.

■ Local antibiograms and infectious disease specialist consult are recommended in choosing initial antibiotic therapy. For initial therapy, use the IDSA/ATS consensus guidelines (see Table 6.12).

■ **Response to treatment:** Antimicrobial therapy initiated within **4 to 8 hours** of presentation is associated with improved outcomes.

■ **Early conversion** from parenteral to oral therapy is appropriate once a patient has improved clinically, is hemodynamically stable, and is able to take oral medication.

■ **Tailor antibiotic therapy** to the narrowest coverage possible per available bacteriologic results (culture, specific serologies) to limit future resistance.

■ **Duration of treatment** varies by organism and setting, but 5 to 7 days is adequate for most cases of pneumonia including HAP/VAP. Patient must be at least 48 to 72 hours afebrile and stable before discontinuing antibiotics.

KEY FACT

CURB-65: If score = 2, admit to hospital. If score ≥3, admit to ICU
Confusion (acute change in mental status)
Urea >7 mmol/L
Respiratory rate ≥30 breaths/min
Blood pressure: systolic <90 mm Hg or diastolic ≤60 mm Hg
Age **65** years or older

TABLE 6.10.   **Scoring System for Risk Class Assignment of CAP (PSI)[a]**

PATIENT CHARACTERISTIC	POINTS ASSIGNED
Demographic factor:	
Age: men	Number of years
Age: women	Number of years minus 10
Nursing home resident	10
Comorbid illnesses:	
Neoplastic disease[b]	30
Liver disease[c]	20
HF[d]	10
Cerebrovascular disease[e]	10
Renal disease[f]	10
Physical examination finding:	
Altered mental status[g]	20
Respiratory rate ≥30 breaths/min	20
Systolic BP <90 mm Hg	
Temperature ≤35°C (95°F) or ≥40°C (104°F)	15
Pulse ≥125 bpm	10
Laboratory or radiographic finding:	
Arterial pH <7.35	30
BUN ≥30 mg/dL	20
Sodium <130 meq/L	20
Glucose >250 mg/dL	10
Hematocrit <30%	10
Arterial Po_2 <60 mm Hg	10
Pleural effusion	10

[a]A total point score for a given patient is obtained by summing the patient's age in years (age minus 10 for women) and the points for each applicable characteristic.

[b]Any cancer except basal or squamous cell carcinoma of the skin that was active at the time of presentation or diagnosed within 1 year before presentation.

[c]Clinical or histologic diagnosis of cirrhosis or another form of chronic liver disease.

[d]Systolic or diastolic dysfunction documented by history, physical examination and CXR, echocardiogram, multigated angiogram (MUGA) scan, or left ventriculogram.

[e]Clinical diagnosis of stroke or TIA or stroke documented by MRI or CT scan.

[f]History of chronic renal disease or abnormal BUN and creatinine concentration documented in the medical record.

[g]Disorientation (to person, place, or time, not known to be chronic), stupor, or coma.

TABLE 6.11.   **Site of Care Recommendations for CAP by Point Score**

POINT SCORE	RECOMMENDED TREATMENT SETTING
≤70	Outpatient
71-90	Outpatient or brief inpatient
>90	Inpatient

TABLE 6.12. Definition of Pneumonia and Initial Antibiotic Therapy

TYPE OF PNEUMONIA	DEFINITION	INITIAL ANTIBIOTIC THERAPY
Community-acquired (CAP)	Dx within 48 hours of admission; does not fit HAP or VAP criteria	Outpatient: macrolide (preferred) or doxycycline If chronic disease, immunocompromised, or antibiotics in last 3 months: respiratory fluoroquinolone or β-lactam + macrolide or doxycycline Inpatient: respiratory fluoroquinolone or β-lactam + macrolide or doxycycline. If concern for pseudomonas use cefepime or piperacillin-tazobactam. If concern for MRSA use vancomycin
Hospital-acquired (HAP)	>2 days acute hospitalization within last 90 days	If no MDR risk factors: monotherapy with β-lactam, ertapenem, or respiratory fluoroquinolone If MDR risk factors: antipseudomonal β-lactam or carbapenem + respiratory fluoroquinolone If MRSA risk factors: add vancomycin, consider consolidation to 2 agents, depending on presumed pathogen (eg, vancomycin + antipseudomonal β-lactam)
Ventilator-associated (VAP)	Develops >48 hours after endotracheal intubation or <48 hours of extubation	Same as above regimen for MDR risk factors
Aspiration	Largely the same therapy for CAP and HAP, but potentially greater risk for anaerobes if severe periodontal disease or macroscopic aspiration event (alcoholism, neuromuscular impairment) Differentiate between pneumonitis (a transient inflammatory infiltrate *not requiring* antibiotics) and pneumonia	No consensus guideline, some expert opinions recommend treating with same antibiotics as above depending on if the patient has CAP or HAP. If there is strong concern for anaerobes, can add on anaerobic coverage. However, in most cases of HAP, the focus should be on the aerobic organism

TABLE 6.13. Criteria for Discharge in Community-Acquired Pneumonia

Clinical stability:

- Improvement in cough/dyspnea
- Adequate O$_2$ saturation (>90%)
- Afebrile (temperature <37.8°C [100°F])
- Resolution of tachycardia (<100 bpm)
- Resolution of tachypnea (RR <24)
- Resolution of hypotension (SBP >90 mm Hg)
- No evidence of complicated infection (eg, extrapulmonary or pleural involvement)
- Ability to tolerate oral medications

- If response after 48 to 72 hours is inadequate, consider resistance, an alternative pathogen (atypical or rare bacteria, virus, fungi), a complicated pneumonia (abscess or empyema), or an alternative diagnosis.
- **Repeat chest imaging is not required** during hospitalization, except when complications are suspected (eg, ongoing fever, hypoxia, clinical deterioration).
- Consider CXR in 4 to 8 weeks in patients with risk factors for persistent infection or underlying malignancy (eg, smokers and patients >65 years of age).
- Patients may be discharged without delay at the time of conversion to oral therapy if they meet specific criteria (Table 6.13).

Complications

- Severe pneumonia can progress to **sepsis**, **ARDS**, shock, and multiorgan failure. If shock (eg, hypotension, organ failure), respiratory failure, or CXR consistent with ARDS is present on presentation, the patient should be directly admitted to the ICU, with critical care consultation as appropriate.
- **Pleural effusion/empyema/lung abscess:** Approximately 40% of patients with CAP have an effusion on CXR/CT. Thoracentesis should be performed if the effusion is impairing oxygenation or ventilation or if the patient is septic or is not responding to antimicrobial therapy. For empyema, complicated parapneumonic effusions, or

a lung abscess, consultation with pulmonology, interventional radiology, or thoracic surgery should be obtained for percutaneous or surgical drainage.

- **Necrotizing pneumonia:** Destruction of the lung parenchyma and airspaces due to infection and inflammation; can lead to fibrosis and chronic lung disease. Consult with a pulmonologist.
- **Recurrent pneumonia:** Recurrent CAP in the same anatomic location within 2 years may be due to an obstruction (ie, mass or foreign body). If recurrence is in a new location, consider an immunodeficiency workup and a chest CT to rule out bronchiectasis or obstructive lesion.

Prevention

- Smoking cessation is key to improving mucociliary clearance and to ↓ risk of COPD and lung malignancy.
- Administer the pneumococcal vaccine to patients >65 years of age, and earlier to patients with chronic disease such as diabetes or cardiopulmonary disease, and to asplenic patients.
- Basic infection control (eg, frequent hand hygiene and sterilization of ventilation equipment) is paramount, as the mortality rate for HAP and VAP may reach 40%.

TUBERCULOSIS

The largest single cause of infectious disease morbidity and mortality worldwide. A slow-growing, acid-fast bacillary infection caused by *Mycobacterium tuberculosis* (mTB). TB can affect nearly any system in the body, most commonly the lungs, and is transmitted by airborne respiratory droplets from patients with active pulmonary disease. TB can cause **primary, latent, and reactivation infection** (Figure 6.12). Symptoms and capacity for transmission depend on location and activity of disease.

Symptoms/Exam

- Symptoms vary, depending on location and type of infection.
- In **latent tuberculosis infection (LTBI)**, patients are asymptomatic. The lifetime risk of acquiring reactivation TB with LTBI is roughly 10% to 20%, with 2% to 5% developing active TB in the first 2 years (see the Community and Preventive Medicine chapter for a discussion of LTBI).
- In **active pulmonary TB,** patients may experience cough, hemoptysis, night sweats, shortness of breath, weight loss, and pleuritic chest pain.

Differential

Depends on location. In pulmonary disease, TB can mimic pneumonia, fungal infection, malignancy, postinfectious scar, autoimmune disease (sarcoidosis, granulomatosis with polyangiitis [Wegener], etc), and pulmonary fibrosis.

Diagnosis

- Imaging studies to evaluate patients with suspected mTB disease should be guided by symptoms and may include **CXR or CT scan** (Figure 6.13).
- Findings on imaging, especially in pulmonary TB, are highly variable and nonspecific:
  - 1° pulmonary infection can display segmental or lobar consolidation, hilar or mediastinal lymphadenopathy, effusion, or atelectasis. **CXR is normal in approximately 15%** of patients with 1° pulmonary TB.
  - Individuals with latent TB often have the classic Ghon complex (a peripheral calcified nodule and hilar lymphadenopathy).

KEY FACT

Tuberculin skin test, purified protein derivative (PPD): Size of wheal is considered positive in specific populations:
- ≥5 mm: Patient with HIV, patient has a close contact who has active TB, immunosuppression, CXR that is consistent with healed TB.
- ≥10 mm: Children <4 years of age, comorbities such as diabetes mellitus or chronic kidney disease, intravenous drug use, some malignancies, recent immigration, some GI surgeries (ie, gastrectomy), residents and employees in high-risk setting (eg, homeless shelters, prison, long-term-care facilities, hospitals).
- ≥15 mm: No known risk factors (kids >4 years of age with no known risk factors).

QUESTION

A 36-year-old man from Burma presents to his primary care doctor with ↑ cough over the last 6 weeks, associated with a 15-pound weight loss and night sweats. He moved to the United States 9 months ago and had a 20-mm PPD skin test during his first primary care visit. On exam, he is febrile to 38.4°C (101.2°F) and has ↓ breath sounds and scattered supraclavicular and axillary lymphadenopathy. What is your next step?

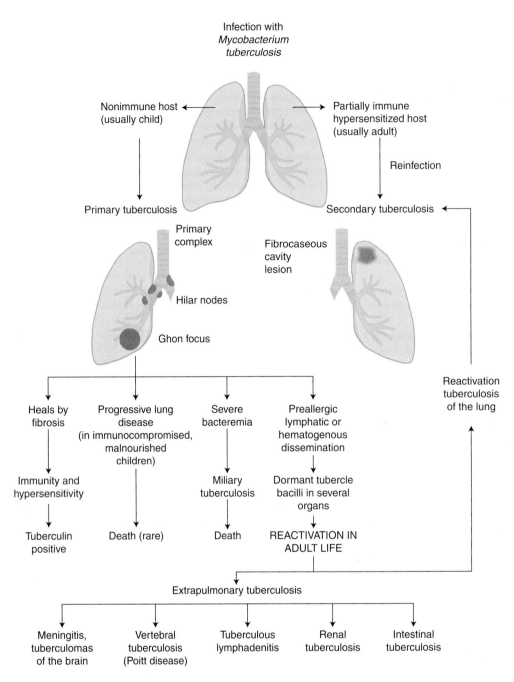

FIGURE 6.12. Evolution of pulmonary tuberculosis. (Reproduced with permission from Chandrasoma P, Taylor CR. *Concise Pathology,* 2nd ed. Originally published by Appleton & Lange. Copyright © 1995 by The McGraw-Hill Companies, Inc.)

ANSWER

Place a mask on the patient and have him wait in an isolation room, ideally with a negative pressure system. All staff in the area should wear appropriately sized N95 respirator masks. Order a CXR and contact your area TB controller for diagnostic and treatment recommendations.

- Reactivation disease in immunocompetent individuals, including HIV-positive patients with CD4+ cell count >400 cells/mm³, usually causes upper lung zone disease with apical cavitation.
- Immunocompromised patients, including those with AIDS with CD4+ cell count <200 cells/mm³, have variable manifestations such as diffuse disease with miliary, lower lung zone, or hilar/mediastinal foci.
- For potential foci of extrapulmonary TB (more common in immunocompromised patients), imaging and sample/biopsy must be guided by the location and probability of disease.

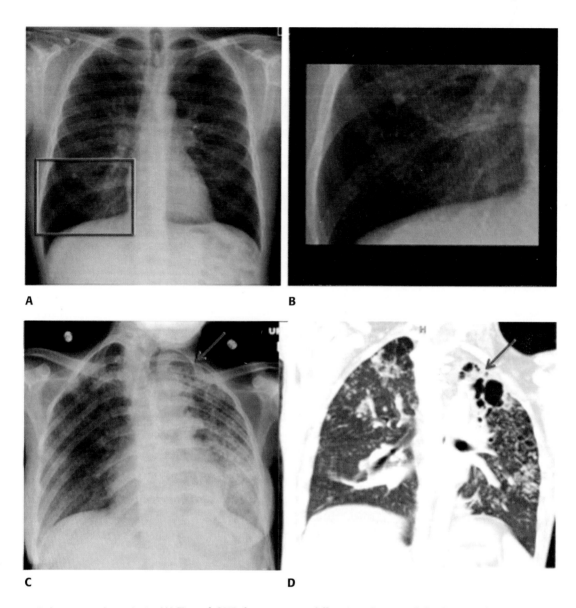

FIGURE 6.13. Pulmonary tuberculosis. (A) Frontal CXR demonstrating diffuse 1- to 2-mm nodules due to miliary TB. **(B)** A zoomed-in view corresponding to the area delineated by the red box in Image A. **(C)** Frontal CXR demonstrating left apical cavitary consolidation (arrow) and patchy infiltrates in the right and left lungs in a patient with reactivation TB. **(D)** Coronal reformation from a noncontrast chest CT in the same patient as Image C, better demonstrating left apical cavitary consolidation (arrows) and other areas of parenchymal abnormality corresponding to the endobronchial spread of TB. (Reproduced with permission from USMLE-Rx.com.)

Diagnosis

- In suspected pulmonary TB, sputum analysis should include an initial (early morning sample preferred) sample sent for Nucleic Acid Amplification Testing (NAAT) and another sent for microscopy with AFB smear. A ⊕ NAAT still warrants confirmation or exclusion of TB with three AFB smears.
- Sputum cultures must be ⊖ × 3 for 8 weeks to definitively rule out growth of TB in the sample. Because of the variable appearance of TB on imaging, a ⊖ CXR or CT should not be used to rule out active pulmonary TB. It is possible to have culture ⊖ TB.
- Presumptive diagnosis while awaiting culture results: one sputum smear ⊕ on both AFB and NAAT OR two or more samples ⊕ with NAAT.
- Patients without cough may have sputum induced by inhalation of hypertonic saline.
- In young children, early-morning gastric aspirates can substitute for sputum samples.

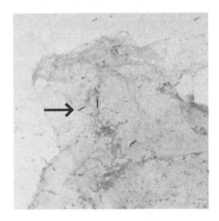

FIGURE 6.14. *Mycobacterium tuberculosis* **on AFB smear.** (Reproduced from the Centers for Disease Control and Prevention, Atlanta, GA.)

KEY FACT

Culture-positive pulmonary TB is not ruled out until three sputum cultures are negative for 8 weeks. Negative chest radiography does not rule out active pulmonary TB.

- In an intubated patient, samples can be obtained by tracheal aspirations performed 8 hours apart.
- If sputum or gastric samples are unobtainable, bronchoscopy can be performed for washings ± biopsies.
- All samples need to be sent specifically for mycobacterial culture (Figure 6.14). mTB may take up to 8 weeks to grow in a traditional mycobacterial culture, although it often grows in 2 to 3 weeks.
- Evidence of infection can be demonstrated with PPD skin testing (false ⊖ possible in patients with immunocompromise, and false ⊕ possible in **recent** BCG vaccination recipients) or with quantiferon (interferon gamma release assay) serology, which is more specific than PPD. These tests, when ⊕, show that an individual has TB infection but do not differentiate between latent and active disease.

Management

- All inpatients with concern for active pulmonary TB must be isolated in an individual room with a negative pressure system. Persons who enter the room must wear N95 masks to minimize chance of infection.
- All newly diagnosed cases of TB should be **reported to the local health department** or TB controller. The reporting requirements vary by location.
- In high-risk individuals (positive history/physical/radiographic findings, active immunocompromise including AIDS with CD4+ cell count <200 cells/ mm^3, exposure in TB-endemic areas, history of homelessness or incarceration), treatment should be started on the first day of care.
- TB therapy is typically a four-drug regimen of rifampin, isoniazid, pyrazinamide, and ethambutol (RIPE) for 2 months, followed by an additional 4 months of rifampin and isoniazid.
- Individuals at high risk for neuropathy (eg, diabetes, vascular disease) should take vitamin B$_6$ (pyridoxine) while on isoniazid to prevent worsening neuropathy.
- Therapy depends on the risk of MDR or extensively drug-resistant (XDR) TB, and consult with the local TB controller before beginning anti-TB therapy for all patients.
- For patients with extrapulmonary TB, therapy is determined by the site and complications of disease, and appropriate specialty consultation should be used.

Extrapulmonary Tuberculosis

Includes miliary TB, tuberculous lymphadenitis, skeletal TB, and tuberculous meningitis. TB can also lead to ocular disease, renal disease, pericarditis, salpingitis, peritonitis, and intestinal TB. HIV-infected patients are at particularly high risk of developing extrapulmonary TB.

- **Skeletal TB** symptoms include bone pain, arthritis of affected joints, pathologic fracture in advanced disease, and paralysis in 50% of patients with undiagnosed vertebral tuberculosis (Pott disease).
- **Miliary TB** is disseminated hematogenous spread of *M tuberculosis*. Risk is ↑ with older age and patients with comorbidities that alter cellular immunity (eg, diabetes, HIV, renal failure).
- Other sites include the GI and GU tracts, lymph nodes (called scrofula in the cervical nodes), skin, eyes, and CNS (causing various manifestations, most commonly a basilar meningitis resulting in headache, altered mental status, possible cranial nerve abnormalities, and potential for cerebrovascular accident).

Diagnosis

Perform TST as the first step in diagnosis, if not already done. Remember, a ⊖ PPD (especially in HIV-infected patients) does not exclude the diagnosis.

KEY FACT

Extrapulmonary TB is more likely to occur in HIV-⊕ patients with CD4 counts <100-300 cells/μL.

Management

Treat with a 6-month, four-drug regimen of the **antitubercular agents** used for pulmonary TB. This is sufficient for most manifestations of extrapulmonary TB. Consider an extension to 9 to 12 months in miliary, meningeal, or skeletal TB, as well as in immunocompromised hosts (as recommended by many experts).

Miliary Tuberculosis

The disseminated hematogenous spread of *M tuberculosis*. Risk is ↑ with older age and comorbidities that alter cellular immunity (eg, diabetes, HIV, renal failure).

Symptoms/Exam

Presentation is highly variable, ranging from fevers, night sweats, and failure to thrive/generalized malaise to specific organ system dysfunction (Table 6.14).

Diagnosis

- CBC reveals hematologic derangements in either direction. ↑ ESR and hyponatremia are also common.
- A miliary pattern is seen on CXR in more than two-thirds of cases (Figure 6.15).
- Obtain an AFB smear and culture of accessible and suspicious body fluids.

Tuberculous Lymphadenitis

- Commonly **presents** as a single swollen nontender lymph node—most often cervical, which is known as scrofula (Figure 6.16).
- Obtain an **FNA or excisional biopsy.** The latter is also a necessary aspect of treatment.

Skeletal Tuberculosis

Symptoms/Exam

- About one-half of cases involve the spine (Pott disease), but other common manifestations include tuberculous arthritis and extraspinal tuberculous osteomyelitis.
- Patients commonly present with progressive localized pain over weeks to months, sometimes associated with muscle spasm and rigidity. Fewer than 40% have constitutional symptoms.

TABLE 6.14. Organ System Involvement in Miliary Tuberculosis

ORGAN SYSTEM	CLINICAL MANIFESTATIONS
GI	Abnormal LFTs, hepatomegaly, cholestatic jaundice, pancreatitis, cholecystitis, peritonitis
CNS	Meningitis, tuberculomas
Skin	Tuberculosis cutis miliaris disseminate
Cardiovascular	Pericarditis (rare)
Adrenal	Adrenal insufficiency (rare)
Renal	Sterile pyuria
Breast	Hard lump, often mimics a breast abscess (rare)

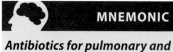

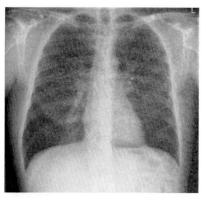
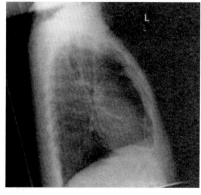

FIGURE 6.15. Miliary tuberculosis. A 32-year-old man from western China presented with cough and fever. Anteroposterior (**A**) and lateral (**B**) CXR shows innumerable scattered 1- to 2-mm pulmonary nodules, many of which are calcified. (Reproduced with permission from USMLE-Rx.com.)

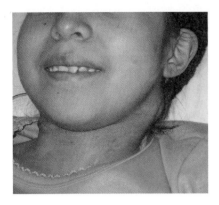

FIGURE 6.16. **Tuberculosis adenopathy.** Bilateral cervical adenopathy (scrofula) in a Peruvian child with documented TB. Cervical adenopathy in a child in highly endemic areas is strongly suggestive, and is the most common form of extrapulmonary TB. (Reproduced with permission from Knoop KJ, et al. *The Atlas of Emergency Medicine,* 3rd ed. New York: McGraw-Hill, 2010, Fig. 21.56. Photo contributors: Seth W. Wright, MD and Universidad Peruana Cayetano Heredia, Lina, Peru.)

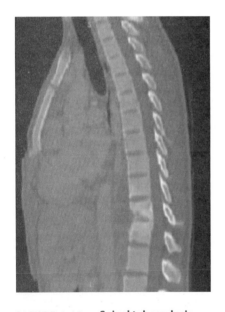

FIGURE 6.17. **Spinal tuberculosis (Pott disease).** CT of dorsolumbar spine bone window and sagittal reconstruction showing a vertebral destruction at T10-11. (Reproduced with permission from USMLE-Rx. com.)

KEY FACT

The most common cause of infectious diarrhea in US children is rotavirus. Noroviruses are the most common cause overall.

Diagnosis

- Obtain vertebral plain films to look for osteolytic lesions (Figure 6.17).
- Further imaging with CT or MRI can be useful.
- Refer for CT-guided biopsy of infected lesions. For tuberculous arthritis, biopsy of the synovium or periarticular bone is necessary.

Management

Refer for evaluation for early surgical intervention to ↓ morbidity. Conservative medical management is often successful as well. Treatment for uncomplicated disease is usually 6 months, extended to 9 to 12 months for more complicated disease.

Complications

Cord compression can occur during the active phase of the infection, which may result in paraplegia.

Tuberculous Meningitis

- Patients may **present** with headache, fevers, meningismus, vomiting, and other neurologic signs.
- Obtain an **AFB stain and culture of CSF.** Hydrocephalus is noted in a minority of patients on CT scan.
- Give **corticosteroids** for the first 6 to 8 weeks of therapy to ↓ mortality in both children and adults.

Gastrointestinal Infections

GASTROENTERITIS AND COLITIS

An acute infection of the gastrointestinal tract with multiple pathogenic etiologies (Table 6.15), primarily characterized by diarrhea and vomiting. Globally, diarrheal illnesses are the second leading cause of death behind cardiovascular disease and are the leading cause of death in children. However, most cases are mild and self-limited. Enteric pathogens are transmitted via the fecal-oral route, and risk factors for acquisition include travel, AIDS/immunocompromise, institutional care, and recent antibiotic use. Historical clues and diarrhea descriptions can be helpful in determining the etiologic agent.

Symptoms

- **Noninflammatory diarrhea:** Pathogens act primarily in the **small intestine** to induce fluid secretion. Patients have **large-volume, watery diarrhea** and nausea, vomiting, cramping, and minimal fever. Most common causes in the United States are viruses (rotavirus, norovirus, adenovirus), *Salmonella,* and *E coli.*
- **Inflammatory diarrhea:** Pathogens induce inflammation in the **colon** via invasion or cytotoxins. Patients present with fever, **small-volume stools containing blood or mucus,** tenesmus, and lower abdominal cramping. Most common causes in the United States are *Shigella, Campylobacter,* and enterohemorrhagic *E coli.*

Exam

- Signs of dehydration, abdominal tenderness, and distention are commonly seen.
- Fever >38.5°C (101.3°F), abdominal guarding or rigidity (acute abdomen), and systemic signs (hypotension, tachycardia, altered mental status) are seen in severe illness.

TABLE 6.15. **Microbiology of Infectious Diarrhea**

INFLAMMATORY DIARRHEA	NONINFLAMMATORY DIARRHEA	GROSSLY BLOODY DIARRHEA	DIARRHEA IN HIV/AIDS PATIENTS	TRAVELER'S DIARRHEA
Bacteria:	**Bacteria:**	**Bacteria:**	**Bacteria:**	**Major causes:**
▪ *Campylobacter jejuni*	▪ *S aureus*	▪ Enterohemorrhagic *E coli*	▪ *Campylobacter jejuni*	▪ Enterotoxigenic *E coli*
▪ *Shigella* spp	▪ *Bacillus cereus*	▪ *Shigella* spp	▪ *Shigella* spp	**Less common causes:**
▪ Enterohemorrhagic *E coli*[a]	▪ *Clostridium perfringens*	▪ *Campylobacter jejuni*	▪ *Salmonella* spp	▪ *Campylobacter jejuni*
▪ *C difficile*	▪ Enterotoxigenic *E coli*	**Protozoa:**	▪ *C difficile*	▪ *Shigella* spp
▪ *Vibrio parahaemolyticus*[b]	▪ *Vibrio cholerae*	▪ *Entamoeba histolytica*	▪ Enteroaggregative *E coli*	▪ *Salmonella* spp
▪ *Listeria monocytogenes*	▪ *Mycobacterium avium* complex		▪ *Mycobacterium avium* complex	▪ Rotavirus
▪ *Yersinia enterocolitica*	▪ *Aeromonas hydrophila*		**Viruses:**	▪ Norwalk virus
▪ Enteroinvasive *E coli*	▪ *Plesiomonas shigelloides*		▪ CMV	▪ *Vibrio parahaemolyticus*
▪ Enteroaggregative *E coli*	**Viruses:**		▪ Enteric adenovirus	▪ *Entamoeba histolytica*
Viruses:	▪ Rotavirus		▪ Caliciviruses	▪ *Giardia lamblia*
▪ CMV	▪ Enteric adenovirus		▪ HIV enteropathy	▪ *Cryptosporidium parvum*
Protozoa:	▪ Caliciviruses		**Protozoa:**	▪ *Cyclospora cayetanensis*
▪ *Entamoeba histolytica*	▪ Norwalk virus		▪ *Cryptosporidium parvum*	
	▪ CMV		▪ *Isospora belli*	
	Protozoa:		▪ *Cyclospora cayetanensis*	
	▪ *Cryptosporidium parvum*		▪ *Microsporidia* spp	
	▪ *Giardia lamblia*			
	▪ *Cyclospora cayetanensis*			
	▪ *Isospora belli*			
	▪ *Microsporidia* spp			

[a]Cases can have no fever or focal leukocytes.

[b]May also cause a noninflammatory syndrome.

Reproduced with permission from Wilson WR. *Current Diagnosis & Treatment in Infectious Diseases*, 1st ed. New York: McGraw-Hill, 2001:261.

Differential

Noninfectious causes include drugs, food allergies, irritable bowel syndrome, malabsorption, and motility disorders.

Diagnosis

▪ The history and physical exam are paramount and are usually sufficient to guide management.
▪ Further evaluation is indicated in the setting of severe symptoms and signs, bloody diarrhea, immunocompromise, age >70 years, or severe dehydration.
▪ Initial tests to help guide severity and management if above risk factors present: **Blood tests** (CBC, electrolytes).
▪ Additional tests to consider: **Stool studies**. Leukocytes (when present, suggest colonic inflammation and inflammatory diarrhea; when absent with bloody diarrhea, may point toward amebiasis), lactoferrin (another marker of colonic inflammation), O&P (in recent travelers or immunocompromised patients), *Giardia* antigen, *C difficile* toxin, bacterial culture, amoeba serologies. Let the lab know of suspected causative bacteria, as different media are required for the various possibilities.
▪ **Endoscopy:** Flexible sigmoidoscopy or colonoscopy with biopsy for chronic diarrhea or in select cases of unclear acute infection. Notable findings in *C difficile* colitis include pseudomembrane formation (Figure 6.18).

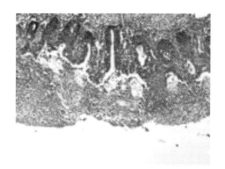

FIGURE 6.18. **Pseudomembranous colitis.** Destruction and eventual necrosis of the superficial crypts under light microscopy with resultant formation of a "pseudomembrane" on the luminal surface, which is composed of neutrophils, mucus, fibrin, and necrotic debris. (Reproduced with permission from USMLE-Rx.com.)

Management

- **Mild diarrhea:**
  - Oral rehydration therapy with oral glucose-electrolyte solutions.
  - A **BRAT** diet (**B**ananas, **R**ice, **A**pplesauce, **T**oast) is recommended but is not evidence based.
  - **Antidiarrheals:** Loperamide. Use with caution in infectious diarrhea, as it may prolong the duration of symptoms, lead to toxic megacolon, and ↑ the risk of hemolytic-uremic syndrome (HUS). Not recommended in children.
  - Oral probiotics may shorten the course of viral diarrhea in children.
- **Severe diarrhea:** Oral or IV rehydration. Consider hospital admission.
- **Antibiotics:**
  - Use only in the presence of fever, tenesmus, bloody stool (unless enterohemorrhagic *E coli* [EHEC] is suspected), fecal leukocytes, or cultures/antigen tests ⊕ for bacteria or protozoa.
  - Empiric treatment for bacterial enteritis/colitis consists of ciprofloxacin 500 mg PO BID or 400 mg IV BID × 3 days.
  - Antibiotics **are** recommended for *Campylobacter* infection, shigellosis, cholera, extraintestinal salmonellosis, severe traveler's diarrhea, *C difficile* colitis (stop other antibiotics if possible and start metronidazole or vancomycin), giardiasis (metronidazole), amebiasis (metronidazole), and AIDS-related infectious diarrhea.
  - Antibiotics **are not** recommended for nontyphoidal *Salmonella* (may prolong shedding), *Aeromonas*, *E coli* O157:H7 (may cause HUS), or *Yersinia* infections.

Prevention

- For infectious gastroenteritis or colitis, frequent hand washing with soap and water is critical, especially for care providers, as well as appropriate cleaning of fomites. (Note: *C difficile* spores are not killed by alcohol-based hand sanitizers. However, in other circumstances, hand gels are more effective than soap and water in ↓ bacterial colony counts on the hands.)
- Avoid excessive or unnecessary antibiotic use: *C difficile* is largely an iatrogenic infection.
- Vaccinate appropriate neonates against rotavirus, a two- or three-dose series given in the first 6 months of life. Notable rare complication of intussusception with vaccination. See ACIP guidelines from 2009 for full details.

Complications

- Volume depletion and electrolyte abnormalities are common.
- **HUS** is seen with **EHEC.** Patients present with renal failure, microangiopathic hemolytic anemia, and thrombocytopenia. Antibiotics and antimotility agents may ↑ the risk. Risk of HUS is greatest in children and the elderly.
- Guillain-Barré syndrome is a potential complication of *C jejuni* and presents with ascending paralysis.
- In severe *C difficile* colitis, the bowel mucosa can be compromised, leading to peritonitis requiring surgical management.
- Some enteroviruses can cause encephalitis (see discussion of encephalitis in the Central Nervous System Infections section above).

Special Situations

- **Diverticulitis** is a bacterial infection of preexisting diverticulosis (small outpouchings) of the colon, most commonly the sigmoid.
  - Mild disesase may be treated in the outpatient setting: clears with or without antibiotics for 2 to 3 days.

KEY FACT

Incidence of **community-acquired** *C difficile* diarrhea is ↑.

MNEMONIC

To prevent traveler's diarrhea:

Remind your patients to use the **5 P's** when choosing food to eat: Make sure it is:

Peeled
Piping hot
Packaged
Purified or
Pasteurized

MNEMONIC

HoUSe RAT:

Hemolytic **U**remic **S**yndrome leads to **R**enal failure, **A**nemia, and **T**hrombocytopenia.

- If disease is severe (ie, peritonitis, inability to tolerate PO, or suspect complications), hospitalize and treat with IV antibiotic coverage for gram-negative and anaerobic organisms. In patients with a severe or complicated case (perforation, sepsis) or multiple (usually more than three) uncomplicated cases, interval surgical resection (when the patient is not infected) is indicated for preventing recurrent severe disease.
- **Appendicitis** is a bacterial infection of the appendix coli (see Figure 12.2 in the Surgery chapter).
    - **History and exam:** Hallmarks are anorexia, nausea, fever, and initial periumbilical pain that localizes to the RLQ (specifically, two-thirds the distance from umbilicus to the right anterior superior iliac spine, called the **McBurney point**). The patient may have peritoneal signs.
    - **Initial test** is CBC.
    - **Best test** to confirm is CT imaging. **Can also use** ultrasound or MRI if CT is contraindicated.
    - **Treatment is surgical,** with interval antibiotics if surgery is delayed.

HEPATIC DISEASE

Hepatitis A

Most common in developing countries. The infection occurs sporadically or in epidemics associated with **seafood, especially shellfish.** HAV is **transmitted via the fecal-oral route** and causes acute hepatitis. Although rare, it can cause severe disease, including fulminant hepatic failure, especially in immunocompromised patients and pregnant women. Severe disease is more common in individuals with HCV coinfection. Symptoms and mortality vary with patient age.

Symptoms/Exam

- Adults present with flulike illness, RUQ pain, jaundice, and pruritus. Children may be asymptomatic.
- Physical exam reveals jaundice and RUQ tenderness.

Differential

- **Viral infections:** HAV, HCV, mononucleosis (EBV), CMV, HSV.
- **Nonviral infections:** Spirochetal disease (leptospirosis, syphilis), rickettsial disease (Q fever), acute bacterial gastroenteritis.
- **Noninfectious causes:** Autoimmune hepatitis, alcoholic hepatitis, fatty liver disease, hemochromatosis, Wilson disease, gallbladder disease.

Diagnosis

Anti-HAV IgM will be $\oplus$ in acute infection, whereas IgG will be $\oplus$ in prior infection or immunization.

Management/Prevention

- Treatment is supportive. Patients with severe symptoms such as dehydration from GI losses or signs of liver failure should be hospitalized and appropriate diagnostic and treatment measures given.
- Vaccination (a series of two) should be given to travelers going to endemic regions, men who have sex with men (MSM), people who inject drugs, people living with HIV (PLHIV), patients with chronic liver disease, food handlers, and day care center workers. HAV vaccine is a formalin-killed vaccine. This is now a routine vaccine for children.

Traveler's diarrhea caused by enterotoxigenic *E coli*.

KEY FACT

Serologic markers for HBV (ie, HBsAg, HBeAg, anti-HBe) can change over time. If there is concern for infection, markers should be monitored periodically along with ALT and HBV DNA viral load.

- Anti-HAV immune globulin may be given to household contacts of infected patients and to those who have eaten uncooked food prepared by an infected individual. However, in many circumstances, HAV vaccine can be used for postexposure prophylaxis in place of immune globulin.

Hepatitis B

Chronic infection with HBV is present in > 400 million people worldwide. **Transmission occurs via exposure to infected body fluids**—ie, blood and semen. Although most individuals clear the infection, 5% to 10% of infected people will become chronic HBV carriers. Of all patients with chronic HBV, 15% to 20% will develop cirrhosis and 10% to 15% will develop hepatocellular carcinoma (HCC). In mothers with acute HBV or those who carry HBsAg and HBeAg, the rate of transmission to the infant is about 90%. Risk of developing a chronic infection is associated with the age at which the person was exposed to the virus. More than 90% of infections become chronic if patient is exposed during infancy (unless hepatitis B immune globulin [HBIG] is given), 30% if during childhood, and <5% if exposed during adulthood. Coinfection with HDV is associated with a worse prognosis.

Symptoms/Exam

- **Acute HBV:** Often asymptomatic. Symptoms, if present, are nonspecific, flulike symptoms such as malaise, anorexia, weakness, low-grade fever, nausea, and vomiting. RUQ pain and jaundice will also be present.
- **Chronic HBV:** Usually asymptomatic.
- **Extrahepatic manifestations:** Serum sickness–like rash, polyarteritis nodosa, glomerulonephritis.
- **Acute HBV:** Scleral icterus, jaundice, RUQ tenderness, arthralgias.
- **Chronic HBV:** Stigmata of cirrhosis, such as spider angiomata, palmar erythema, gynecomastia, caput medusae, and ascites.

Differential

See the differential for HAV above.

Diagnosis

- Best and most accurate test: Serologic markers are the gold standard (Table 6.16).
- Check LFTs to assess disease progress: ↑ transaminases, bilirubin, and PT/PTT.
  - **HBsAg:** Surface antigen. Indicates **acute** or chronic HBV infection.

TABLE 6.16. **Commonly Encountered Serologic Patterns of HBV**

HBSAG	ANTI-HBS	ANTI-HBC	HBEAG	ANTI-HBE	INTERPRETATION
+	–	IgM	+	–	Acute or chronic HBV atitis B
+	–	IgG[a]	+	–	Chronic hepatitis B with active viral replication
+	–	IgG	–	+	Chronic hepatitis B with low viral replication
+	+	IgG	+ or –	+ or –	Chronic hepatitis B with heterotypic anti-HBs
–	–	IgM	+ or –	–	Acute hepatitis B
–	+	–	–	–	Vaccination (immunity)
–	–	IgG	–	–	False ⊕; infection in remote past and anti-HBs has waned; window period; low-level chronic infection

[a]Low levels of IgM anti-HBc may also be detected.

- **Anti-HBs:** Antibody to surface antigen. Serves as the **protective** antibody and indicates past viral infection or immunization.
- **Anti-HBc:** Antibody to core antigen. IgG indicates **prior or current HBV infection.** IgM indicates acute infection.
- **HBeAg:** Envelope antigen. Proportional to the quantity of intact virus—a sign of infectivity.
- HBV DNA: Can be used to measure active replication.
- Liver biopsy is not routinely needed but should be considered if the diagnosis is in question or to rule out other processes.

Management

There is no cure, however it is possible for the body to clear the virus on its own. For those who cannot clear the virus, the goal is to suppress the virus to prevent progression of liver disease.

- **Acute exposure/postexposure prophylaxis:** If the source has hepatitis B and the exposed patient is unvaccinated, the CDC recommends that HBIG be given as soon as possible, ideally within 7 days, along with the first dose of vaccine to start the immunization process. Babies born to infected women should receive HBIG and HBV vaccine in the first 24 hours of life, followed by three doses of the vaccine in the first 6 months of life (prevents infection in 85%-95% of infants exposed).
- **Chronic active HBV:** The AASLD/IDSA published a consensus guideline in *Hepatology* (2009) for consideration of HBV treatment. The risk-to-benefit ratio of treatment depends on the presence of HBeAg, viral load, transaminitis, and liver biopsy results, with recommendations to treat patients who show persistent elevation in viral load, transaminitis, or parenchymal damage without an alternative cause on liver biopsy. For those with cirrhosis, treat if the HBV DNA viral load is >2000 IU/ml and always treat if there is decompensated cirrhosis. For those without cirrhosis, consider treatment for the following:
  - HBeAg ⊕, elevated ALT, and HBV DNA viral load >20,000 IU/mL.
  - HBeAG ⊖, elevated ALT, HBV DNA viral load >2000 IU/mL.
  - **Antiviral agents:** First-line therapy in most cases. Lamivudine given PO is well tolerated but resistance develops when used as monotherapy. Adefovir, entecavir, telbivudine, and tenofovir are alternatives for 1° therapy and may have activity against lamivudine-resistant virus. Treatment should not have HIV activity if there is coinfection of HIV and patient is not on antiretroviral medication.
  - Pegylated **interferon-α:** Given SQ for 4 to 6 months. Confers long-term benefit in 33% of cases but has many adverse effects and is contraindicated in some cases (eg, advanced cirrhosis, decompensated psychiatric disease).
  - **Corticosteroids:** Not indicated for viral hepatitis.
  - **Liver transplant:** Consider in eligible patients with decompensated cirrhosis.
  - Chronic carriers should be encouraged to avoid hepatotoxic agents, including EtOH and high-dose acetaminophen.
- The risk of HCC is very high in chronic HBV carriers. They should be screened for HCC with imaging every 6 to 12 months with or without an α-fetoprotein test.

Prevention

- 1° prevention is accomplished by the HBV vaccine, a recombinant vaccine. A series of three vaccines provides detectable HBsAb levels in >95% of individuals.
- Patients with known HBV should be vaccinated against HAV.

Complications

- HCC can develop **before** cirrhosis in patients with HBV (this is not the case in HCV).
- Approximately 0.1% of patients develop fulminant hepatic failure.

Hepatitis C

Generally transmitted via blood. Before screening, HCV was the most common cause of posttransfusion hepatitis, accounting for 90% of all such cases. Today, most infections occur due to shared needles (60% in the United States), but occupational exposure as well as sexual and vertical transmission may also be seen. Chronic HCV infection occurs in about 75% of those exposed; the remaining patients clear the virus without sequelae. Approximately 20% of carriers develop cirrhosis within 20 years. HCC risk is 1% to 4% per year of cirrhosis. Rates of coinfection with HIV in high-risk populations can exceed 50%, and HIV coinfection accelerates the risk of cirrhosis and HCC.

The CDC recommends screening everyone born between 1945 and 1965 at least once, as well as people who inject drugs, use intranasal drugs, are on long-term hemodialysis, and received tattoos from unregulated places.

Symptoms/Exam

- **Acute HCV:** Generally asymptomatic or symptoms are very mild and nonspecific such as fatigue, abdominal pain, and anorexia.
- **Chronic HCV:** Mostly asymptomatic as well, but may include renal failure, vasculitic skin rash, and arthralgias, all caused by cryoglobulinemia and sicca syndrome.
- Symptoms of cirrhosis may also be seen.
- Exam findings same as in HBV.

Differential

See the HAV differential above.

Diagnosis

- Best **initial test:** HCV antibody.
- After diagnosis, check: LFTs, coagulation, HBV/HAV immunity, HCV genotype, and viral load. Signs of cirrhosis on exam warrant liver ultrasound.
- **HCV antibody** will be present 8 to 12 weeks after infection and will remain ⊕ even after treatment or clearance. HCV viral load can be used to detect viremia to confirm an acute infection. A ⊕ HCV viral load in an antibody ⊖ patient may indicate chronic infection in an immunocompromized patient. If qualitative PCR is used, antibody may appear as soon as 2 weeks postinfection. Use HCV viral load to check for reinfection or for those with recent exposure (<6 months).
- Liver biopsy can be used to determine the extent of cirrhosis, giving prognostic information. Biopsy is not required before initiating therapy.

Management

- Now curable!
- Prior to treatment, check viral genotype and evaluate for advanced fibrosis with imaging, serology, or biopsy.
- Treatment is indicated for all patients except for those with short life expectancies due to a condition that will not improve with HCV or liver transplant. No longer is treatment restricted to those who are not using drugs or alcohol.
- **First-line treatment:**
  - Highly effective HCV protease inhibitor therapy (ie, ledipasvir/sofosbuvir, elbasvir/grazoprevir). Treatment is generally 12 weeks, with >99% of patients achieving a sustained virologic response. Treatment depends on the genotype and may be extended up to 48 weeks depending on genotype/cirrhosis. Can add pegylated interferon and ribaviron in certain genotypes.
  - Those with HCV infection be immunized for HAV and HBV unless s/he has already demonstrated immunity.

ANSWER

Hepatitis serologies, including a hepatitis C antibody, HIV antibody, LFTs, CBC, and coagulation profile. Obtain abdominal imaging and ensure follow-up for further evaluation and treatment.

Hepatic Abscess

The liver is the most common organ for abscess development, aside from the skin. Pyogenic liver abscesses are generally polymicrobial and can develop through bacterial invasion from the biliary tree (most common), portal vein, or hepatic artery as well as through direct trauma or adjacent bacterial infection. Approximately 15% to 40% of abscesses have no known cause and are termed **cryptogenic.** Predisposing factors include advanced age, male gender, diabetes, malignancy, inflammatory bowel disease, and a history of diverticulitis or cirrhosis. Common organisms include *E coli*, *Klebsiella pneumoniae*, *Proteus vulgaris*, *Enterobacter aerogenes*, and other gram-negative and anaerobic organisms. Streptococci may also be present. Consider other etiologies as well, eg, *Entamoeba histolytica* in immigrants and travelers or *Candida* spp in neutropenic hosts.

Symptoms/Exam

- Onset is generally insidious. **Fever** is the most common presenting symptom.
- RUQ/epigastric pain, chills, nausea/vomiting, and weight loss are additional symptoms. Referred right shoulder pain occurs as well.
- Fever, jaundice, RUQ tenderness.

Differential

Cholelithiasis, cholecystitis, cholangitis, hepatitis, gastritis, pancreatitis.

Diagnosis

- **Best initial step: Labs:** CBC, LFTs (nonspecific elevations, but alkaline phosphatase is ↑ in 70% of patients), and blood cultures (⊕ in 33% to 100% of cases). Also check CRP and serology for *E hisotolytica*.
- **Next best step: Imaging:** Abdominal CT with contrast has high sensitivity for diagnosis and is the imaging modality of choice, but ultrasound, MRI, and/or tagged WBC scan can detect hepatic abscesses as well (Figure 6.19).

Management

- Depends on if it is a pyogenic liver abscess versus an amoebic liver abcess.
- Pyogenic liver abscess: prompt drainage and antibiotics for at least 2 to 6 weeks. Aim to cover gram-negative organisms and anaerobes—ie, use a third-generation cephalosporin and metronidazole or a carbapenem. Treatment should be initiated

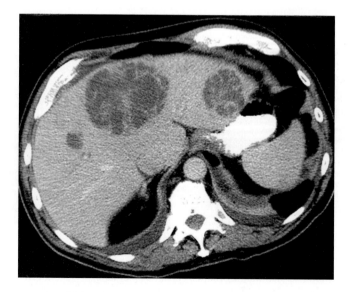

FIGURE 6.19. **Multiple pyogenic liver abscesses.** L = liver; S = spleen. (Reproduced with permission from Brunicardi FC, et al. *Schwartz's Principles of Surgery,* 9th ed. New York: McGraw-Hill, 2010, Fig. 31-19.)

by IV, start broad and then narrow using cultures from drainage. Treatment is often continued until radiographic resolution for bacterial liver abscesses.

- Amoebic liver abscess: treat with PO antibiotics alone, metronidazole × 7 to 10 days followed by paromomycin × 7 days. Clinical response is usually prompt, but imaging improvement/resolution lags and should not lead to prolonged or repeated treatment.

BILIARY INFECTIONS: CHOLECYSTITIS, CHOLANGITIS

Infections of the biliary tree are most commonly caused by gram-negative enteric pathogens in the setting of biliary obstruction (gallstones, biliary, or pancreatic mass). **Cholecystitis** is an acute or chronic purulent infection of the gallbladder, causing surrounding pericholecystic inflammation. **Cholangitis** is a purulent infection of the biliary tree, specifically the common bile duct, and is associated with a higher degree of morbidity and mortality.

Symptoms/Exam

- In cholecystitis, classic symptoms include RUQ/epigastric pain worst immediately postprandial (due to contraction of an inflamed gallbladder), fever/rigors, and nausea/vomiting. Jaundice may be present, and pain may be referred to the right shoulder due to the phrenic nerve.
- **Classic findings in severe ascending cholangitis** are termed **Reynolds pentad** (fever, RUQ pain, jaundice, altered mental status, and hypotension).
- **Charcot triad** in cholangitis: Fever, jaundice, RUQ tenderness.

Differential

Cholelithiasis, hepatitis, gastritis, pancreatitis, hepatic abscess.

Diagnosis

- **Labs:** CBC, LFTs, blood cultures, CRP.
- **Imaging:** Best initial imaging is ultrasound. MRCP is more sensitive and may help plan for either ERCP or surgery. CT with contrast, or nuclear medicine HIDA scan can be used to visualize the gallbladder and biliary tree (Figure 6.20).

Management

- **Antibiotics:** Initial coverage should include activity against gram-negative and anaerobic pathogens (β-lactam or cephalosporin or fluoroquinolone plus metronidazole; or monotherapy with carbapenem).

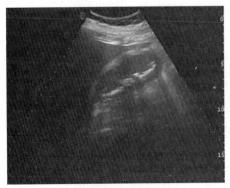
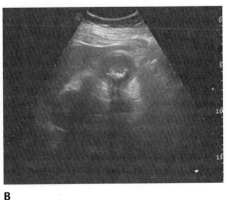

A   B

FIGURE 6.20. **Cholecystitis.** Longitudinal (**A**) and transverse (**B**) ultrasound images of a distended gallbladder containing mobile echogenic debris with posterior shadowing (gallstones), gallbladder wall thickening, and pericholecystic fluid. (Reproduced from Mazzei MA, et al. The role of US examination in the management of acute abdomen. *Crit Ultrasound J.* 2013;5(Suppl 1):S6.)

- ERCP with sphincterotomy may be used to allow passage of obstructing gallstones and infected bile. If abscess is present and not relieved by endoscopic intervention, it may be drained by percutaneous cholecystostomy and, less commonly, open surgical approaches. If duct stenosis is present, biopsies and brushings via ERCP are often taken to rule out malignancy as the cause of stenosis.
- Admission to ICU for patients with hypotension or evidence of shock or concomitant organ failure.
- Patients with acute infection should have a surgical consult for cholecystectomy. In cholangitis, cholecystectomy can be performed after drainage. Early cholecystectomy (within 24-72 hours) is preferred for cholecystitis. However, if there is severe inflammation or organ dysfunction, choleycstecomy can be delayed.

Complications

- Abscess or necrosis of the biliary tree, including biliary extravasation into the peritoneum requiring surgical exploration and wash-out.
- Severe sepsis and ARDS, more commonly in the setting of ascending cholangitis ± concomitant pancreatitis.

Genitourinary Disorders

URINARY TRACT INFECTION

Infection along the urinary tract, from the renal parenchyma to urethra. Commonly divided into cystitis (when isolated to the bladder and distal structures) and pyelonephritis (when affecting the kidneys ± other structures). Generally more common in women. A UTI in a man should prompt a urologic workup. UTIs can be classified as complicated or uncomplicated:

- **Uncomplicated:** Cystitis in a young, healthy, nonpregnant woman. The most common organisms are *E coli* and *Staphylococcus saprophyticus*. Less common are *Proteus mirabilis*, *Klebsiella* spp, and *Enterococcus* spp.
- **Complicated:** Defined as cystitis in anyone else—eg, male, elderly, hospitalized, and pregnant patients; or pyelonephritis in any patient. Complicating factors may include an indwelling catheter, recent catheterization, anatomic abnormalities, recent antibiotics, symptoms >1 week, immunosuppression, diabetes, recurrent UTI, or a history of resistant UTI. Culture data will be important for treatment, and duration of therapy should be longer.

Symptoms/ Exam

- **Cystitis** commonly presents with a triad of dysuria, frequency, and urgency. Gross hematuria, fever, or suprapubic pain may also be present.
- **Pyelonephritis** presents with flank or back pain and fever. These are usually accompanied by one or more of the symptoms of cystitis, beginning 1 to 2 days prior. Patients may also have nausea, vomiting, abdominal pain, and/or diarrhea.
- In cystitis, suprapubic tenderness may be present; **fever is uncommon.**
- Pyelonephritis findings include fever, CVA tenderness, mild to severe abdominal tenderness, and, in severe cases, hypotension and organ failure.
- Perform a pelvic exam in sexually active women if STIs are being considered in the differential.
- Perform a rectal exam in men to rule out prostatitis; however, vigorous prostate massage can lead to bacteremia and should be avoided.

QUESTION 1

A 43-year-old woman presents to the ED with acute onset of fever, chills, and right shoulder pain. She reports vomiting an hour ago after eating lunch. Her exam is remarkable for fever of 39°C (102.2°F), BP of 105/60 mm Hg, ⊕ Murphy sign, and rigors. What is your next step?

KEY FACT

Usually the same species that caused the prior UTI is responsible for subsequent infections. You do not have to reculture with each subsequent UTI unless you suspect treatment failure.

QUESTION 2

A 24-year-old woman presents with fever, nausea, and mild dysuria. She says that she has had two bladder infections in the past, but she adds that this feels "a little different." On exam, her temperature is 38.0°C (100.4°F), and she has mild epigastric pain and moderate CVA tenderness on the right side. UA shows ⊕ leukocyte esterase, 20 to 50 WBCs, and more than three bacteria. What would be the most appropriate choice of antibiotic for this patient?

Differential

- **Prostatitis:** In acute prostatitis, men present with fever, chills, dysuria, frequency, and perineal and low back pain. Exam will reveal an exquisitely tender prostate. Although it is most often caused by *E coli*, other Enterobacteriaceae are common as well. Treatment should continue for 4 weeks.
- **Other:** Pyelonephritis, epididymitis, STIs, vaginitis (including atrophic), nephrolithiasis, interstitial cystitis, "bubble-bath" urethritis, and bladder tumors.

Diagnosis

- **Best initial test:** UA. UA typically shows leukocyte esterase, protein, blood, WBCs, and RBCs. With infection due to ammonia splitting bacteria, such as *E coli*, nitrites may be positive. Urine microscopy will show ↑ WBC, ↑ RBC, and bacteria. ↑ Squamous cells suggests a contaminated specimen.
- **Most accurate test:** Urine culture. A person with symptomatic UTIs should have at least one episode with a urine culture to help guide treatment and to confirm diagnosis. At least 100,000 colony-forming units of a pathogenic single organism should be present, although less than this may be significant in men, in a specimen obtained through catheter, or in complicated UTI in women.
- Additional tests may include focused STI testing, wet mount, and KOH if there is a concern for vaginitis.
- Need for other laboratory evaluation in UTI depends on severity of illness.

Management

- **Outpatient:** For **uncomplicated cystitis**, treatment options are the following: 3 days of treatment with trimethoprim-sulfamethoxazole (TMP-SMX) or a fluoroquinolone, a single dose of fosfomycin or nitrofurantoin for 5 days. **Phenazopyridine** can be used for symptomatic treatment of severe dysuria for up to 2 days.
  - **Pregnancy:** Nitrofurantoin is safe in pregnancy. Note that fluoroquinolones are contraindicated in pregnancy and TMP-SMX is not recommended in the first and third trimesters.
  - In **complicated UTI** in outpatients, fluoroquinolone × 7 to 14 days can be used. Second-line therapy consists of either amoxicillin/clavulanate or TMP-SMX for the same duration. Susceptibility results should be confirmed.
- **Inpatient:** Patients may require hospitalization if they are unable to tolerate PO treatment, if signs of urosepsis are present, or if pregnant. Antibiotic therapy should be initiated early and guided by local antibiotic sensitivities.
  - IV ceftriaxone is a reasonable empiric choice for most patients; however, resistance is developing, especially among *E coli* (ESBL strains; see Emerging Antibiotic Resistance section).
  - Add ampicillin if **enterococcus** is suspected.
- Radiologic evaluation for complications may be necessary in patients who are severely ill, are immunocompromised, or are not responding to treatment, as well as for patients in whom complications are likely (eg, pregnant patients, patients with diabetes, and those with nephrolithiasis, reflux, transplant surgery, or other GU surgery).
- Plain films can detect radiopaque stones (uric acid and indinavir stones are radiolucent), some masses, and abnormal gas collections.
- Ultrasound can examine the ureters and kidneys for fluid collections and stones. Ultrasound and voiding cystoureterography can evaluate patients suspected of having reflux disease.
- CT with and without contrast is most sensitive but may be contraindicated in those with impaired renal function.

Complications

- Perinephric abscess should be considered in patients who remain febrile 2 to 3 days after appropriate antibiotics (Figure 6.21). Patients with large abscesses or those who have failed antibiotics alone are treated by percutaneous or surgical drainage.
- Intrarenal abscess (eg, infection of a renal cyst) <5 cm usually responds to antibiotics alone.
- Patients with diabetes may develop emphysematous pyelonephritis. This condition once required urgent nephrectomy because of its high mortality rate, but now it is often treated medically with percutaneous drainage.
- In pregnant patients, pyelonephritis is associated with ↑ risk of preterm delivery and maternal complications.
- **Recurrence:**
  - Any patient with new symptoms of a UTI >2 weeks after resolution of a prior UTI has a recurrence. Patients with two or more recurrences in a 6-month period may need suppression. There are several antibiotics of choice for recurrent UTI, including daily nitrofurantoin or TMP-SMX. Postcoital antibiotics are an option for sexually active women. Antibiotic prophylaxis may ↓ recurrence but may ↑ resistance. May offer antibiotic prescriptions for patients to self initiate treatment if they have recurrent UTIs.
  - In patients with recurrent complicated UTIs, consider discussion with a urologist and imaging with IVP, renal ultrasound, or CT to rule out anatomic abnormalities or nephrolithiasis, which may act as a nidus for infection. Struvite stones (staghorn calculi) are associated with recurrent UTIs due to urease-producing bacteria (*Proteus, Pseudomonas,* and *Klebsiella*).

Prevention

Patients with recurrent UTIs are commonly instructed to clean themselves away from the urethra and to void immediately after intercourse. Although limited, data suggest that these maneuvers are not helpful. Drinking cranberry juice, which ↓ bacterial adherence to the uroepithelium, has been shown to be helpful in some studies. Diaphragm and spermicide use and douching in women should be avoided. Topical estrogen can be considered in postmenopausal women. There is ↑ frequency of UTIs in uncircumcised infant males.

KEY FACT

Risk factors for recurrent UTIs in premenopausal women include: sexual intercourse ≥3 times/wk, spermicide use, new or multiple partners, or a previous UTI prior to the age of 15 years.

KEY FACT

Asymptomatic bacteria should not be treated unless the patient is pregnant or is pre-op for a traumatic urologic procedure (ie, TURP).

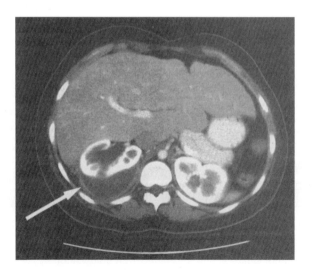

FIGURE 6.21. Perinephric abscess. Acute right pyelonephritis complicated by right perinephric abscess (arrow). (Reproduced with permission from McAninch JW, Lue TF. *Smith's General Urology.* 18th ed. New York, NY: McGraw-Hill; 2013, Fig. 14-4.)

Skin, Soft Tissue, and Orthopedic Infections

CELLULITIS AND SKIN ABSCESS

Common skin and soft tissue infections (SSTIs) of the dermis, either diffusely infiltrative in cellulitis or creating a loculated purulent focus in abscess. The two can coexist and are usually due to bacterial entry into a laceration, abrasion, or irritated skin without a macroscopic defect. SSTIs are most commonly due to *S aureus* and group A streptococci (*S pyogenes*). Other causes of SSTIs are erysipelas and impetigo, most common in children, and human and animal bite wounds.

Symptoms/Exam

- Pain, warmth, and redness of the skin. Swelling or pus drainage from the skin. Fever indicates a complicated case with systemic illness.
- Erythema (reticular pattern in mild cases, circumferential in more severe cases, sometimes tracking via lymphangitic spread), induration, warmth; in abscess, fluctuance may be found. Regional lymphadenopathy is common.
- **Erysipelas,** due to group A streptococci, typically displays a well-demarcated, tender, intensely erythematous plaque, with possible lymphangitic spread. It is most commonly found on the face and in one-third of cases follows streptococcal pharyngitis.
- **Impetigo** typically causes one or more demarcated plaques or ulcers, with a "honey-colored" crust. It can cause bullae, which rupture and form plaques. Often found around the external nares and mouth of children. Impetigo may be caused by *S aureus* or group A streptococcus.
- Pain out of proportion to exam, crepitus, systemic toxicity, or rapidly progressive exam findings should prompt consideration of **necrotizing fasciitis,** requiring hospital admission with emergent surgical consult. Imaging may show subcutaneous gas and fluid in the fascial planes (Figure 6.22).

Differential

Burns, dermatitis (atopic, contact, photosensitivity), chronic stasis dermatitis (in lower extremities), erythema multiforme, and varicella. Streptococcal and staphylococcal toxic shock syndromes create diffuse erythema (erythroderma). Although gangrene and necrotizing fasciitis are much less common, they have much greater morbidity and mortality and need to be considered in appropriate settings.

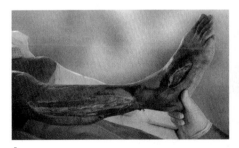
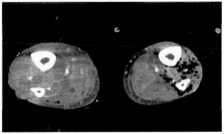

A   **B**

FIGURE 6.22.   **Necrotizing fasciitis.** (A) Gangrenous limb from necrotizing fasciitis after fasciotomy. (B) Contrast-enhanced lower extremity with fluid within the fascial planes and subcutaneous gas consistent with necrotizing fasciitis. (Reproduced from Spadaro S, et al. *Aeromonas sobria* necrotizing fasciitis and sepsis in an immunocompromised patient: a case report and review of the literature. *J Med Case Rep.* 2014;8:315.)

Diagnosis

- Cellulitis, abscess, and associated skin infections are clinical diagnoses.
- **Most accurate test:** Skin biopsy can be obtained in cases with unclear diagnosis.
- Consider x-ray or MRI if there is suspicion for osteomyelitis.
- Culture of cellulitis is not helpful; however, with an abscess, deep wound culture in the setting of incision and drainage, carefully obtained without skin flora contamination, can help tailor antibiotic therapy.
- Common etiologies are group A streptococcus and *S aureus* (*S aureus* is more common for purulent cellulitis and abscess). In most communities, MRSA is common enough that **all staph infections should be treated empirically** as MRSA until proven otherwise. In immunocompromised hosts, gram-negative flora are a possible cause (see section on Diabetic Foot Infections). In neonates, group B streptococci are a possible cause and can present with sepsis. β-hemolytic streptococci other than GAS (most commonly, group B streptococci and group G streptococci) may cause SSTI in older persons or those with underlying illness. Rarely, fungus or other atypical bacteria can cause skin and soft tissue infection. Risk factors for SSTI include immunocompromise, homelessness, severe tinea pedis, and frequent skin trauma, as in injection drug use.

KEY FACT

If you diagnose bilateral cellulitis, it is probably a misdiagnosis. Cellulitis is rarely bilateral. Consider broadening your differential.

Management

- **Uncomplicated cellulitis** can be treated with oral antibiotic therapy to cover streptococci and staphylococci, such as cephalexin or penicillin. Because of the rising prevalence of MRSA, if there are risk factors for a staph infection (ie, penetrating wound, purulent drainage), antibiotics with MRSA coverage such as TMP-SMX, doxycycline, or clindamycin should be strongly considered based on local antibiogram. TMP-SMX and doxycycline do not have adequate coverage for group A streptococci.
- **Uncomplicated abscess** is treated definitively by incision and drainage and does not require antibiotics, unless complicated by surrounding cellulitis or systemic symptoms.
- **Erysipelas** and **impetigo** are effectively treated with similar medications, which have activity against streptococcal and staphylococcal bacteria (again, consider agents with activity against MRSA). Mild cases of impetigo can be treated with topical antibiotics, such as mupirocin, and polymyxin B plus neomycin.
- Infected animal or human **bite wounds** are typically polymicrobial and include aerobic and anaerobic flora. While the specific biting organism's oral flora may differ (humans include *Eikenella corrodens*; dogs and cats include *Pasteurella multocida*, among others), the initial antibiotic coverage is largely similar: oral amoxicillin/clavulanate or intravenous ampicillin/sulbactam or carbapenems. For patients with severe penicillin allergy, a fluoroquinolone plus clindamycin is generally recommended.
- Treatment of immunocompromised hosts may require broader-spectrum coverage (eg, coverage of both gram-positive and gram-negative flora).
- Current guidelines for necrotizing fasciitis recommend broad antibiotic coverage (ie, vancoycin or linezolid plus piperacillin-tazobactam or a carbapenem). If group A strep is known to be the cause, treat with penicillin and clindamycin. **Surgical debridement** must be accomplished urgently and thoroughly, and sometimes amputation is required.

Complications

If not properly treated, superficial SSTIs can progress by lymphatic or hematogenous spread to cause gangrene, necrotizing fasciitis, or sepsis.

Prevention

General good hygiene should be practiced and regular examinations of the extremities performed, particularly in patients with neuropathy. It is important to treat and control for risk factors such as obesity, eczema, and foot hygiene (ie, fungus, fissures, macerated skin). Although evidence is weak, one can consider prophylactic antibiotic therapy for patients who have three or more episodes of cellulitis per year.

SEPTIC ARTHRITIS

KEY FACT

If a young, sexually active patient presents with acute monoarticular joint pain, think about disseminated gonococcal disease.

An infection of the joint space that is usually spread by hematogenous seeding from another site. Risk factors for infection include trauma, diabetes, rheumatoid arthritis (RA), malignancy, frequent glucocorticoid injections, prior joint surgery, and IV drug use. The most common organism is *S aureus*, but other etiologic agents include *H influenzae*, gram-negative bacilli, *S pneumoniae*, β-hemolytic streptococci, and *N gonorrhoeae*.

Symptoms/Exam

- Presents with acute onset of a painful, warm, swollen joint. Fever, chills, ↓ ROM, and skin rash may be seen.
- Although monoarticular more common, may be polyarticular. Most commonly involves the knee and hip; less commonly involves the shoulder, elbow, and small joints. If the sacroiliac or sternoclavicular joints are involved, screen the patient for **IV drug use** (the most common risk factor for these sites).
- Findings include fever, warmth, intra-articular effusion, ↓ ROM, tenderness to palpation, and erythema.
- Tenderness to palpation of bones beyond the region of erythema suggests possible osteomyelitis.

Differential

- **Infectious:** Osteomyelitis, cellulitis, Lyme disease, fungal infection.
- **Rheumatologic:** Gout, pseudogout, SLE, RA, psoriatic arthritis.
- **Other:** Degenerative joint disease, arthritis due to serum sickness, reactive arthritis, or poststreptococcal infection (may be a manifestation of rheumatic fever).

Diagnosis

- **Arthrocentesis: Best initial step** is to obtain a joint aspirate and send for cell count, synovial fluid culture, crystal microscopy, and Gram stain (typically ⊖ in *N gonorrhoeae* septic arthritis) (Table 6.17). **Most accurate test** is synovial culture. A joint aspirate that shows WBC >50,000/mm³ suggests infection but can also be seen in gout. Check for crystals using microscopy to rule out gout.
- **Labs:** Also draw CBC; consider ESR and CRP (serial monitoring of CRP provides evidence of response to treatment); obtain blood cultures (⊕ in <30% of cases).
- Imaging is not diagnostic.
- **Imaging:** Plain films may show soft tissue swelling but are otherwise unhelpful, except in excluding other diagnoses. Consider bone scan or MRI if there is concern for osteomyelitis.
- **Other:** Urethral/cervical testing for *N gonorrhoeae*.

Management

- Joint infection:
  - Drainage can be accomplished by open surgical wash-out (preferred by many orthopedists), arthroscopic wash-out, or percutaneous needle drainage. Surgical wash-out is usually necessary only once, but repeated procedures may be needed. Preferred method of drainage is not clearly established.

TABLE 6.17. **Examination of Synovial Fluid**

	NORMAL	NONINFLAMMATORY	INFLAMMATORY	SEPTIC
Clarity	Transparent	Transparent	Cloudy	Cloudy
Color	Clear	Yellow	Yellow	Yellow
WBC/μL	<200	<200-2000	200-50,000	>50,000
PMNs (%)[a]	<25	<25	>50	>50
Culture	Negative	Negative	Negative	>50% positive
Crystals	None	None	Multiple or none	None
Associated conditions		Osteoarthritis, trauma, rheumatic fever	Gout, pseudogout, spondyloarthropathies, RA, Lyme disease, SLE	Nongonococcal or gonococcal septic arthritis

[a]WBC count and percent PMNs are affected by a number of factors, including disease progression, affecting organism, and host immune status. The joint aspirate WBC and PMNs should be considered part of a continuum for each disease, particularly septic arthritis, and should be correlated with other clinical information.

Reproduced with permission from Tintinalli JE, et al. *Emergency Medicine: A Comprehensive Study Guide*, 6th ed. New York: McGraw-Hill, 2004:1795.

- Start empirical antibiotics after cultures have been sent. Ideally, treat parenterally for 2 to 4 weeks.
- Empirical antimicrobial choice depends on the age of the patient, regardless of sexual activity and Gram stain results.
- Vancomycin ± a third-generation IV cephalosporin is appropriate first-line therapy.
- Because of the rising prevalence of fluoroquinolone-resistant gonococcal disease, agents such as ciprofloxacin and levofloxacin **are no longer recommended** unless susceptibility is confirmed. For N *gonorrhoeae* arthritis, ceftriaxone plus azithromycin can be used as initial therapy, and can be transitioned after 48 to 72 hours of improvement to oral cephalosporins, such as cefpodoxime or cefixime. All individuals with N *gonorrhoeae* arthritis should be tested and treated for *Chlamydia* infection because of the high rate of coinfection.
- **Special situations:** Patients with **prosthetic joints** require surgical intervention.

ACUTE OSTEOMYELITIS

In adults, 80% of osteomyelitis cases result from contiguous spread. These cases often become chronic. This is seen in patients with diabetes, prosthetic joints, decubitus ulcers, trauma, and recent surgery. In 20% of cases, the infection is hematogenous in origin. Risk factors include IV drug use, sickle cell disease, and advanced age. Etiologies are as follows:

- **Common organisms:** S *aureus* (most common), coagulase-negative staphylococci (prosthetic joints or postoperative infections), streptococci and anaerobes (bites, diabetic foot infections, decubitus ulcers), *Pasteurella* spp (animal bites), *Eikenella corrodens* (human bites), P *aeruginosa* (injection drug use and nail punctures).
- **Other causes:** S*almonella* spp (sickle cell patients), M *tuberculosis* (HIV, exposure outside United States), *Bartonella* spp (HIV), *Brucella* spp (unpasteurized dairy products).
- **By most common location:** P *aeruginosa* affects the sternoclavicular joint and symphysis pubis (in IV drug use); *Brucella* spp affect the sacroiliac joint, knee, and hip; and TB affects the lower thoracic vertebrae (Pott disease).

QUESTION

A 54-year-old man presents to the urgent care center with a very painful right knee. The day before, he was cleaning his house and cut his knee with a nail while kneeling on the floor. The knee became painful, warm, and swollen over the last 24 hours. On exam, you find ↓ and exquisitely painful ROM, tenderness, warmth, and erythema of the skin. No other joints are affected, and he has no prior history of these symptoms. What should you do?

Symptoms/Exam

- Localized pain and swelling of the affected extremity or area. Fever is more common in acute osteomyelitis.
- Fever, tenderness, erythema, and swelling over the affected bone. May present as a chronic draining wound that tracks to bone. Ulcers that probe to bone should be assumed to be associated with osteomyelitis.

Differential

Cellulitis, RA, osteoarthritis, diskitis, bone cyst/tumor, septic arthritis, simple skin ulcer.

Diagnosis

- **Labs:** Most accurate test is bone culture, although it often can be negative. CBC, ESR, CRP (serial monitoring of CRP may provide evidence of response to treatment), and blood cultures ($\oplus$ in 10%-50% of cases where hematogenous spread in suspected). Serology for atypical causes can be ordered on an individual basis.
- **Imaging:** Most accurate imaging: **MRI**, especially for vertebral osteomyelitis. **Plain films** are frequently normal but may reveal periosteal elevation or bony erosions especially earlier in the disease course.
- **Bone biopsy and culture:** The gold standard and will in some cases reveal an etiologic agent. Very helpful if $\oplus$, but frequently $\ominus$. Swabs of exposed bone are generally not helpful, as the organisms isolated do not correlate well with organisms in the bone. May be used to determine if S *aureus* is present.

Management

- Empiric antibiotics such as vancomycin plus a third-generation cephalosporin should be started **after** all cultures have been obtained. The regimen should be directed toward the most likely organism(s). After culture results are received, therapy may be narrowed.
- IV antibiotics should be given for 4 to 6 weeks, although some patients may be treated with PO regimens, as guided by culture results.
- Surgery is indicted for spinal cord decompression, bony stabilization, removal of necrotic bone, and reestablishment of vascular supply.
- Complications include epidural abscess and diskitis (with vertebral osteomyelitis). Most osteomyelitis that has invaded contiguous foci is chronic by the time it is diagnosed.
- Chronic osteomyelitis requires longer courses of treatment and is generally not cured without **surgical debridement of infected bone.**

DIABETIC FOOT INFECTIONS

Because of neuropathy, abnormal blood flow, and poor biomechanics of the feet, patients with diabetes are prone to foot ulcers and infections, including osteomyelitis. Although most infections are polymicrobial, common organisms include S *aureus*, streptococci (often group B), gram-negative aerobes, and anaerobic bacteria.

Symptoms/Exam

- May be asymptomatic because of neuropathy or may present with significant pain. Ulcer with eschar is frequently present.
- Exam reveals an ulcer on the foot that may have indurated edges, erythema, swelling, and/or drainage. The plantar surface of the foot is the most common site of infection. Fever is possible.

Differential

Cellulitis, noninfected ulcer, peripheral artery disease, venous stasis ulcer.

ANSWER

Obtain a joint aspirate, call for an orthopedic consult, and begin empiric antibiotics for septic arthritis.

Diagnosis

- **Labs:** CBC, ESR, CRP, HbA_{1c}.
- **Specimen:** Most accurate lab: Culture taken from a debrided ulcer or bone.
- **Imaging:** Plain films are of some use but an **MRI** is more sensitive and specific. Arterial flow to the foot should be assessed with the ankle-brachial index (ABI), especially if pedal pulses are diminished.

Management

- **Wound care:** Can range from daily dressing changes to bedside or intraoperative debridement.
- **Antibiotics:** Mild infections can be treated on an outpatient basis with PO amoxicillin/clavulanate. More extensive infections should be treated with hospitalization and IV antibiotics such as cefepime, piperacillin/tazobactam, or carbapenems. Given the risk of MDR organisms in patients with chronic illness or in long-term care facilities, strongly consider coverage for MRSA, resistant gram-negative rods, and vancomycin-resistant *Enterococcus* (VRE). Typically, 1 to 2 weeks of therapy is sufficient for mild to moderate infection (with IV switched to PO after 48-72 hours) and 2 to 4 weeks in patients with severe or complicated infection.

Prevention

In addition to reasonable glycemic control: frequent foot exams, proper footwear, and routine monofilament neuropathy screening.

Complications

Osteomyelitis, sepsis, need for surgical debridement.

Human Immunodeficiency Virus

Since the initial cases in 1981, more than 78 million people have been infected with HIV and more than 39 million people have died from AIDS and related complications. The CDC estimates there are 1.2 million people living with HIV (PLHIV) in the United States and the WHO estimates there are 36.9 PLHIV globally. In the United States, HIV prevalence rates disproportionally affect people of color, with African Americans having a 6-fold higher prevalence rate than their Caucasian counterparts.

The virus targets and destroys CD4+ T lymphocytes, which leads to AIDS, a state of immunocompromise causing ↑ vulnerability to infection and malignancy. HIV, even in the absence of AIDS, results in noninfectious complications such as metabolic disorders, ↑ rates of coronary heart disease, and endocrinopathies.

HIV is transmitted via percutaneous or mucosal exposure to contaminated body fluids. Fluids such as tears, saliva, urine, and stool are not considered to be infectious unless it is grossly bloody. Markers used to measure progression are **CD4+ count and HIV RNA viral load.** The CD4+ count measures the degree of immunocompromise and predicts the risk of opportunistic infections. Viral load measures HIV replication rate, and genotypic and phenotypic resistance testing can predict the efficacy of specific antiretrovirals.

With antiretroviral therapy (ART), infected individuals can have similar life expectancies as those without the diagnosis and the demographic is aging. However, individual patient outcomes in HIV/AIDS remain largely determined by economics; according to UNAIDS, only two of five PLHIV have access to ART.

QUESTION 1

While you are finishing nursing home rounds, a nurse asks you to inspect a male patient's foot. As you approach the man, you note that he is one of your colleague's elderly patients with diabetes. Exam reveals an erythematous 1.5-cm foot ulcer. The ulcer is draining yellow, foul-smelling material. Pulses in the foot are palpable, but monofilament testing reveals peripheral neuropathy. The patient has been afebrile. What is the most appropriate management of this patient's infection?

QUESTION 2

A 35-year-old man with a 6-year history of HIV comes into your clinic for a routine follow-up. In the last 2 months he has had worsening dysphagia with both solids and liquids. On exam, you notice a moderate amount of thrush on his tongue and oropharynx. In addition to treating his candidal infection, you check a CD4+ cell count, which has ↓ to 150 cells/mm³ and his viral load is 6000. Which chemoprophylactic agents should be started today?

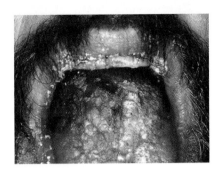

FIGURE 6.23. **Oral thrush in an HIV-positive patient.** (Reproduced from the CDC/Drs. John Molinari and Sol Silverman, Jr.)

Symptoms/Exam

- **1° HIV infection:**
  - Often asymptomatic or may present with **acute retroviral syndrome,** which consists of fever, sore throat, lymphadenopathy, and a truncal maculopapular rash or mucocutaneous ulceration occurring 2 to 6 weeks after initial infection.
  - Other signs and symptoms include myalgias, arthralgias, diarrhea, headache, nausea, vomiting, weight loss, and thrush.
- **Chronic HIV infection:**
  - Suspect and test for in patients with thrush (Figure 6.23), oral hairy leukoplakia, herpes zoster, seborrheic dermatitis, oral aphthous ulcers, or recurrent vaginal candidiasis. Signs and symptoms of opportunistic infections and HIV/AIDS-related malignancy are variable; see the section on AIDS and Opportunistic Infections.
  - Other symptoms may be vague and may include fatigue, fevers, night sweats, diarrhea, dysphagia, dyspnea, persistent lymphadenopathy, weight loss, and altered mental status.

Differential

- Acute retroviral syndrome resembles viral URI, influenza, infectious mononucleosis, acute CMV infection, aseptic meningitis, and syphilis.
- Depending on the manifestation, chronic HIV infection may resemble malignancy, subacute bacterial endocarditis, connective tissue disease, depression, eating disorders, IBD, or malabsorption syndromes.

Diagnosis

- The CDC now recommends HIV testing of all persons 13 to 64 years of age at least once in their lifetimes and at least once in each pregnancy. Separate written consent is not required but patients may opt out of testing.
- People at higher risk of HIV should be offered more frequent testing.
- **Testing:** Fourth-generation antigen/antibody combination immunoassay detects both HIV-1 and HIV-2 antibodies as well as the HIV-1 p24 antigen. This test has replaced most third-generation tests that included the ELISA/confirmatory Western blot. If the fourth-generation test is positive, a monospot immunoassay should be sent to differentiate between HIV-1 and HIV-2. If the monospot is nonreactive or indeterminate, HIV-1 viral load should be measured to confirm the diagnosis. If the HIV-1 viral load is not detected, then the result is a false positive unless there is concern for HIV-2 infection (seen only in West Africa). There are only a few laboratories in the United States that can test for HIV-2. The fourth-generation testing can detect infection as early as 2 weeks after exposure (Figure 6.24).
- CD4+ cell count should **not** be used for screening, as it can be ↓ in many conditions other than HIV, including acute illness.
- **HIV-1 RNA viral load** (PCR, or nucleic acid amplification testing [NAAT]) determination may be used when the monospot immunoassay is indeterminate. False-positive results do occur. It is not a first-line test for HIV diagnosis.

Management

- Decisions regarding treatment of HIV are complex, and a comprehensive discussion is outside the scope of this review. Early initiation of treatment **regardless of CD4+ cell count** should be offered for all patients. Treatment guidelines differ by locale, including resource-rich versus resource-poor settings. The main goals of treatment are to suppress viremia, **prevent transmission,** and prevent immunosuppression and other HIV-related systemic complications, such as malignancy and noninfectious dysregulatory sequelae.
  - Before treatment is started, additional tests should be obtained, including CBC and complete metabolic panel (hepatic and renal function), HIV viral load, HIV genotype/resistance testing, hepatitis/syphilis/toxoplasmosis, and

ANSWER 1

All patients presenting with a diabetic foot infection should have an x-ray to look for bony abnormalities and soft tissue gas. If there is still diagnostic uncertainty, obtain an MRI to rule out osteomyelitis. If no osteomyelitis is found, start a first-generation cephalosporin and metronidazole or amoxicillin/clavulanate. The patient should be serially examined, and, if no improvement is seen, admitted to the hospital for debridement and IV antibiotic therapy.

ANSWER 2

TMP-SMX for PCP prophylaxis. Given that your patient is taking antiretroviral medication, you consider the possibility of resistance or nonadherence. First, discuss adherence with the patient and test for viral load and genotyping/resistance pattern. If resistance is found, modify the current antiretroviral therapy.

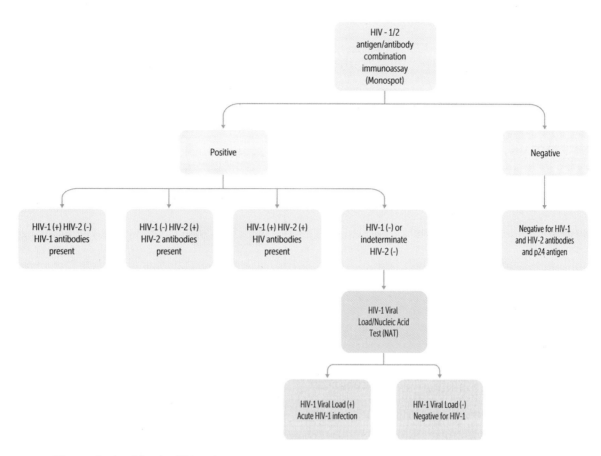

FIGURE 6.24. **Diagnostic algorithm for HIV testing.** (Adapted from CDC guidelines; courtesy of USMLE-Rx.com.)

HLA-B5701 serotype (for abacavir hypersensitivity if abacavir use is planned). If not already obtained, check a PPD skin test or quantiferon serology for TB. Syphilis, gonococcal, and chlamydial (three sites: urine/vaginal, throat, and anal) testing should be used as appropriate.

- For HIV-positive adult and adolescent treatment-naive patients, the 2014 IAS-USA guidelines recommend initiation with a dual nucleoside reverse transcriptase inhibitor (NRTI) such as tenofovir/emtricitabine or abacavir/lamivudine and a third agent, a nonnucleoside reverse transcriptase inhibitor (NNRTI) such as efavirenz; a ritonavir-boosted protease inhibitor (PI) such as atazanavir, darunavir, fosamprenavir, or lopinavir; or an integrase inhibitor (INST) such as raltegravir, or dolutegravir.
  - The targets of HIV therapy are shown in Figure 6.25. Table 6.18 is a brief summary of ART mechanisms, side effects, and considerations.
  - During **pregnancy,** HIV-positive women should be offered standard therapy as above for infected adults/adolescents. While there are medications with more safety data in pregnancy, the best regimen is the one that will suppress viral load most effectively. Women who are already on ART should continue treatment. Women who are not already on ART should start treatment as soon as they are diagnosed to ↓ the rate of perinatal infection to their infant.
  - **Intrapartum, all HIV-positive women with an HIV viral load >1000 at time of delivery or with an unknown viral load should receive IV zidovudine infusion to prevent transmission.** In the United States, women who have HIV-1 RNA >1000 copies/mL should have a planned cesarean delivery at 38 weeks' gestation to ↓ the risk of intrapartum transmission.
- **Strict adherence** to ART is crucial. Patients should be counseled regarding the importance of adherence.
- **ART failure** (demonstrated by ↑ viral load or ↓ CD4+ cell count, despite medication adherence) or **reinitiation of ART** after discontinuation requires **HIV specialty**

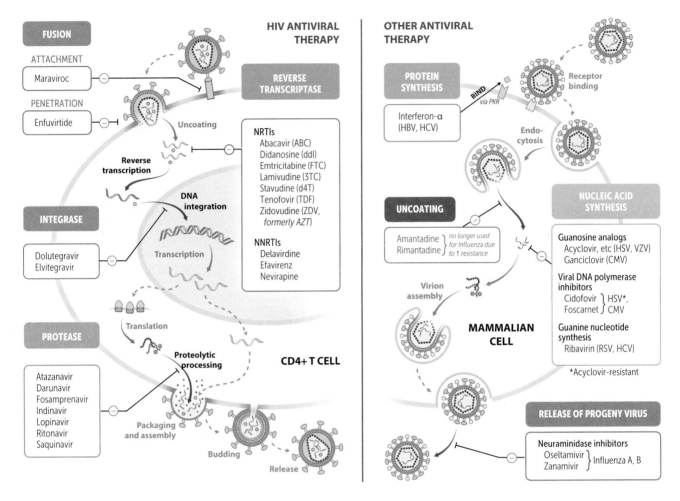

FIGURE 6.25.   Targets of HIV therapy. (Reproduced with permission from USMLE-Rx.com.)

consultation because of the risk of ↑ medication resistance and the complexity of medication choice.

■ Primary care management of PLHIV on ART includes routine assessment of renal function and cardiovascular risk. Pap smears (cervical and anal) are annual versus every 3 years and bone mineral density screening is earlier than for people without HIV. PLHIV should also receive pneumococcal vaccinations.

Prevention

■ **Prevention counseling:** Preexposure prophylaxis (PrEP); needle exchange programs for people who inject drugs; safe sex practices; universal **HIV testing and linkage to care;** universal precautions for health care workers.

■ **Preexposure prophylaxis (PrEP):** Daily dosing of the combination pill of tenofovir and emtricitabine dramatically reduces HIV transmission. It should be offered to those at high-risk for HIV (ie, partners of PLHIV, persons engaging in high-risk sexual practices, people who inject drugs). **Adherence is key!**

■ **Postexposure prophylaxis (PEP):** Rapid initiation of PEP and nonoccupational postexposure prophylaxis (nPEP) are paramount to ↓ the risk of infection. PEP is a three-drug regimen of raltegravir, tenofovir, and emtricitabine. For maximum benefit it should be taken within 72 hours of exposure and continued for 28 days. Check HIV tests at baseline and at 6 weeks and 4 months after exposure. Individualized treatment should be formulated for high-risk exposures to highly resistant viruses.

TABLE 6.18. ARV Medications in HIV Treatment

ANTIRETROVIRAL CLASS	METHOD OF ACTION	EXAMPLES	COMMON SIDE EFFECTS	SPECIFIC CONSIDERATIONS
Nucleoside reverse transcriptase inhibitors	Malfunctioning substrate for HIV reverse transcriptase, preventing viral DNA formation	Zidovudine (AZT), lamivudine, didanosine, stavudine, abacavir, and emtricitabine (tenofovir = nucleotide reverse transcription inhibitor)	Peripheral neuropathy, GI (anorexia, diarrhea), pancreatitis; these are drug specific	Abacavir can cause a fatal hypersensitivity syndrome; check for risk with HLA-B5701 test
Nonnucleoside reverse transcriptase inhibitors	Bind directly to reverse transcriptase, preventing viral DNA formation	Delavirdine, efavirenz, and nevirapine	Rash, vertigo, myalgia	Efavirenz causes vivid dreams and may exacerbate underlying psychiatric illness
Protease inhibitors	Interfere with viral maturation by preventing cleavage of viral protein precursors	Indinavir, darunavir, nelfinavir, ritonavir (used for boosting other protease inhibitors), saquinavir, fosamprenavir, atazanavir, tipranavir, and lopinavir + ritonavir	Metabolic abnormalities and GI side effects, including diarrhea	
Integrase inhibitors	Prevent insertion of HIV genome into host DNA by integrase	Raltegravir, dolutegravir	Diarrhea, nausea, headache, fever	
CCR5 inhibitors	Prevent HIV virus binding to CD4 cell surface by coreceptor CCR5	Maraviroc	Diarrhea, nausea, headache	HIV strains divide into R5 (susceptible) and x4 classes (resistant); must do tropism assay before using
Fusion inhibitors	Prevent fusion of the virus to CD4 cell membrane	Enfurtivide (SQ injection)	Injection-site reactions, GI upset	

AIDS AND OPPORTUNISTIC INFECTIONS

Patients with HIV, especially those with AIDS, are vulnerable to complications of immunosuppression, including infections atypical in the immunocompetent host, metabolic complications, and a higher rate of certain types of malignancy. This section provides a short description of such complications of advanced HIV and AIDS.

AIDS is defined as HIV infection and a CD4+ cell count <200 cells/mm³ or the presence of any AIDS-defining condition (ADC)—one of 20 infectious, degenerative, or malignant diseases. Some of the most common ADCs are discussed below.

Diagnosis/Management

- Depends on disease process and exam findings. A guiding principle is that ART and the maintenance of an undetectable viral load and high CD4+ cell count largely prevent the following complications, even when a patient has previously been diagnosed with AIDS.
- See Table 6.19 for prophylaxis and testing/treatment guidelines for AIDS-related opportunistic infections.

 QUESTION

A 45-year-old woman returns from visiting her relatives in Cape Cod, Massachusetts. On her trip, she went camping and mountain biking in a state park. She presents today for left knee pain and swelling. She recently had a target-shaped rash on her leg, which has disappeared. On ROS, you elicit a history of fatigue and subjective fevers. On exam, her temperature is 37.7°C (99.8°F) and her left knee is erythematous, with a moderate effusion and mild tenderness to palpation. What do you do?

TABLE 6.19. **Prophylaxis Against AIDS-Related Opportunistic Infections**

PATHOGEN	INDICATION FOR PROPHYLAXIS	MEDICATION	COMMENTS
Pneumocystis jiroveci pneumonia (PCP)	CD4+ cells < 200/mm³ or a history of oral thrush; prophylaxis may be stopped if CD4+ cells >200/mm³ for ≥3 months on HAART	TMP-SMX or dapsone ± pyrimethamine or pentamidine nebulizers or atovaquone	Single-strength tablets of TMP-SMX are effective and may be less toxic than double-strength tablets
Mycobacterium avium complex	CD4+ cells <50/mm³. Prophylaxis may be stopped if CD4+ cells > 100/mm³ for ≥3 months on HAART	Azithromycin or clarithromycin or rifabutin	Azithromycin can be given once weekly; rifabutin can ↑ hepatic metabolism of other drugs
Toxoplasma	CD4+ cells <100/mm³ and *Toxoplasma* IgG ⊕; prophylaxis may be stopped if CD4+ cells > 100-200/mm³ for ≥3 months on HAART	TMP-SMX or dapsone ± pyrimethamine or atovaquone	Covered by all PCP regimens except pentamidine
Mycobacterium tuberculosis	PPD >5 mm; history of ⊕ PPD that was inadequately treated; close contact to a person with active TB	INH sensitive: INH × 9 months (include pyridoxine)	For INH-resistant strains, use rifampin or rifabutin ± pyrazinamide
Candida	Frequent or severe recurrences	Fluconazole or itraconazole	
HSV	Frequent or severe recurrences	Acyclovir or famciclovir or valacyclovir	
Pneumococcus	All patients	Pneumococcal vaccine. Repeat when CD4+ cells >200/mm³	Some disease may be prevented with TMP-SMX, clarithromycin, and azithromycin
Influenza	All patients	Influenza vaccine	
HBV	Generally, all susceptible patients; depends on immune status	Hepatitis B vaccine (3 doses)	
HAV	All susceptible patients at ↑ risk for HAV infection or with chronic liver disease (eg, chronic HBV or HCV)	Hepatitis A vaccine (2 doses)	IV drug users, MSM, and hemophiliacs are at ↑ risk

ANSWER

Send anti-Lyme IgM and IgG tests, and if ⊕, order a confirmatory Western blot. (If ⊖, it may be too early for a serologic result.) Consider an ECG and begin early doxycycline for a presumptive diagnosis of Lyme disease. Check CSF if there is neurologic involvement and synovial fluid analysis if arthritis is suspected. Consider IV antibiotics with a third-generation cephalosporin if there is carditis or neuritis.

- Notable opportunistic infections include:
  - **Candidiasis:** Although common in infants and in localized candidal dermatitis in immunocompetent hosts, AIDS can predispose patients to esophageal and diffuse oropharyngeal candidiasis. Treat with antifungal medication such as fluconazole.
  - ***Pneumocystis jiroveci* pneumonia** (still called PCP for *Pneumocystis* pneumonia): A rapidly progressive fungal pneumonia, typified by severe hypoxemia, dry or no cough, and elevated LDH. Diagnose via induced sputum (50%-90% sensitive) or bronchioalvoeolar lavage (90% sensitive). Treat with TMP-SMX and, if the hypoxia is severe, steroids such as prednisone.
  - **Toxoplasmosis:** An infection, usually reactivation in the CNS, by *Toxoplasma gondii*, a protozoan parasite. Exam findings include fever, altered mental status, and focal neurologic deficits. Diagnosis is made by antitoxoplasmosis IgG serology and CT, showing ring-enhancing lesions in the brain parenchyma (Figure 6.26). Treat with pyrimethamine + sulfadiazine and leucovorin. Treatment nonresponders after 7 to 14 days (diagnosed by reimaging of CNS) require a brain biopsy for further evaluation (rule out lymphoma, TB, bacterial abscess, atypical cryptococcosis, other parasites).

- **Cryptococcal meningitis:** An infection of the CNS by the fungus *Cryptococcus neoformans.* Presents with fever and progressively worsening headache. Diagnose with lumbar puncture sent for CSF cryptococcal antigen and culture. Serum cryptococcal antigen also aids in diagnosis. ↑ ICP is common and is associated with worse outcomes. Treat with ICP management (serial LP or, rarely, a drainage device) and antifungal therapy with amphotericin or amphotericin B and flucytosine, followed by fluconazole suppression until adequate immune reconstitution, or if this does not occur, indefinitely.
- **Cytomegalovirus:** Infection, usually reactivation, of a human herpesvirus (HHV-5), leading to colitis and chorioretinitis, with other manifestations somewhat less common. Treat with ganciclovir, valganciclovir, or foscarnet (cidofovir is a second-line agent). Occurs at low CD4+ counts (<50 cells/mm³).
- **TB:** See section on TB.
- **Viral hepatitis:** Coinfection of HIV and hepatitis is common and is associated with worse outcomes from HBV- and HCV-related complications. Vaccination for HAV and HBV are indicated, and prevention/risk reduction is imperative.

- **Notable AIDS-related malignancies include:**
  - **Kaposi sarcoma:** A vascular lymphatic tumor, rare except in Mediterranean and African populations before HIV disease; due to unchecked infection with HHV-8. Lesions are reddish purple, vascular-appearing nodules, typically found on the mouth and skin (Figure 6.27), but can affect the respiratory and GI tracts. Many patients respond to ART alone; also consider local therapy (radiation, cryotherapy, retinoids) or systemic therapy, including interferon and chemotherapy.
  - **Lymphoma:** Related to immune dysregulation and susceptibility to oncogenic viruses; patients with HIV disease have ↑ susceptibility to lymphoma, especially diffuse large B cell lymphoma.
  - **Invasive anogenital cancer** (including cervical cancer): ↑ prevalence and progression of squamous cell carcinoma caused by human papillomavirus (HPV) due to ↓ immune surveillance and ↓ endogenous antineoplastic capability. Treat with surgical excision, chemotherapy, and radiation therapy, depending on staging and location. PLHIV should have annual Pap smears, including anal pap smears for MSM and women who have anal sexual intercourse.
- **Notable metabolic disorders promoted by immune dysregulation in HIV include:**
  - **HIV wasting syndrome:** A hypermetabolic state, characterized by anorexia, leading to muscle atrophy and weight loss, often worsened by GI complications of advanced HIV. Treatment options include nutritional counseling, appetite stimulants, and recombinant human growth hormone.
  - Metabolic syndrome/dyslipidemia.
  - Advanced coronary atherosclerosis.

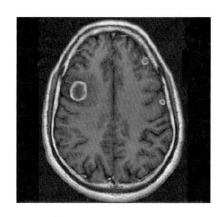

FIGURE 6.26.   Toxoplasmosis. Contrast-enhanced MRI of the brain shows peripherally enhancing lesions with surrounding edema in an immunocompromised patient. (Reproduced from Agrawal A, et al. Multiple-ring enhancing lesions in an immunocompetent adult. *J Glob Infect Dis.* 2010;2(3):313-314.)

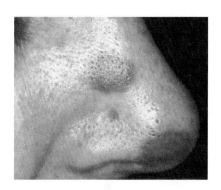

FIGURE 6.27.   HIV-associated Kaposi sarcoma. Characteristic violaceous plaques on the alar and tip of the nose in an HIV-positive female patient. (Reproduced from Sand M, et al. Cutaneous lesions of the nose. *Head Face Med.* 2010;6:7.)

Vector-Borne Infections

MOSQUITO-BORNE INFECTIONS

Table 6.20 lists common types of mosquito-borne infections.

TICK-BORNE INFECTIONS

Table 6.21 outlines the presentation of tick-borne zoonoses.

Lyme disease: Number of cases has tripled over the past 20 years, and the geographic area where the ticks carrying the disease are found has expanded. Typical erythema

TABLE 6.20.   Mosquito-Borne Zoonotic Infections

DISEASE	CLINICAL FEATURES	GEOGRAPHIC DISTRIBUTION	COMMENTS
Malaria (*Plasmodium* spp)	Fever, hemolysis, meningoencephalitis	Worldwide, largely in para-equatorial distribution Highest mortality in sub-Saharan Africa and Southeast Asia	Causes 1-3 million deaths yearly, predominantly in underresourced nations Artemisinin derivatives now standard of care for antimalarial therapy in most settings Widespread resistance to older agents, such as choloroquine Prophylaxis recommended for travel in endemic areas
Dengue fever (flaviviruses)	Two common presentations: "breakbone fever" = myalgia, fever, headache, petechial rash; and less commonly, hemorrhagic fever, with thrombocytopenia, spontaneous hemorrhage, and shock	Central and South America, sub-Saharan Africa, Southeast Asia	Endemic in >100 countries No cure; treatment is supportive
Yellow fever (flavivirus)	Most cases 3- to 4-day self-limited febrile illness; second phase with jaundice due to hepatitis Can cause acute hemorrhagic illness, accounting for majority of mortality	Tropical and subtropical areas of Africa and South America	Vaccine is available WHO estimates 200,000 cases and 30,000 deaths yearly in unvaccinated populations Treatment is supportive
Zika virus	Nonspecific symptoms (fever, rash, joint pain, conjunctivitis) Can cause microcephaly if infected during pregnancy	South and Central America Prior outbreaks seen in Africa, Southeast Asia, and the Pacific Islands	Evolving at the time of this writing Check CDC for most recent guidelines
ENCEPHALITIC ALPHAVIRUSES			
Eastern equine	Encephalitis, peripheral neuropathy	United States (Atlantic and Gulf coasts), Caribbean, South America	Children are usually affected; mortality is 50%-75%; neurologic sequelae are common
Western equine	Encephalitis	Western and central United States, South America	Infants and adults >50 years of age are usually affected; mortality is 5%-15%; neurologic sequelae are uncommon, except in infants
Venezuelan equine	Encephalitis	Florida, southwestern United States, Central and South America	Adults are usually affected; mortality is 1%; neurologic sequelae are rare
FLAVIVIRUSES			
Japanese B	Encephalitis	China, Southeast Asia, India, Japan	A vaccine is available
St. Louis	Encephalitis	United States (rural western and mid-western states, New Jersey, Florida, Texas), Caribbean, Central and South America	Adults >50 years of age are most often affected; mortality is 2%-20%; neurologic sequelae occur in about 20% of cases
West Nile	Encephalitis, polymyelitis-like, peripheral neuropathy	Middle East, Afric, Europe, Central Asia, United States	

Adapted with permission from Aminoff MJ, et al. *Clinical Neurology*, 6th ed. New York: McGraw-Hill, 2005:28.

TABLE 6.21. **Tick-Borne Zoonotic Infections**

DISEASE	VECTOR	ANIMAL RESERVOIR	CLINICAL FEATURES	ANTIBIOTIC TREATMENT	GEOGRAPHIC DISTRIBUTION
Babesiosis	*Ixodes scapularis, Ixodes pacificus*	Cattle, horses, dogs, cats, rodents, deer	Fatigue, malaise, anorexia, nausea, headache, sweats, rigors, abdominal pain, emotional lability, depression, dark urine, hepatomegaly, fever, petechiae, ecchymosis, occasionally rash and pulmonary edema	For the seriously ill, atovaquone and azithromycin, or quinine plus clindamycin	Coastal areas of Massachusetts, Rhode Island, and New York; also in Maryland, Virginia, Minnesota, Wisconsin, Georgia, Washington, and Mexico
Colorado tick fever	*Dermacentor andersoni*	Deer, marmots, porcupines	Fever, chills, headache, myalgias, nausea, vomiting, photophobia, abdominal pain, and occasional sore throat; also may have conjunctivitis, lymphadenopathy, hepatosplenomegaly, stiff neck, retro-orbital pain, weakness, and lethargy	Supportive care	Western and northwestern United States and southwestern Canada
Human granulocytic anaplasmosis	*Ixodes scapularis*	Dogs, deer, other mammals	Fevers, chills, malaise, headache, nausea, muscle aches, cough, sore throat, and pulmonary infiltrates (especially in children)	Doxycycline or tetracycline	Japan, Malaysia, and the eastern, northeastern, and north central United States; some cases in western United States
Human monocytic ehrlichiosis	*Amblyomma americanum* (Lone Star tick) and *D variabilis*	Dogs, deer, other mammals	Fevers, chills, malaise, headache, nausea, muscle aches, cough, sore throat, and pulmonary infiltrates (especially in children)	Doxycycline or tetracycline	Japan, Malaysia, and southern United States
Lyme disease (*Borrelia burgdorferi*)	*Ixodes dammini*	Deer, sheep, deer mice	Erythema migrans (see Figure 6.28), meningitis, encephalitis, neuropathy, and joint and heart symptoms	Doxycycline, amoxicillin, cefuroxime, erythromycin, ceftriaxone, or cefotaxime	Atlantic central and north central United States, occasionally in western United States; separate species in Europe

(continues)

TABLE 6.21.   Tick-Borne Zoonotic Infections (continued)

DISEASE	VECTOR	ANIMAL RESERVOIR	CLINICAL FEATURES	ANTIBIOTIC TREATMENT	GEOGRAPHIC DISTRIBUTION
Rocky Mountain spotted fever (*Rickettsia rickettsii*)	*Dermacentor andersoni* (wood tick) and *D variabilis* (dog tick)	North American mammals	Petechiae, purpura, pulmonary infiltrates, jaundice, myocarditis, hepatosplenomegaly, meningitis, encephalitis, and lymphadenopathy	Doxycycline or chloramphenicol	Most of the continental United States; more prevalent in the southeastern and south central United States
Relapsing fever (*Borrelia* spp)	*Ornithodoros* spp (actually human body lice, not ticks)	Wild rodents	Fever, chills, headache, myalgias, and arthralgias; pain, nausea, vomiting, and hypotension	Erythromycin or doxycycline	Worldwide
Tularemia (*Francisella tularensis*)	*Dermacentor* spp and *Amblyomma* spp	Rabbits, deer, dogs	Pneumonia, regional lymphadenopathy and HA, cough, myalgias, arthralgias, nausea, vomiting, ulceration at inoculation site, and ocular findings	Tobramycin or gentamicin; chloramphenicol for meningitis	United States (except Hawaii) and Canada

Reproduced with permission from Tintinalli JE, et al. *Emergency Medicine: A Comprehensive Study Guide*, 6th ed. New York: McGraw-Hill, 2004:372.

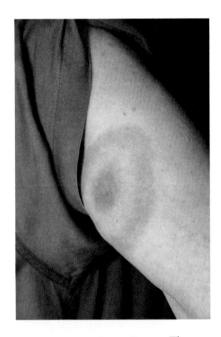

FIGURE 6.28.   Lyme disease. The classic "target" or "bull's-eye" lesion of erythema migrans is seen. (Reproduced from CDC/James Gathany.)

migrans rash is not always apparent (Figure 6.28), and symptoms can be misleading. Prevention of tick bites and early antibiotic treatment are key in management.

- Early Lyme disease treatment:
    - Doxycycline 100 mg BID (adults).
    - Doxycycline 2 mg/kg, max 100 mg (children ≥8).

OR

- Amoxicillin 500 mg TID (adults).
- Amoxicillin 50 mg/kg TID (children).

- To prevent Lyme disease give a single dose of antibiotics within 72 hours of tick removal:
    - Doxycycline 200 mg × 1 (adults).
    - Doxycycline 4 mg/kg, max 200 mg (children ≥8).

Special Topics

SEPSIS AND INFECTIONS IN THE CRITICAL CARE SETTING

In 2016, a task force comprised of members of the Society of Critical Care Medicine and the European Society of Intensive Care Medicine redefined sepsis in an effort to differentiate it from an uncomplicated infection. They defined sepsis as "life-threatening organ dysfunction caused by a dysregulated host response to infection." This new definition eliminates the term "severe sepsis" as all sepsis is considered to have end organ damage. Septic shock continues to fall under the umbrella of sepsis with severe metabolic abnormalities that is not responsive to fluid resuscitation alone.

Diagnosis

Although we continue to use the previous definition of sepsis as meeting two or more systemic inflammatory response syndrome (SIRS) criteria and a suspicion for infection, we are moving towards using the quick Sequential Organ Failure Assessment (qSOFA) as the initial score to identify those with early sepsis and poor outcomes. The full SOFA score is more in-depth than the qSOFA but can be useful to help predict mortality. A change in the SOFA score by two or more ↑ the risk of in-hospital mortality by 10%.

- qSOFA score:
  - Is the patient in the ICU?
  - Does the patient have altered mentation?
  - Is the respiratory rate ≥22 breaths per minute?
  - Is the SBP ≤100 mm Hg?
- SIRS criteria include:
  - Core temperature >38.0°C (100.4°F) or <36°C (96.8°F).
  - Heart rate >90 bpm.
  - Respiratory rate >20, P_{CO_2} <32 mm Hg, or need for mechanical ventilation.
  - WBC >12,000/mm³ or <4000/mm³, or >10% bands.

Management

- Successful treatment of sepsis depends on early, aggressive fluid resuscitation and early infectious source control. Once a patient is fluid replete, if they are still hypotensive, vasopressors and inotropes can be used.
- The organisms causing infections in critically ill patients may differ, depending on length of hospitalization, antecedent hospitalizations, risk factors for MDR organisms, indwelling devices, and immunocompromise, among other variables. Consideration of MDR organisms should occur (see next section) and may influence choice of empirical antibiotic coverage.

KEY FACT

To identify patients with suspected sepsis and a higher risk of poor outcomes, use qSOFA (score ≥2 indicates worse outcomes).

KEY FACT

Whether in the ICU setting or in the outpatient or medical/surgical ward setting, the same types of infections occur, and the same principles of selecting and tailoring antimicrobial coverage apply.

EMERGING ANTIBIOTIC RESISTANCE

Development of antibiotic resistance is not a new phenomenon, but because of the ↑ availability of many types of antimicrobial agents, you must **carefully consider the choice and spectrum of agent and length of therapy** to both ensure coverage and limit resistance.

Brief descriptions of four common MDR organisms are presented here.
- **MRSA:**
  - MRSA is present in both nosocomial and community settings (CA-MRSA, usually with the strain USA-300). Primarily responsible for SSTIs, MRSA can also cause pneumonia (especially in patients post-influenza, with a history of smoking methamphetamine, and in the critical care setting, especially mechanically ventilated patients). The following antibiotics may be used, depending on local resistance profiles and degree of illness: clindamycin, TMP-SMX, ciprofloxacin (if susceptibility confirmed) + rifampin, tetracycline derivatives, linezolid, vancomycin, and daptomycin.
  - Carriage of MRSA occurs in the nares and other skin sites; however, studies examining the efficacy of decolonization have been disappointing. In patients with a history of severe or recurrent MRSA infection, decolonization may be attempted with intranasal mupirocin and chlorhexidine-containing body washes.
- **VRE:**
  - VRE infections are primarily found in nosocomial settings among patients who have previously received antibiotics. Enterococci are part of the gastrointestinal flora and have both endogenous and acquired antibiotic resistance.

QUESTION

A 64-year-old man with diabetes is brought to the ED by ambulance. His wife found him in bed this morning, delirious and sweating, and called 911. EMS arrived to find an obtunded, obese man, GCS 10 in bed, diaphoretic, and with mottled skin. BP en route was 85/palpation, and his pulse was 125 bpm. Peripheral IV access was established prehospital. The patient's wife notes that he was complaining of fever and malaise yesterday but had no other specific complaints. After a focused physical exam, including assessment of airway, breathing, and circulation, you feel that infection is the most likely cause. What do you do?

- VRE strains, most commonly *E faecium*, are responsible for infections of the urinary tract, catheter-related infections, endocarditis, intra-abdominal and wound infections, among others.
- Risk factors for VRE infection include recent antibiotic use, critical illness, immunocompromise (organ transplant, hematologic malignancy, corticosteroid use, neutropenia, chemotherapy), prior VRE colonization, and parenteral nutrition. Before treatment, all indwelling devices (eg, urinary catheters) should be removed and any abscesses drained.
- Antibiotics should be tailored by antibiogram and culture results, as the susceptibility of VRE strains is variable. Linezolid, daptomycin, and tigecycline are commonly used. Infectious disease consultation is advised.

- *Pseudomonas aeruginosa:*
  - A gram-negative rod, *Pseudomonas* is an opportunistic microbe common in nosocomial infections of the urinary tract, lungs (especially in mechanically ventilated patients), and CNS and in bacteremia among patients with or without indwelling devices. It is typically found after >7 days of hospitalization and in patients who are immunocompromised.
  - Other than its presence as a nosocomial pathogen, *Pseudomonas* has been a long-treated microbe in patients with cystic fibrosis and in otitis externa.
  - Often produces a blue-green pigment, leading to the blue purulent exudate sometimes found in infected tissue (not a sensitive finding).
  - Treatment for *Pseudomonas* coverage varies by severity and site of infection. Outpatient treatment is appropriate in non–life-threatening infections. For hospitalized patients, single coverage with an antipseudomonal agent (β-lactams such as ticarcillin and piperacillin; cephalosporins such as cefepime; or fluoroquinolones such as ciprofloxacin) is usually adequate. Double coverage is not indicated in most circumstances. When given, use a β-lactam with an aminoglycoside or with an antipseudomonal fluoroquinolone (either ciprofloxacin or levofloxacin).

- **Extended-spectrum beta-lactamase (ESBL)–producing bacteria:**
  - ESBL bacteria are found in gram-negative organisms (ie, *Klebsiella, E coli*) that have resistance to commonly used β-lactam antibiotics such as penicillins and cephalosporins.
  - Although generally found in hospitalized patients, its prevalence in the community is ↑. Risk factors include longer hospital/ICU stays, emergent abdominal surgery, hemodialysis, and presence of urinary or central venous/arterial catheters. ESBL infections are associated with ↑ mortality and longer hospital stays.
  - The best treatment option is a carbapenem. High doses of cefepime may be acceptable, although it is not considered first-line treatment. Other cephalosporins are associated with treatment failure.

ANSWER

Begin aggressive intravenous rehydration with isotonic fluids, obtain labs (including CBC, chemistry panel, and a lactate), blood and urine cultures, and CXR, and begin empirical broad-spectrum antibiotics. If his mental status does not improve after hydration or the source of infection is unclear, consider an LP.

THE ASPLENIC PATIENT

Patients who have undergone splenectomy are at ↑ risk for serious bacterial infections, especially with encapsulated organisms such as *S pneumoniae, N meningitidis,* and *H influenzae*. The highest risk is in the first 3 years after splenectomy. The most feared complication is overwhelming **postsplenectomy sepsis.** Patients present after a short viral-like prodrome that is followed by abrupt decompensation and shock. Vaccination against pneumococcus, *H influenzae,* and *N meningitidis* should be given 2 weeks prior to elective splenectomy or at hospital discharge for emergent cases.

All splenectomized patients should be counseled that new fever is a medical emergency and that they should seek attention immediately. Penicillin prophylaxis is controversial, given that the only data are based on sickle cell anemia patients with functional asplenia. Recommendations are strongest for children <5 years old in the first year postsplenectomy, and those with additional underlying immunodeficiency. Penicillin prophylaxis is not routinely recommended in adults. These patients are also at ↑ risk for parasitic infections, specifically, babesiosis and malaria.

COMMON FUNGAL INFECTIONS

Table 6.22 lists the presentation and treatment of common fungal infections.

TABLE 6.22.   **Clinical Presentation and Treatment of Selected Fungal Infections**

FUNGUS	GEOGRAPHY	MANIFESTATION	TREATMENT	NOTES
Candida spp	Common yeast on the skin worldwide	Thrush, esophagitis, intertrigo, vaginitis, candiduria, hepatosplenic candidiasis (in post–neutropenic chemo patients), disseminated candidiasis	Topical antifungals for mucosal disease; oral fluconazole for esophagitis; IV or PO fluconazole, amphotericin formulation, or echinocandin for disseminated disease Remove vascular catheters	*Candida glabrata* is frequently resistant to azole therapy
Aspergillus spp	Widespread in soil, water, compost, potted plants, and ventilation ducts	Allergic bronchopulmonary aspergillosis; aspergilloma of the lung or sinuses; invasive aspergillosis	Voriconazole, echinocandin, or amphotericin for invasive disease (combination therapy is sometimes used); surgical excision of aspergilloma in the setting of hemoptysis	A common infection in neutropenic patients or posttransplant
Cryptococcus	Worldwide in bird droppings (especially pigeons)	Meningitis, especially in HIV patients with CD4+ cells <100 mm^3 and in atypical pneumonia	For meningitis, amphotericin and 5-flucytosine, followed by fluconazole; fluconazole for mild lung disease	Cryptococcal antigen on CSF and serum
Coccidioides	Soil of the southwestern United States and San Joaquin Valley	"Valley fever," flulike syndrome, pneumonia. Disseminated disease in 1%-5%	Supportive therapy for valley fever; fluconazole or amphotericin for disseminated disease	Check for *Coccidioides* antibody titer
Histoplasma	Bird and bat droppings in the Mississippi and Ohio River valleys and in Central America	Pulmonary infection, disseminated disease	Supportive therapy for lung disease; itraconazole or amphotericin for disseminated disease	Risk factors include spelunking and contact with chicken coops
Blastomyces	Upper Midwest and Great Lakes region	Most commonly pneumonia; occasionally skin infections, osteomyelitis, and epididymitis/prostatitis	Itraconazole or amphotericin	Risk factor is exposure to forests and streams
Sporothrix	Found in soil, especially rose bushes	Most commonly SSTI; can also cause disseminated disease	Itraconazole for mild disease; amphotericin for severe disease	

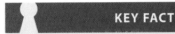

CATHETER-RELATED INFECTIONS

A category of infections that includes catheter-related bloodstream infections as well as exit-site, tunnel, and pocket infections. The most commonly isolated etiologic agents are coagulase-negative staphylococci, *S aureus*, *Enterococcus* spp, and *Candida* spp. In the United States, 5 million central venous catheters (CVCs) are placed per year, and more than 200,000 nosocomial bloodstream infections occur per year. Risk of infection varies by type and site of catheter, with CVC first (1.6-6.8 infections/1000 catheter days), then PICC (peripherally inserted central catheter), then peripheral IV (0.2/1000 catheter days). Among CVCs, risk of infection is lowest with subclavian lines, and risk of infection in femoral = internal jugular CVCs.

Symptoms/Exam

- Clinical findings are **unreliable.**
- Fever and chills are sensitive but not specific.
- Inflammation and purulence around the catheter are specific but not sensitive.

Diagnosis

- Most accurate: **Blood cultures:** Obtain two sets of cultures, at least one set drawn percutaneously.
- **Catheter tip culture:** Should be performed if line sepsis is suspected.

Management

- **Catheter removal:** Used in most cases of nontunneled catheters. For tunneled catheters and implantable devices, consider removal in the presence of severe illness or documented infection (especially *S aureus*, gram-negative rods, or *Candida* spp) or if complications occur.
- **Initial antibiotic choice:** Empirical treatment should include vancomycin to cover *S aureus* (including MRSA) and coagulase-negative staphylococci until culture data are available.
- **Duration of therapy:** Patients with uncomplicated bacteremia should be treated for 10 to 14 days. Patients with complicated infections (eg, those with persistently ⊕ blood cultures after catheter removal, endocarditis, or septic thrombophlebitis should be treated for 4 to 6 weeks. Adults with osteomyelitis should be treated for 6 to 8 weeks.

Complications

Septic thrombophlebitis, infective endocarditis, septic pulmonary emboli, osteomyelitis, or other complications due to septic emboli.

Prevention

Recent trials have shown that good practices at the time of insertion ↓ CVC-associated bloodstream infection: Use gloves, gown, mask, full drape, and cap, with hand hygiene at the time of insertion. Inpatients with a CVC should be assessed daily to see if a central line is still necessary.

FEVER OF UNKNOWN ORIGIN IN ADULTS

A temperature >38.3°C (100.9°F) for ≥3 weeks that remains undiagnosed despite evaluation over three outpatient visits or three hospital days. Common etiologies include infection (25%-40%), cancer (25%-40%), and autoimmune disease (10%-15%). Infection is more likely if the patient is older or from a developing country, as well as in cases of nosocomial, neutropenic, or HIV-associated fever of unknown origin (FUO). Adverse reactions to medications resulting in a fever should also be considered. In approximately 10% to 15% of cases, no diagnosis will be discovered, and the fever will resolve spontaneously.

Symptoms/Exam

- Fever; otherwise variable, but a careful history should be taken on serial visits to elucidate any clues to a diagnosis.
- Repeated physical exams may yield subtle findings in the fundi, conjunctivae, sinuses, temporal arteries, and lymph nodes. Heart murmurs, splenomegaly, and perirectal or prostatic fluctuance/tenderness should be assessed.

Differential

- **Infectious: TB, endocarditis,** and **occult abscesses** are the most common infectious causes of FUO in immunocompetent patients. Consider 1° HIV infection or opportunistic infections due to unrecognized HIV. In rare cases, the cause is babesiosis or other tick-borne diseases.
- **Neoplastic: Lymphoma** and **leukemia** are the most common cancers causing FUO. Other causes include hepatoma, renal cell carcinoma, and atrial myxoma.
- **Autoimmune:** Adult Still disease, SLE, cryoglobulinemia, polyarteritis nodosa, and temporal arteritis (especially in elderly patients).
- **Other:** Drug fever, thyroiditis, granulomatous hepatitis, sarcoidosis, Crohn's disease, Whipple disease, familial Mediterranean fever, recurrent pulmonary embolism, retroperitoneal hematoma, factitious fever.

Diagnosis

- Ask about HIV risk factors, cardiac valve disorders, drug use, travel, exposure to animals/insects, occupational history, recent medications, sick contacts, and a family history of fever.
- Initial steps: Obtain routine labs and CXR. Blood cultures should be drawn off of antibiotics and held for 2 weeks. Place a PPD (or check a gamma interferon release assay). If indicated, obtain cultures of other body fluids (sputum, urine, stool, CSF). If travel history is present, obtain a blood smear (malaria, babesiosis). Do an HIV test.
- Perform echocardiography to look for vegetations. If neoplasm or abscesses are suspected, order a CT/MRI.
- Use other tests selectively (ANA, rheumatic fever, viral cultures, antibody/antigen tests for viral and fungal infections).
- Invasive procedures are generally low yield except for temporal artery biopsy in the elderly, liver biopsy in patients with LFT abnormalities, and bone marrow biopsy in patients with HIV with pancytopenia.

Management

- If no other symptoms are present, treatment may be deferred until a definitive diagnosis is made.
- Give broad-spectrum antibiotics if the patient is severely ill or neutropenic.
- Ten percent to 15% of cases will spontaneously resolve.

ACUTE RHEUMATIC FEVER

A postinfectious autoimmune complication of GAS pharyngitis. Acute rheumatic fever (ARF) was once a common cause of acquired valvular disease but is now rare in the era of antistreptococcal antibiotics, with an incidence of 0.5% to 1.0.%. Antibiotic treatment for GAS is the 1° method of preventing ARF.

Diagnosis

The Jones criteria are used for the diagnosis of ARF (Table 6.23). **Two major criteria** or **one major criterion plus two minor criteria** must be present.

TABLE 6.23.   **The Jones Criteria for Rheumatic Fever**

MAJOR CRITERIA	MINOR CRITERIA
Carditis	Clinical:
Migratory polyarthritis	Fever
Sydenham chorea	Arthralgia
Subcutaneous nodules	Laboratory:
Erythema marginatum	Elevated acute-phase reactants
	Prolonged PR interval

Plus:

Supporting evidence of a recent group A streptococcal infection (eg, a $\oplus$ throat culture or rapid antigen detection test and/or an elevated or $\uparrow$ streptococcal antibody test).

Management

A course of penicillin; NSAIDs for inflammation, preferably salicylates; bed rest for cardiac complications; IV immunoglobulin for severe inflammatory states; and anti-epileptics, specifically, valproic acid for severe chorea. ARF has high probability of recurrence leading to worsening valvular disease, stroke, and premature death. Lifelong prophylaxis with benzathine penicillin should be offered.

CHAPTER 7

Hematology/Oncology

Jennifer Karlin, MD, PhD

Anemia

APPROACH TO ANEMIA

Definition: Low oxygen-carrying capacity of blood, shown by low level of hemoglobin (Hb) or low number of circulating RBCs in blood.
- Hematocrit (adult): <41%.
- Hemoglobin: <13.5 g/dL in men and <12 g/dL in women.

Symptoms/Exam

Depends on acuity, severity, and patient age:
- Acute anemia: Symptoms of hypovolemia—**tachycardia** (first sign), **postural hypotension** (second sign), and shock.
- Chronic anemia: Often asymptomatic if mild and chronic; **fatigue, dyspnea on exertion, postural lightheadedness, pallor, headache, systolic ejection murmur** if moderate to severe.
- Elderly patients may exhibit worsening angina, claudication, and possibly HF.

Diagnosis

Workup: Begin by categorizing the possible causes by MCV. Next, look at reticulocyte count (hyper- or hypoproliferative). The etiology is often multifactorial, but the basic algorithm and possible causes are shown in Figure 7.1.

MICROCYTIC ANEMIA

Iron Deficiency Anemia (IDA)

Etiologies generally include blood loss (eg, GI losses, surgical blood loss, menstrual blood loss, GI parasites), malabsorption (eg, gastrectomy, gastritis and *Heliobacter pylori*, bariatric surgery, celiac disease), ↑ demand for iron (hemodialysis, pregnancy, rapid growth coupled with inadequate diet).

KEY FACT

- Assume GI bleed for men and postmenopausal women until proven otherwise!
- Menstrual blood loss is the most common cause in premenopausal women.
- Iron deficiency due to nutritional deficiency is most common in children (especially with excessive cow's milk intake).

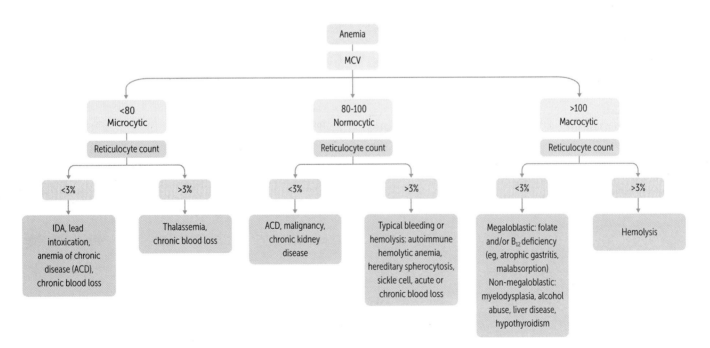

FIGURE 7.1. Algorithm for categorizing anemia. (Reproduced with permission from USMLE-Rx.com.)

Symptoms/Exam

The following symptoms are not sensitive or specific; lab studies should be done to diagnose IDA.

- Mostly asymptomatic if mild.
- If severe: Fatigue, pallor, ↓ exercise capacity.
- If severe and prolonged:
  - **Angular cheilosis:** Fissures at the corners of the mouth.
  - **Atrophic glossitis.**
  - **Pica:** Craving for nonnutritive substances.
  - **Koilonychia:** Spooning of the fingernails and brittle nails.
  - **Plummer-Vinson syndrome:** Esophageal webs and atrophic glossitis, leading to dysphagia.

Diagnosis

- CBC with smear: ↓/normal MCV, ↑ RDW, microcytic, hypochromic RBCs, and variation in RBC size (anisocytosis) or shape (poikilocytosis). No target cells!
- Iron studies: ↓ serum iron, ↑ transferrin iron-binding capacity (TIBC), ↓ transferrin saturation, and ↓ serum ferritin.

Differential Diagnosis

See Table 7.1.

Management

If possible, correct the underlying cause (eg, GI bleed, malabsorption).

- **Oral iron replacement:** Adequate for ↑ physiologic needs, inadequate dietary iron intake, or pregnancy. Ineffective in GI malabsorption. Poor response in continuing blood loss, end-stage renal disease (ESRD), inflammatory illness, or damaged marrow. Generally takes 1 to 2 months to return Hb to normal but 6 months of treatment is required to replete iron stores. Reticulocyte count should ↑ 3 to 4 days after the initiation of treatment and peaks at about 10 days. Goal is 150 to 200 mg/day elemental iron. ↑ absorption with vitamin C rich foods. ↓ absorption with ↑ pH foods, such as milk.
- **Parenteral iron therapy:** Use to adequately deliver iron for patients unable to tolerate PO iron or unable to correct iron deficiency with PO iron because of malabsorption, IBD, severe iron deficiency, and ongoing blood loss, and to reduce the risk of blood transfusion.

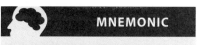

MNEMONIC

Causes of microcytic anemia:
TICS

Thalassemia
Iron deficiency
Chronic disease
Sideroblastic anemia

KEY FACT

Always order a smear for the diagnosis of microcytic anemia.

KEY FACT

↑ HbA2 on electrophoresis is diagnostic of α-thalassemia.

TABLE 7.1.   Distinguishing Factors of Microcytic Anemias

	MCV	RDW	IRON	TIBC	FERRITIN	TRANSFERRIN SATURATION	TRANSFERRIN	SMEAR	ELECTROPHORESIS
IDA	↓/normal	↑	↓	↑	↓	↓	↑	Hypochromia	Normal
ACD	↓/normal	Normal	↓	Normal/↓	Normal/↑	Normal	Normal	Normal	Normal
Thalassemia	↓	Normal	Normal/↑	Normal	Normal	Normal	Normal	+ target cells, microcytosis, hypochromia	↑ HbA2
Sideroblastic anemia	↓/normal (congenital) ↑/normal (aquired)	↑	Normal/↑	Normal	↑	↑	Normal	Siderocytes	Normal

Sideroblastic Anemia

Defective heme biosynthesis in RBC precursors, leading to impaired erythropoiesis, which in turn leads to accumulation of iron in mitochondria and "ringed sideroblasts."

- **Hereditary:** X-linked or autosomally inherited. Manifests in infancy.
- **Acquired:** see the mnemonic "Anemia Loses Its Clinical Color."

Diagnosis

- Variable RBC morphology and MCV.
- Peripheral smear with siderocytes: Hypochromic RBCs with basophilic stippling that stains $\oplus$ for iron (ie, Pappenheimer bodies).
- Bone marrow with ringed sideroblasts (pathognomonic).
- ↑ iron, transferrin saturation, and ferritin (iron overload).

Management

- Treat any reversible causes.
- Transfuse periodically for severe anemia.
- Supplement pyridoxine for some hereditary forms.
- Iron chelation or therapeutic phlebotomy for iron overload.

NORMOCYTIC ANEMIA

Anemia of Chronic Disease (ACD)

Caused by multiple factors usually ↓ erythropoietin (EPO) production/release or inflammation. In anemia of inflammation, hepcidin production is ↑ and inhibits iron absorption. This accounts for the defining feature of this condition: Sequestration of iron in macrophages.

Diagnosis

↓/normal MCV, normal RDW, ↓ reticulocyte (does not respond to iron repletion), ↓ iron and TIBC, normal/↓ transferrin saturation, normal (in renal disease) or ↑ (in inflammation) ferritin. Table 7.1 outlines the distinguishing factors of ACD and other types of anemia. Usually, Hb does not fall below 8 g/dL except in ESRD due to ↓ EPO.

Management

- Treat the underlying cause, if possible.
- Give EPO for ACD in renal disease if iron stores replete and Hb <10 g/dL. Consider EPO for patients with inflammatory ACD with adequate iron stores if ↓ serum EPO levels and symptomatic.
- Give transfusion if symptomatic or Hb <7 to 8 g/dL.

Hemolytic Anemia

Premature destruction of RBCs before their normal life span of 90 to 120 days. Various causes:

- **Intrinsic factors:** RBC interior abnormalities leading to shortened RBC life span.
- **Extrinsic/membrane factors:** RBCs are normal, but are destroyed due to infections, antibodies, metabolic or oxidative stress, toxins, or other external mechanisms.

Symptoms/Exam

- General symptoms of anemia (such as fatigue) plus jaundice, red-brown urine (hemoglobinuria) ± splenomegaly.
- **Labs:** ↑ reticulocytes, ↑ indirect bilirubin (up to 5 mg/dL), ↓ haptoglobin, ↑ LDH. (*Note:* No urine bilirubin.)

■ Hemolytic anemia can be classified as extravascular or intravascular, based on the site of RBC destruction (Table 7.2).

■ Major causes of hemolytic anemia:

- ■ **Autoimmune hemolytic anemia (warm AIHA):** An acquired disorder in which an IgG autoantibody binds to the RBC membranes, causing RBC destruction by macrophages or spleen. Spherocytosis and reticulocytosis are seen on the peripheral smear. ⊕ direct Coombs test. Indirect Coombs test may be ⊕ or ⊖. Fifty percent idiopathic. Other causes: systemic lupus erythematosus (SLE), chronic lymphocytic leukemia (CLL), lymphoma. Ten percent with immune thrombocytopenia (Evans syndrome). Treated with steroids (first line, acutely), immunosuppressants (first line chronically), rituximab, and splenectomy.

- ■ **Cold agglutinin disease (cold AIHA):** Acquired hemolytic anemia due to an IgM autoantibody, which occurs only in cooler parts of the body such as fingers, nose, and ears. IgM binds to RBC and fixes complement. Lysis is rare. RBCs with complement are sequestered by Kupffer cells in the liver. Mostly idiopathic. Other cases associated with lymphoproliferative disorders, nonlymphoid malignancies, and acute infections (mycoplasmal pneumonia, infectious mononucleosis). ⊕ direct Coombs test for complement only.

- ■ **Microangiopathic hemolytic anemia:** Intravascular destruction of RBCs, with RBC fragmentation. ⊕ hemoglobinemia, hemoglobinuria, and methemalbuminemia if severe. ⊖ Coombs test. ⊕ schistocytes, helmet cells on the peripheral smear (Figure 7.2). Etiologies include thrombotic thrombocytopenic purpura (TTP), disseminated intravascular coagulation (DIC), malignant hypertension, HELLP syndrome, and prosthetic cardiac valves.

- ■ **Glucose-6-phosphate dehydrogenase (G6PD) deficiency:** X-linked, recessive. ↑ susceptibility of RBCs to oxidative stress, causing episodic hemolytic anemia in response to oxidant drugs (dapsone, sulfonamides, antimalarias, nitrofurantoin), acute infections, or foods (fava beans). ⊕ Heinz body (precipitants formed by denatured oxidized hemoglobin) and "bite cells" on the peripheral smear. Seen in 10% to 15% of African American men. Remember that testing G6PD levels during acute hemolysis episode may yield false ⊖ results since G6PD deficient cells are often destroyed, leaving only healthy RBCs to test.

- ■ **Paroxysmal nocturnal hemoglobinuria (PNH):** Acquired disorder in stem cell, leading to ↑ RBC sensitivity to complement and episodes of intravascular hemolysis and hemoglobinuria. Patients are prone to thrombosis (especially

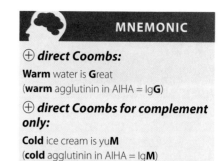

MNEMONIC

⊕ *direct Coombs:*

Warm water is **G**reat
(**warm** agglutinin in AIHA = Ig**G**)

⊕ *direct Coombs for complement only:*

Cold ice cream is yu**M**
(**cold** agglutinin in AIHA = Ig**M**)

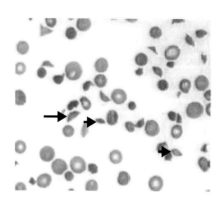

FIGURE 7.2.   Disseminated intravascular coagulation. Peripheral blood smear shows numerous fragmented (short arrows) and some helmet-shaped (long arrow) red blood cells, known as schistocytes. (Reproduced with permission from USMLE-Rx.com.)

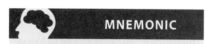

MNEMONIC

Medications causing hemolysis in G6PD deficiency:

SNIP
Sulfonamides
Nitrofurantoin
Isoniazid
Primaquine (quinine, chloquinine)

TABLE 7.2.   **Extravascular Versus Intravascular Hemolytic Anemia**

	EXTRAVASCULAR	INTRAVASCULAR
Site of RBC destruction	Macrophage (spleen, liver)	Blood vessels
Serum haptoglobin	↓	↓↓
Serum LDH	↑	↑↑
Urine hemosiderin	⊖	⊕
Urine hemoglobin	⊖	⊕ if severe
Peripheral smear	Spherocytes	Schistocytes
Etiologies	Warm AIHA, hypersplenism, delayed hemolytic transfusion reaction, hemoglobinopathies	Cold AIHA, acute hemolytic transfusion reaction, microangiopathic hemolysis, G6PD deficiency, PNH, hemoglobinopathies

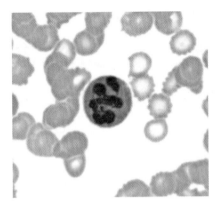

FIGURE 7.3. **Megaloblastic anemia.** Note the hypersegmented neutrophil with a nucleus containing more lobes than normal. (Reproduced with permission from USMLE-Rx.com.)

mesenteric, hepatic, CNS, and skin veins). May precede aplastic anemia, myelodysplasia, or acute myelogenous leukemia (AML). ⊕ urine hemosiderin. WBC and platelets may be ↓.

- **Sickle cell anemia:** See the discussion of hemoglobinopathies below.

MACROCYTIC, MEGALOBLASTIC ANEMIA

Results from impaired DNA synthesis caused by vitamin B_{12} or folate deficiency or bone marrow suppression (Figure 7.3).

Diagnosis

- Anemia and ↑ MCV are usually found but are not required for diagnosis. Pancytopenia may be seen with severe disease.
- ↑ LDH and indirect bilirubin from ineffective erythropoiesis.
- ↑ homocysteine (in both vitamin B_{12} and folate deficiency) and methylmalonic acid (vitamin B_{12} deficiency only) resulting from ↓ rate of metabolism.
- Hypersegmented neutrophils, macro-ovalocytes, and megaloblasts in the peripheral smear (see Figure 7.3).

VITAMIN B_{12} DEFICIENCY

Vitamin B_{12} is found in animal products and binds to intrinsic factor (IF) secreted by gastric parietal cells. The complex is absorbed in the terminal ileum.

- **Pernicious anemia:** Most common cause. ⊕ autoantibody against IF and gastric parietal cells, leading to chronic atrophic gastritis and ↓ production and function of IF. This can lead to ↑ **risk of gastric cancer and carcinoid tumors.**
- Other causes may include:
    - Malnutrition in individuals following a strict vegan diet.
    - ↓ **absorption:** Abnormal GI tract (including after bariatric surgery), metformin use, and PPI use.
    - ↑ competition for vitamin B_{12}, as seen in **fish tapeworm infestation** or bacterial overgrowth of the terminal ileum.

Symptoms/Exam

- **Symmetric peripheral neuropathy** with paresthesias and **ataxia**, leading to severe weakness, spasticity, and clonus, poor position and vibration sense, ⊕ Babinski reflex.
- Memory loss, **personality changes,** and **dementia.**
- **Glossitis,** vaginal atrophy, and malabsorption.

Diagnosis

- ↓ serum cobalamin (vitamin B_{12}). In subclinical cases when levels are low normal, check methylmalonic acid and homocysteine, which will be elevated in vitamin B_{12}-deficient states.
- Pernicious anemia: ⊕ **anti-IF antibody** (**Schilling test** is not done anymore).

KEY FACT

Neurologic symptoms of vitamin B_{12} deficiency may precede the anemia.

Management

- Give vitamin B_{12} PO in high doses or IM.
- Neurological abnormalities may not be reversible if present >6 months.

FOLATE DEFICIENCY

Folate is found in animal products and in leafy vegetables. In the United States and many other countries, flour and grains are supplemented with folic acid. Causes of deficiency include:

- **Malnutrition,** especially common in **alcohol use disorder.**
- **Malabsorption:** Due to celiac disease, IBD.
- **Drugs:** Methotrexate, trimethoprim, phenytoin.
- ↑ **requirements:** Pregnancy, lactation, chronic hemolysis, and **psoriasis.**

Diagnosis

↓ serum or RBC folate.

Management

Give PO folate for 1 to 4 months or until the underlying condition resolves.

Hemoglobinopathies

THALASSEMIAS

Normal adult Hb (HbA) consists of one pair of α and β chains each ($\alpha_2\beta_2$). Thalassemias are hereditary disorders caused by ↓ **production of globin chains (α or β)** of Hb. This leads to ↓ Hb synthesis, which in turn leads to hypochromic microcytic anemia. Abnormal RBCs are also hemolyzed.

- **α-chain disorders:** Most commonly found in patients from **Southeast Asia** and **China,** and less commonly in those of African descent (Table 7.3).
- **β-chain disorders:** Most commonly found in patients of **Mediterranean** origin and sometimes in Asians and those of African descent (Table 7.4).

SICKLE CELL DISEASE

An autosomal-recessive disease due to a defect in the β-chain, leading to an unstable form of Hb (hemoglobin S, HbS). Deoxygenation of HbS leads to ↓ solubility, causing aggregation into long strands, which are the "sickled"-appearing RBCs. The sickled RBCs are stiff and less able to pass through microvasculature.

Symptoms/Exam

Common manifestations are as follows (see also Figure 7.4 and Table 7.5):
- **Sickle cell crisis:**
  - The most common manifestation among patients >2 years of age.
  - Most commonly affects the back and long bones of the extremities; lasts for days.
  - Often presents with fever, swelling, tenderness, hypertension, tachypnea, and nausea/vomiting. **Note: This cannot be diagnosed with labs.**

QUESTION

A 29-year-old man presents with a 6-week history of dyspnea on exertion and recurrent fevers and sweats. He has a 7-year history of drinking one liter of hard alcohol per day and smokes 10 cigarettes per day; otherwise healthy with no significant medical or family history. He takes no medications. Hb, 8.6 g/dL, and MCV, 120. What is the next step in your evaluation?

TABLE 7.3.   α-Chain Disorders

ALLELES	DISEASE	CLINICAL RESULT
(−/−)	Hydrops fetalis	Incompatible with life outside the uterus
(a-/−)	Hemoglobin H disease	Moderate to severe hemolytic anemia; splenomegaly; may require occasional transfusions
(a-/a-)(aa/−)	Thalassemia minor or α-thalassemia-1 trait	Mild microcytic anemia with a normal life expectancy
(aa/a-)	Carrier/ α-thalassemia-2 trait	Patients are clinically normal

KEY FACT

Acute chest is the most common cause of death in sickle cell disease.

A ANSWER

Evaluate for vitamin B_{12} deficiency, then start folate, as folate replacement may mask the hematologic manifestation of vitamin B_{12} deficiency while allowing neurologic damage to progress.

TABLE 7.4. **β-Chain Disorders**

β-CHAIN SYNTHESIS	DISEASE	CLINICAL RESULT
Near absence	β-thalassemia major	Severe anemia dependent on **lifelong transfusions** **Bony changes** due to bone marrow expansion Hepatosplenomegaly Manifests during the first year of life as hemoglobin F (HbF) declines Patients typically die in the third or fourth decade because of sequelae of **iron overload**
Moderate	β-thalassemia intermedia	Mild bony changes and hepatosplenomegaly; may require transfusions
Near normal	β-thalassemia minor	Mild anemia but overall asymptomatic

- **Acute chest syndrome:**
  - **New pulmonary infiltrate** in at least one whole lung segment; **chest pain, fever, and tachypnea, wheezing, or cough.**
  - Usually due to vaso-occlusion; may also be caused by infarction, embolism, or bacterial pneumonia.

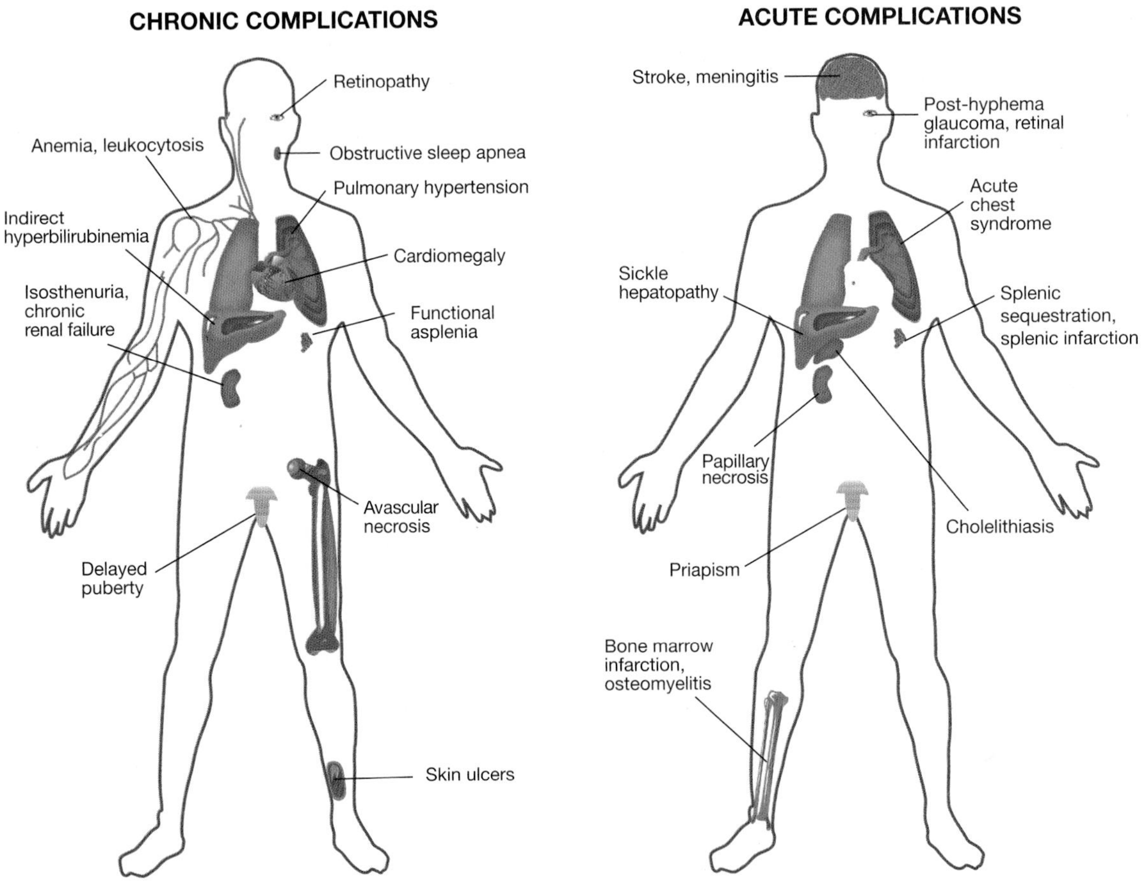

FIGURE 7.4. **Complications of sickle cell disease.** (Reproduced with permission from Hall JB, et al. *Principles of Critical Care,* 3rd ed. New York: McGraw-Hill, 2005, Fig. 108-1.)

TABLE 7.5. **Complications of Sickle Cell Disease by Etiology**

ACUTE VASO-OCCLUSIVE COMPLICATIONS	CHRONIC VASO-OCCLUSIVE COMPLICATIONS	CHRONIC HEMOLYTIC ANEMIA COMPLICATIONS
Acute pain crisis	Retinopathy	Cholelithiasis
Acute chest syndrome	Splenic infarction	**Aplastic crisis** (precipitated by **parvovirus B19** infection)
Splenic sequestration	Avascular necrosis of the femoral or humeral head	
Priapism		
Stroke	Chronic renal failure	
Dactylitis (the most common initial symptom)		
Acute hepatic crisis		

- Splenic sequestration crisis:
  - Vaso-occlusion within the spleen leads to pooling of RBCs and ↓ peripheral hemoglobin concentration.
  - Massive splenomegaly.
  - Risk of hypovolemic shock.
  - Usually occurs in younger patients, as their spleens have not yet fibrosed.
  - **Ten percent to 15% mortality rate** and a **high rate of recurrence:** Recommended treatment is a splenectomy after the first episode.

Diagnosis

- Diagnosis made by hemoglobin electrophoresis.
- CBC shows normocytic anemia and reticulocytosis.
- Remember to check peripheral smear: Sickle cells, Howell-Jolly bodies, and target cells (see Figure 7.5).

Management

- Chronic treatment:
  - Give pneumococcal vaccine (↑ risk of infection from encapsulated organisms due to functional asplenism).
  - Screen for retinopathy annually.
  - Supplement folic acid 1 mg PO daily.
  - Consider chronic hydroxyurea treatment to ↓ frequency of crises in patients with >3 crises/year requiring hospitalization; this will ↑ production of HbF.

> **KEY FACT**
>
> Patients with sickle cell disease have functional asplenia and are at ↑ risk for infection, especially from encapsulated organisms, such as *Streptococcus pneumoniae*, *Haemophilus influenzae* type b, and *Neisseria meningitidis*. As such, it is important to immunize against these organisms.

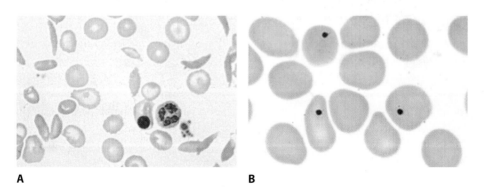

A   B

FIGURE 7.5.   **Sickle cell anemia.** (**A**) Sickle and target cells. (**B**) Howell-Jolly bodies in a thin blood smear stained with Giemsa. (Image A reproduced with permission from USMLE-Rx.com; image B reproduced from the CDC.)

- **Acute treatment:**
  - Start with hydration, O_2, and analgesia.
  - Transfusion for aplastic or hemolytic crises. Consider exchange transfusion for acute vaso-occlusive crises (ie, intractable pain crises, acute chest syndrome, stroke, or recurrent priapism).
  - Because of racial bias, African American patients are at ↑ risk for having their acute pain undertreated. Be sure to adequately treat the pain of sickle cell crisis.

Complications

Patients have ↓ life expectancy, with the median age of death in the fifth decade. The most common causes of death include acute chest infection and splenic sequestration.

Platelet Disorders

THROMBOTIC THROMBOCYTOPENIC PURPURA

Platelet aggravation and microthrombi formation in the microvasculature, leading to thrombocytopenia and microangiopathic hemolytic anemia. TTP and hemolytic-uremic syndrome (HUS) are similar and likely two variants of the same disease, with TTP more strongly associated with CNS involvement and HUS more strongly associated with renal involvement **without neurologic changes**. Both may be associated with the following conditions:
- **Pregnancy** and postpartum state.
- **HIV.**
- **Medications: Estrogens,** quinine, ticlopidine, clopidogrel, bleomycin, cisplatin, cyclosporine, tacrolimus.
- **Autoimmune disorders:** SLE, antiphospholipid antibody syndrome (APS), scleroderma.
- **Enterohemorrhagic** *E coli* **(O157:H7).**

Symptoms/Exam

All of the **five classic features** are present in only 25% of patients:
- **Microangiopathic hemolytic anemia,** leading to schistocytes (see Figure 7.2), ↑ LDH and total bilirubin.
- **Thrombocytopenia,** leading to purpura, petechiae, and/or bleeding.
- **Fever.**
- **Acute renal insufficiency.**
- **Neurologic abnormalities:** Usually confusion or headache; occasionally seizures, aphasia, or hemiparesis.

Differential

Other causes of ↓ platelets include DIC, idiopathic thrombocytopenic purpura (ITP), HIV, SLE, heparin-induced thrombocytopenia (HIT), microangiopathies, mechanical destruction, hypersplenism, bone marrow suppression, drug-induced thrombocytopenia, and platelet clumping.

Diagnosis

Made clinically: Thrombocytopenia and microangiopathic hemolytic anemia without an obvious underlying cause.

Management

- Initiate urgent **plasma exchange** of fresh frozen plasma (FFP) or solvent/detergent plasma to reverse platelet consumption (mortality >95% if untreated). This is a medical emergency and is almost always fatal if appropriate treatment is not initiated promptly.
- Do not transfuse platelets unless there is life-threatening bleeding and only after plasmapheresis is under way because ↑ platelets can speed up TTP process and lead to rapid consumption of platelets.
- Do not delay treatment while awaiting results of ADAMTS13 activity levels.
- Consider **corticosteroids** for inadequate response to plasmapheresis.
- Consider **splenectomy** for recurrent cases.

Complications

- Survival with plasma exchange: 80% at 6 months.
- High rate of relapse after remission (especially in the first year).
- About 25% of patients develop chronic renal failure.
- Complications of treatment: Local infection, bacteremia, hypotension, and urticaria.

HEMOLYTIC-UREMIC SYNDROME

Commonly associated with diarrheal illnesses with shiga toxin–producing bacteria (eg, *E coli* O157:H7, O154:H4, *Shigella*, *Campylobacter*). Characterized by microangiopathy, ↑ LDH, and **renal failure.** Supportive care and renal replacement therapy as needed for uremic symptoms.

IDIOPATHIC THROMBOCYTOPENIC PURPURA

An autoimmune platelet disorder in which antibodies against platelets lead to platelet clearance and ↓ platelet production in the bone marrow, resulting in thrombocytopenia. Most commonly affects women <40 years of age (female-to-male ratio is 3:1). An acute form may develop in children after a viral infection.

Symptoms/Exam

Related to bleeding due to thrombocytopenia:
- **Petechiae, purpura,** and ecchymoses.
- **Mucosal bleeding** (epistaxis, gingival bleeding, menorrhagia).
- Rarely, GI bleeding and gross hematuria may be seen.

Diagnosis

- Exclude other differential diagnoses by history, physical, and tests. This is a diagnosis of exclusion.
- CBC with smear: **Isolated thrombocytopenia** and **large platelets.**
- Order ANA to rule out SLE.
- Also consider abdominal ultrasound to rule out sequestration in liver or spleen as cause of low platelets.
- Order tests for hepatitis, CMV, EBV, toxoplasma, and HIV if hepatic or splenic enlargement, lymphadenopathy, or atypical lymphocytes.
- Order HIV test.
- A bone marrow examination should be done in patients >60 years of age to rule out myelodysplasia.

 QUESTION

A 27-year-old woman has had frequent nosebleeds during the last week. She denies any gingival or GI bleeding, easy bleeding or bruising, or family history of such symptoms. Her last menses may have been heavier than normal. Exam reveals petechiae over her lower legs bilaterally, no splenomegaly. Platelet count is 9000; CBC is otherwise normal. Her peripheral smear shows isolated thrombocytopenia and occasional megathrombocytes. What is the most likely diagnosis?

Management

- Acute symptoms (platelets <20,000-30,000 or if significant bleeding): **Corticosteroids.**
- Refractory to steroids:
    - **IVIG.** Platelet transfusions may also be tried for life-threatening bleeding. Also consider Rho (D) immune globulin for Rh+ patients.
    - A **splenectomy** may be necessary for patients with more serious manifestations refractory to treatment.
    - Rituximab can also be considered. Optimal sequence of therapy to try has not been determined.
- Treatment of chronic symptoms (for cases that last >3 months and are refractory to splenectomy): Danazol, cyclophosphamide, azathioprine, or vincristine/vinblastine.

Complications

Fatalities are rare. Most patients achieve remission with corticosteroids. Cerebral hemorrhage is a rare but the most serious complication.

HEPARIN-INDUCED THROMBOCYTOPENIA

Acquired disorder caused by formation of IgG antibodies to heparin-platelet factor 4 (PF4) complexes: IgG antibodies bind to platelets, leading to activation of platelets, which results in thrombocytopenia and a prothrombotic state. Affects 3% of patients on unfractionated heparin and 0.6% of patients on low-molecular-weight heparin (LMWH).

Symptoms/Exam

- A ↓ in platelet count within **5 to 10 days** of exposure to heparin.
- **Venous and arterial thrombosis,** especially DVT, is common.

Diagnosis

- **New-onset** thrombocytopenia of ≥50% from the baseline platelet count within 5 to 10 days of exposure to heparin.
- **Rapid-onset HIT** can occur in patients previously (last 100 days) exposed to heparin who formed heparin-PF4 antibodies within 1 to 4 days of reexposure.
- **Confirmation:** Clinical diagnosis, supported by ⊕ **heparin-PF4** antibody by ELISA, functional assay (serotonin release assay).

Management

- Immediately **stop all heparin** products, including flushes and LMWH.
- Begin treatment with direct thrombin inhibitor (eg, **lepirudin** or **argatroban**) to prevent possible thrombosis.
- Perform Doppler ultrasound of lower extremities to rule out subclinical thrombosis if indicated.
- Do not start warfarin until the patient is on direct thrombin inhibitor and platelet count >100,000, as it may transiently worsen hypercoagulability. Continue warfarin for at least 30 days, even after platelet recovery, and for 3 months if documented thrombosis.

MNEMONIC

The 4 T's of HIT:

Timeliness of platelet fall: 5 to 10 days
Thrombocytopenia
Thrombosis (venous or arterial)
No o**T**her causes of thrombocytopenia

ANSWER

In the absence of a history and exam suggesting another alternative, the probable diagnosis is idiopathic thrombocytopenic purpura.

Bleeding Disorders

HEMOPHILIA A AND B

X-linked recessive disorders that cause excessive bleeding due to clotting factor deficiencies. Severity depends on the extent of the deficiency.

- **Hemophilia A: Factor VIII deficiency.**
- **Hemophilia B** (also called **Christmas disease**): **Factor IX deficiency.**

MNEMONIC

Hemophilia clotting factor deficiencies:

A8 (factor **VIII**)
B9 (factor **IX**)

Symptoms/Exam

- Patients typically become symptomatic by 2 years of age.
- Many patients are diagnosed by excessive bleeding following a circumcision.
- Common sites of spontaneous bleeding: Joints (80% of hemorrhage), muscles, and GI tract.
- **Spontaneous hemarthrosis: Stiffness,** warmth, pain, and swelling, often in knees or ankles.
- Excessive bleeding following invasive procedures or injuries may be the initial manifestation in patients with mild or moderate disease.

Diagnosis

- Isolated, reproducibly low factor VIII or factor IX activity level (without other conditions). Severe: <1%; moderate: 1% to 5%; mild: >5% activity.
- Normal platelet count, normal PT, typically ↑ **APTT** (especially in severe hemophilia), which is **corrected when mixed with normal plasma,** unless an inhibitor is present.
- Many cases are diagnosed on the basis of family history but **one-third of patients have no family history.**

Management

- Administer purified or recombinant **factor VIII or IX concentrate** during acute bleeding or prophylactically before invasive procedures (or FFP if specific factor concentrate is unavailable). Children with severe disease receive regular, long-term infusions to prevent recurrent joint bleeding.
- Patients with mild hemophilia A may respond to **DDAVP (desmopressin),** which ↑ release of factor VIII from endothelial storage, leading to ↑ circulating factor VIII level.
- **Antifibrinolytic therapy (such as aminocaproic acid)** can be used to stabilize mucosal bleeding and is usually used adjunctively.
- **Chronic treatment:** Avoid high-impact activities or surgical risks for trauma. Screen for hepatitis and HIV because of frequent transfusions. Advise vigilant preventive dental care. COX-2 selective NSAIDs, acetaminophen, and opioids can be used for joint pain but other NSAIDs and aspirin should be used selectively because of the ↑ risk of bleeding.

Complications

- **Hemophiliac arthropathy:** Synovitis and joint destruction, leading to chronic pain and ↓ ROM. Usually avoided in patients who have received long-term prophylaxis with factor concentrate in childhood.
- Blood-borne infections from factor concentrates (hepatitis C and HIV in the 1980s).
- Development of antibodies inhibiting the deficient factor (**inhibitors**), leading to ↓ response to factor concentrates.

QUESTION

A 24-year-old woman describes a history of easy bruising, with frequent epistaxis as a child that resolved in adolescence. Her menses are moderately heavy, and her dentist has told her that she bleeds somewhat more than the typical patient. Her father and aunt also have easy bleeding. Initial laboratory work is significant for a slightly ↑ PTT. Her platelet count and INR are normal. What do you suspect?

VON WILLEBRAND DISEASE

The **most common inherited bleeding disorder.** Characterized by ↓ production or activity of von Willebrand factor (vWF), produced by megakaryocytes and endothelial cells. vWF forms a platelet plug and acts as a carrier protein for factor VIII, prolonging the half-life of factor VIII. vWF is the only clotting factor not synthesized by the liver.

- Usually inherited but may be acquired:
    - **Inherited:** Three major types; the most common type is a quantitative deficiency of vWF that is inherited in an autosomal-dominant pattern, causing mild to moderate disease.
    - **Acquired:** Could be caused by an autoimmune disease, a mechanical valve, hypothyroidism, or certain medications, such as valproic acid or the ciprofloxacin.

Symptoms/Exam

- Bleeding patterns similar to those seen in platelet disorders: **Easy bruising, mucosal bleeding,** heavy menses, and excessive bleeding after trauma or dental or surgical procedures.
- **Bleeding following aspirin or NSAID use** is common.

Diagnosis

- **Screening tests:** Variable plasma vWF antigen levels, depending on the type, ↓ plasma vWF activity (ristocetin cofactor activity), ↓ factor VIII activity, ↑ or normal PTT. Bleeding time is rarely performed anymore.
- Send vWF multimer analysis and ristocetin-induced platelet aggregation for subtyping.

Management

- **Desmopressin (DDAVP)** indirectly ↑ the release of vWF from endothelial storage and can be used prophylactically before invasive procedures or during acute bleeding episodes. The effect is variable, depending on disease type and subtype.
- **vWF replacement therapy** via **recombinant vWF** or **factor VIII concentrates** rich in vWF can be used in patients with more severe disease.

Prognosis

Good. Severe disease is rare and can be managed with replacement therapy.

DISSEMINATED INTRAVASCULAR COAGULATION

Consumptive coagulopathy that occurs as a complication of an underlying illness, leading to **bleeding and thrombosis.** Common underlying illnesses include sepsis, transfusion reaction, neoplasia, trauma, and obstetric complications.

Symptoms/Exam

- **Bleeding:** Petechiae, ecchymoses, oozing from wounds and IV sites, and mucosal bleeding.
- **Thrombosis:** DVT, migratory thrombophlebitis, digital ischemia, renal cortical necrosis.
- **End-organ damage:** Acute renal failure (ARF), hepatic dysfunction, and CNS dysfunction can occur as a result of microthrombi, hypotension, and sepsis.

ANSWER

Von Willebrand disease. Diagnosis can be confirmed by checking plasma von Willebrand factor antigen and factor VIII activity.

Diagnosis

- ↑ fibrin split product, D-dimer, and PT/PTT.
- ↓ fibrinogen, platelets, and hematocrit.
- Don't forget to check the peripheral smear for schistocytes.

Management

- Correct the underlying disease.
- If no serious bleeding or thrombosis is present or anticipated, then no specific coagulopathy treatment is required.
- **Transfuse platelets** for platelet counts <20,000 or <50,000 with serious bleeding.
- Consider **cryoprecipitate** to maintain a fibrinogen concentration >100 mg/dL.
- Give **activated protein C** for patients with severe sepsis.
- In patients with thrombotic manifestations, **heparin** can be used to achieve a goal PTT of about 45 seconds.

Prognosis

Varies widely, depending on the ability to correct the underlying disease.

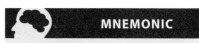

MNEMONIC

Causes of DIC:
STOP Making New Thrombi
Sepsis
Trauma
Obstetric complication
Acute **P**ancreatitis
Malignancy
Nephorotic syndrome
Transfusion

Clotting Disorders

APPROACH TO THROMBOPHILIA

The differential diagnoses of clotting disorders are outlined in Table 7.6. Consider inherited hypercoagulability in patients with the following:

- Idiopathic venous thrombosis at <50 years of age.
- Recurrent thrombosis.
- A first-degree relative with idiopathic thromboembolism at <50 years of age.
- Thrombosis associated with pregnancy or OCPs.
- Thrombosis in an unusual location.
- Arterial thrombosis.

Diagnosis

- Perform **CBC with peripheral smear** to evaluate for myeloproliferative disorders and thrombotic microangiopathies.
- Check **PTT** to screen for antiphospholipid antibody syndrome.
- Order age-appropriate malignancy screening.

TABLE 7.6. **Differential Diagnoses of Clotting Disorders**

ARTERIAL AND VENOUS	VENOUS ONLY	ARTERIAL ONLY
Malignancy	Factor V Leiden	Atherosclerosis
HIT syndrome	Prothrombin 20210 mutation	Vasculitis
Hyperhomocysteinemia	Protein C or S deficiency	
Paroxysmal nocturnal	Antithrombin III deficiency	
hemoglobinuria	Hormonal	
Myeloproliferative disease	Postsurgical, pregnancy,	
APS	immobilization	

- **Screen for inherited hypercoagulability:** Strong family history of VTE (one first-degree relative with documented VTE before the age of 45 years), <45 years with recurrent thrombosis, **thrombi in unusual places** (patients with portal, hepatic, mesenteric, or cerebral vein thromboses should be tested for all five inherited thrombophilias), warfarin skin necrosis, and arterial thrombosis.
    - **Factor V Leiden** mutation.
    - **Homocysteine level** for hyperhomocysteinemia.
    - **Antiphospholipid antibody tests,** including anticardiolipin antibody test and lupus anticoagulant antibody assays.
    - **Prothrombin 20210 (Factor II) mutation** for deficiency.
    - If an inherited thrombophilia is strongly suspected, include **functional assays for protein C, protein S, and antithrombin III activity** as well. These tests should be done **2 weeks after completion of anticoagulation therapy.**

FACTOR V LEIDEN DEFICIENCY

A mutation in the gene for clotting factor V leads to a gene product called factor V Leiden, which is resistant to cleavage by activated protein C, leading to slower inactivation. It is the most common cause of inherited hypercoagulability in white populations (3%-5% of persons of northern European descent). Heterozygotes have a 7-fold ↑ risk of thrombosis, and homozygotes have a 50- to 80-fold ↑ risk.

Symptoms/Exam

DVT, PE, cerebral vein thrombosis, and unexplained pregnancy loss.

Diagnosis

Order genotyping for **factor V Leiden mutation.**

Management

- Avoid smoking and OCPs.
- Anticoagulation after the first thrombotic event:
    - Heterozygotes should be treated with the same anticoagulation algorithm as noncarriers.
    - Homozygotes should be considered for lifelong anticoagulation.

Prognosis

Despite the ↑ risk of thromboembolic events, there is no evidence of ↑ mortality.

ANTIPHOSPHOLIPID ANTIBODY SYNDROME

Characterized by thrombosis and/or pregnancy morbidity associated with antibodies to plasma proteins that are bound to phospholipids. APS may be associated with SLE or other rheumatic diseases.

Symptoms/Exam

- May present with arterial and venous thrombosis, thrombocytopenia, recurrent spontaneous abortions, livedo reticularis, and hemolytic anemia.
- Catastrophic APS presents with widespread thrombotic disease, with multiorgan failure.

Diagnosis

Diagnostic criteria are as follows:

- **Thrombosis OR pregnancy morbidity AND**
- **Anticardiolipin antibody OR lupus anticoagulant** present in serum on two or more occasions at least 6 weeks apart.
- Other lab findings include: ↑ PTT (not corrected by mixing the patient's plasma with normal plasma), biological false-positive syphilis test.

Management

- Start anticoagulation with **LMWH,** since **PTT** cannot be used to titrate unfractionated heparin.
- Simultaneously intiate warfarin anticoagulation and continue for a minimum of 6 months after the first thrombotic event. Consider lifelong therapy. Use aspirin if warfarin is discontinued (eg, in pregnancy).
- Continue lifelong anticoagulation with warfarin in patients with recurrent thrombotic events.
- **Goal INR: 2 to 3.**
- For asymptomatic, nonpregnant, non–aspirin-allergic patients, start **prophylactic aspirin therapy** (81 mg/day), particularly if concomitant SLE or history of miscarriage.

Prognosis

APS is associated with premature death from thromboembolic disease as well as from associated comorbidities.

KEY FACT

Only a small proportion of patients ⊕ for lupus anticoagulant will develop **SLE;** however, patients with SLE are more likely to develop a lupus anticoagulant than the general population.

Transfusion Medicine

BLOOD PRODUCTS

Table 7.7 compares the categories of blood products used in transfusion medicine.

PRETRANSFUSION TESTING

- **Type and screen:** Obtained when transfusion is possible. An indirect Coombs test on a **standardized reference RBC** panel to test for reactivity from recipient plasma.
- **Type and cross:** Obtained when transfusion is imminent/expected. The recipient's blood and the donor's blood are crossmatched (via indirect Coombs test) for reactivity from recipient plasma.
- Weigh the need for transfusion against the risks:
  - Transfusion reactions (Table 7.8).
  - **Risk of infection** in ↓ order of risk: **CMV, HBV, HCV,** and **HIV.**

TRANSFUSION REACTIONS

Manage transfusion reactions as follows (see also Table 7.8):
- Immediately discontinue the transfusion.
- Alert the blood bank and check for clerical errors.
- From the **other arm, draw blood** for CBC, direct antiglobulin test, plasma free Hb, LDL, haptoglobin, indirect bilirubin, and PT/PTT. Repeat type, crossmatch, and blood culture.
- Save a **urine sample** for UA and urine Hb.
- Send all untransfused blood with attached tubing back to the blood bank.

QUESTION

A 46-year-old man becomes febrile 14 hours after a transfusion of two units of packed RBCs. He then develops chills, flank pain, and hypotension. His urine appears brown and is negative for nitrites and leukocyte esterase, and no bacteria are seen. What is the appropriate treatment?

TABLE 7.7.   Types of Blood Products

PRODUCT AND DESCRIPTION	COMMENTS
Whole blood	Provides volume expansion; used in patients with **acute massive blood loss**
Packed RBCs	Concentrated; each unit should ↑ hematocrit by 3%-4%
Washed RBCs	Removes the small amount of residual plasma from packed RBCs; used for the following: ▪ Patients with a history of severe or recurrent allergic **transfusion reactions** ▪ Patients with IgA deficiency if RBCs from IgA-deficient donors are unavailable ▪ Patients with complement-dependent AIHA
Irradiated RBCs	Prevents donor T lymphocytes from dividing in the recipient; used in **immunodeficient or immunosuppressed patients at risk for graft-versus-host disease**
Leukocyte-depleted RBCs	Used because WBCs lead to **HLA** alloimmunization and cytokine release and carry **CMV;** used for the following: ▪ Patients who are **chronically transfused** ▪ Potential **transplant recipients** ▪ Patients with a history of febrile nonhemolytic transfusion reactions ▪ Patients in whom CMV-seronegative components are desirable but not available
Pooled random donor platelets	Used for the following: ▪ Prophylactic transfusion for platelet counts <20,000 ▪ Transfusions for platelet counts <50,000 in bleeding patients or those undergoing major surgery
Single-donor platelets	Used in patients refractory to random donor platelets caused by alloimmunization
FFP	Contains all coagulation factors; used for the following: ▪ Patients with documented **coagulation factor deficiencies** who are actively bleeding or are scheduled for an invasive procedure ▪ **Reversal of warfarin** anticoagulation if significant bleeding or risk of bleeding is present ▪ Treatment of **TTP**
Cryoprecipitate	Prepared from plasma and containing fibrinogen, vWF, factor VIII, factor XIII, and fibronectin; used for the following: ▪ Patients with significant **hypofibrinogenemia** (<100 mg/dL) who are actively bleeding or are scheduled for an invasive procedure ▪ Replacement of factor VIII or vWF when specific factor concentrates are unavailable

Myeloproliferative Disorders

POLYCYTHEMIA VERA

A clonal proliferation of myeloid cells distinguished by ↑ RBC mass.

Symptoms/Exam

ANSWER

This clinical history is consistent with an acute hemolytic transfusion reaction. Aggressive hydration should be initiated to prevent acute tubular necrosis.

- Symptoms related to ↑ blood volume and ↑ blood viscosity: Headache, dizziness, tinnitus, blurred vision, fatigue.
- Other symptoms include: **Pruritus** (due to histamine from basophilia), epistaxis (mucosal engorgement and platelet dysfunction), **erythromelalgia** (burning pain in feet or hands, with erythema, pallor, and cyanosis), PUD, **acute gouty arthritis.** Can be associated with venous or arterial thrombosis, including unusual locations such as splenic or mesenteric vein thrombosis, or Budd-Chiari syndrome.
- ↑ risk of MI due to cardiac artery thrombosis.
- Exam: **Plethora (flushing), engorged retinal vein, splenomegaly, HTN.**

TABLE 7.8. **Types of Transfusion Reactions**

TYPE	RISK	CLINICAL FEATURES	TREATMENT	CAUSE	COMMENTS
Febrile nonhemolytic reactions	1/100	Fever, chills, mild dyspnea within 6 hours of transfusion	Antipyretics ; if severe, meperidine for rigors	Antibodies against donor WBCs and cytokine buildup	The **most common reaction**
Allergic reactions	1/100				
Urticaria		Hives	Diphenhydramine	Allergic reaction to plasma proteins	
Anaphylaxis		Bronchospasm, angioedema, hypotension; occurs within seconds to minutes	Epinephrine	Anti-IgA antibodies in **IgA-deficient patients**	
Delayed hemolytic transfusion reaction	1/1000	Fever, ↓ hematocrit, hyperbilirubinemia, spherocytosis within 2-10 days of transfusion	Supportive care Evaluate for new alloantibody and avoid in the future	An anamnestic response to undetected alloantibodies against minor antigens	Occurs with re-exposure to an antigen encountered during prior transfusion, transplantation, or pregnancy
Transfusion-related acute lung injury (TRALI)	1/5000	Noncardiogenic pulmonary edema, ARDS, hypotension, and fever, usually within 6 hours of transfusion	Supportive care as in ARDS ▪ O_2 ▪ May require intubation ▪ Diuresis	Donor antibodies to recipient WBCs in pulmonary capillaries	Recovery is usually complete within 96 hours
Acute hemolytic transfusion reaction	1/250,000	Fever, chills, flank pain, red or brown urine, hypotension, and tachycardia within 24 hours of transfusion DIC if severe	Vigorous hydration to prevent ATN Maintain urine output with diuretics, mannitol, or dopamine	Preformed antibodies against donor RBCs Usually 2/2 ABO incompatibility	Usually due to an error

Differential

- Distinguish from reactive erythrocytosis, which can be caused by hypoxia, smoking, COPD, high altitude, sleep apnea, and renal and liver lesions.
- Other myeloproliferative diseases (eg, chronic myelogenous leukemia [↑↑ WBC]), myelofibrosis (abnormal RBC morphology), essential thrombocytosis (↑ platelets only).

KEY FACT

Polycythemia vera can be distinguished from 2° causes of erythrocytosis by ↑ RBC mass in the setting of normal O_2 saturation and low EPO.

Diagnosis

- Must meet both major criteria and one minor criterion OR the first major criterion and two minor criteria (2008 WHO criteria):
    - **Major criteria:**
        - Hemoglobin >18.5 g/dL (men) or >16.5 g/dL (women) or other evidence of ↑ RBC volume.
        - **JAK2 mutation** (JAK2V617F or similar mutation): ⊕ in nearly all patients.

- Minor criteria:
    - **Bone marrow biopsy:** Hypercellularity for age with trilineage growth (panmyelosis), with ↑ erythroid, granulocytic, and megakaryocytic proliferation.
    - ↓ serum EPO.
    - Endogenous erythroid colony formation in vitro.
- Other lab findings include ↑ WBC, ↑ platelets, eosinophilia, iron deficiency, ↑ vitamin B_{12}, ↑ uric acid.

Management

- Perform **serial phlebotomy** to maintain hematocrit <45% in men and <42% in women (avoid iron supplementation, even if iron deficiency develops).
- Recommend low-iron diet.
- Give **low-dose daily ASA** in all patients to prevent thrombosis.
- Give **hydroxyurea** in patients at ↑ risk for thrombosis: >60 years of age, prior thrombosis, CVD risk factors, or platelet count >1,500,000. (Avoid alkylating agents, as they may ↑ conversion to acute leukemia.)
- Consider **anagrelide** in patients with platelet count >1,500,000 and refractory to hydroxyurea.
- Use **allopurinol** in patients with symptomatic ↑ uric acid or ↑ risk of uric acid calculi (↑ uric acid excretion).

Complications

- Venous or arterial **thrombosis** (due to ↑ viscosity and abnormal platelet function).
- Hemorrhage (due to abnormal platelet function).
- Transformation to **AML/myelodysplastic syndromes** in 5% of cases.
- Transformation to **myelofibrosis/myeloid dysplasia** in 15% of cases. Risk ↑ with disease duration and most commonly occurs after 10 years.

Prognosis

Indolent disease course. The median survival is 10 to 15 years. The major cause of morbidity and mortality is arterial thrombosis.

MYELOFIBROSIS

A clonal proliferative disorder of myeloid cells that leads to reactive bone marrow fibrosis, causing extramedullary hematopoiesis. Seen in adults >50 years of age.

Symptoms/Exam

- **Ineffective erythropoiesis,** leading to cytopenias, causing **fatigue and bleeding.**
- **Extramedullary hematopoiesis** (may occur in any organ but often is in liver, spleen, and lungs):
    - **Massive splenomegaly** leads to abdominal fullness and abdominal pain (splenic infarction) and early satiety.
    - Hepatomegaly leads to abdominal fullness and portal HTN, ascites, esophageal varices.
- Bone pain (especially in the upper legs).
- Transverse myelitis (due to myelopoiesis in the epidural space).
- Tumor bulk and ↑ cell turnover lead to **constitutional "B" symptoms** (fever, night sweats, and weight loss).

Diagnosis

There are no uniformly accepted criteria, but the 2008 WHO criteria state that patients must meet all three major criteria and two minor criteria:

- **Major criteria:**
  - Megakaryocyte proliferation and atypia on bone marrow smear, usually with reticulin and/or collagen fibrosis, or if ⊖, significant reticulin fibrosis; the megakaryocyte changes must have ↑ bone marrow cellularity, characterized by granulocytic proliferation and often ↓ erythropoiesis (ie, prefibrotic cellular-phase disease).
  - Not meeting WHO criteria for polycythemia vera, BCR-ABL1+ chronic myelogenous leukemia, myelodysplastic syndromes, or other myeloid neoplasms.
  - Demonstration of JAK2V617F or other clonal marker (eg, MPLW515L/K), or if ⊖ clonal marker, no evidence that the bone marrow fibrosis or other changes are caused by infection, autoimmune disorder, or other chronic inflammatory condition; hairy cell leukemia or other lymphoid neoplasm; metastatic malignancy; or toxic (chronic) myelopathies.
- **Minor criteria:**
  - Leukoerythroblastosis (nucleated RBCs and immature WBCs).
  - ↑ serum LDH.
  - Anemia.
  - Splenomegaly.
- Other findings include:
  - Peripheral smears: Poikilocytosis, **teardrop cells** (Figure 7.6), and giant granulated platelets.
  - Bone marrow aspirate: A **"dry tap."**

Management

- Treat anemia with androgens, periodic transfusions, and EPO.
- Use thalidomide or lenalidomide ± steroids.
- Consider splenectomy for symptomatic splenomegaly and anemia requiring frequent transfusions.
- Allogenic stem cell transplantation (ASCT) provides the only potential cure and may be considered for young patients with an appropriate donor available.

Prognosis

- Median survival: 5 years. Three-year survival rate: 50%.
- Transformation into AML <5%, with a much worse prognosis.
- Common causes of death: Bleeding (due to thrombocytopenia) and liver failure (due to liver hematopoiesis and subsequent portal HTN).

ESSENTIAL THROMBOCYTHEMIA

Marked proliferation of megakaryocytes in the bone marrow, leading to nonreactive ↑ platelets. Median age 50 to 60 years.

Symptoms/Exam

- Often asymptomatic at presentation and diagnosed incidentally.
- May present with thrombosis and hemorrhage.
- Vasomotor symptoms: Headache, lightheadedness, atypical chest pain, acral paresthesia, and erythromelalgia (erythema, warmth, and burning of the hands and feet).
- Palpable splenomegaly may be present on exam.

QUESTION

A 70-year-old woman with 900,000 platelets and an arterial clot presents with dyspnea on exertion for the last 6 months, fatigue, heart palpitations, and one episode of syncope. After obtaining an echocardiogram, you find that her pulmonary artery pressure is significantly elevated. Why?

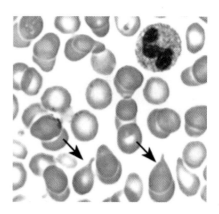

FIGURE 7.6. Myelofibrosis. Blood smear shows teardrop red blood cells (arrows). (Reproduced with permission from USMLE-Rx.com; courtesy of Dr. Kristine Krafts.)

Diagnosis

Must meet all four criteria (2008 WHO criteria):

- Sustained platelet count ≥450,000.
- Bone marrow biopsy specimen showing ↑ of the megakaryocytic lineage with ↑ enlarged, mature megakaryocytes. No significant ↑ or left shift of neutrophil granulopoiesis or erythropoiesis.
- Not meeting WHO criteria for polycythemia vera, 1° myelofibrosis, BCR-ABL1-positive chronic myelogenous leukemia (discussed below in the Chronic Leukemia secion), myelodysplastic syndromes, or other myeloid neoplasms.
- ⊕ JAK2V617F or other clonal marker, or if JAK2V617F-negative, no evidence of reactive thrombocytosis (due to iron deficiency, splenectomy, surgery, infection, inflammation, connective tissue disease, metastatic cancer, or lymphoproliferative disorders).

Management

- Patients <60 years of age with no history of thrombosis or hemorrhage and platelet count <1,500,000: Follow-up only or treat with low-dose ASA.
- Patients >60 years of age or those with history of thrombosis: Treat with **hydroxyurea** (preferred) or **anagrelide.**

Prognosis

Survival does not greatly differ from that of the control population. Rate of transformation to leukemia or other myeloid disorder increases in second decade after diagnosis (3%-10% in first decade and 6%-30% in second decade).

Miscellaneous Hematologic Disorders

MULTIPLE MYELOMA

A neoplastic clonal proliferation of B cells, producing a monoclonal IgG and IgA. Median age of patients with multiple myeloma is 65 years.

Symptoms/Exam

- The most common complaints are **bone pain** (especially back or ribs), weakness, fatigue, and weight loss.
- **Anemia, hypercalcemia, renal insufficiency, and lytic bone lesions.**
- Symptoms of hyperviscosity: Mucosal bleeding, vertigo, nausea, visual disturbances, altered mental status.
- Neurologic disease may lead to radiculopathy, peripheral neuropathy, cord compression, and CNS involvement (vertebral fracture).
- Amyloidosis, leading to enlarged tongue, neuropathy, HF, or hepatomegaly.
- ↑ infection.

Diagnosis

- Must meet the following three criteria:
    - A **bone marrow aspirate or biopsy with clonal plasma cells ≥10%** or the presence of a plasmacytoma (Figure 7.7).
    - **Monoclonal protein** level in serum (≥3 g/dL) or in urine (≥300 mg/24 hr) on electropheresis.
    - Evidence of 2° organ or tissue impairment such as lytic bone lesions, renal insufficiency, anemia, or hypercalcemia.
- **Skeletal survey reveals lytic lesions in the majority of patients** (Figure 7.8). The lesions will not be seen on bone scan, as they are not osteoblastic.

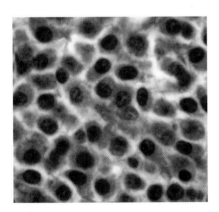

FIGURE 7.7. Multiple myeloma bone marrow aspirate. (Reproduced with permission from USMLE-Rx.com.)

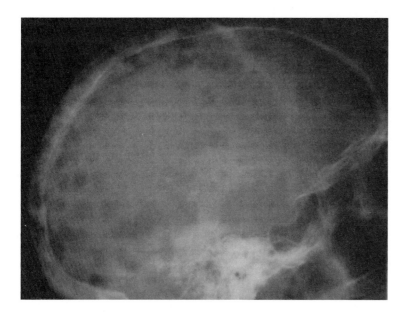

FIGURE 7.8. **Radiographic appearance of multiple myeloma.** (Reproduced with permission from USMLE-Rx.com.)

- Check β_2-microglobulin and albumin levels for staging.
- β_2-microglobulin usually ↑. Higher values = more advanced staging (poorer prognosis).
- The presence of monoclonal protein <3 g/dL, with <10% clonal plasma cells in the bone marrow.
- Multiple myeloma without organ or tissue impairment is called monoclonal gammopathy of undetermined significance (MGUS).
- Periodic follow-up is recommended, as MGUS can progress at 1%/year to multiple myeloma or a related B-cell disorder, such as macroglobulinemia, amyloidosis, or lymphoma.

Management

No treatment for smoldering multiple myeloma (ie, no end-organ damage). The main options for therapy include:

- Chemotherapy: **Melphalan, doxorubicin.**
- Immune modulators: **Thalidomide, lenalidomide,** and bortezomib. These agents may be used in combination with standard chemotherapy agents and steroids.
- **Corticosteroids** such as prednisone or dexamethasone.
- **Stem cell (bone marrow) transplantation.**
- Regimens and combinations are chosen based on the risk of the disease and whether bone marrow transplantation is a possibility.
- Prevention and treatment of complications, including:
  - **Hypercalcemia:** Hydration, prednisone, or a bisphosphonate.
  - **Skeletal lesions: Bisphosphonates,** chemotherapy, local radiation, or surgical fixation.
  - **Infection:** Immunization with pneumococcal and influenza vaccines and aggressive treatment of bacterial infections. Consider prophylactic antibiotics and IVIG for recurrent infections.
  - **Renal failure:** Hydration, prednisone, allopurinol, avoidance of NSAIDs and IV contrast, and plasmapheresis for acute failure.
  - **Hyperviscosity syndrome:** Plasmapheresis.
  - **Anemia:** EPO.

KEY FACT

Lytic lesions associated with multiple myeloma will not light up on bone scan (vs those due to osteoblastic bony metastases).

Prognosis

Median survival is 4 to 6 years, depending on the level of tumor burden and the availability of stem cell transplantation. Newer combinations of agents can often show >90% response rates.

WALDENSTRÖM MACROGLOBULINEMIA

Lymphoplasmacytic lymphoma in the bone marrow and an IgM monoclonal gammopathy in the blood. The median age at diagnosis is 60 years. Most cases are sporadic, and 20% are familial. Etiology is unknown. Symptoms are mainly related to lymphoplasmacytic infiltration and IgM monoclonal gammopathy.

Symptoms/Exam

- Anemia, leading to fatigue, weakness, pallor.
- Constitutional symptoms such as weakness, fatigue, weight loss, fever, night sweats.
- Lymphadenopathy and/or organomegaly.
- Oronasal and GI bleeding from engorged blood vessels and platelet dysfunction.
- Hyperviscosity in serum, leading to vision change, headache, ataxia, dementia, stroke, or coma.
- Peripheral neuropathy.
- Fundoscopic abnormalities: "Sausage link appearance" of retinal veins seen in 34% of patients.

Diagnosis

- Must meet the following three criteria:
    - A bone marrow biopsy sample with >10% **plasmacytic lymphocytes.**
    - An IgM monoclonal gammopathy in the serum (any size).
    - The bone marrow infiltrate shows the typical immunophenotype.
- Other labs include anemia, neutropenia, thrombocytopenia, ↑ LDH, ↑ β_2-microglobulin, ↑ ESR, ↑ serum viscosity.
- Smear typically shows rouleaux formation.

Management

- Asymptomatic patients: No treatment is indicated.
- Symptomatic patients: Standard treatment is not established. Treat hyperviscosity with plasmapheresis emergently. For tumors, many experts have incorporated rituximab into the initial treatment, alone or in combination with other chemotherapeutic agents. Hematopoietic cell transplantation is also considered.

Prognosis

Median survival is approximately 5 years from the time of diagnosis. Poor prognostic factors are older age, cytopenias, and an elevated β_2 microglobulin level.

APLASTIC ANEMIA

Hypoplastic or aplastic bone marrow (with no dysplasia), leading to pancytopenia. Biphasic distribution, with a peak in adolescent and elderly years. May be congenital (rare) or acquired. Etiologies of acquired diseases are as follows:

- **Idiopathic (most common** and probably autoimmune).
- Cytotoxic drugs and radiation.
- Idiosyncratic drug reactions to chloramphenicol, NSAIDs, and sulfa drugs.
- **Viral infections:** Parvovirus B19, EBV, HIV.
- **Immune disorders:** SLE, GVHD, thymoma.
- Paroxysmal nocturnal hemoglobinuria.
- Pregnancy.

Symptoms/Exam

- Anemia, leading to fatigue, weakness, pallor.
- Neutropenia, leading to recurrent infections.
- Thrombocytopenia, leading to mucosal and skin bleeding, purpura, petechiae.
- What should **not** be present: hepatosplenomegaly, lymphadenopathy, or bone tenderness.

Diagnosis

- Labs: **Pancytopenia** and **absolute reticulocytopenia.**
- Bone marrow: **Hypocellular,** with morphologically normal residual hematopoietic precursor cells.
- For severe disease, at least three of the following four values must be present: Neutrophils <500; platelets <20,000, reticulocytes <1%, and bone marrow cellularity <20%.

Management

- Mild: Supportive care (RBC and platelet transfusions as needed).
- Hematopoietic cell (bone marrow) transplantation is the only definitive therapy (for children and young patients).
- Immunosuppression with antithymocyte globulin, cyclosporine, or prednisone for patients >50 years of age or those without HLA-matched donors.

Prognosis

Prognosis depends on the severity of the pancytopenia and the patient's age. In severe forms, the median survival without treatment is 3 months, and 1-year survival is 20%. If treated, the 5-year survival rate is 20% to 80%.

Acute Leukemia

Neoplastic disorder characterized by proliferation of immature hematopoietic precursor cells in the bone marrow and later in the peripheral blood and other organs and tissues. If untreated, death usually occurs within 6 months of diagnosis. ↑ **risk** is associated with the following:

- **Congenital disorders:** Down syndrome, Bloom syndrome, Fanconi anemia, ataxia-telangiectasia.
- **Acquired disorders:** Myeloproliferative disorders, myelodysplastic syndromes, aplastic anemia.
- **Environmental exposure:** Alkylating agents, radiation, cigarette smoke, benzene, organic solvents.

Symptoms/Exam

Common presenting symptoms due to anemia, thrombocytopenia, and neutropenia: Fatigue, fever, easy bruising and purpura/petechiae, and infection.

Diagnosis

- **Peripheral smear:** ↑ circulating blasts (90% of patients), anemia, and thrombocytopenia.
- **Bone marrow:** ↑ blasts (>20%).
- Immunohistochemistry, cytogenetics, and flow cytometry should also be done to aid in diagnosis, classification, and risk stratification.
- An **LP** on all patients with acute lymphocytic leukemia (ALL) and any AML patients with **CNS symptoms.**

ACUTE LYMPHOCYTIC LEUKEMIA

Seen predominantly in children (the most common cancer in children). Bimodal distribution, with peaks at 3 to 7 years and 65 years of age. Classified as follows:

- Clonal cells may be B cells (75%) or T cells.
- Test patients with T-cell ALL for **HTLV-1.**
- **Burkitt leukemia:** Subtype of ALL with ↑ B cells. **t(8;14) translocation** is universally seen, leading to aberrant expression of the **c-myc oncogene.**

Symptoms/Exam

Findings that are more common in ALL than in AML include the following:

- **Bone pain.**
- **Lymphadenopathy:** Occurs in >50% of patients with ALL.
- **Hepatosplenomegaly:** Occurs in 66% of patients with ALL.
- **CNS involvement.**

Management

- Remission induction with combination chemotherapy to prevent resistance.
- **CNS prophylaxis** with **intrathecal chemotherapy** for all patients to prevent CNS relapse.
- Prolonged **postremission therapy** (1-3 years) to eliminate residual disease.

Complications

- Long-term disease-free survival rate: **30% for adults, 66% to 85% for children.**
- Common sites of **solitary relapse (sanctuary sites): CNS and testes** (due to poor penetration of chemotherapy).

ACUTE MYELOGENOUS LEUKEMIA

Represents 80% of all acute leukemia cases in adults. Most patients are >65 years of age, and the incidence ↑ with age.

Symptoms/Exam

Findings that are more common in AML than in ALL include the following:

- **Leukostasis:** Sludging of blasts in the microvasculature, which occurs when the blast count in the peripheral blood >100,000/mm³. Commonly leads to CNS symptoms **(somnolence, seizure, stroke)** and pulmonary symptoms **(dyspnea).**
- **DIC:** Commonly associated with the promyelocytic subtype.
- **Leukemia cutis:** Violaceous raised lesions of the skin due to infiltration of leukemic cells; associated with monocytic subtypes.

Diagnosis

Auer rods are pathognomonic for AML (Figure 7.9).

Management

- **Induction chemotherapy** with anthracycline (daunorubicin or idarubicin) + cytarabine.
- **Postremission therapy** options include:
  - **Consolidation chemotherapy.**
  - **Allogenic or autologous HSCT** may be considered, especially for patients with poor-risk cytogenetics or those who fail to achieve a complete remission or who relapse.

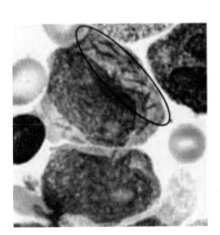

FIGURE 7.9. **Auer rods.** (Reproduced with permission from USMLE-Rx.com; courtesy of Dr. Robert W. Novak.)

Prognosis

Although approximately 60% to 80% of patients (<60 years of age) achieve complete remission, the overall 5-year survival rate is 10% to 35%. The cure rate for older patients is very low (10%-15%).

ACUTE PROMYELOCYTIC LEUKEMIA

- M3 subtype of AML caused by somatic mutation consisting of t(15;17) translocation that produces fusion gene protein PML-RARα (retinoic acid receptor-α).
- Commonly associated with DIC.
- **Management:** Anthracycline + *all*-trans retinoic acid induces complete remission in 90% of patients. For high-risk patients, the addition of arsenic trioxide may be beneficial.

Chronic Leukemia

CHRONIC LYMPHOCYTIC LEUKEMIA

A monoclonal proliferation of immunologically **incompetent mature B cells.** CLL is the **most common adult leukemia** in the Western world, representing 30% of all cases of leukemia. The median age of onset is 65 years.

Symptoms/Exam

- CLL is an **indolent** disease.
- Many patients are **asymptomatic at diagnosis.**
- Presenting symptoms include fever, night sweats, weight loss, fatigue, and weakness.
- **Generalized lymphadenopathy** and **hepatosplenomegaly** are common.
- Note ↑ incidence of autoimmune diseases, including AIHA, autoimmune thrombocytopenia, and pure red cell aplasia.

Diagnosis

- **Peripheral smear shows isolated lymphocytosis.** Lymphocytes appear small and mature and are **monoclonal on flow cytometry.**
- **Smudge cells** are common on peripheral smear and occur when fragile malignant lymphocytes are disrupted during preparation of the smear (Figure 7.10).

Management

- **Treatment is palliative.**
- Asymptomatic patients may be followed without treatment.
- **Alkylating agents** (chlorambucil or fludarabine) are the mainstay of therapy for symptomatic patients and those with rapidly progressive disease or complications.
- **Monoclonal antibodies** such as rituximab and alemtuzumab are options.
- Use **corticosteroids** for treatment of AIHA or autoimmune thrombocytopenia.
- **Radiation therapy** for large, bulky lymphoid masses.
- Nonmyeloablative **allogeneic bone marrow transplant** is being studied as an option.

Prognosis

New therapies are changing the prognosis of CLL. The early-stage disease has a median survival of 10 to 15 years. For more advanced diseases, the 2-year survival has improved to >90%.

KEY FACT

The most important prognostic factor in AML is **cytogenetics,** or the chromosomal structure of the leukemic cell. AML arising from preexisting **myelodysplastic syndromes** or **myeloproliferative disease** has a worse prognosis, as does treatment-related AML after chemotherapy for a previous malignancy.

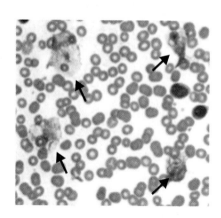

FIGURE 7.10. Chronic lymphocytic leukemia. Peripheral blood smear shows ↑ lymphocyte count with smudge cells. (Reproduced with permission from USMLE-Rx.com.)

CHRONIC MYELOGENOUS LEUKEMIA

A myeloproliferative disorder characterized by proliferation of myeloid cells that are capable of differentiation. Median age at presentation is 55 years. The clinical course may be divided into three phases, defined by the number of blasts:

- **Chronic phase:** Blasts <10%.
- **Accelerated phase:** Blasts 10% to 20%.
- **Blast phase:** Blasts >20%.

Symptoms/Exam

- **Approximately 85% of patients present in the chronic phase and are typically asymptomatic.**
- Patients become ↑ symptomatic as they progress through the accelerated and blast phases.
- Common symptoms include fatigue, weight loss, night sweats, LUQ pain, early satiety, and bone pain.
- Hepatosplenomegaly is common.
- Symptoms of leukostasis (blurred vision, respiratory distress, priapism) may be seen in the blast phase.

Diagnosis

- Peripheral smear shows ↑↑ WBC (with a left-shift, ie, blast predominance) and may show anemia, thrombocytopenia (but could be ↑ before blast phase), basophilia, and eosinophilia.
- As noted above, **the number of blasts seen determines the phase.**
- **Leukocyte alkaline phosphatase is low** (in contrast to other myeloproliferative disorders).
- The **Philadelphia chromosome t(9;22)**, producing the **fusion gene BCR/ABL,** is present in **95% of patients** and may be diagnosed via cytogenetics or PCR for the *BCR-ABL* gene product.

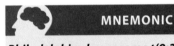

Management

- **Imatinib mesylate** is an oral **tyrosine kinase inhibitor** targeted to the fusion gene product. It is first-line treatment. It is associated with a 95% rate of complete hematologic remission.
- **Allogenic ASCT** is the only curative treatment and should be considered in the **chronic phase** for patients who are not responding to imatinib and have a suitable donor available.
- Dasatinib and nilotinib are second-generation inhibitors that compare favorably to imatinib mesylate.
- Interferon-α (IFN-α) plus cytarabine may be tried in patients who do not respond to imatinib, but is associated with greater toxicity and fewer treatment responses.

Prognosis

CML used to have a poor prognosis, with a median survival of 4 to 6 years. However, with imatinib mesylate and other molecular targeted agents, >80% of patients remain alive and without disease progression at 7 years.

MYELODYSPLASTIC SYNDROMES

A group of malignant stem cell disorders characterized by cytopenia, dysplastic changes in the marrow, morphologic and cytogenetic abnormalities, and a variable risk of transformation to acute leukemia. Risk of developing a myelodysplastic syndrome increases with age, with the median age >65 years. Consider in any patient, particularly the elderly patient, with unexplained cytopenia(s) or monocytosis.

Symptoms/Exam

Nonspecific; many patients are asymptomatic. Common presentations when patients
are symptomatic include:

- Symptoms of anemia, including fatigue, weakness, dizziness, angina.
- Pallor from anemia, petechia, and/or purpura are relatively common.
- Infection, easy bruising, or bleeding is less commonly seen.
- Fever, night sweats, and weight loss are uncommon.

Diagnosis

- Perform peripheral blood smear and bone marrow aspiration to define the subtypes.
  Many subtypes exist, including refractory anemia, refractory anemia with ringed
  sideroblasts, refractory anemia with excess blasts, chronic myelomonocytic anemia,
  and refractory anemia with excess blasts in transformation.
- Common findings include macrocytic red cells, ↓ reticulocyte percentage, ↓ neutrophil lobulation, and pancytopenia.
- Check vitamin B_{12} and folate levels to rule out megaloblastic anemia, which can
  show similar morphologic abnormalities of blood cells.

Management

- Due to the advanced age and comorbidities of most patients, supportive care is the
  mainstay of treatment, including antibiotics for infections, transfusion, and hematopoietic growth factors.
- Depending on the subtype, patient age, functional status and prognostic scores,
  hematopoietic growth factors (EPO, G-CSF), immunosuppressive agents (antithymocyte globuline, cyclosporine), or other chemotherapeutic agents such as lenalidomide, cytarabine, or azacitidine may be used. Hematopoietic stem cell transplantation may also be considered. The isolated deletion of 5q subtype is particularly
  responsive to lenalidomide.

Prognosis

The risk of transformation to AML depends on the percentage of blasts in the bone
marrow. Survival could range from <1 year to many years. Infection, transfusion re-
fractoriness, and transformation to acute leukemia are common reasons for death.

Lymphoma

HODGKIN LYMPHOMA

A clonal **B-cell** malignancy in which **Reed-Sternberg cells** are the malignant cells
(Figure 7.11). Bimodal age distribution, with peaks among patients in their 20s and in
those >50 years of age.

Symptoms/Exam

Common presentations include the following:

- A painless, enlarged, rubbery lymph node (70% of patients).
- A mediastinal mass on CXR, with possible retrosternal chest pain, cough, or short-
  ness of breath.
- **B symptoms:** Fever, night sweats, and weight loss.
- Hepatosplenomegaly and pruritus are common.
- Pain in the affected lymph node after EtOH consumption is uncommon but
  suggestive.

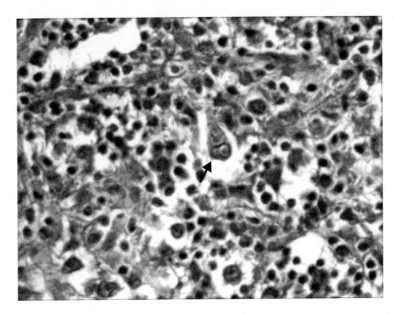

FIGURE 7.11. **Hodgkin lymphoma.** Lymph node mixed inflammatory infiltrate, including eosinophils, as well as binucleate Reed-Sternberg cell (arrow) with prominent nucleoli from a 20-year-old woman with lymphadenopathy. (Reproduced with permission from USMLE-Rx.com.)

Diagnosis

- Perform **excisional lymph node biopsy** for definitive diagnosis (see Figure 7.11).
- Staging studies include CXR and CT of the chest, abdomen, and pelvis.
- Labs that may affect choice of therapy or staging include CBC with differential, ESR, LFTs, albumin, LDH, and calcium.
- Bone marrow biopsy.

Management

- Treat with irradiation and/or ABVD (adriamycin, bleomycin, vincristine, dacarbazine), depending on the stage and on whether bulky mediastinal disease is present.
- Treat relapsed disease with conventional chemotherapy or high-dose chemotherapy plus autologous ASCT.

Prognosis

The 10-year survival rate of patients with stage IA or IIA disease treated by radiotherapy is >80%. Patients with disseminated disease (stage IIB, IV) have 5-year survival rates of 50% to 60%.

NON-HODGKIN LYMPHOMA

Heterogeneous cancers of B and T cells. A number of different classification systems exist for lymphoma. The **WHO classification** defines five large groups (Table 7.9) organized by cell type (ie, the normal cell type that most resembles the tumor), defining phenotype, and molecular or cytogenetic characteristics.

Some major examples with the typical disease course are:
- **Indolent:** Typically not curable, but even if left untreated, survival is measured in years. Patients may have prolonged survival, even with partial treatment response.
  - **Follicular lymphoma:** Patients are typically middle-aged or older and present with painless peripheral lymphadenopathy.

- **Mucosa-associated lymphoid tissue (MALT) lymphoma:** A form of marginal zone lymphoma. Gastric tumors have been linked to *H pylori* infection, and the majority of patients regress with antimicrobial therapy. Patients with gastric tumors may present with PUD or abdominal pain.
- **Aggressive:** Typically curable, but survival is measured in months if untreated.
  - **Diffuse large B-cell lymphoma:** Patients are typically middle-aged or older and often present with a rapidly enlarging neck or abdominal mass.
- **Highly aggressive:** Typically curable, but survival is measured in weeks if untreated. There is a high risk of tumor lysis syndrome.
  - **Burkitt lymphoma:** Exists in endemic, sporadic, and immunodeficiency-related forms. It is endemic in Africa, with up to 90% of cases related to EBV infection; presents as a tumor of the jaw or facial bone. Of sporadic cases, only about 20% are related to EBV infection. Typically presents as bulky abdominal disease.

Symptoms/Exam

- B symptoms, including fever, weight loss, and sweats.
- Systemic lymphadenopathy is seen ± hepatosplenomegaly.

Diagnosis

- **Excisional lymph node biopsy** is preferable for definitive diagnosis and staging.
- Staging studies include CXR, CT of the chest/abdomen/pelvis, and bone marrow biopsy.
- Labs that may affect choice of therapy or staging include **LDH,** CBC with differential, peripheral smear, LFTs, chem 10, and serum protein electrophoresis.

Management

- **Indolent:** Treatment is aimed at alleviation of symptoms.
  - Early, asymptomatic disease may be observed or treated with locoregional or extended-field radiation therapy.
  - Options for more advanced disease include single-agent chemotherapy with chlorambucil, cyclophosphamide, or fludarabine; combination chemotherapy with CVP (cyclophosphamide, vincristine, and prednisone).
  - Monoclonal antibody therapy with rituximab used for B-cell lymphomas.
  - Radioimmunotherapy with yttrium-90 ibritumomab tiuxetan or iodine 131 tositumomab may also have a role in treatment.
- **Aggressive:** Treatment is aimed at cure.
  - Treat early disease with CHOP (cyclophosphamide, doxorubicin, vincristine, and prednisone), possibly followed by involved-field radiation.
  - Treat advanced disease with CHOP or a CHOP-like regimen.
  - Rituximab is used for aggressive B-cell lymphomas.
- **Highly aggressive:** May benefit from autologous ASCT early in the course.
- **Special forms of lymphoma:**
  - Burkitt lymphoma, lymphoblastic lymphoma: Require specific regimen tailored to each type.
  - Mantle cell lymphoma: Intensive initial chemotherapy, including autologous ASCT or reduced-intensity allogeneic HSCT.
  - MALT lymphoma: Eradicate *H pylori* with antibiotics.

Prognosis

The median survival with indolent lymphomas has been 6 to 8 years. Factors for poor prognosis are age >60 years, ↑ serum LDH, stage III or IV disease, and poor performance status.

TABLE 7.9.   WHO-Proposed Classification of Non-Hodgkin Lymphoma

Precursor B
  B-cell lymphoblastic lymphoma
Mature B
  Diffuse large B-cell lymphoma
  Mediastinal large B-cell lymphoma
  Follicular lymphoma
  Small lymphocytic lymphoma
  Lymphoplasmacytic lymphoma
  Mantle cell lymphoma
  Burkitt lymphoma
  Marginal zone lymphoma
    MALT type
    Nodal
    Splenic
  Mucosal tissue associated
Precursor T
  T-cell lymphoblastic lymphoma
Mature T (and NK cell)
  Anaplastic T-cell lymphoma
  Peripheral T-cell lymphoma

KEY FACT

Burkitt lymphoma and Burkitt leukemia are considered manifestations of the same disease.

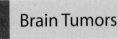

Brain Tumors

1° BRAIN TUMORS

Classified by predominant cell type:

- **Meningiomas:** Arise from cells in the arachnoid membrane. The vast majority are benign, but morbidity is caused by their mass effect (Figure 7.12A).
- **Gliomas:** Tumors derived from glial cells—the most common 1° brain tumor (50%). Classified according to grade (glioblastomas are the highest/worst; Figure 7.12B). Various genetic syndromes may lead to a predisposition to these tumors, including tuberous sclerosis, neurofibromatosis type 1, and Li-Fraumeni syndrome.
- **Medulloblastomas:** Embryonal tumors, most often seen in children.

Symptoms/Exam

- Present with headaches, seizures, nausea and vomiting, syncope, disturbance in memory or mood, personality changes, muscle weakness, sensory deficits, and aphasia.
- Headache suggestive of a possible brain tumor: A change in a prior headache pattern, an abnormal neurologic exam, positional changes, and associated nausea and vomiting.

Diagnosis

- **MRI** (preferred) or CT (diagnostic for meningioma), both ± contrast.
- Tissue biopsy for histologic confirmation is often obtained at the time of resection or may be done via stereotactic biopsy in cases where resection will not improve survival.

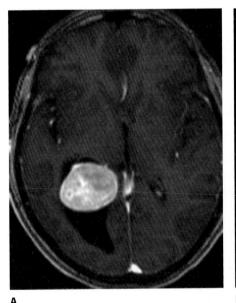
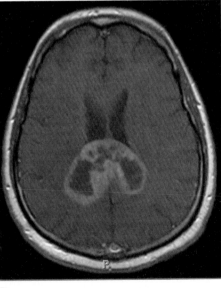

A   B

FIGURE 7.12.   **Meningioma (A) and glioblastoma multiforme (B). (A)** Postcontrast axial T1-weighted sequence in a 62-year-old woman with headaches demonstrates a large, homogeneously enhancing mass within the trigone of the right lateral ventricle associated with ventricular dilatation. Histology was that of a meningioma (grade I). **(B)** Transaxial contrast-enhanced image shows an enhancing intra-axial mass with central necrosis crossing the corpus callosum ("butterfly glioma"). (Image A reproduced from Watts J, et al. Magnetic resonance imaging of meningiomas: a pictorial review. *Insights Imaging.* 2014;5(1):113-122; image B reproduced with permission from USMLE-Rx.com.)

Management

- Choose treatment depending on the type and location of the tumor and the condition of the patient.
- Monitor asymptomatic meningiomas with serial neuroimaging every 3 to 6 months. If symptomatic, expanding, infiltrative, or associated with significant surrounding edema, resect the lesion. Adjuvant radiation therapy may be offered for patients with high-grade lesions or incomplete resection.
- Stereotactic radiosurgery may be used instead of surgical excision for small tumors in sites where complete excision is difficult.
- Give corticosteroids for cerebral edema before surgery. Treat herniation with dexamethasone and IV mannitol. Give anticonvulsants for seizures. Place shunt for obstructive hydrocephalus.

BRAIN METASTASES

Represent **>50% of intracranial tumors** in adults. Approximately 10% to 15% of patients with solid tumors develop brain metastases.

Symptoms/Exam

Same as 1° brain tumors.

Diagnosis

- **MRI and CT (± contrast)** with characteristic findings suggesting metastasis, including multiple lesions, circumscribed margins, vasogenic edema out of proportion to the size of the lesion, and location at the gray-white matter junction.
- Brain biopsy if the diagnosis is in doubt.
- LP for patients with suspected carcinomatous meningitis.
- **CXR** to look for pulmonary metastasis or to establish a 1° site if it is unknown. About 60% of patients with brain metastases have either a lung 1° or pulmonary metastases from their 1° tumor.
- Don't forget mammography in women if 1° unknown.

Management

- Patients with a **favorable prognosis** include those <65 years of age with a high-performance status, a controlled 1° tumor, and no extracranial metastases. Median survival is about 7 months. Aggressive treatment with **surgical resection or stereotactic radiosurgery** followed by **whole-brain radiation therapy** may be recommended.
- Patients with a **poor prognosis** have a poor performance status and a median survival of about 2 months. The following treatments are recommended:
  - Whole brain radiation therapy to improve neurologic deficits and prevent further neurologic deterioration.
  - Corticosteroids to control symptoms related to edema.

MNEMONIC

Tumors that commonly metastasize to the brain:
Pounds (LBS) Kilos (K)

Lung
Breast
Skin (melanoma)
Kidney

Squamous Cell Carcinoma of the Head and Neck

Most commonly associated with tobacco and alcohol use. Other risk factors include radiation, occupational exposures, and chronic viral infection (with EBV, HPV, HSV, or HIV).

Symptoms/Exam

- Neck mass.
- Ulcers or exophytic lesions in the nose, lips, mouth, or throat.
- Nasal obstruction, hoarseness, dysphagia, odynophagia, cervical lymphadenopathy, globus sensation, otalgia.

KEY FACT

Physical exam: Make sure to include bimanual palpation of the tongue and the floor of the mouth and palpation of the neck.

Diagnosis

- Ulcer(s) or exophytic lesion(s) on bimanual palpation of the tongue or floor of the mouth, or on palpation of the neck.
- Panendoscopy: Perform laryngoscopy, bronchoscopy, and esophagoscopy to visualize the extent of tumor involvement.
- Check CT or MRI to determine the size/extent and location of lesions and nodes.
- Perform fine-needle aspiration of suspicious neck nodes (or of the visible tumors when scoped).

Management

Determine treatment by the resectability of the lesion and the extent of advancement. Treat early lesions with radiotherapy or surgery alone and more advanced lesions with concomitant chemotherapy.

NASOPHARYNGEAL CARCINOMA

- Cancer of the nasopharynx—squamous cell carcinoma (SCC) is the most common.
- Rare in the West and associated with tobacco and alcohol, as with other SCCs of the head and neck. Endemic in southern China and associated with EBV, genetic predisposition, and dietary factors such as nitrates, salted fish, and Chinese herbs. There are endemic areas in Southeast Asia and the Mediterranean as well.

Symptoms/Exam

Neck mass, nasal obstruction, epistaxis, and otitis media.

Diagnosis

Same as for other SCCs of the head and neck; possible role for PET scan in staging. ↑ IgA to EBV.

Management

Concomitant chemoradiation with cisplatin and fluorouracil is commonly used. Selected cases of locally recurrent nasopharyngeal carcinoma may be treated with repeated irradiation or surgery. Other SCCs are treated with a combination of surgery (when resectable) and irradiation.

Genitourinary Cancers

BLADDER CANCER

Second most common GU cancer after prostate cancer. Affects men more than women. Mean age at diagnosis: 65 years. Risk factors for bladder cancer include cigarette smoking (60%), exposure to industrial dyes or solvents (15%), arsenic exposure, chronic cystitis, schistosomiasis, radiation, and cyclophosphamide use. In order of prevalence: urothelial cell carcinoma (90%), SCC (7%), and adenocarcinoma (2%).

Symptoms/Exam

- **Hematuria** is the most common presenting symptom (85%-90%). Typically, is gross, painless, and throughout micturition.
- Irritative or obstructive voiding symptoms may be seen.
- Flank pain, suprapubic pain, hypogastric pain, and perineal pain may all result from invasive or metastatic disease.

Diagnosis

- Assume hematuria in a patient >40 years of age is urothelial cancer until proven otherwise and investigate with **cystourethroscopy, urine cytology,** and **CT with urography** or **IVP with renal ultrasound!**
- A CXR and bone scan may be used for screening patients with documented bladder cancer who are at high risk for metastasis.

Management

- **Superficial bladder cancer** (superficial to the muscularis propria):
  - Cystoscopic resection of visible tumor (**transurethral resection of the bladder tumor**).
  - If the superficial cancer is high risk based on histology, number of lesions or recurrences, or failure to completely resect, then intravesical therapy with BCG (live attenuated *Mycobacterium bovis*) or other chemotherapeutic agents is recommended.
  - Aggressive posttreatment surveillance with urine cytology and cystoscopy is recommended.
- **Invasive bladder cancer:**
  - **Radical cystectomy** with bilateral pelvic lymph node dissection.
  - **Neoadjuvant or adjuvant chemotherapy** is superior to radical cystectomy alone:
    - Gemcitabine plus cisplatin.
    - MVAC (methotrexate, vinblastine, doxorubicin, and cisplatin).

RENAL CELL CARCINOMA

Risk factors include smoking, obesity, hypertension, and ESRD. Hereditary clear cell renal carcinoma is associated with von Hippel–Lindau syndrome and the von Hippel–Lindau gene mutation on chromosome 3.

Symptoms/Exam

- Remember: The classic triad—**flank pain, hematuria,** and a **palpable abdominal mass**—is found in only 10% to 15% of patients.
- Increasingly diagnosed in asymptomatic patients during incidental abdominal imaging.

Diagnosis

- Abdominal ultrasound is useful for distinguishing a benign cyst from a complex cyst or tumor.
- CT of the abdomen will show a multilocular mass, with thickened, irregular walls and septae, enhanced with contrast (Figure 7.13).
- Percutaneous biopsy is occasionally used if imaging is not clear.

Management

- Patients with disease limited to the kidney (stages I and II) should undergo partial or radical (preferred if the condition allows) nephrectomy.
- Patients with limited invasion (stage III) should undergo radical nephrectomy; those with extensive invasion or metastasis (stage IV) may have palliative nephrectomy.
- No chemotherapeutic regimen has been consistently shown to be effective in metastatic RCC.
- **Immunotherapy with IFN-α** or **interleukin-2** has been shown to induce an immune response against tumor cells and can be considered for metastatic RCC.
- The vascular endothelial growth factor receptor tyrosine kinase inhibitors **sorafenib** and **sunitinib** are approved by the FDA for the treatment of patients with advanced

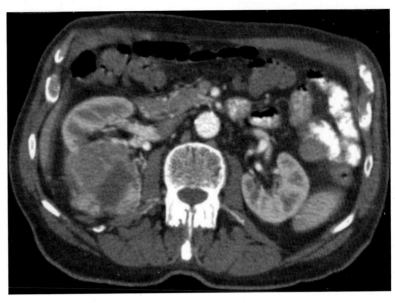

FIGURE 7.13.   Renal cell carcinoma. Large heterogenous mass within the right kidney. (Reproduced from Schnoeller TJ, et al. Partial nephrectomy using porcine small intestinal submucosa. *World J Surg Oncol.* 2011;9:126.)

RCC and the treatment of metastatic kidney cancer that has progressed after a trial of immunotherapy, respectively.

■ Many other targeted agents may benefit, including bevacizumab and others in clinical trials.

Complications

Fever, erythrocytosis, hypercalcemia, anemia, hepatopathy, and amyloidosis are all paraneoplastic syndromes associated with RCC.

Breast Cancer

The most common cancer among women of all races and the second leading cause of cancer death in women, after lung cancer. See the Community and Preventive Medicine chapter for recommendations on screening and prevention of breast cancer.

Symptoms/Exam

Palpable mass on exam, with or without abnormality on mammography.

Diagnosis

Made by biopsy after suspicious lesion localized on imaging. Staging by TNM (tumor, node, metastasis) system.

Pathology

■ **Ductal carcinoma in situ (DCIS):** Proliferation of abnormal cells confined within the mammary ductal system. A precursor to invasive breast cancer.
■ **Invasive breast carcinoma:** Infiltrating ductal carcinoma is the most common type of invasive breast cancer; infiltrating lobular carcinoma is the second most common; less common histologies include tubular, mucinous, and medullary carcinoma.
■ **Inflammatory breast cancer:** Rare but very aggressive form of breast cancer with diffuse dermatologic erythema and edema (peau d'orange). Often presents with

breast pain, breast enlargement, itching, or fast-growing lump. On presentation, almost all women have lymph node involvement, and approximately one-third have distant metastases. Presents at a younger age than other breast cancers. It is critical to obtain a biopsy within days if the diagnosis is suspected.

Management

- **Early stage:** Includes patients with clinical stage I, IIA, or a subset of stage IIB disease (T2N1):
    - Start with surgery (lumpectomy or mastectomy) and test lymph nodes.
    - Remove lymph nodes, if needed, with or without radiation therapy.
    - Following definitive local treatment, adjuvant systemic therapy may be offered depending on tumor size, grade, number of involved lymph nodes, the status of estrogen and progesterone receptors, and expression of the human epidermal growth factor 2 (HER2) receptor.
- **Locally advanced:** For some patients with clinical stage IIB disease (T3N0) and stage IIIA to IIIC disease, management involves **neoadjuvant systemic therapy.** Goal is to reduce tumor size before surgery and enable breast conservation.
- If HER2-positive, a HER2-specific agent is added (eg, trastuzamab).
- After neoadjuvant therapy, all patients should have **surgery,** even if the tumor seems resolved. Either breast-conserving surgery or mastectomy may be appropriate depending on tumor and patient characteristics. During surgery, lymph nodes can be assessed for removal.
- The use of **postoperative (adjuvant) systemic therapy** is guided by the patient's clinical status and tumor characteristics.
- See the Surgery chapter for more on breast cancer management.
- **Posttreatment surveillance:** Annual mammograms for patients who had breast-conserving therapy. Breast MRI, whole-breast ultrasound, lab testing, and whole-body imaging are not recommended.

KEY FACT

If you see what looks like mastitis (often referred to as peau d'orange or an orange peel appearance) in a non-breastfeeding woman, think **inflammatory breast cancer** and obtain a biopsy immediately.

Carcinoma of Unknown Primary

A term used when patients present with a metastatic site and initial evaluation fails to identify a 1° tumor. Represents 2% to 5% of all cancer diagnoses. Classified in one of five histologic categories, based on light microscopy of biopsied tissue:
- Adenocarcinoma.
- SCC.
- Neuroendocrine carcinoma.
- Poorly differentiated carcinoma.
- Poorly differentiated neoplasm (the pathologist cannot differentiate between carcinoma and other cancers).
- **Exam and diagnosis:**
    - Begin with a complete history and physical (including genital and rectal exams).
    - Include a CBC and UA in the initial labs. Fecal immunochemical test, Pap smear, and mammogram as indicated.
    - Initial imaging: CXR and CT of the chest, abdomen, and pelvis.
- Biopsy with pathologic evaluation guides further studies. Examples:
    - Poorly differentiated carcinoma: Human chorionic gonadotropin, α-fetoprotein.
    - Adenocarcinoma: Prostate-specific antigen (PSA), mammography, endoscopy.
    - SCC of cervical nodes: CT of the head and neck, laryngoscopy, nasopharyngoscopy, PET scan.

Management

Table 7.10 outlines the treatment options for carcinoma of unknown primary.

TABLE 7.10.   **Empiric Treatment for Carcinoma of Unknown Primary**

PATIENTS WITH:	TREAT AS:
SCC in cervical lymph nodes	Advanced head and neck cancer
SCC in inguinal nodes	Do a careful exam of the anal canal and genitalia and consider lymphadenectomy and postoperative radiation ± chemotherapy
Women with peritoneal carcinomatosis	Advanced ovarian cancer
Women with adenocarcinoma in axillary lymph nodes	Stage II breast cancer
Men with bone metastases or an ↑ PSA	Advanced prostate cancer
Young men with poorly differentiated carcinoma and a midline tumor	Extragonadal germ cell tumor
Poorly differentiated carcinoma	Treat with empiric platinum/paclitaxel
Poorly differentiated neuroendocrine carcinoma	Treat with empiric platinum/etoposide ± paclitaxel

Chemotherapeutic Agents

Chemotherapeutic agents interfere with the cell cycle. They are divided into two categories based on kinetics:

- Cell-cycle-specific (CCS) drugs: Act specifically on cells that are cycling and are usually most active in one specific phase of the cycle.
- Cell-cycle-nonspecific (CCNS) drugs: Act on cells whether they are cycling or resting.

CLASSES OF CHEMOTHERAPEUTIC AGENTS

Drug classes are as follows:

- **Alkylating agents:** CCNS agents that alkylate nucleic acid bases, thus causing cross-linking, abnormal pairing, and breakage of DNA/RNA strands. Examples include busulfan, chlorambucil, cyclophosphamide, ifosfamide, cisplatin, carboplatin.
- **Antimetabolites:** CCS agents that act primarily in the S phase of the cell cycle. They antagonize folate or nucleic acid bases, thus interfering with DNA/RNA synthesis. Examples include methotrexate, mercaptopurine, thioguanine, cytarabine, fluorouracil, fludarabine, cytarabine, cladribine, gemcitabine, hydroxyurea.
- **Plant alkaloids:** CCS agents that are naturally occurring nitrogenous bases. Many act by inhibiting the mitotic spindle. Examples include **vinblastine, vincristine,** etoposide, paclitaxel.
- **Antibiotics:** CCNS agents that intercalate adjacent nucleotides, thus causing DNA strand breaks. Examples include doxorubicin, daunorubicin, bleomycin, mitomycin.
- **Hormonal agents:** Not directly cytotoxic, but they downregulate hormonally stimulated growth. Examples include tamoxifen, anastrozole, letrozole, exemestane, leuprolide, goserelin, fulvestrant.
- **Immunotherapeutic agents:** Examples include rituximab and other similar agents, IFN-α.

KEY FACT

Vinblastine treats solid tumor, leukemias, and lymphomas.

KEY FACT

Vincristine and vinblastine prevent formation of microtubles into spindles and paclitaxel prevents breakdown of microtubles.

TOXICITIES

Selected toxicities of chemotherapeutic agents include the following:
- **Cardiomyopathy:** Doxorubicin, daunorubicin.
- **Pulmonary fibrosis:** Bleomycin.
- **Hemorrhagic cystitis:** Alkylating agents, especially cyclophosphamide and ifosfamide.
- **Peripheral neuropathy:** Paclitaxel, vincristine, vinblastine.

Acute Complications of Cancer Therapy

TUMOR LYSIS SYNDROME

A syndrome of metabolic disarray that results from rapid lysis of cancer cells. Typically induced by chemotherapy or radiation, but may rarely be caused by spontaneous necrosis. Most commonly associated with poorly differentiated lymphomas (eg, Burkitt lymphoma) and with leukemias, especially ALL. Rare in solid tumors.

KEY FACT

Risk factors for tumor lysis syndrome:
- Hyperuricemia (pretreatment)
- Renal insufficiency
- Hypovolemia
- Chemosensitivity
- High tumor cell turnover
- Elevated LDH (pretreatment)

Diagnosis

- Suspect the diagnosis in at-risk patients who develop ARF, ↑ uric acid, ↑ phosphate, and/or ↑ potassium.
- Laboratory diagnosis may be based on two of the following: 25% ↑ from baseline in uric acid, potassium, or phosphate; or 25% ↓ from baseline in calcium.

Management

- Pretreat patients at high risk for tumor lysis syndrome before (as well as during and after) chemotherapy or radiation with allopurinol and fluids to maintain urine output >2 to 3 L/day.
- Treatment includes management of electrolyte abnormalities, aggressive hydration, and diuretics to ↑ urine output.
- Hemodialysis may be needed for hyperkalemia, hyperphosphatemia, ARF, or fluid overload.

NEUTROPENIC FEVER

Defined as a single temperature >38.3°C (101°F) or sustained temperature >38°C (100.4°F) for 1 hour in a patient with an ANC <500. Etiologies are as follows:
- **Gram-positive bacteria** are the most common causes of infection in neutropenic patients, but **gram-negative bacteria (eg, *Pseudomonas aeruginosa*)** are generally associated with the most serious infections.
- Fungal infections, especially *Candida* and *Aspergillus,* are commonly found with prolonged and severe neutropenia and prolonged antibiotic use.
- Viral infections also occur, especially with **human herpesviruses.**

Symptoms/Exam

Perform a thorough review of systems and exam to localize the source of fever. Remember to examine the skin, mucous membranes, oropharynx, sinuses, and perirectal area.

Diagnosis

- **Labs:** CBC with differential, chem 7, a hepatic panel, and UA.
- **Microbiology workup:** Obtain blood cultures through each line and one peripheral culture; urine Gram stain and culture. LP if indicated (headache, change in mental status, neurologic symptoms, clinical manifestations on exam); although will need platelets >100 to safely perform LP.
- **Imaging:** CXR; further imaging as indicated.

Management

- Start empiric antibiotic therapy:
  - **Monotherapy:** Antipseudomonal β-lactams cefepime, carbapenem, or piperacillin-tazobactam.
  - **Combination therapy:** Aminoglycosides can be added to the above if hypotensive or resistance is suspected.
  - **Vancomycin** should be added in certain situations (eg, patients with a history of MRSA colonization or with hypotension, mucositis, possible skin or catheter site infection, or recent quinolone prophylaxis). Discontinue if cultures are ⊖ at 72 hours.
  - In patients with neutropenia and unexplained fever persisting for 5 to 7 days, an antifungal agent should be started.
  - **Low-risk** adult patients can be discharged on oral ciprofloxacin + amoxicillin/clavulanate after an initial IV dose, provided they are observed carefully and have access to medical care 24/7; ANC >100; monocyte count >100; normal CXR; normal LFTs and creatinine; no clinical IV site tunnel/exit site infection; temperature <39.0°C (102.2°F); no abdominal pain; evidence of impending bone marrow recovery; no comorbidities; and neutropenia expected to last <10 days.
- **Duration:**
  - If the source is known, complete a standard course of treatment, even after ANC recovery.
  - For an unknown source:
    - Continue empiric antibiotics until afebrile with ANC >500 for at least 1 day and the patient is afebrile for 2 days, or complete a minimum of a 7-day course.
    - If the patient becomes afebrile but remains neutropenic, consider completing a 14-day course.
    - Persistent fever: If ANC >500, discontinue antibiotics 4 to 5 days after ANC >500 and reassess. If ANC <500, continue for 14 days and reassess.

GRAFT-VERSUS-HOST DISEASE

A syndrome that is caused by immunocompetent cells from a graft targeting the receiving patient's cell antigens. Occurs most often after an allogeneic bone marrow transplantation. Rates of GVHD are 30% to 40% among related donors and recipients and 60% to 80% between unrelated donors and recipients. The greater the mismatch between donor and recipient, the greater the risk of GVHD.

There are two categories of disease:

- **Acute GVHD:** Presents within the first 100 days after transplantation and usually manifests in the skin, GI system, liver, and hematopoietic system.
- **Chronic GVHD:** Onset is >100 days from the transplantation and usually manifests in the skin, GI system, liver, and lungs.

Symptoms/Exam

- **Acute:**
  - The most common presenting symptom is a **maculopapular rash** that may become confluent or form bullous lesions with diffuse desquamation.
  - Profuse watery or bloody **diarrhea, crampy abdominal pain,** nausea, vomiting, anorexia, and dyspepsia are also seen.
- **Chronic:**
  - Skin changes resemble those in scleroderma or SLE.
  - Also presents with dry oral mucosa with ulceration and pain, dysphagia, diarrhea, and weight loss.
  - Dyspnea and nonproductive cough are also seen.

Diagnosis

- Labs show **hyperbilirubinemia** and ↑ alkaline phosphatase if the liver is involved.
- You can make a clinical diagnosis in patients with a characteristic presentation.
- Biopsies of affected organ systems can confirm.

Management

- Give **prophylaxis with methotrexate and cyclosporine** ± T-cell depletion of the graft.
- Use **corticosteroids for treatment.** For chronic disease, cyclosporine or tacrolimus may be used as well.

Oncologic Emergencies

SPINAL CORD COMPRESSION

Usually caused by metastasis to the vertebral bodies. The prostate, breast, and lung are the most common 1° sites.

Symptoms/Exam

- Consider the diagnosis in any patient with cancer who complains of **back pain.** It is usually the earliest symptom and may ↑ with recumbency, movement of the spine, or Valsalva maneuver.
- Note that functional deficits typically occur later and are progressive. They include weakness, sensory loss, and bowel and bladder dysfunction.
- There may be tenderness to palpation over the spine at the level of the lesion.
- Patients may be hyper- or hypotonic and hyper- or hyporeflexic, depending on the acuity of the lesion.

Diagnosis

- Order **MRI** of the entire spine. Plain films cannot rule out compression.
- Bone scan may be useful for screening if the back pain symptoms are nonspecific.
- Neurologic status at the time treatment is initiated is the most important prognostic factor, so evaluation in symptomatic patients should be prompt.

Management

- Give urgent **dexamethasone** 10 to 100 mg IV, followed by 4 to 6 mg IV or PO every 6 hours. (Patients with paraparesis or paraplegia may be given 100 mg, followed by 24 mg every 6 hours.) Treatment should be started before the MRI if neurologic deficits are present.

QUESTION 1

A 45-year-old man presents with complaints of hardened skin. He has lost 30 lbs since his last visit 6 months ago, right after he received an ASCT for multiple myeloma. What do you suspect and how do you proceed?

QUESTION 2

A 63-year-old man presents with thoracic back pain 6 months after completing RCC treatment. He believes the pain started about 4 weeks ago. He notices the pain more when he lies down in bed at night. He is afebrile, and UA is unremarkable. Thoracic spine films show mild disk degeneration but are otherwise unremarkable. What is the next step?

QUESTION 3

A 32-year-old male smoker presents with a complaint of a red face. On exam, you note distended neck veins in addition to his facial plethora. He denies dyspnea, and his O_2 saturation is 98% on room air. CXR shows a widened mediastinum, and contrast chest CT shows a mediastinal mass compressing the superior vena cava as well as suspicious mediastinal nodes. What is the next step?

MNEMONIC

Tumors that commonly metastasize to bone:

BLT with Mayo, Mustard, and Kosher Pickle

Breast
Lung
Thyroid
Multiple **M**yeloma
Kidney (renal cell)
Prostate

ANSWER 1

Suspect GVHD (chronic). Check liver enzymes and ask about GI symptoms. Rule out drug eruption, and effects viral exanthem, radiation dermatitis, infectious causes. Treat with corticosteroids.

ANSWER 2

An MRI of the spine should be immediately obtained. Plain films cannot rule out spinal cord compression. If any new neurological deficits present, treat with dexamethasone 10-100 mg IV, followed 6 hours later with 4-6 mg IV or PO before MRI.

ANSWER 3

If there is no evidence of airway obstruction, treatment can be delayed until a definitive tissue diagnosis is established.

- Perform emergent neurosurgical evaluation for possible surgical decompression and biopsy if the 1° cancer is unknown, followed by radiation therapy or radiation therapy alone if the patient is not a surgical candidate.
- Chemotherapy is occasionally used for sensitive tumors.

SUPERIOR VENA CAVA SYNDROME

Defined as compression of the superior vena cava (SVC) that is mainly caused by malignancy (non–small cell lung cancer, 50%; small cell lung cancer, 25%; lymphoma, 10%; and metastatic lesions, 10%) and thrombosis or nonmalignant conditions (35% of cases). Commonly associated with intravascular devices such as catheters or pacemakers. Mediastinitis from infections (syphilis, TB) or aneurysm can also be rare causes.

Symptoms/Exam

- Typical presentation includes facial/neck/arm swelling, plethora (leading to edema that can cause cyanosis), headache, dizziness, visual disturbances, syncope (congestion and cerebral edema), dyspnea, and cough (edema of the larynx/pharynx). Symptoms are usually worse when patient is supine or bends over.
- Venous distention of the neck and chest wall is also seen.

Diagnosis

- CXR may show mediastinal widening and a pleural effusion (⊕ in two-thirds of cases).
- **Contrast chest CT** is the study of choice (Figure 7.14).
- Perform biopsy of a peripheral lesion (such as lymph nodes), sputum cytology, thoracentesis, and pleural effusion cytology (50% diagnostic yield).
- Bronchoscopy (50%-70% diagnostic yield), transthoracic needle aspiration biopsy (75% diagnostic yield), mediastinoscopy/mediastinostomy (>90% diagnostic yield).

Management

- SVC syndrome is a true **emergency only if central airway obstruction** is present. Otherwise, treatment may be delayed while an oncologic diagnosis is established, as chemoradiation may complicate subsequent diagnosis.
- Chemotherapy ± radiation therapy is used for treatment-responsive tumors.

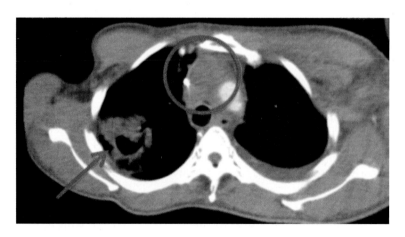

FIGURE 7.14. **Superior vena cava obstruction.** Right upper lobe lung cancer (arrow) with associated superior mediastinal mass (circled), which obstructs the SVC. (Reproduced with permission from USMLE-Rx.com.)

An endovascular stent may be used for palliation in patients who are not good candidates for chemoradiation.

■ Corticosteroids and loop diuretics are frequently used for symptomatic relief but have not been shown to be effective.

Paraneoplastic Syndromes

Table 7.11 outlines common paraneoplastic syndromes and their causes.

HYPERCALCEMIA

Affects 20% to 30% of cancer patients—the most common paraneoplastic syndrome (see Table 7.11). The most common causes are myeloma, breast cancer, and non–small cell lung cancer ± bone metastasis. Also related to PTH-related protein (PTHrP).

Symptoms/Exam

Depends on the rate and degree of hypercalcemia.
■ **Early:** Anorexia, nausea, fatigue, constipation, polyuria.
■ **Late:** Muscular weakness, hyporeflexia, confusion, psychosis, tremor, lethargy, coma.

TABLE 7.11.   **Paraneoplastic Syndromes**

SYNDROME	ASSOCIATED NEOPLASM	CAUSES	CLINICAL MANIFESTATION/DIAGNOSIS
Lambert-Eaton syndrome	Small cell lung cancer, thymoma	Autoantibodies against presynaptic calcium channels at the neuromuscular junction	Neuromuscular junction transmission disorder. Manifests primarily with muscle weakness (proximal > distal); alteration in gait or difficulty rising from a chair or climbing stairs; may have aching or stiff muscles Diagnosis confirmed by electrodiagnostic studies and antibodies to voltage-gated calcium channel (VGCC)
Erythrocytosis	RCC, hepatocellular carcinoma	EPO	HCT is >48 in women or >52% in men Hb >16.5 in women or >18.5 g/dL in men
Cushing syndrome	Small cell lung cancer, adrenal cancer, thymoma	ACTH precursors	Hypercortisolism causing centripetal obesity, adominal striae, facial plethora, glucose intolerance, weakness, proximal myopathy, acne, bruisability
SIADH	Small cell lung cancer, intracranial neoplasms, pancreatic cancer	ADH or atrial natriuretic factor	Elevated ADH → impaired water excretion. Free water retention → hyponatremia, hypoosmolality, and urine osmolality >100 mOsmol/kg
Hypercalcemia	Breast cancer, non–small cell lung cancer, and other solid tumors metastatic to bone Multiple myeloma, lymphoma Lymphoma, squamous cell lung cancer	Local osteolysis by tumor cells Osteoclast activating factors PTHrP	May manifest with personality or mood changes, cognitive dysfunction, stupor, polyuria, GI symptoms, bone pain, and shortened QT

Diagnosis

- ↑ calcium (correct with the serum albumin level or check the ionized/free calcium).
- When calcium >12 mg/dL, ↑ risk of arrhythmia or sudden cardiac death. Check ECG (shortening of QT).

Management

- Hydrate immediately with NS at 100 to 200 mL/hr.
- Use bisphosphonate if normal kidney function: Pamidronate 60 to 90 mg IV for 2 to 4 hours, or zoledronic acid 4 mg IV for several minutes.
- Treat underlying cancer if possible.
- For refractory hypercalcemia: Calcitonin, corticosteroids (with myeloma and lymphoma).

CHAPTER 8

Pulmonary

Jocelyn Young, DO, MS

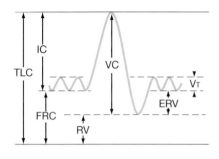

FIGURE 8.1. **Lung volumes shown by spirogram tracing.**

Diagnostics in Pulmonary Medicine

LUNG VOLUMES

Used to assess for restrictive lung disease, to show evidence of hyperinflation in obstructive lung disease, and to interpret the diffusing capacity for carbon monoxide (DLco).

Common definitions pertinent to the measurement of lung volume are as follows (see also Figure 8.1):

- **Residual volume (RV):** Air in the lung at maximal expiration.
- **Expiratory reserve volume (ERV):** Air that can be exhaled after normal expiration.
- **Tidal volume (V_T):** Air entering and exiting the lungs during normal respirations.
- **Inspiratory reserve volume (IRV):** Air in excess of V_T that enters the lungs at full inspiration.
- **Functional residual capacity (FRC):** RV + ERV.
- **Inspiratory capacity (IC):** V_T + IRV.
- **Total lung capacity (TLC):** RV + ERV + V_T + IRV.

PULMONARY FUNCTION TESTS

Assessing lung function is important in pulmonary disease, and pulmonary function tests (PFTs) may aid significantly in diagnosis. The components of PFTs include spirometry, measurement of lung volume (as discussed above), and quantification of diffusing capacity. PFTs can be used to evaluate several pulmonary diseases or can be used to screen for disease presence in patients with a risk factor, such as smoking (see Tables 8.1 and 8.2). Examples of use include:

- Evaluation of chronic persistent cough, wheezing, dyspnea, or exertional cough/ chest pain.
- Objective assessment of bronchodilator therapy.
- Evaluation of work exposures.
- Assessment of risk before major surgery.
- Objective assessment of impairment/disability.

Spirometry

Spirometry is the most useful and readily available of the PFTs. It includes measurement of forced expiratory volume in 1 second (FEV_1) and forced vital capacity (FVC). It may also include slow vital capacity (SVC), a measure that is useful when FVC is ↓, as slow exhalation causes less airway narrowing, and lung volumes are normal (which can screen for possible restrictive disease).

TABLE 8.1.   **Diagnostic Applications of PFTs**

MODALITY	MEASURES	PATIENT SELECTION
Spirometry	FEV_1, FVC, SVC	All smokers >45 years of age to screen for COPD
Forced inspiratory maneuvers	FIVC	Stridor heard over the neck or unexplained dyspnea
Postbronchodilator spirometry	FEV_1, FVC	Obstruction on spirometry or suspicion of asthma
Lung volumes	TLC	Interstitial lung disease
Diffusing capacity	DLco	Restrictive/obstructive disease

TABLE 8.2. PFT Results in Common Settings

SETTING	FEV$_1$/FVC	TLC	DL$_{CO}$
Asthma	Normal/low	Normal	Normal/high
COPD	Low	High/normal	Low
Fibrotic disease	Normal/low	Low	Low
Extrathoracic restriction	Normal	Low	Normal

- **Forced inspiratory maneuvers** (ie, forced inspiratory vital capacity [FIVC]) can help detect variable airway obstruction, as is seen with vocal cord paralysis or dysfunction (Figure 8.2).
- **Postbronchodilator spirometry** refers to the use of albuterol during initial workup. If baseline spirometry indicates obstruction or if asthma is suspected, albuterol can be administered, followed by repeat spirometry testing. An ↑ in FVC$_1$ >12% and at least >0.2 L indicates acute bronchodilator responsiveness and raises concern for asthma.
- **Methacholine challenge test** describes use of the cholinergic to trigger bronchospasm; this is used for diagnosis as well as to test effectiveness of asthma treatment.

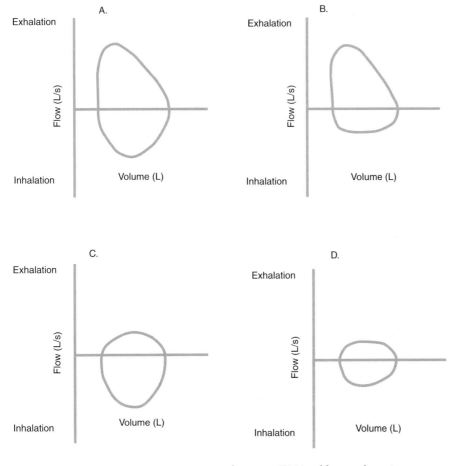

FIGURE 8.2. Flow volume loops. (A) Normal pattern. **(B)** Variable extrathoracic obstruction. **(C)** Variable intrathoracic obstruction. **(D)** Fixed obstruction.

Diffusing Capacity

Diffusion capacity refers to the measurement of single-breath DLco. Most useful in evaluating restrictive lung disease to distinguish intrinsic lung disease (DLco is ↓) from other causes of restriction in which DLco is typically normal. In obstructive disease, diffusing capacity helps differentiate COPD (characterized by a low DLco) from other causes of chronic airway obstruction.

Pulmonary Physiology

HYPOXEMIA

- **Hypoxia** is defined as **insufficient delivery of O_2 to the tissues.**
- **Hypoxemia** is defined as an **abnormally low arterial O_2 tension.** Generally, a Pao_2 of <80 mm Hg is considered hypoxemic (normal range: 80-100). With age, this number ↓ according to the formula: $80 - [(age - 20)/4]$. Under most conditions, hypoxemia is the cause of hypoxia. This can change if cardiac output is abnormal.

Hypoxemia is the result of any combination of five separate mechanisms:
- **Hypoventilation:**
    - Many causes—including oversedation from medications and obesity-related hypoventilation—and responds well to O_2 therapy.
    - ↓ in **minute ventilation** (V_T × breaths/minute) causes an ↑ in $Paco_2$ and a **normal** alveolar-arterial (A-a) O_2 gradient.
- **Right-to-left shunt:**
    - Blood bypasses the ventilated lung (eg, vascular malformations or intracardiac shunts) or perfuses a nonventilated lung (eg, pulmonary consolidation or pulmonary atelectasis) before returning to systemic circulation. Also seen with massive pulmonary embolism (PE), patent foramen ovale, or patent ductus arteriosus.
    - Always involves an ↑ in the A-a O_2 gradient. $Paco_2$ may be low because of hyperventilation.
    - Characteristically, levels will not improve with supplemental O_2, as blood is flowing past the nonventilated lung. Will respond to positive pressure ventilation.
    - Definitive treatment of a right-to-left shunt requires removal of the underlying cause.
- **Ventilation-perfusion (V/Q) mismatch:**
    - Failure to perfuse a ventilated lung (eg, in PE, asthma, COPD, pneumonia).
    - Associated with an ↑ A-a O_2 gradient. Hypoxemia usually **improves** with supplemental O_2 (↑ Fio_2 [the fraction of inspired O_2] in the ventilated lung will ↑ O_2 diffusion in the blood).
- **Diffusion impairment:**
    - Occurs when there is a ↓ in the diffusion of gas across the alveolar-capillary membrane and is associated with a very low DLco, such as occurs in interstitial lung disease or parenchymal disease.
    - Associated with an ↑ A-a O_2 gradient; hypoxemia improves with supplemental O_2.
- **Low inspired O_2:**
    - ↓ ambient O_2 pressure leads to hypoxemia.
    - Seen at high altitudes—ie, with lowered atmospheric pressure but preserved Fio_2 (21%). May also be seen in closed-space rescues or structural fires.
    - Characteristically has a normal A-a gradient and responds to O_2 supplementation.

Symptoms/Exam

- Neurologic findings of hypoxemia include agitation, headache, somnolence, coma, and seizures. Motor dysfunction may also be seen.
- Tachypnea and ↑ work of breathing are frequent signs, may also have complaints of pleuritic chest pain. Unlikely to see cyanosis in adult patients.
- With chronic hypoxemia, polycythemia and pulmonary cachexia (weight loss as a result of ↑ energy requirements unbalanced by dietary intake) may be present. At very low values of Pao_2 (<20 mm Hg), depression of the central respiratory drive is seen, and death usually results from respiratory failure.

Diagnosis

- Start with pulse oximetry, important to remember that it does not assess ventilation status.
- Obtain an ABG to know the true arterial oxygen percentage and help differentiate causes.
- Would also obtain a CXR to further elucidate potential causes.
- Narrow the differential by calculating the A-a O_2 gradient.
    - Normal A-a: Hypoventilation is the cause.
    - High A-a: Shunting or impaired diffusion—think V/Q mismatch or alveolar membrane disease.

Management

Treat with supplemental oxygen, repositioning, bronchodilators (if indicated). If possible, treat the underlying condition. In some cases, long-term O_2 therapy may be warranted:

- If there is evidence of cor pulmonale, right heart failure, or polycythemia (hematocrit >55%), patients who have a Pao_2 of 56 to 59 mm Hg or an Sao_2 of 89% should also receive long-term O_2.
- If sleep or exercise causes O_2 desaturation as above, O_2 therapy is warranted. This can be evaluated by an overnight sleep study or ambulatory oxygen test.

KEY FACT

Patients are eligible for (and should be treated with) long-term O_2 therapy when their arterial **Pao_2** is **≤55 mm Hg** or their arterial O_2 saturation (Sao_2) is **≤88%.**

KEY FACT

Tactile fremitus is ↑ in pneumonia if it is alveolar; it is ↓ in bronchoalveolar pneumonia, as bronchial mucous plugs dampen the tactile fremitus to make it softer.

KEY FACT

When you hear a high-pitched "bleating" sound on auscultation, think **egophony.** This is compression of the lung tissue by consolidation or effusion.

LUNG PHYSICAL FINDINGS

Table 8.3 outlines physical findings commonly associated with various lung conditions.

TABLE 8.3. **Physical Findings Associated With Common Lung Conditions**

	COPD	PNEUMONIA	ATELECTASIS	PNEUMOTHORAX	PLEURAL EFFUSION	TUMOR
Barrel chest (AP diameter > transverse)	+	–	–	–	–	If associated COPD
Retractions	+	±	–			–
Tracheal deviations	–	Ipsilateral	Ipsilateral	Contralateral	Contralateral (if large)	–
Fremitus	↓	↓↑	↓	↓	↓	↑
Percussion	Hyperresonant	Dull	Dull	Resonant to hyperresonant	Dull	Dull
Breath sounds	Distant	Bronchial	↓	↓ or absent	↓ or absent (based on size)	↓
Egophony	–	Ipsilateral	–	–	+ or –	–

TABLE 8.4.   Infiltrates Found on CXR

ACUTE ALVEOLAR INFILTRATE

Pulmonary edema

Aspiration

Hemorrhage

Pneumonia

UPPER LOBE DISEASE

Ankylosing spondylitis

2° TB

Eosinophilic granulomatosis

Silicosis

OPACIFIED HEMITHORAX

Atelectasis

Pleural effusion

Pneumonia

Postpneumonectomy

INTERSTITIAL DISEASE

Bronchiectasis

Aspiration

Dermatomyositis/polymyositis

Asbestosis

Sickle cell disease

Sarcoidosis

Pulmonary Imaging Modalities

CHEST X-RAY

Chest x-ray (CXR) has high clinical utility for identifying pulmonary infiltrates (such as pneumonia, atelectasis, and pulmonary edema; see Table 8.4) and masses. To a lesser extent can show mediastinal masses (see the Mnemonic and Figure 8.3) and hilar abnormalities.

- Generally includes both PA and lateral views.
- Lateral decubitus views are used to look for free-flowing pleural fluid, and apical lordotic views visualize the lung apices more effectively than the standard PA view.
- Portable views for acutely ill or otherwise bed-bound patients yield an AP view.

COMPUTED TOMOGRAPHY

Advantages of CT over standard CXRs include:

- Cross-sectional images show fluid collections, distinguish soft tissue structures, eliminate overlap, and define mediastinal structures.
- CT scan can show detailed imaging of airways, vasculature, and parenchyma, including bronchiectasis, emphysema, and interstitial lung disease.
- CT angiography is the **gold standard** to assess for the presence of a PE. This has replaced pulmonary angiography as a tool, given its convenience.

Disadvantages include cost, radiation exposure, and adverse reactions to IV contrast media.

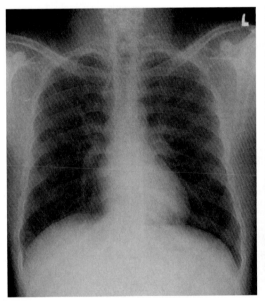

A

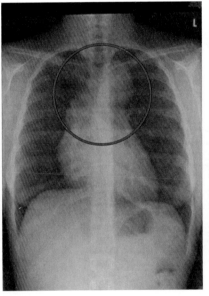

B

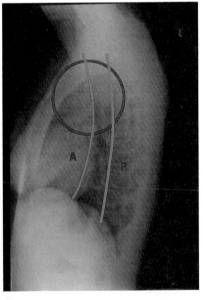

C

FIGURE 8.3.   **Chest x-rays.** Normal mediastinum **(A)**. PA **(B)** and lateral **(C)** views demonstrate predominantly anterior and middle superior mediastinal masses (circles) found to be lymphoma. On the lateral radiograph **(C)**, the anterior "A" and middle "M" compartments are separated by a line anterior to the trachea and the middle "M" and posterior "P" compartments are separated by a line passing 1 cm posterior to the anterior border of the vertebral bodies. (Image A reproduced from Karippacheril JG, et al. Negative pressure pulmonary oedema and haemorrhage, after a single breath-hold: Diaphragm the culprit? *Indian J Anaesth.* 2010;54(4):361-363; images B and C reproduced from Ellis AK, et al. Hodgkin's lymphoma presenting with markedly elevated IgE: a case report. *Allergy Asthma Clin Immunol.* 2009;5(1):12.)

VENTILATION/PERFUSION SCAN

Uses radioactive isotopes that bind to albumin and lodge in the pulmonary capillaries showing the distribution of blood flow in the lung. Radiolabeled xenon gas can be inhaled to demonstrate the distribution of ventilation. In PE, defects in perfusion are not accompanied by a corresponding defect in ventilation and are thus called **mismatched defects.**

PULMONARY ANGIOGRAPHY

Rarely used in clinical practice, pulmonary angiography was considered the gold standard for the diagnosis of PE—CT angiography has replaced this. Its main use is in cases of hemoptysis to identify an occult pulmonary arteriovenous malformation (AVM) or to embolize a known AVM.

Radiopaque contrast medium is injected into the pulmonary artery, allowing visualization of **filling defects** (defects in the lumen of a vessel) or an abrupt termination ("**cutoff**") of the vessel. The **disadvantage** is that it is invasive.

BRONCHOSCOPY

Bronchoscopy allows for evaluation of the airway/bronchial tree through direct visualization. Types include:
- **Flexible bronchoscopy:** Performed on awake but sedated patients; can identify endobronchial pathology (eg, tumors, granulomas, bronchitis, foreign bodies, bleeding sites) up to the level of subsegmental bronchi.
- Samples can be obtained via washing, brushing, needle aspiration endobronchial biopsy, and transbronchial biopsy.
- **Bronchoalveolar lavage** can reach the more distal pulmonary parenchyma and can recover organisms or cancer cells from the alveolar spaces.
- **Rigid bronchoscopy:** Requires general anesthesia and is performed for massive bleeding and for the removal of large foreign bodies, blood clots, and tumors that may be obstructing airways.

Complications stemming from bronchoscopy include hemorrhage, fever, transient hypoxemia, and pneumothorax.

Common Respiratory Complaints

COUGH

Cough is one of the most common reasons patients visit their physicians. Healthy individuals rarely cough because mucociliary mechanisms are sufficient to clear normal bronchial secretions. Cough is useful for clearing foreign bodies and secretions from the respiratory tract; however, it can spread illness through droplets and contamination of objects or be a sign of underlying disease.

Differential

Findings that may help narrow the differential include:
- Digital clubbing: Think chronic pulmonary disease.
- Boggy nasal mucosa and cobblestoning of the posterior oropharynx: Upper airway cough syndrome (UACS).

MNEMONIC

To remember anterior mediastinal masses on CXR—

T's

Teratoma
Thymoma
Thymolipoma
Thymic carcinoma/carcinoid
Thymic cyst
Thoracic thyroid
Terrible lymphoma

To remember posterior mediastinal masses on CXR—
BAC"K"

Bronchial cysts and **B**one marrow expansion (extramedullary haematopoiesis)
Abscess and **A**denopathy of lymph nodes
Cysts: Enterogenic and Peri**C**ardial (plasmacytoma)
"K":"Most common" posterior mediastinal masses = neurogenic tumors

- Wheeze or cough on forced exhalation: Asthma.
- Crackles or rhonchi: HF or pneumonia.
- Elevated JVP, peripheral edema: HF.

Diagnosis

Evaluation is broken down by duration of cough. Common causes are listed in Table 8.5.

Management

Acute cough:
- Start treatment with first-generation antihistamine and decongestant.
- If cough persists: Consider asthma and treat with inhaled corticosteroids and β-agonists.

Chronic cough:
- Consider tobacco use, angiotensin-converting enzyme inhibitor (ACEI) use, environmental irritants: First step is to stop these exposures.
- If no toxic/drug exposure present: Obtain CXR.
- Normal CXR can help exclude TB, malignancy, sarcoidosis, and bronchiectasis.
- If cough is unresolved and no underlying disease is present: Continue any partially effective treatments and begin sequential treatment for the three most common causes of chronic cough:
  - UACS (also known as postnasal drip syndrome): First-generation antihistamine and decongestant. If clinically suspicious for UACS but without adequate response to treatment, the most likely cause is sinusitis and may be treated as such.
  - Asthma: Empiric treatment with inhaled corticosteroids and β-agonist. Consider PFTs and pulmonology referral if there is no response to treatment.
  - GERD: PPI or H_2-blocker with diet and lifestyle modifications.
- If cough remains: Will require additional testing and referral.

Complications

Persistent and recurrent cough can lead to posttussive syncope, retinal vessel rupture, persistent headache, chest wall and abdominal muscle strain (causing abdominal wall hernias or dehiscence after surgery), and rib fractures. Severe chronic cough can significantly impact quality of life, potentially restrict social activities, disrupt family life, and—in rare cases—lead to attempted suicide.

KEY FACT

In patients with normal CXR and no other clinical signs/symptoms, treatment focus should be on UACS, asthma, and GERD before moving on to less common causes of chronic cough.

TABLE 8.5.   **Evaluation of Cough**

	ACUTE COUGH <3 WEEKS	SUBACUTE COUGH 3-8 WEEKS	CHRONIC COUGH >8 WEEKS
More common causes	Viral URTI	Postinfectious origin	UACS (formerly postnasal drip syndrome)
	COPD exacerbation		
	Asthma		Asthma
	Allergic rhinitis		GERD
	Irritant exposure		
Less common causes	Pneumonia	Asthma	ACEIs
	HF	Bacterial sinusitis	Chronic bronchitis
	PE	*Bordetella pertussis*	Irritant exposure
			Psychogenic cough
			TB
			Malignancy

DYSPNEA

Defined as a feeling of difficulty breathing that is disproportionate to the stimulus and thus abnormally uncomfortable. Patients with dyspnea often report feeling "breathless" or "short of breath." Consider dyspnea out of proportion to exertion a marker of disease. The causes of dyspnea create a wide differential diagnosis and can be of neurogenic, respiratory, or cardiac origin.

Differential

Most common causes: asthma, HF, MI, COPD, interstitial lung disease, pneumonia, and psychogenic disorders.

- Intermittent symptoms particularly postprandial or recumbent: Consider GERD.
- Sudden onset: Consider MI, pneumothorax, PE, or asthma exacerbation.
- Insidious onset: Consider COPD, heart failure, pulmonary hypertension, and interstitial lung disease.
- Fever: Consider infection, inflammation, or neoplasm.
- Recent immobility, prolonged travel, and history of malignancy: Consider thromboembolic disease leading to pulmonary hypertension.

Exam findings:
- Tachycardia: Possibilities include anemia, recent use of albuterol inhaler, PE, and decompensation related to HF.
- ↓ breath sounds with wheezing: Suspect COPD, HF, or asthma.
- ↓ or muffled heart sounds: Suspect obesity-related condition or cardiac tamponade.
- Signs of fluid overload (jugular venous distention, hepatomegaly, ascites, hepatojugular reflux, or lower extremity edema): Suspect right-sided heart failure or pulmonary hypertension.
- Clubbing: Suspect chronic process, such as lung cancer or pulmonary fibrosis.

Diagnosis

- CXR: Look for cardiomegaly or pulmonary edema (HF, see Figure 8.4), nodules (malignancy), ↑ lung volumes (COPD), consolidation (pneumonia).
- ECG: Look for dysrhythmia, ischemia, LVH, or atrial fibrillations (think new HF).
- Spirometry:
  - ↓ FEV_1/FVC ratio: obstructive—COPD, chronic bronchitis, asthma.
  - Normal or ↑ FEV_1/FVC: restrictive—interstitial lung disease.
- Labs:
  - CBC: Specifically looking for anemia or polycythemia to show chronic hypoxia.

> **KEY FACT**
>
> The most common causes of chronic dyspnea are asthma, COPD, interstitial lung disease, and cardiomyopathy.

> **KEY FACT**
>
> A history of atrial fibrillation increases the likelihood of developing HF—look for atrial fibrillation in the patient's history and on physical exam.

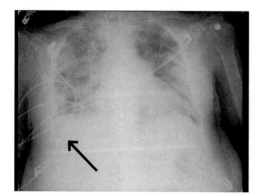

FIGURE 8.4. **Heart failure.** CXR demonstrates diffuse bilateral interstitial infiltrates and a small right-sided small pleural effusion (arrow) in the setting of cardiomegaly. (Reproduced from Robin J, et al. Multiple myeloma presenting with high-output heart failure and improving with anti-angiogenesis therapy: two case reports and a review of the literature. *J Med Case Reports.* 2008;2:229.)

- Basic metabolic panel: CO_2 retention would indicate COPD or advanced interstitial lung disease.
- B-type natriuretic peptide: If elevated, could indicate HF.
- D-dimer: ⊖ test in patients with ↓ pretest probability can rule out PE.

HEMOPTYSIS

The coughing up of blood that **originates below the vocal cords,** hemoptysis, can range from trivial to massive in scope. **Massive hemoptysis** defined as any amount of blood that is hemodynamically significant or impairs respiratory function. Volume may range from 100 cc to >600 cc in a 24-hour period.

Differential

Most common causes include acute URTI, COPD, bronchiectasis, lung cancer, bronchitis, and pneumonia. In patients traveling or immigrating from countries where TB is endemic, TB should be in the differential.

According to the American Academy of Family Physicians, **findings** that may help determine the cause of hemoptysis include:

- Anticoagulant use: Coagulopathy.
- Cough: Bronchiectasis, COPD, foreign body, pneumonia, TB.
- Fever: Bronchitis, lung abscess, neoplasm, pneumonia, PE, TB.
- Sputum production: Bronchiectasis, COPD, pneumonia, TB.
- Trauma: Airway trauma, PE.
- Weight loss: COPD, neoplasm, TB.

Diagnosis

Most important step is to determine the **anatomic location** of the bleeding (Table 8.6). Figure 8.5 outlines the evaluation of nonmassive hemoptysis (<600 cc in 24 hours).

Patient age may also point to the cause of hemoptysis:

- In patients <**40 years of age,** think bronchiectasis (if there is a history of recurrent pneumonia) or **mitral stenosis** (if a diastolic murmur is present).
- In a young person, a URTI prodrome and a benign exam may suggest bronchitis.
- In patients >**40 years of age,** consider **malignancy,** especially with a history of tobacco use, cachexia, and weight loss.

> **KEY FACT**
>
> CXR is the initial step in the diagnosis of hemoptysis.

> **KEY FACT**
>
> Mitral stenosis is an often overlooked cause of hemoptysis, as it is associated with elevated pulmonary capillary pressure.

TABLE 8.6.   Differential Diagnosis of Hemoptysis by Anatomic Location

AIRWAYS	PULMONARY VASCULATURE	PULMONARY PARENCHYMA	IATROGENIC
Bronchitis	LV failure	Pneumonia	Transbronchial lung biopsies
Bronchogenic carcinoma	Mitral stenosis	Inhalation of crack cocaine	Anticoagulation
Bronchiectasis	Pulmonary emboli AVMs	Autoimmune disease: Goodpasture syndrome; granulomatosis with polyangiitis (Wegener)	Pulmonary artery rupture from balloon-tipped catheter placement

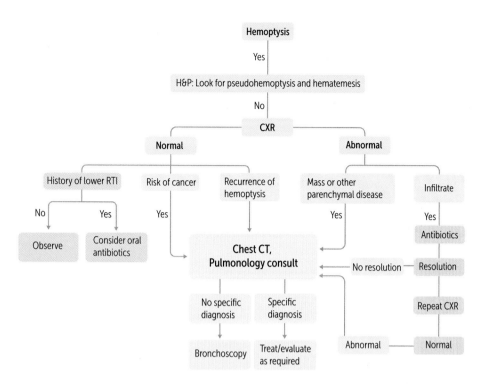

FIGURE 8.5.   **Evaluation of hemoptysis.** (Reproduced with permission from USMLE-Rx.com; data from Earwood JS, et al. Hemoptysis: evaluation and management. *Am Fam Physician.* 2015;91(4):243-249.)

Management

Treatment of hemoptysis is two-fold:

- **Supportive care:** Bed rest, supplemental O_2, and blood products, if needed. Place patient bleeding side down. Ensure ventilation with airway protection and intubate if necessary to achieve this. Avoid antitussives to allow blood clearance from airways, but consider suppression of the cough reflex if not actively bleeding.
- **Definitive treatment:**
  - **Nonmassive hemoptysis:** Identify and treat the specific cause (see Figure 8.5).
  - **Massive hemoptysis:** A life-threatening condition; the treatment goal is to bring a rapid end to the bleeding; cases of massive hemoptysis usually require surgical involvement. Treatment can include bronchoscopy and angiography to embolize bleeding vessels.

KEY FACT

In a patient with dyspnea, hemoptysis, and renal failure, think Goodpasture syndrome.

WHEEZE

A wheeze is an adventitious, "musical" lung sound produced by airflow through central and distal airways. Wheezes can be single toned or polyphonic and can occur on inspiration or expiration. Wheezing is not pathognomonic of an airway obstruction, and patients who have airway obstruction may not wheeze. With severe obstruction there is not always enough air movement to generate sound.

Differential

Table 8.7 outlines a differential for wheezing based on the location of the obstruction. The sound of the wheeze can help determine the location:

- Polyphonic wheeze with multiple notes: Indicates dynamic compression of larger, more central airways.
- Monophonic wheeze: Points to small airway disease.

Diagnosis

PFTs with flow volume loops (see Figure 8.2) can be used to distinguish intrathoracic from extrathoracic obstruction.

TABLE 8.7. Differential Diagnosis of Wheezing

UPPER AIRWAY OBSTRUCTION	LOWER AIRWAY OBSTRUCTION
Extrathoracic	Asthma
Vocal cord dysfunction	Allergic bronchopulmonary aspergillosis (ABPA)
Postnasal drip	Aspiration
Laryngeal edema	Bronchiolitis
Malignancy	Bronchiectasis
Relapsing polychondritis	Cystic fibrosis
Granulomatosis with polyangiitis (formerly	COPD
Wegener granulomatosis)	HF
	Parasitic infections
Intrathoracic	Pulmonary embolus
Tracheal stenosis	
Foreign body	
Benign tumors	
Tracheomalacia	
Malignancy	

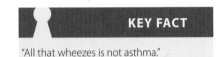

KEY FACT

"All that wheezes is not asthma."

Management

Treatment choices should be based on the specific cause of the wheeze. Response to treatment helps confirm the diagnosis. Conversely, a lack of response should prompt the alteration of therapy (vs looking for other potential causes).

Upper Respiratory Tract Disorders

OBSTRUCTIVE SLEEP APNEA

Obstructive sleep apnea (OSA) is the cessation of breathing during sleep caused by repetitive, partial, or complete obstruction of the airway by pharyngeal structures. Ultimately, clinical sequelae result from chronic sleep deprivation and recurrent oxyhemoglobin desaturation.

 Apnea: A temporary absence or cessation of breathing (airflow) during sleep, traditionally defined as **10 seconds** for adults.

 Hypopnea: Essentially "underbreathing." Unlike in apnea, breathing is slower or more shallow than normal.

Symptoms/Exam

Excessive daytime sleepiness and waking up coughing or gasping tend to be initial complaints. Other pieces of the H&P may include: physically restless sleep, morning dry mouth or sore throat, impotence, nocturia, and morning headache. Patients' bed partners may report loud snoring or witness apneic events.

On exam, patients appear fatigued and often have ↑ BMI; collar size is frequently >17 inches for men and >16 inches for women.

 Hypertension is present in **50% of cases** and this can present as isolated 2° hypertension without other symptoms.

 Airway crowding may be present as a result of adenotonsillar hypertrophy or redundant soft tissue of the soft palate, together with an elongated uvula.

Differential

If your patient complains of excessive daytime sleepiness, also consider:

- Chronic sleep deprivation shift work or schedule disorders.
- Narcolepsy.
- Depression.
- Alcohol use.
- Severe restrictive lung disease.
- Drug use.
- Periodic restless leg syndrome.
- Chronic pain or discomfort.

Diagnosis

- Polysomnography (sleep study) is the first-line study for diagnosis.
- Results are reported in terms of the **apnea-hypopnea index** (AHI, or the number of episodes of apnea/hypopnea in an hour), also known as the respiratory disturbance index (RDI). Table 8.8 outlines the interpretation of AHI scores.

Management

- **Conservative measures** (for patients with an AHI <20): Avoid EtOH, avoid sleeping on the back, and trial intranasal steroids; encourage weight loss.
- **Continuous positive airway pressure (CPAP):** The **gold standard** for treatment; delivers constant air pressure through the nostrils to maintain a patent airway. Significantly improves quality of life and ↓ complications. Oral appliances can be used as an alternative to CPAP.
- **Surgical treatment** (for patients with severe sleep apnea who cannot tolerate CPAP):
  - Uvulopalatopharyngoplasty increases the pharyngeal lumen by removing redundant tissue.
  - Nasal surgery for septal deviation repair, turbinectomy, or polypectomy.

Complications

Patients have a two- to three-fold ↑ risk of motor vehicle accidents.

Cardiovascular complications:

- Contributes to refractory systemic hypertension and often pulmonary hypertension.
- Significantly ↑ risk of stroke or death from any cause, independent of other risk factors, including hypertension.

NASAL POLYPS

Pale, edematous masses that are covered by mucosa and are frequently encountered in patients with allergic rhinitis (Figure 8.6). Nasal polyps arise from the sinuses (eg, the **ethmoid sinuses**) and obstruct airflow by extending into the nasal cavity.

Symptoms/Exam

- H&P may include nasal obstruction, diminished sense of smell, chronic rhinorrhea, or recurrent bacterial sinusitis.
- Ask about a history of asthma, as up to 20% to 30% of asthmatic patients with nasal polyps have a sensitivity to aspirin (and the use of aspirin in these subjects may precipitate bronchospasm).
- On physical exam, polyps appear as pale, gelatinous, rounded masses in the nasal cavity and are insensitive to pain.

QUESTION

A 44-year-old obese man comes to your office complaining of snoring and ↑ daytime sleepiness. His wife has reportedly witnessed apneic events while the patient sleeps. You suspect OSA. What vital sign is most likely to be abnormal?

TABLE 8.8. AHI Results

SCORE	INTERPRETATION
<5	Normal
5-15	Mild OSA
16-30	Moderate OSA
>30	Severe disease

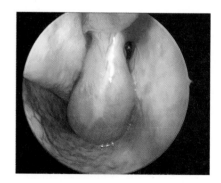

FIGURE 8.6.   Nasal polyp. (Reproduced with permission from Brunicardi FC, et al. *Schwartz's Principles of Surgery,* 9th ed. New York: McGraw-Hill, 2010, Fig. 18-3.)

KEY FACT

The Samter triad consists of nasal polyps, asthma, and aspirin sensitivity.

Differential

Chronic allergic rhinitis, sinusitis, Samter triad, cystic fibrosis, eosinophilic granulomatosis with polyangiitis (formerly Churg-Strauss syndrome), allergic fungal sinusitis.

Management

- Intranasal corticosteroids block growth and may cause regression.
- Systemic corticosteroids may cause regression that can then be maintained with nasal steroids.
- Surgical removal may be necessary to relieve symptoms in severe cases (eg, those with intolerable nasal obstruction or recurrent sinusitis requiring multiple courses of antibiotics).

Complications

Recurrence rate is high, making preventive measures—including controlling allergen exposure and maximizing medial therapy—essential.

EPISTAXIS

Defined as bleeding from the nose, most commonly caused by rupture of small vessels (Kiesselbach plexus) in the mucosa overlying the anterior aspect of the nasal septum.

Symptoms/Exam

Bleeding can occur from the anterior nasal cavity (95% of the time) as a product of the Kiesselbach plexus or from the posterior cavity, which is a product of the sphenopalatine artery or carotid artery. With posterior bleeds, there may be associated hemoptysis or hematemesis and these are typically a surgical emergency due to the risk of aspiration and rate of blood loss.

When conducting the exam:
- If possible, examine the patient sitting upright to prevent ingestion or aspiration of blood. Wear protective eyewear and clothing.
- Use a nasal speculum to examine both nares for bleeding sites and to see whether septum is intact.
- Examine the posterior oropharynx for at least 15 seconds: Look for fresh blood flowing down the back wall, suggestive of posterior site.
- If exam is difficult due to amount of bleeding, consider use of topical 4% cocaine or a topical decongestant plus a topical anesthetic (eg, oxymetazoline and tetracaine, respectively), applied as a spray or on a cotton strip, to halt bleeding.

Differential

Nasal trauma (eg, nose picking, foreign body, forceful nose blowing), rhinitis, dry nasal mucosa, deviated septum, chronic sinusitis, inhaled steroids, cocaine use, alcohol use, antiplatelet medications, thrombocytopenia, hemophilia, leukemia, granulomatosis with polyangiitis (formerly Wegener granulomatosis), nasal neoplasm, Osler-Weber-Rendu disease, von Willebrand disease, or a bleeding diathesis.

Diagnosis

- Diagnose by exam as above. Obtain baseline vitals and monitor accordingly.
- Obtain CBC and coagulation studies to assess for acute blood loss anemia, thrombocytopenia, or other sites of coagulopathy.

Management

Anterior epistaxis:

- Continuous pressure to the nasal alae for 10 minutes: Have the patient sit upright and lean forward.
- Topical nasal decongestants such as a phenylephrine solution may be beneficial.
- Silver nitrate or electrocautery can cauterize the bleeding site.
- Anterior packing if bleeding persists.

Posterior epistaxis: Usually calls for a referral. Treatment options include posterior pack placement to occlude choanae, followed by anterior packing. Endovascular embolization or surgical ligation of the nasal arterial supply may be necessary.

Lower Respiratory Tract Disorders

ASTHMA

Asthma is defined as **inflammation of airways that causes ↑ airway secretions and contraction of smooth muscles.** May be idiopathic or triggered by allergies or environmental factors.

- **Acute inflammation** leads to an asthma exacerbation.
- **Chronic inflammation** can lead to long-term narrowing and remodeling of the airways (Figure 8.7).

Symptoms/Exam

- Presents with episodic or chronic dyspnea, cough, wheezing, and chest tightness that sometimes worsens at night or in the early morning (Figure 8.8).
- Precipitants may be allergens such as dust mites, cockroaches, cat dander, or pollen. Nonallergic precipitants include exercise, cold air, URTIs, stress, GERD, and secondhand smoke.
- Inquire about a history of atopy (the association is more common in younger patients).
- Exam may reveal prolonged expiration, tachypnea, tachycardia, hyperresonance, accessory muscle use, and diffuse wheezes.

KEY FACT

Ask about this classic triad: **A**topy, **A**sthma, **A**llergic rhinitis.

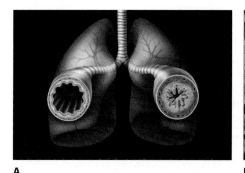
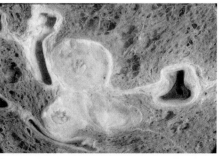

A   **B**

FIGURE 8.7.   Remodeling of the airways in asthma. (A) Normal bronchial airway (left airway) compared with diffuse thickening (right airway) seen in asthma. **(B)** Gross pathology of the airway demonstrating mucus plugging of the thickened airway. (Reproduced from Jeffery PK, et al. Allergic rhinitis and asthma: inflammation in a one-airway condition. *BMC Pulm Med.* 2006;6(Suppl 1):S5.)

  QUESTION

A 23-year-old woman with a history of asthma previously managed by albuterol alone has needed to use an inhaler more for the last several months. She is coughing 3 days a week and has nighttime cough approximately once per week. What would be the next step in her asthma management?

INITIAL VISIT: CLASSIFYING ASTHMA SEVERITY AND INITIATING THERAPY
(in patients who are not currently taking long-term control medications)

Level of severity (Columns 2–5) is determined by events listed in Column 1 for both impairment (frequency and intensity of symptoms and functional limitations) and risk (of exacerbations). Assess impairment by patient's or caregiver's recall of events during the previous 2–4 weeks; assess risk over the last year. Recommendations for initiating therapy based on level of severity are presented in the last row.

Components of Severity	Intermittent			Persistent								
				Mild			Moderate			Severe		
	Ages 0–4 years	Ages 5–11 years	Ages ≥12 years	Ages 0–4 years	Ages 5–11 years	Ages ≥12 years	Ages 0–4 years	Ages 5–11 years	Ages ≥12 years	Ages 0–4 years	Ages 5–11 years	Ages ≥12 years
Impairment — Symptoms	≤2 days/week			>2 days/week but not daily			Daily			Throughout the day		
Nighttime awakenings	0	≤2x/month		1–2x/month	3–4x/month		3–4x/month	>1x/week but not nightly		>1x/week	Often 7x/week	
SABA* use for symptom control (not to prevent EIB*)	≤2 days/week			>2 days/week but not daily	>2 days/week but not daily and not more than once on any day		Daily			Several times per day		
Interference with normal activity	None			Minor limitation			Some limitation			Extremely limited		
Lung function		Normal FEV$_1$ between exacerbations	Normal FEV$_1$ between exacerbations									
➜ FEV$_1$* (% predicted)	Not applicable	>80%	>80%	Not applicable	>80%	>80%	Not applicable	60–80%	60–80%	Not applicable	<60%	<60%
➜ FEV$_1$/FVC*		>85%	Normal†		>80%	Normal†		75–80%	Reduced 5%†		<75%	Reduced >5%†
Risk — Asthma exacerbations requiring oral systemic corticosteroids‡	0–1/year			≥2 exacerb. in 6 months, or wheezing ≥4x per year lasting >1 day AND risk factors for persistent asthma	≥2/year	*Generally, more frequent and intense events indicate greater severity.* →						

Generally, more frequent and intense events indicate greater severity. →

Consider severity and interval since last asthma exacerbation. Frequency and severity may fluctuate over time for patients in any severity category. Relative annual risk of exacerbations may be related to FEV$_1$.*

Recommended Step for Initiating Therapy (See "Stepwise Approach for Managing Asthma Long Term," page 7)	Step 1			Step 2			Step 3	Step 3 medium-dose ICS* option	Step 3	Step 3	Step 3 medium-dose ICS* option or Step 4	Step 4 or 5

The stepwise approach is meant to help, not replace, the clinical decisionmaking needed to meet individual patient needs.

Consider short course of oral systemic corticosteroids.

In 2–6 weeks, depending on severity, assess level of asthma control achieved and adjust therapy as needed.
For children 0–4 years old, if no clear benefit is observed in 4–6 weeks, consider adjusting therapy or alternate diagnoses.

* **Abbreviations:** EIB, exercise-induced bronchospasm; FEV$_1$ forced expiratory volume in 1 second; FVC, forced vital capacity; ICS, inhaled corticosteroid; SABA, short-acting beta$_2$-agonist.

† Normal FEV$_1$/FVC by age: 8–19 years, 85%; 20–39 years, 80%; 40–59 years, 75%; 60–80 years, 70%.

‡ Data are insufficient to link frequencies of exacerbations with different levels of asthma severity. Generally, more frequent and intense exacerbations (e.g., requiring urgent care, hospital or intensive care admission, and/or oral corticosteroids) indicate greater underlying disease severity. For treatment purposes, patients with ≥2 exacerbations may be considered to have persistent asthma, even in the absence of impairment levels consistent with persistent asthma.

FIGURE 8.8. Classification of asthma severity. (Reproduced from the US Department Health and Human Services; National Institutes of Health. NIH Publication No. 12-5075; Revised September 2012.)

MNEMONIC

Remember the medications for ASTHMA exacerbation:

Albuterol
Steroids
Theophylline
Humidified O$_2$
Magnesium
Antileukotriene

ANSWER

This patient meets the criteria for mild persistent asthma and thus requires a controller medication. The current preferred long-term controller treatment in mild persistent asthma is a low-dose inhaled corticosteroid.

Differential

HF (cardiac asthma), GERD, PE, vocal cord dysfunction, Churg-Strauss syndrome, conversion disorder.

Diagnosis

- CXR: Needed to rule out other causes of dyspnea or cough. May show hyperinflation, or possible infiltrate as the cause of an asthma exacerbation.
- Obtain PFTs: Most helpful to also obtain PFTs after administration of a short-acting bronchodilator.
- Look for significant reversibility of obstruction after bronchodilator use.
- Try methacholine challenge test to provoke bronchospasm.
- ↑ of 12% or 200 mL in FEV$_1$ or an ↑ of 15% and 200 mL in FVC.

In patients in the ED or admitted for an asthma exacerbation:
- ABG will likely have respiratory alkalosis with an ↑ in the A-a O$_2$ gradient.
- In severe exacerbations, hypoxemia will develop.
- ↑ Paco$_2$ and respiratory acidosis are warning signs of impending respiratory failure due to loss of ability to compensate.
- CBC may show eosinophilia.

Management

Figure 8.9 details a stepwise approach to the management of asthma in youths and adults aged ≥12 years; for younger children, see the Child and Adolescent Medicine chapter.

- Rescue treatment consists of a short-acting β-agonist with or without a short course of oral corticosteroids.
- Step up if asthma is not well controlled and you have checked for good inhaler technique, adherence, adaptable environmental factors, and comorbidities. May want to consider using a spacer with inhalers to improve technique.
- Can consider a trial of stepping down if asthma is well controlled for > 3 months.
- Evidence of good control of asthma includes:
  - Symptoms ≤2 days per week.
  - Nighttime awakenings ≤2 times per month.
  - Use of short-acting β-agonist ≤2 days per week.
  - No interference with normal activity.
  - ≤1 exacerbation requiring oral corticosteroids per year.
- **Make sure your asthma patients receive influenza and pneumococcal vaccines.**

QUESTION

A 69-year-old woman presents to the hospital with severe COPD along with a history of multiple hospital admissions, 30-step dyspnea on exertion, weight loss, weakness, and a resting Pao_2 of 59 mm Hg. Which intervention will most likely affect her survival?

STEPWISE APPROACH FOR MANAGING ASTHMA LONG TERM

The stepwise approach tailors the selection of medication to the level of asthma severity (see page 5) or asthma control (see page 6). The stepwise approach is meant to help, not replace, the clinical decisionmaking needed to meet individual patient needs.

ASSESS CONTROL:

STEP UP IF NEEDED (first, check medication adherence, inhaler technique, environmental control, and comorbidities)

STEP DOWN IF POSSIBLE (and asthma is well controlled for at least 3 months)

At each step: Patient education, environmental control, and management of comorbidities

≥12 years of age

	STEP 1	STEP 2	STEP 3	STEP 4	STEP 5	STEP 6
	Intermittent Asthma	**Persistent Asthma: Daily Medication** Consult with asthma specialist if step 4 care or higher is required. Consider consultation at step 3.				
Preferred Treatment†	SABA* as needed	low-dose ICS*	low-dose ICS* + LABA* **OR** medium-dose ICS*	medium-dose ICS* + LABA*	high-dose ICS* + LABA* **AND** consider omalizumab for patients who have allergies††	high-dose ICS* + LABA* + oral corticosteroid§§ **AND** consider omalizumab for patients who have allergies††
Alternative Treatment†,‡		cromolyn, LTRA,* or theophylline§	low-dose ICS* + either LTRA,* theophylline,§ or zileuton‡‡	medium-dose ICS* + either LTRA,* theophylline,§ or zileuton‡‡		
		Consider subcutaneous allergen immunotherapy for patients who have persistent, allergic asthma.**				
Quick-Relief Medication	▪ SABA* as needed for symptoms. The intensity of treatment depends on severity of symptoms: up to 3 treatments every 20 minutes as needed. Short course of oral systemic corticosteroids may be needed. ▪ Caution: Use of SABA >2 days/week for symptom relief (not to prevent EIB*) generally indicates inadequate control and the need to step up treatment.					

* **Abbreviations:** EIB, exercise-induced bronchospasm; ICS, inhaled corticosteroid; LABA, inhaled long-acting $beta_2$-agonist; LTRA, leukotriene receptor antagonist; SABA, inhaled short-acting $beta_2$-agonist.

† Treatment options are listed in alphabetical order, if more than one.

‡ If alternative treatment is used and response is inadequate, discontinue and use preferred treatment before stepping up.

§ Theophylline is a less desirable alternative because of the need to monitor serum concentration levels.

** Based on evidence for dust mites, animal dander, and pollen; evidence is weak or lacking for molds and cockroaches. Evidence is strongest for immunotherapy with single allergens. The role of allergy in asthma is greater in children than in adults.

†† Clinicians who administer immunotherapy or omalizumab should be prepared to treat anaphylaxis that may occur.

‡‡ Zileuton is less desirable because of limited studies as adjunctive therapy and the need to monitor liver function.

§§ Before oral corticosteroids are introduced, a trial of high-dose ICS + LABA + either LTRA, theophylline, or zileuton, may be considered, although this approach has not been studied in clinical trials.

FIGURE 8.9. **Asthma management in youths and adults ≥12 years.** (Reproduced from the US Department Health and Human Services; National Institutes of Health. NIH Publication No. 12-5075; Revised September 2012.)

KEY FACT

Chronic lower respiratory disease, primarily COPD, was the **third leading cause of death** in the United States in 2014, and smoking is the most important risk factor.

KEY FACT

α_1-Antitrypsin deficiency is a rare genetic abnormality that can lead to early-onset emphysema COPD, and liver disease. Think of this in panacinar emphysema and concomitant cirrhosis.

KEY FACT

The absolute risk of COPD among active, nonsmokers is at least 25%.

CHRONIC OBSTRUCTIVE PULMONARY DISEASE

An inflammatory pulmonary disease state characterized by **irreversible airflow limitation** that progresses. The definition of COPD is no longer limited to **emphysema** (destruction of the alveolar-capillary membrane and enlargement of lung alveoli) and **chronic bronchitis** (chronic cough and phlegm for ≥3 months for 2 consecutive years). Remember that other pathologic changes are also seen in those with COPD. Chronic airflow obstruction must be present to make the diagnosis; not all patients with chronic bronchitis will have this component. This disease state also causes destruction of lung parenchyma, leading to a decline in elastic recoil, resulting in air trapping.

- Pathophysiology: Chronic airway inflammation leads to ↑ mucus production and ↓ mucociliary function that results in symptoms of sputum production and coughing.
- Risk factors: 1° is smoking. Other risk factors include advancing age, secondhand smoke exposure, chronic exposure to environmental pollutants, α_1-**antitrypsin deficiency,** childhood history of chronic recurrent respiratory infections, and family history of COPD.

Symptoms/Exam

- Hallmark symptoms are cough, ↑ sputum production, and dyspnea—classically in a patient with a smoking history.
- Less common presenting features include wheezing, chest tightness, weight loss, and nocturnal awakenings.
- Physical exam in early stages of COPD may be normal.
- Later in the disease course as right-sided heart pressure increases from worsening pulmonary damage, signs of cor pulmonale (peripheral edema, jugular venous distention, hepatomegaly) may develop.
- Signs of ↑ work of breathing associated with COPD include the use of respirator accessory muscles, paradoxical abdominal movement, ↑ expiratory time, and pursed lip breathing (the result of blowing off carbon dioxide).
- As the prognosis worsens, most patients will develop chronic weight loss and cachexia from ↑ metabolic usage to maintain saturation.

Differential

Acute bronchitis, asthma, bronchiectasis, lung mass, HF.

Diagnosis

- **CXR:** May have findings suggestive of COPD and can help rule out other causes of presenting symptoms. Shows flattening of the diaphragm, ↓ lung markings, and an enlarged retrosternal space (Figure 8.10).
- **Spirometry:** The key test for diagnosing COPD, use results to determine the severity in the WHO's Global Initiative for Chronic Obstructive Lung Disease (GOLD criteria). Obstructive lung disease will have FEV_1/FVC <70%.
  - Stage I (mild): FEV_1 ≥80% predicted value.
  - Stage II (moderate): FEV_1 50 to 79% of predicted value.
  - Stage III (severe): FEV_1 30 to 49% of predicted value.
  - Stage IV (very severe): FEV_1 <30% of predicted value.
- **Labs:** CBC should be normal. If leukocytosis, consider infectious cause or steroid use. Presence of anemia can suggest alternate cause of dyspnea.
- Pulse oximetry: Should be done to assess for hypoxemia and determine the need for supplemental oxygen.
- **ABGs:** Reveal chronic hypoxemia and hypercarbia with metabolic compensation for the chronic respiratory acidosis.

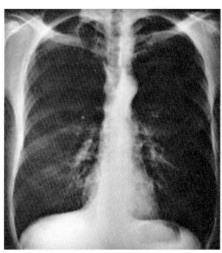
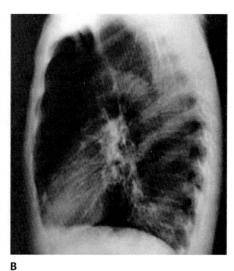

A   **B**

FIGURE 8.10. **CXR in a patient with chronic obstructive pulmonary disease.** Note the flattened diaphragms, large retrosternal space, and minimal lung markings on AP (**A**) and lateral (**B**) CXR. (Reproduced with permission from Stobo JD, et al. *The Principles and Practice of Medicine,* 23rd ed. Stamford, CT: Appleton & Lange, 1996:135.)

Management

Includes a combination of nonpharmacologic and pharmacologic interventions. Make sure your COPD patients receive influenza and pneumococcal vaccines.

Nonpharmacologic: The most important intervention is **smoking cessation,** as it improves lung function initially and slows annual loss of FEV_1. Hypoxemic patients should receive **supplemental O_2.** Exercise and pulmonary rehabilitation can ↓ pulmonary symptoms and improve exercise tolerance.

Pharmacologic:

- **Inhaled anticholinergics** (eg, ipratropium): Fewer side effects and better response than inhaled β-agonists. **Tiotropium** is a long-acting anticholinergic that should be the bronchodilator of choice.
- Additional therapy: Intermittent use of a **β-agonist inhaler** can be beneficial. Long-acting β-agonists may be useful as well, as they last through the night.
- **Antibiotic therapy** may play a role in patients with COPD exacerbations who have ↑ volume or a purulent appearance to their sputum. The optimal choice of antibiotic and length of treatment has not been determined but should be based on local antibiotic resistance patterns.
- Inhaled **corticosteroids** can provide symptomatic relief as symptoms worsen, and oral steroid bursts during exacerbations can also ↓ symptoms.

BRONCHIECTASIS

An abnormal and permanent **dilatation of medium-sized airways** that is either focal or diffuse and is the result of repeated cycles of infection, leading to pooling of secretions in the dilated airways and thus continued bronchial destruction. Caused by **cystic fibrosis, 1° ciliary dyskinesia, and other conditions that damage the airways.**

Symptoms/Exam

- Persistent or recurrent cough with purulent sputum production, **hemoptysis.** Symptoms may be insidious or may occur after an initial severe pneumonia.
- Auscultation may reveal a combination of crackles, rhonchi, and wheeze.
- With long-standing disease may also see clubbing of nailbeds.

Differential

COPD, asthma, bronchiolitis, allergic bronchopulmonary aspergillosis.

Diagnosis

The following studies can help diagnose and/or clarify the underlying cause of bronchiectasis:

- **CXR:** Findings are fairly nonspecific but may reveal **"tram tracks,"** which are dilated airways crowded in parallel because of atelectasis. In cross-section, these produce **"ring shadows."**
- **High-resolution CT:** Offers good sensitivity for detecting bronchiectatic airways (Figure 8.11). May show ring shadows or tram tracks, depending on the CT plane of section.
- Sputum sample for bacterial and mycobacterial culture.
- PFTs may show airflow **obstruction** from diffuse bronchiectasis.
- Sweat chloride levels for cystic fibrosis in cases of extensive lung involvement.
- Skin testing/serology/sputum culture for *Aspergillus* if ABPA can be considered.

Management

Treatment has three goals:

- Treat/eliminate the underlying condition causing bronchiectasis.
- Control infection with **antibiotics:** Used in exacerbations when there is an ↑ in sputum quantity and purulence. Empiric coverage may include amoxicillin, TMP-SMX, or quinolone with an aminoglycoside if *Pseudomonas aeruginosa* is present. Chronic cases may warrant more prolonged courses or may benefit from intermittent but regular courses of single or rotating antibiotics.
- Improve clearance of secretions:
  - **Airway clearance techniques:** Chest physical therapy, flutter devices (which produce oscillatory positive pressure to assist the clearance of sputum), and percussive vests. Mucolytic agents to thin secretions are controversial (eg, **DNase,** a medication that reduces mucus viscosity from DNA from degenerating neutrophils, is appropriate for cystic fibrosis but not for idiopathic bronchiectasis).

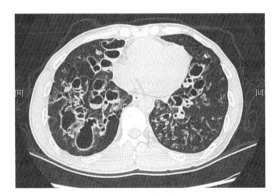

FIGURE 8.11.   Bronchiectasis. Chest CT scan shows markedly dilated segmental and subsegmental bronchi secondary to recurrent infection in the lower lobes with associated mucus plugging. (Reproduced from King P. *Haemophilus influenzae* and the lung (*Haemophilus* and the lung). *Clin Transl Med.* 2012;1:10.)

- **Bronchodilators:** Can improve obstruction and aid in the clearance of secretions.
- **Surgical resection:** Less commonly done; may be indicated with severe focal disease.

CYSTIC FIBROSIS

The most common lethal autosomal-recessive disorder in whites, affecting one in every 3200 births; one in 25 is a carrier. It is caused by mutations affecting a sodium/chloride exchange channel (the cystic fibrosis transmembrane conductance regulator [CFTR]) that leads to multisystem dysfunction. Although CF is usually found in childhood, 7% of cases are diagnosed in adulthood, and because of improvements in therapy, >38% of patients are now adults.

Symptoms/Exam

- Look for a history of failure to thrive, especially with recurrent infections of the airways (eg, with *Pseudomonas*).
- Suspect CF in infants with meconium ileus or intussusception.
- Patients may have a history of pancreatic insufficiency, recurrent pancreatitis, sinusitis, intestinal obstruction, chronic hepatic disease, vitamin (fat-soluble) deficiencies, male urogenital/infertility problems, or bronchiectasis. Symptoms include chronic or recurrent cough, sputum production, dyspnea, and wheezing.
- Exam may reveal digital clubbing, ↑ AP chest diameter, and apical crackles.

Differential

COPD, asthma, α_1-antitrypsin deficiency, celiac disease, chronic sinusitis.

Diagnosis

Because of the large number of CF mutations, 1° diagnosis is typically made on the basis of clinical criteria and laboratory analysis of sweat Cl⁻ values.
- **PFTs** may show a mixed obstructive and restrictive pattern.
- **ABGs** reveal hypoxemia with compensated respiratory acidosis in advanced disease.
- Sweat Cl⁻ concentrations >60 mEq/L help distinguish CF from other lung diseases.
- Genotyping, measurement of nasal membrane potential difference, semen analysis, and assessment of pancreatic function aid in diagnosis.
- Sputum cultures frequently show *Staphylococcus aureus* or *Pseudomonas aeruginosa* infections.
- CXR may show hyperinflation early; other findings include peribronchial cuffing, mucous plugging, bronchiectasis (seen effectively on high-resolution CT), and ↑ interstitial markings (Figure 8.12).

Management

- **Acute exacerbations:** Treat with bronchodilators, DNase to thin sputum, antibiotics (at least two with antipseudomonal coverage), and chest physical therapy.
- **Long-term therapy:**
  - Includes aerobic exercise, flutter devices, and external percussive vests to help with airway clearance.
  - Give pancreatic enzymes and the fat-soluble (A, D, E, and K) vitamins for malabsorption.
  - Nebulized DNase.
  - The only definitive treatment is double lung transplantation.

MNEMONIC

Presentation of cystic fibrosis:
CF PANCREAS

Chronic cough and wheezing
Failure to thrive
Pancreatic insufficiency (symptoms of malabsorption such as steatorrhea)
Alkalosis and hypotonic dehydration
Neonatal intestinal obstruction (meconium ileus)/**N**asal polyps
Clubbing of fingers/**C**hest radiograph with characteristic changes
Rectal prolapse
Electrolyte elevation in sweat; salty skin
Absence or congenital atresia of the vas deferens
Sputum with *Staphylococcus* or *Pseudomonas* (mucoid)

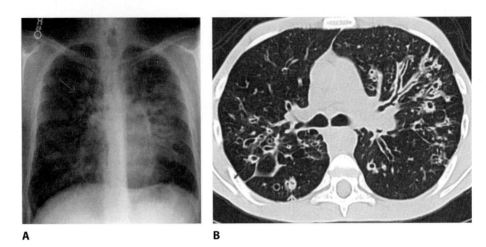

A   B

FIGURE 8.12. **Cystic fibrosis. (A)** Frontal CXR showing central cystic bronchiectasis (arrow) in a patient with CF. **(B)** Transaxial CT image showing cystic bronchiectasis (red arrow), with some bronchi containing impacted mucus (yellow arrow). (Reproduced with permission from USMLE-Rx.com.)

INTERSTITIAL LUNG DISEASE

Interstitial lung disease (ILD) refers to more than 200 conditions that are characterized by diffuse parenchymal lung involvement (Figure 8.13), often with significant morbidity and mortality. Conditions can be categorized as those that are predominantly inflammatory and fibrotic (eg, idiopathic pulmonary fibrosis) or those that are predominantly granulomatous (eg, sarcoidosis).

Symptoms/Exam

- Progressive **exertional dyspnea** or a persistent, nonproductive **cough.**
- Fatigue and weight loss are often seen. Chest pain, wheeze, and hemoptysis may be present but are less common. Clubbing with advanced disease.

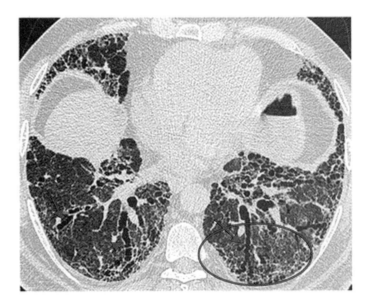

FIGURE 8.13. **Interstitial lung disease.** Chest CT scan shows extensive reticulation and honeycombing (circle) with traction bronchiectasis (arrows) seen in interstitial lung disease in a patient with rheumatoid arthritis. (Modified from Walsh SLF, et al. Relationship between fibroblastic foci profusion and high-resolution CT morphology in fibrotic lung disease. *BMC Med.* 2015;13:241.)

■ Insidious presentations are much more common than acute presentations that develop over days to weeks.
■ Exam findings may reveal tachypnea and **bibasilar end-inspiratory dry crackles** (seen in inflammatory ILD but less often in granulomatous states).
■ **"Inspiratory squeaks"** are late inspiratory high-pitched rhonchi heard in bronchiolitis.

KEY FACT

Important history includes smoking, occupational/environmental exposures, travel history, and a family history of lung conditions.

Differential

■ **Inflammation/fibrosis:** Think about asbestosis, silicosis, and other pneumoconioses; drug reaction (eg, amiodarone or chemotherapy), radiation exposure, idiopathic interstitial pneumonias, connective tissue diseases (eg, RA, SLE), ulcerative colitis/Crohn's disease, heritable diseases (eg, neurofibromatosis, tuberous sclerosis).
■ **Granulomatous disease:** Hypersensitivity pneumonitis, sarcoidosis, granulomatosis with polyangiitis (formerly Wegener granulomatosis), eosinophilic granulomatosis with polyangiitis (formerly Churg-Strauss syndrome).

Diagnosis

■ **Labs:** Assess for connective tissue or autoimmune conditions.
■ **Imaging:** Presence of reticular or nodular opacities, volume loss, and honeycombing (caused by small cystic spaces and progressive fibrosis) indicates a poor prognosis.
  ■ **CXR:** Most often nonspecific.
  ■ **High-resolution CT:** Effective for early detection or confirmation of suspected ILD. Also demonstrates the extent of disease (see Figure 8.13).
■ **PFTs:** Restrictive pattern, with a ↓ TLC, FRC, and RV. The FEV_1/FVC ratio is usually normal or ↑. DLco is commonly ↓.
■ **ABGs:** May be normal or reveal hypoxemia and respiratory alkalosis.
■ **Lung biopsy:** The gold standard for disease confirmation and assessing disease activity; can be transbronchial with fiberoptic bronchoscopy or open.

Management

Disease specific. The goals of treatment include permanent removal of the offending agent when known and suppression of the inflammatory process to limit further lung damage.
■ O_2 for hypoxemia (Pao_2 <55 mm Hg) at rest and/or with exercise.
■ **Corticosteroids:** Although no evidence of benefit due to irreversible scarring, may still be trialed in patients.
■ **Immunosuppressive agents** such as cyclophosphamide and azathioprine are used with variable success.
■ Lung transplantation is considered in severe and nonresponsive cases.

ACUTE RESPIRATORY DISTRESS SYNDROME

Acute respiratory failure accompanied by refractory hypoxemia caused by diffuse alveolar capillary damage (Figure 8.14), leading to ↓ lung compliance and noncardiogenic pulmonary edema. ARDS has the potential to progress to extrapulmonary multisystem organ failure.

Symptoms/Exam

■ Presents with an acute onset (12-48 hours) of tachycardia, dyspnea, fever, cyanosis, ↑ work of breathing, and hypoxia refractory to O_2 therapy in the setting of a systemic disorder (sepsis, brain trauma) or direct lung injury (pneumonia, tuberculosis, diffuse alveolar hemorrhage, or aspiration).
■ No signs of fluid overload on exam such as JVP elevation, lower extremity edema, S3 on heart sound.

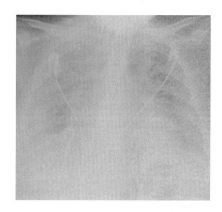

FIGURE 8.14. Acute respiratory distress syndrome (ARDS). Diffuse bilateral consolidation in an intubated 21-year-old patient with a history of aspiration pneumonia. Echocardiogram had demonstrated normal left atrial pressures and good cardiac output, distinguishing this entity from cardiogenic pulmonary edema. (Reproduced with permission from USMLE-Rx.com.)

Differential

Pneumonia, asthma, COPD, HF, *Pneumocystis jiroveci* (previously *Pneumocystis carinii*) pneumonia, multisystem organ failure, sepsis, toxic shock syndrome.

Diagnosis

- Clinically: Acute onset of respiratory distress refractory to oxygen supplementation.
- Pulmonary artery wedge pressure of <18 mm Hg, without evidence of cardiac origin.
- Pao_2:Fio_2 ratio ≤200.
- Bilateral infiltrates on CXR (see Figure 8.14).

Management

- Treat the underlying cause of ARDS.
- High Fio_2.
- Typically requires mechanical ventilation with adequate sedation and analgesia to tolerate high positive end expiratory pressure.
- Maintaining low tidal volumes has been shown to be superior to traditional tidal volumes.

PLEURAL EFFUSION

Defined as a fluid collection in the pleural space caused either by ↑ pleural fluid formation or ↓ removal by the lymphatic system. The fluid may be **transudative** or **exudative** (Table 8.9).

- **Transudative effusion:** ↑ production of pleural fluid due to ↑ hydrostatic or ↓ oncotic pressures. Found in HF, PE, cirrhosis, and nephrotic syndrome.
- **Exudative effusion:** ↑ production due to abnormal capillary permeability or ↓ lymphatic clearance of fluid. Found in malignancy, pneumonia, TB, PE, pancreatitis, esophageal rupture, collagen vascular disease, and chylothorax.

Symptoms/Exam

- May be asymptomatic or patient may complain of dyspnea, pleuritic pain, and cough.
- On exam, crackles, dullness to percussion, ↓ fremitus, and ↓ breath sounds may be found on the affected side. Patients may show symptoms of their underlying disease process (cancer, pneumonia, HF, cirrhosis).

Diagnosis

- **CXR:** On upright PA and lateral films, blunting of costophrenic angles may be present with effusions >250 mL. Decubitus films can differentiate pleural fluid from pleural scarring and can help determine if the fluid is loculated (Figure 8.15).
- Diagnostic thoracentesis is recommended if the cause of the effusion is unknown. More emergent thoracentesis is performed in cases of respiratory or cardiac decompensation. Protein and lactate dehydrogenase are used for Light's criteria to differentiate transudative from exudative processes. Gram stain, culture and cell count can help to identify a causative pathogen. In some cases a pH, fungal and mycobacterial

TABLE 8.9. **Pleural Effusion Classification**

	PLEURAL-TO-SERUM PROTEIN (RATIO)	PLEURAL-TO-SERUM LDH (RATIO)	PLEURAL FLUID LDH
Transudative	<0.5, and	<0.6, and	<200
Exudative	>0.5, or	>0.6, or	>200

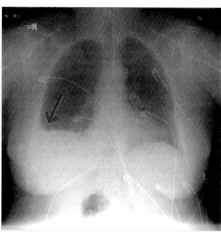
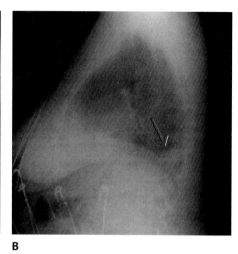

A   B

FIGURE 8.15. **Pleural effusion.** PA (**A**) and lateral (**B**) CXRs show blunting of the right costophrenic sulcus (arrows). (Reproduced with permission from USMLE-Rx.com.)

cultures, and cytology can be obtained. Grossly purulent fluid represents empyema while milky fluid may be indicative of a chylothorax.

- **Hemothorax:** A pleural hematocrit-to-peripheral hematocrit ratio >0.5.
- **Pancreatitis, pancreatic pseudocyst, adenocarcinoma of lung, or esophageal rupture:** ↑ pleural fluid amylase.
- **Malignancy:** Cytology is only 50% to 60% sensitive for detection. pH less than 7.30 may point toward malignant effusion as well.
- Pleural biopsy can help diagnose TB or cancer.

Management

- **Transudative effusion:** Treat the underlying cause, and consider therapeutic thoracentesis if symptomatic. No further workup is required.
- **Exudative effusion:**
  - **Parapneumonic:** Give appropriate antibiotics for infections; insert a chest tube for drainage if complicated (eg, if pH <7.2 **or** glucose <60 mg/dL) or if empyema is present.
  - **Malignant:** Treat the underlying malignancy; further thoracentesis procedures may be done for symptom relief and pleurodesis can help to ↓ reaccumulation of fluid.
  - **Hemothorax:** Rapid drainage via a large-bore chest tube to prevent fibrothorax.
  - **Tuberculous:** Usually resolves with treatment of TB.

KEY FACT

Any untreated pleural effusion can become infected, leading to empyema. Loculations also occur over time, requiring video-assisted thoracoscopic surgery (VATS) drainage or surgical decortication.

PNEUMOTHORAX

The presence of air in the pleural space. Can be **spontaneous** (occurring without prior trauma to the thorax), **traumatic** (caused by penetrating or nonpenetrating chest injuries), **iatrogenic**, or **tension** (pressure in the pleural space is ⊕ throughout the respiratory cycle, as in mechanical ventilation or resuscitative efforts). In tension pneumothorax, ventilation is severely compromised and venous return can be ↓, reducing cardiac output and leading to a medical emergency. There are two types of spontaneous pneumothorax:

- **1°:** Occurs in individuals without clinically apparent lung disease (typically in tall, thin males 10-30 years of age, with smoking frequently a factor).
- **2°:** Found in patients with underlying lung disease such as COPD, asthma, CF, TB, *P jiroveci*, and ILD.

Symptoms/Exam

- Patients may complain of acute onset of unilateral chest pain dyspnea and cough. Mild cases could be asymptomatic.
- Exam may be normal; possible findings include tachycardia, unilateral chest expansion, ↓ tactile fremitus, hyperresonance, and diminished breath sounds. Think tension pneumothorax if severely decompensated, hypotensive, or cyanotic.

Differential

Costochondritis, rib fracture, PE, infectious pneumonia, viral pleuritis, empyema, MI.

Diagnosis

- On upright PA CXR, look for a thin visceral pleural line on expiration and loss of normal pulmonary interstitial markings (Figure 8.16). In difficult or equivocal cases with a high degree of clinical suspicion, CT may be necessary.
- ABGs, if obtained, may show hypoxemia and acute respiratory alkalosis.

In a tension pneumothorax, there will be tracheal deviation toward the side of the pneumothorax.

Management

Depends on the severity and nature of underlying disease:
- Small (<15% of a hemithorax), stable pneumothoraces may resolve spontaneously. Supplemental O_2 may hasten resolution. Treat the associated pain with either NSAIDs or morphine.
- Larger (>30% of a hemithorax), spontaneous 1° pneumothoraces: Respond to simple aspiration drainage of pleural air with a small-bore catheter or a larger small-bore chest tube with a 1-way valve. Follow patients with a daily CXR. Recurrent pneumothoraces may require pleurodesis.
- **2° spontaneous pneumothorax,** large pneumothorax, tension pneumothorax, or those with severe symptoms: Chest tube placement under water-seal drainage. Suction should be applied until the lung expands, and the chest tube should then be removed after cessation of the air leak.
- Recurrence/treatment failure: Thoracoscopy or open thoracotomy may be necessary in recurrences of spontaneous pneumothorax, bilateral pneumothorax, and failure of tube thoracostomy. Surgery allows for the resection of blebs as well as for pleurodesis by mechanical abrasion and insufflation of talc.

KEY FACT

If there is clinical suspicion of tension pneumothorax, initiate immediate needle decompression or tube thoracostomy with a 14- to 16-gauge needle in the second intercostal space at the midclavicular line or the fourth intercostal space in the midaxillary line. In an unstable patient, do not wait for x-ray confirmation. Tension pneumothorax will lead to ↓ venous return, causing hypotension and then circulatory collapse.

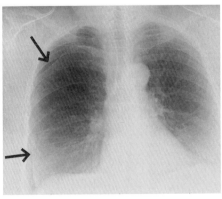

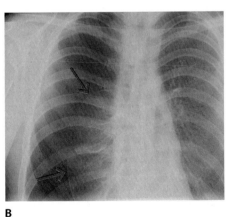

A   B

FIGURE 8.16.   **Pneumothorax. (A)** Small right pneumothorax. **(B)** Right tension pneumothorax, with collapse of the right lung and shifting of mediastinal structures to the left. Arrows denote pleural reflections. (Reproduced with permission from USMLE-Rx.com.)

PULMONARY EMBOLISM

An obstruction of the pulmonary vasculature that most commonly results from a deep venous thrombosis (DVT) that has embolized. Rarely, other substances can cause an obstruction, such as air, fat, and amniotic fluid. Symptoms can range from mild to complete circulatory collapse and death. Risk factors include **hypercoagulable states,** including malignancy; recent trauma; immobility (eg, postsurgery or long flights); pregnancy; and coagulation disorders such as factor V Leiden mutation and protein C, protein S, or antithrombin III deficiencies. **Venous stasis** and **endothelial damage** also predispose to DVT formation.

Symptoms/Exam

- Most common symptom is acute dyspnea. Other symptoms include pleuritic pain, cough, and hemoptysis. Tachycardia is the most common sign on exam. Patients may appear anxious but otherwise well.
- Patients may also exhibit low-grade fever, JVD, or a loud P2. With a massive PE, the presentation could include syncope, hypotension, or cyanosis.

Differential

MI/acute coronary syndrome, pneumonia, pericarditis, HF, pleuritis, pneumothorax, pericardial tamponade, rib fracture, anxiety.

Diagnosis

Accurate diagnosis remains difficult, so PE should be high on the differential for any patient presenting with sudden chest pain, dyspnea, and tachycardia in the setting of a normal CXR. The Wells criteria can aid in predicting the probability of PE (Figure 8.17). Diagnostic modalities are as follows:

- D-**dimer:** Elevated in >90% of patients with PE, has low specificity and can be elevated in cases of cardiopulmonary disease and most systemic illnesses. Has a high ⊖ predictive value and can help to exclude the diagnosis.
- **ABGs:** In PE, both Po_2 and Pco_2 will often be ↓. Respiratory alkalosis and an ↑ A-a O_2 gradient may also be seen.
- **ECG:** Frequently reveals sinus tachycardia; less often shows a new-onset atrial fibrillation/flutter. Presence of a pulmonary embolus can lead to right ventricular strain, which manifests as T wave inversion in leads V_1-V_4 (Figure 8.18).

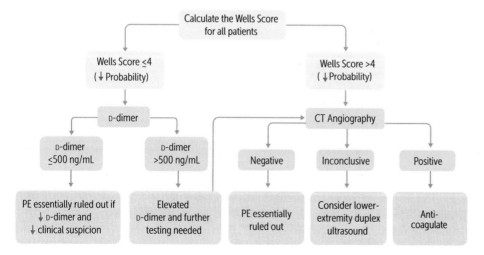

FIGURE 8.17. **Diagnostic algorithm for PE using the modified Wells criteria.** (Reproduced with permission from USMLE-Rx.com.)

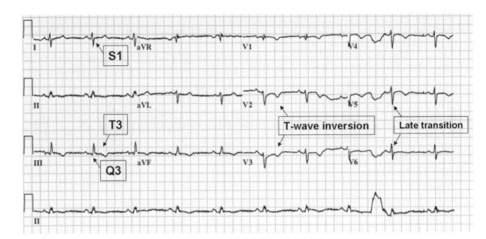

FIGURE 8.18. **Pulmonary embolism on ECG.** Note the right axis deviation with S1Q3T3 pattern seen in right heart strain. (Reproduced from Todd K, et al. ECG for the diagnosis of pulmonary embolism when conventional imaging cannot be utilized: a case report and review of the literature. *Indian Pacing Electrophysiol J.* 2009;9(5):268-275.)

- **CXR:** A normal CXR in a dyspneic patient may suggest PE. **Westermark sign** (an area of lucency related to the abrupt tapering of the pulmonary vessel from the embolus, leading to vasoconstriction in the affected lobe), **Hampton hump** (a peripheral wedge-shaped density from the pulmonary infarct), pleural effusion, or atelectasis may be present.
- **Lower extremity ultrasound:** In suspected cases of PE, a finding of DVT establishes the need for CT angiography to assess for presence of PE. Of all patients with PE, >50% will not have evidence of DVT with imaging, and workup for PE should continue if there is a high clinical suspicion with a ⊖ ultrasound.
- **V/Q scan:** May show segmental regions of V/Q mismatch; results are expressed as normal-low, intermediate, and high probability for PE. This test has fallen out of favor in light of CT angiography.
- **Spiral CT with contrast:** Diagnostic test of choice, also referred to as CT angiogram. Effective for the diagnosis of most PEs (Figure 8.19). Can detect peripheral thrombi up to fifth order branches. In patients without PE, lung parenchymal images may reveal other diagnoses that may explain the presenting symptoms. It cannot reliably exclude PE in patients with a high probability.
- **Pulmonary angiography:** The **gold standard,** but very rarely performed due to its invasiveness and risks.

Management

Options for treatment include anticoagulation to prevent further embolism, clot lysis with thrombolytic agents, and surgical removal of the clot.

- **Warfarin:** Should be started at the onset of anticoagulation therapy and requires bridging with a heparin product or fondaparinux. Continue the additional agents until INR is at goal of 2 to 3. Total treatment duration is typically 6 months for a first episode when there is a reversible risk factor; 12 months after a first-episode idiopathic thrombus; and 6 to 12 months to indefinitely in those with recurrent disease or nonreversible risk factors.
- **Unfractionated heparin:** Associated with heparin-induced thrombocytopenia (HIT), and requires inpatient stay due to IV dosing.
- **Low-molecular-weight heparin (LMWH):** Equally safe and effective as unfractionated heparin with lower risk for HIT and can be used at home.

FIGURE 8.19. **Pulmonary embolism on CT.** Contrast-enhanced CT shows a clot (arrows) within bilateral proximal pulmonary arteries, consistent with a saddle PE. (Reproduced from Minet C, et al. Venous thromboembolism in the ICU: main characteristics, diagnosis and thromboprophylaxis. *Crit Care.* 2015;19(1):287.)

Ⓐ ANSWER

Obtain a CT angiogram if kidney function allows, given his history of immobilization, lack of an alternative diagnosis, and heart rate.

- **Fondaparinux:** Given subcutaneously, only affects factor Xa with no effect on thrombin. Recommended for patients with a contraindication to LMWH.
- **Novel anticoagulants** have been approved for use:
  - Dabigatran, direct thrombin inhibitor, contraindicated if creatinine clearance <15 mL/min and need for rifampin therapy.
  - Rivaroxaban and apixaban are factor Xa inhibitors. Rivaroxaban is contraindicated if creatinine clearance <30 mL/min or severe liver disease is present. Apixaban is contraindicated with severe liver disease.
- **IVC filters:** May be useful in patients in whom anticoagulation has failed or those who cannot be safely anticoagulated. Filters are associated with a higher risk of recurrent DVT.
- **Thrombolytic agents:** Reserved for patients with documented large central PE and hemodynamic instability.

KEY FACT

Onset of skin lesions characterized by demarcated purpura and necrosis can occur in the first few days of warfarin therapy, known as warfarin-induced skin necrosis. This is associated with protein C deficiency.

PULMONARY ARTERY HYPERTENSION

An abnormal elevation in pulmonary artery pressure; defined as a resting pulmonary artery mean pressure of >25 or >30 mm Hg with exercise is called pulmonary artery hypertension (PAH). It can occur in isolation (idiopathic or 1° pulmonary hypertension) or may be caused by a range of disorders, including connective tissue disease, advanced parenchymal lung disease, OSA, congenital heart disease, advanced liver disease, HIV, chronic thromboembolic disease, and drug use. It is generally seen as a marker of advanced disease. 1° pulmonary hypertension is rare and occurs mostly in young to middle-aged women.

Symptoms/Exam

- Difficult to recognize in the early stages because symptoms and signs may be attributed to underlying disease. Patients may complain of dyspnea initially on exertion and progress to dyspnea at rest. Dull, substernal chest pain may be present. Fatigue and syncope on exertion may occur.
- On exam there may be splitting of S2, with a loud P2 best heard at the apex on auscultation. In advanced cases, tricuspid and pulmonary valve insufficiency and signs of right heart failure and cor pulmonale can be seen.

Differential

LV systolic failure, LV diastolic dysfunction, causes of 2° pulmonary hypertension (see above).

Diagnosis

- **Echocardiography:** May be the first test suggesting the presence of PAH. Most commonly reveals enlargement of the right ventricle and atrium, with tricuspid regurgitation. Allows for the estimation of pulmonary artery pressure as well as the evaluation of LV function, valvular disorders, and congenital heart disease.
- **Lab findings:** Presence of polycythemia may point to chronic severe hypoxemia. Can evaluate for connective tissue diseases with targeted testing such as ANA, ESR, and RF.
- **ABGs:** May show hypoxemia with respiratory alkalosis.
- **ECG:** Look for RVH, rightward axis, RV strain, and right atrial enlargement.
- **CXR:** Reveals cardiomegaly with enlarged central pulmonary arteries. May show evidence of parenchymal lung disease such as COPD.

- **CT:** Commonly employed to look for underlying pulmonary parenchymal disease as a cause for PAH.
- **Overnight oximetry:** Should be done to evaluate the need for oxygen supplementation overnight.
- **Sleep study:** Conduct in patients with symptoms consistent with sleep-disordered breathing, as this may potentially reverse PAH.
- **Right heart catheterization:** Less commonly done outside of critical care situations, but obtains definitive pulmonary artery pressure, cardiac output, and pulmonary vascular resistance as well as left-to-right shunts and evidence of left heart dysfunction.

Management

Treatment is disease specific in 2° causes of PAH. Early detection is vital to disrupting the self-perpetuating cycle that can lead to rapid clinical progression.

- **Hypoxemic COPD:** Supplemental O_2 can slow progression.
- **High risk of thromboembolism:** Permanent anticoagulation in patients with chronic thromboembolic disease as a cause of their PAH.
- Vasodilatory agents (eg, calcium channel blockers, hydralazine, nitroglycerin) have yielded disappointing results in the treatment of PAH.
- **1° PAH:** Continuous long-term IV infusion of prostacyclin (via a portable pump) has improved survival.
- **PDE5 inhibitors** (sildenafil, tadalafil, vardenafil): Prolong vasodilatory effect of nitrous oxide, thereby improving pulmonary hemodynamics and exercise capacity in patients with idiopathic, hereditary, congenital, and HIV-related PAH.
- Bilateral lung transplantation may be necessary after failure of medical therapy.

SOLITARY PULMONARY NODULE

Defined as a solitary mass <3 cm in diameter, well circumscribed, and surrounded by normal lung tissue and not associated with atelectasis, infiltrates, or adenopathy. Historically referred to as **"coin lesions."** Often found incidentally when a CXR is obtained for a different purpose. Lesions >3 cm are pulmonary masses and are much more likely to be malignant (Table 8.10).

Symptoms/Exam

- Often these are found incidentally. Some cases may include cough, hemoptysis, and dyspnea. Age, smoking history, environmental/infectious exposures, residence/ travel, cancer history, and previous lung disease should be elicited.

TABLE 8.10.   **Pulmonary Nodule Classification**

CHARACTERISTICS	LIKELY BENIGN	LIKELY MALIGNANT
Nodule	Very fast or no growth on serial imaging 2 years apart **"Bull's eye"** pattern of granulomas, a **"popcorn"** pattern of hamartomas, and a diffuse, dense central core of calcification	>3 cm Spiculation, lesions lacking calcium, or having a stippled appearance Upper lobe location
Patient	Lifelong nonsmoker <30 years of age No history of malignancy	Smoking history >30 years of age Prior diagnosis of cancer

- On exam, lungs may be entirely clear. A localized wheeze may indicate an endobronchial tumor. Look for clubbing and hypoxemia, and check for lymphadenopathy (if localized to the supraclavicular/scalene nodes, it raises concern for cancer; generalized lymphadenopathy suggests lymphoma or an infectious etiology).

Differential

- **Benign:** Infectious granulomas, viral infections (measles, CMV), *P jiroveci* pneumonia, lung abscess, hamartoma, chondroma, pulmonary infarct, AVM, sarcoidosis, pulmonary amyloidosis.
- **Malignant:** Bronchogenic carcinoma, bronchial carcinoid tumors, metastatic tumors (colorectal, breast, renal cell, testicular, malignant melanoma, sarcoma).

Diagnosis

- Start by comparing current CXR or CT findings with prior CXR or CT scans, if available.
- **Chest CT:** Best for further evaluating solitary pulmonary nodules, giving a better indication of size, calcification pattern, and nodule density. IV contrast can further aid diagnosis and can assess for mediastinal adenopathy.
- **PET scans:** Can be used to better evaluate indeterminate lesions; sensitivity and specificity are 85% to 95% and 75% to 85%, respectively.

Management

- **Stable:** If nodule has benign appearance or no change for 2 years, recommend close observation with 3- to 6-month repeat images.
- **Growing:** Nodules noted to have grown on serial imaging tests require cancer workup.
- For a nodule found incidentally with no prior imaging, manage as described in Table 8.11. Lesions with >1 malignant characteristic (eg, smoking history, see Table 8.10) should be further evaluated with CT and then followed with the Fleischner criteria. The larger the lesion, the more likely it is to be malignant (although lesions <1 cm have a 15% chance of malignancy).

TABLE 8.11.   Management of Solitary Pulmonary Nodules

SIZE (MM)	NO RISK FACTORS FOR MALIGNANCY	RISK FACTORS FOR MALIGNANCY
<4	No further imaging needed	Follow-up CT at 12 months; if unchanged, no further follow-up
4-6	Follow-up CT at 12 months, if unchanged, no further follow-up	Initial follow-up CT at 6-12 months, then at 18-24 months if no change
6-8	Initial follow-up CT at 6-12 months, then at 18-24 months if no change	Follow-up CT at 3-6, 9-12, and 24 months, if no change
>8 mm	Follow-up CT in 3, 9, and 24 months, dynamic contrast-enhanced CT, PET, and/or biopsy	Same as for patients with no risk factors

QUESTION 1

A 48-year-old man requires a CXR for a physical exam through his work. He is otherwise healthy and denies smoking. CXR reveals a 1-cm lesion with some central calcification in the left upper lobe. PPD is negative. He has no prior chest films for comparison. What is your next step?

QUESTION 2

A 47-year-old African American woman presents with a several-week history of fatigue and malaise. She complains of low-grade fevers, shortness of breath with exertion, and cough. Her exam is unremarkable. CXR shows bilateral hilar adenopathy. PPD is negative. What is the next step in diagnosis?

SARCOIDOSIS

Defined as a chronic, idiopathic, systemic disease characterized by noncaseating granulomas that disturb tissue architecture. The lung is the most commonly affected organ in sarcoidosis, followed by the liver; skin, eye, and lymph node involvement is also common. Presentations include acute, subacute, and self-limiting, or a chronic waxing and waning disease occurring over many years. In the United States, African Americans are affected more than 10 times as often as whites. The typical age range for onset is 20 to 50 years.

Symptoms/Exam

- Patients may be asymptomatic. Common complaints include fatigue, malaise, weight loss, and fever. Patients presenting with pulmonary disease may also have exertional dyspnea, nonproductive cough, and chest pain.
- Subtypes of sarcoidosis may present with fever, erythema nodosum, polyarthralgias, and hilar lymphadenopathy (Löfgren syndrome) or with uveitis, parotid enlargement, fever, and facial palsy (Heerfordt syndrome).
- Exam findings are usually normal but may include crackles or lymphadenopathy.
- The H&P should focus on occupational and environmental exposures and on organs that are commonly affected, such as the lung, skin, eyes, and lymph nodes.

Differential

TB, lymphoma, histoplasmosis, coccidioidomycosis, idiopathic pulmonary fibrosis, pneumoconiosis, syphilis, HIV, berylliosis.

Diagnosis

Three components to diagnosis:
- Clinical and radiographical presentation that correlates (Figure 8.20A).
- Pathologic evidence of noncaseating granulomas (Figure 8.20B).
- Exclusion of other etiologies. Tissue biopsy is integral to diagnosis to exclude infection or malignancy.

ANSWER 1

Obtain a CT scan. The patient has a solitary pulmonary nodule, which, given its size (1 cm) and appearance (calcification), is likely to be benign. Because he is young at 48 and a nonsmoker, a CT scan is warranted.

ANSWER 2

You suspect sarcoidosis and refer her for bronchoscopy with biopsy of her lesions.

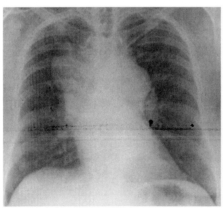
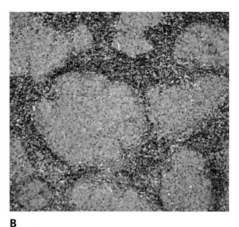

A   **B**

FIGURE 8.20.   **Sarcoidosis. (A)** CXR demonstrates large bilateral hilar and mediastinal lymphadenopathy seen in sarcoidosis. **(B)** Histology slide of an affected lymph node demonstrating the noncaseasting granulomas seen within the organs affected by sarcoidosis. (Image A reproduced from Harris NK. Cough, sarcoidosis and idiopathic pulmonary fibrosis: raw nerves and bad vibrations. *Cough.* 2013;9:9; image B reproduced with permission from USMLE-Rx.com.)

Diagnostic evaluation includes the following:

- CXR staging is based on presence of bilateral hilar lymphadenopathy and pulmonary infiltrates. Pulmonary fibrosis is the most severe radiographic finding. In asymptomatic patients with stage 1 radiographic evidence, tissue biopsy is not warranted given that it will not change the management for monitoring the patient.
- **Fiberoptic bronchoscopy with transbronchial biopsy** most commonly makes the diagnosis, showing a "sarcoid granuloma," which is a **well-formed noncaseating epithelioid cell** granuloma surrounded by a rim of fibroblasts and lymphocytes.
- ACE levels are elevated in 75% of patients, however they are not reliable for diagnostic use or grading severity.
- PFTs, ECG, ophthalmologic evaluation, CBC, a complete metabolic panel, tuberculin skin test, urinalysis, chest radiograph, and 24-hour urine calcium at baseline.
- On follow-up, periodic screening for other organ involvement is appropriate, along with specialist referral as indicated.

Management

Asymptomatic disease: Often nonprogressive and will resolve spontaneously.
Symptomatic and severe disease: Therapy is aimed at ↓ the amount of granulomatous inflammation and end organ damage such as fibrosis and honeycombing. Systemic corticosteroid therapy for 3 to 6 months is the first-line treatment. Refractory cases may be treated with methotrexate, tumor necrosis factor-α inhibitor, and lung transplants.

KEY FACT

In general, an abnormal CXR with a normal exam should make you think sarcoidosis. PFTs show a restrictive or mixed restrictive-obstructive pattern (if granuloma is obstructing airways), with a ↓ DLco.

LUNG CANCER

The leading cause of cancer death in the United States, with a 54% survival rate if caught while localized to lungs. However only 15% are caught prior to becoming metastatic. The various histologic types of bronchogenic carcinoma include **squamous cell carcinoma, adenocarcinoma, large cell carcinoma,** and **small cell carcinoma.** For purposes of staging and treatment, small cell lung cancer (SCLC) is separated from the three other subtypes (labeled together as non–small cell lung cancer [NSCLC]).

- Adenocarcinoma is the most common lung cancer, the most common lung cancer in women, and peripherally located.
- Squamous cell carcinoma starts centrally, may be cavitary, and is associated with hypercalcemia.

KEY FACT

Squamous **c**ell carcinoma and **s**mall **c**ell carcinomas start **c**entrally (think "sssssss"), whereas adenocarcinomas are more peripheral in origin. Large-cell carcinomas can present centrally or peripherally.

Symptoms/Exam

- Major risk factor is tobacco use. Other risk factors include secondhand smoke exposure, radon, and asbestos exposure.
- Up to 15% of patients may be asymptomatic.
- Symptoms may reflect tumor location:
    - With **central tumors,** common complaints include cough, hemoptysis, wheeze, and stridor. In cases where postobstructive pneumonitis or pneumonia are present, symptoms also include dyspnea, fever, and productive cough.
    - **Peripheral** tumors are more likely to present with pleuritic chest pain, cough, and dyspnea.
    - **Regional** spread of tumor may cause further symptoms such as evidence of tracheal obstruction, dysphagia (from esophageal compression), hoarseness, hemidiaphragm elevation with dyspnea, or Horner syndrome (ptosis, miosis, and anhidrosis on the unilateral side of face) from nerve compressions.
    - **Extrathoracic** metastatic disease is common and can affect nearly every organ system.

- The presence of malignant effusions can lead to dyspnea.
- **Paraneoplastic syndromes** can lead to anorexia, cachexia, weight loss, fever, and suppressed immunity, whereas **endocrine syndromes** can lead to symptoms related to hypercalcemia, hypophosphatemia, and hyponatremia.

Diagnosis

- Screening of high-risk individuals with sputum cytology and CXR has not been shown to improve survival rate.
- The USPSTF recommends annual screening for lung cancer with low-dose CT scans in adults aged 55 to 80 years with a 30 pack-year smoking history who currently smoke or smoked within the last 15 years. Tissue biopsy is necessary to confirm a suspected diagnosis.
- A biopsy can be performed with fiberoptic bronchoscopy, mediastinoscopy, surgical resection, percutaneous biopsy of an enlarged lymph node or pleural lesion, FNA under CT guidance, or cytology of a malignant pleural effusion (Figure 8.21).

Management

Based on diagnosis and staging:

- SCLC shows early hematogenous spread and an aggressive course. Surgery is not recommended but chemotherapy and/or radiation may be.
- NSCLC is slower to spread and has a higher chance of being cured with early resection. Higher stages require multimodality therapy with chemotherapy and radiation.
- **Palliative therapy** can take many forms and may assist in relieving symptoms, whether it is photoresection with laser, external beam radiation, resection of brain metastases, or aggressive pain control in advanced disease. Referral to a palliative care specialist is recommended in advanced disease, along with appropriate referral to hospice programs.

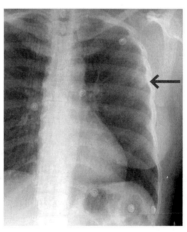

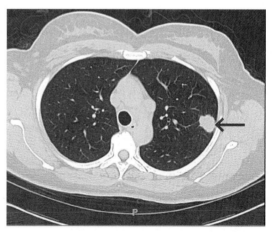

A

B

FIGURE 8.21. **Lung cancer.** Lung cancer (arrows) on (**A**) frontal CXR and (**B**) transaxial CT. (Reproduced with permission from USMLE-Rx.com.)

Nephrology

Richard Giovane, MD

Evaluation of Kidney Disease

In the evaluation of kidney disease, measurement of serum creatinine (Cr) and blood urea nitrogen (BUN) and urinalysis (UA) are often done first as they give a good clinical picture of the patient and they are cost effective. Table 9.1 summarizes the various laboratory tests and imaging that can assist in the diagnosis and treatment of kidney disease. Table 9.2 reviews urinary casts as part of the UA.

T A B L E   9 . 1 .   Diagnostic Tests in the Evaluation of Kidney Disease

DIAGNOSTIC TEST	MEASUREMENTS	INDICATIONS
Serum Cr	Produced in skeletal muscle metabolism and filtered by the kidney Elevated in renal dysfunction Higher in muscular people and lower in elderly patients and pregnant women Can be elevated by medications such as ACEIs, ARBs, cimetidine, trimethoprim, aminoglycosides	First step in evaluating kidney disease Monitor kidney function Used in determination of BUN:Cr ratio, fractional excretion of sodium or urea
BUN	Produced by the liver during the urea cycle and filtered by the kidneys Elevated in renal dysfunction Can be elevated in patients who are bleeding, taking prednisone, and who are dehydrated	First step in evaluating kidney disease, along with serum Cr BUN:Cr ratio can be used to determine kidney function
UA Random specimen, midstream collection ("clean catch"), first morning collection, bladder catheterization	Dipstick testing: specific gravity, pH, protein, hemoglobin, glucose, ketones, bilirubin, nitrite, leukocyte esterase Microscopy: crystals, cells, casts, infecting organisms, and oval fatty bodies	First test + serum Cr in patients with kidney disease Screening in patients with family history of kidney disease To detect infection, dehydration, diabetic ketoacidosis, proteinuria, hematuria, rhabdomyolysis, nephrolithasis
Urine culture Midstream clean catch, bladder catheterization, suprapubic aspiration	>100,000 colony-forming units/mL of one type of bacteria indicates infection in a midstream, clean catch specimen Growth of several types of bacteria indicates contamination Susceptibility testing may guide antibiotic therapy	Infection Usually ordered with UA
24-hr urine collection	Urine protein, Cr, electrolytes, urine volume	Quantitative testing for proteinuria (such as orthostatic proteinuria) Kidney function monitoring for patients with known kidney disease Early detection of kidney damage in the form of proteinuria Other conditions: Diabetic nephropathy, preeclampsia, nephrotic syndrome, multiple myeloma
Spot urine protein to Cr ratio (eg, microalbumin to Cr ratio)	>3.5 g considered nephrotic range proteinuria <0.2 is normal >0.3 g/24 hr or >0.3 protein to Cr ratio in preeclampsia	

(continues)

TABLE 9.1.   Diagnostic Tests in the Evaluation of Kidney Disease *(continued)*

DIAGNOSTIC TEST	MEASUREMENTS	INDICATIONS
Renal ultrasound, Doppler ultrasound of renal arteries and veins	Measures thickness of renal cortex, echogenicity of kidneys, distention of urinary collecting system, kidney size, comparison of bilateral kidneys	Hydronephrosis (Figure 9.1), renal failure of unknown etiology, renal abscess, urinary calculus Identifying and characterizing renal cysts or masses Part of evaluation of malignancy in patients >50 years of age with hematuria Localizing kidney for percutaneous procedures Renal artery stenosis, arterial or venous thrombosis, embolus
Intravenous pyelogram[a]	X-ray of the kidneys, ureters, and bladder before and after administration of IV contrast; less frequently used because of advances in CT technology although has a high sensitivity and specificity for renal stones Characterizes structural disorders	Obstruction such as nephrolithiasis (Figure 9.2), BPH, tumors such as renal cell carcinoma (RCC), polycystic kidney disease, medullary sponge kidney, papillary necrosis
CT Noncontrast and contrast-enhanced[b]	Visualizes anatomy, obstruction, infection, size, growths in the kidneys and the collecting system	**Noncontrast** helical CT scan is the gold standard for detecting renal stones (95% sensitivity and 98% specificity in acute flank pain) Identifying abnormalities found on ultrasound or IVP; eg, simple vs complex cysts Evaluating/staging RCC Part of evaluation for malignancy in patients >50 years of age with hematuria
MRI	Similar to CT scan but superior in soft tissue contrast, which improves detection and characterization of renal lesions	100% sensitive and 96%-98% specific for renal artery stenosis (Figure 9.3); has ↓ the role of renal artery angiography Differentiation of benign lesions from malignant lesions in patients who cannot undergo CT Evaluating/staging RCC
Voiding cystourethrography	Detects abnormalities of the bladder and urethra, vesicoureteral reflux, urine extravasation in bladder ruptures, obstructions or strictures of the urethra	Children with UTI to evaluate for vesicoureteral reflux Bladder obstruction or rupture
Retrograde urethrogram	Insertion of catheter into the fossa navicularis of the distal urethra and injection of contrast under fluoroscopy Detects abnormalities of the anterior urethra, such as stricture or traumatic injury	Suspected anterior urethral stricture or traumatic injury
Renal biopsy[c,d]	Diagnosing unexplained acute or chronic kidney disease	Guiding future treatment in established disease Acute nephritic syndrome Determining renal involvement in systemic diseases; eg, SLE, Goodpasture syndrome, granulomatosis with polyangiitis (Wegener granulomatosis)

[a]Contraindications to IVP: Patients with chronic kidney disease and those with poorly controlled diabetes are not candidates for this study. Also, patients taking metformin should discontinue this medication 48 hours before undergoing IVP. Finally, any patient with a history of a severe allergic reaction to contrast should not have this procedure. Patients with a mild or moderate reaction can be premedicated with antihistamines or corticosteroids.

[b]Contraindications to a contrast CT scan: Any patient who has had a severe allergic reaction to contrast or renal impairment is not a suitable candidate for this procedure. Lastly, patients with hyperthyroidism should avoid iodine-containing contrast as this may induce thyrotoxic crisis.

[c]Contraindications to kidney biopsy: The finding of kidneys <9 cm indicates irreversible changes; multiple bilateral cysts; renal neoplasm; uncorrectable bleeding disorders; severe uncontrolled hypertension; pyelonephritis or abscess.

[d]Complications of kidney biopsy: Bleeding into collecting system, below renal capsule, or into perinephric space. Pain due to obstruction of ureter by a blood clot or renal capsular stretching due to a hematoma. Infection. AV fistulas. "Page kidney," or chronic hypertension with persistent activation of renin-angiotensin system from a large subcapsular hematoma. Consider postprocedure observation for 24 hours, since 90% of complications occur within this time.

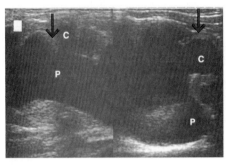
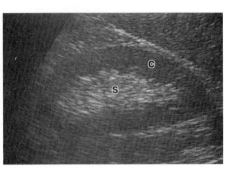

A   **B**

FIGURE 9.1. **Renal ultrasound.** (**A**) Severe hydronephrosis. Renal pelvices are dilated "P." Renal calyces "C." Arrows show severely thinned renal cortices. (**B**) Sagittal ultrasound shows normal-sized kidney with normal-appearing parenchyma and hypoechogenic medullary periods.

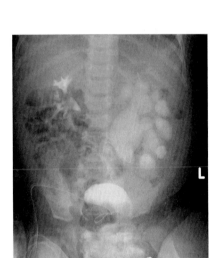

FIGURE 9.2. **Hydronephrosis from ureteropelvic junction obstruction.** Intravenous pyelogram shows markedly enlarged renal collecting system in a child with abdominal mass. (Reproduced with permission from USMLE-Rx.com.)

KEY FACT

A patient with superimposed glomerular injury and a preexisting condition such as CHF will still have an Fe$_{Na}$ of <1%.

KEY FACT

Oliguria is defined as <400 mL urine output in 24 hours and anuria as <100 mL urine output in 24 hours in adults. A urine output of <0.5 mL/kg/hr in children or <1 mL/kg/hr in infants is considered oliguria.

Acute Kidney Injury

Defined as the abrupt loss of kidney function resulting in the retention of urea and dysregulation of electrolytes. The most accepted criteria for AKI is from the Kidney Disease: Improving Global Outcomes (KDIGO):

- ↑ in serum Cr by ≥0.3 mg/dL within 48 hours.
- ↑ in serum Cr to ≥1.5 times baseline within 7 days.
- Urine volume <0.5 mL/kg/h for 6 hours.

Symptoms/Exam

- Review history and medications and rule out any causes that could have precipitated AKI.
- Do a focused physical exam with special attention to the patient's volume status, such as skin turgor, orthostatic changes, body weight, fluid intake, and urine output.
- Obtain UA with microscopy. See Table 9.2 for the significance of various urinary casts in AKI.

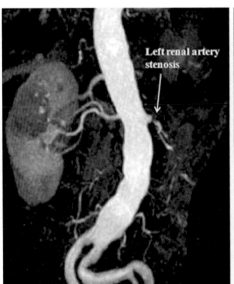
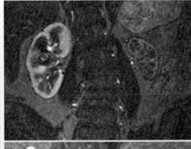
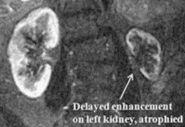

FIGURE 9.3. **Renal artery stenosis.** 3D MRA study of a 66-year-old hypertensive patient with ↑ plasma creatinine on ACE-inhibitor therapy. (Reproduced from Maceira AM, et al. Cardiovascular magnetic resonance in systemic hypertension. *J Cardiovasc Magn Reson.* 2012;14(1):28.)

TABLE 9.2.   **Significance of Specific Urinary Casts**

TYPE	SIGNIFICANCE
Hyaline casts	Concentrated urine, febrile disease, after strenuous exercise, in the course of diuretic therapy (not indicative of renal disease)
RBC casts	Glomerulonephritis
WBC casts	Pyelonephritis, interstitial nephritis (indicative of infection or inflammation)
Renal epithelial cell casts	Acute tubular necrosis, interstitial nephritis
Muddy granular casts	Nonspecific; can represent acute tubular necrosis
Broad, waxy casts	Chronic renal failure (indicative of stasis in enlarged collecting tubules)

Adapted with permission from Tierney LM, et al. *Current Medical Diagnosis & Treatment,* 45th ed. New York: McGraw-Hill, 2006, Table 22-1.

- **If patient is oliguric and *not* using diuretics, determine the fractional excretion of sodium (Fe$_{Na}$):**

$$Fe_{Na} = [(urine_{Na} \times plasma_{Cr}) / (plasma_{Na} \times urine_{Cr})] \times 100$$

- A value <1% suggests prerenal AKI as the kidney is still able to reabsorb sodium; in this case think dehydration or volume depletion.
- A value >3% suggests acute tubular necrosis or post renal damage as the tubular damage.
- A value between 1% and 3% is suggestive of either prerenal, renal, or postrenal disease.
- **If patient is oliguric and using diuretics, determine the fractional excretion of urea (Fe$_{Urea}$):**

$$Fe_{Urea} = [(urine_{Urea} \times plasma_{Cr}) / (urine_{Cr} \times plasma_{Urea})] \times 100\%$$

- A value <35% suggests prerenal AKI. A value >50% suggests acute tubular necrosis.
- If patient has signs and symptoms related to an obstruction, order renal ultrasound.

Diagnosis

See Tables 9.3 through 9.5 for the clinical features and diagnostic tests.

KEY FACT

Casts are specific but not sensitive. When a type of cast is present in the urine, it is usually indicative of the "most likely diagnosis."

KEY FACT

AKI can lead to hyperkalemia, fluid overload, metabolic acidosis and uremia which can lead to platelet dysfunction, mental status change, or pericarditis. Any of these manifestations require urgent dialysis.

MNEMONIC

Indications for emergent dialysis:
AEIOU
Acidosis
Electrolytes (hyperkalemia)
Ingestions
Overload (pulmonary edema)
Uremia

TABLE 9.3.   **Clinical Presentation and Diagnosis of Prerenal AKI**

CAUSES AND SUGGESTIVE CLINICAL FEATURES	UA AND OTHER CONFIRMATORY TESTS
Volume depletion: History of vomiting, diarrhea, ↓ PO intake, diuretic use, hemorrhage, burns	Hyaline casts on microscopy Fe$_{Na}$ <1% Fe$_{Urea}$ <35%
Signs/Symptoms: Thirst, hypotension, tachycardia, dry mucous membranes	BUN:Cr ratio >20:1 Urine specific gravity >1.020
Low-output states: History of CHF, cirrhosis, severe valvular disease, hepatorenal syndrome, sepsis, shock	Urine osmolality >500 mOsm/kg U$_{Na}$ <10 mmol/L
Symptoms: Pulmonary edema, ↑ JVP, ascites	Rapid resolution of AKI with restoration of renal perfusion, such as with fluid bolus or, in the
Medications: NSAIDs, ACEIs, ARBs	case of CHF, diuresis

TABLE 9.4.   **Clinical Presentation and Diagnosis of Intrarenal AKI**

CAUSES AND SUGGESTIVE CLINICAL FEATURES	UA AND OTHER CONFIRMATORY TESTS
TUBULAR	
Acute tubular necrosis (ATN), see Figure 9.4:	Muddy granular casts
90% of intrarenal AKI is due to ATN	Renal epithelial cell casts
Tubular injury is caused by ischemia or nephrotoxins	Fe_{Na} >1%
Ischemic:	Fe_{Urea} >35%
Prolonged prerenal failure, hemorrhage, hypotension, sepsis	Urine Osm <350 mOsm/kg (failure to concentrate urine, even in oliguria)
Toxic:	U_{Na} >30 mmol/L
Nephrotoxic drugs and substances (see Table 9.6), rhabdomyolysis, tumor lysis, multiple myeloma, contrast nephropathy	In rhabdomyolysis: Cola-colored urine, heme-positive urine dipstick with no RBCs on microscopy, ↑ serum creatine kinase, myoglobin
	In tumor lysis: ↑ calcium and uric acid
	In multiple myeloma: SPEP/UPEP
INTERSTITIAL	
Acute interstitial nephritis (AIN), see Figure 9.5:	WBC casts, WBCs on urine microscopy
Due to allergic reaction to drug (see Table 9.6):	Urine eosinophils
Signs/Symptoms: Fever, rash, or arthralgias	Interstitial inflammation on renal biopsy
Due to infection:	Treatment includes withdrawal or eradication of the offending agent and administration of corticosteroids
Pyelonephritis, HIV, CMV, EBV, HBV, HCV	
Due to autoimmune disorders:	
Wegener granulomatosis, sarcoidosis, SLE, Sjögren syndrome	
GLOMERULAR	
Glomerulonephritis/vasculitis:	Finding of RBC casts on urine microscopy is pathognomonic
Signs/Symptoms: Hypertension, hematuria, edema, oliguria	Urine microscopy can also show:
Postinfectious (PIGN):	Granular casts, RBCs and WBCs, dysmorphic red cells, hematuria, proteinuria
Poststreptococcal glomerulonephritis (PSGN): 2-3 weeks after streptococcal pharyngitis or skin infection	⊕ blood cultures and vegetations on echocardiogram for endocarditis
Endocarditis:	Consider the additional tests:
Signs/Symptoms: Fever, new heart murmur	ASO titers (PSGN), complement levels (low in SLE, PIGN/PSGN, MPGN, cryoglobulinemia)
Risk factors: Abnormal heart valve, IV drug use, recent dental procedure	ANA, anti-dsDNA, anti-Smith antibodies (SLE)
Other:	Cryoglobulins, RPR, HCV, HBV, HIV (MPGN)
Goodpasture syndrome	c-ANCA, anti-PR3 (Wegener granulomatosis)
Wegener granulomatosis	p-ANCA, anti-MPO (Churg-Strauss syndrome, PAN)
Churg-Strauss syndrome	Anti-GBM (Goodpasture syndrome)
Polyarteritis nodosa (PAN)	Renal biopsy for definitive diagnosis
SLE	
IgA nephropathy	
Cryoglobulinemia	
Membranoproliferative glomerulonephritis (MPGN)	
Henoch-Schönlein purpura	
Medications: Gold, penicillamine	

(continues)

TABLE 9.4. **Clinical Presentation and Diagnosis of Intrarenal AKI** *(continued)*

CAUSES AND SUGGESTIVE CLINICAL FEATURES	UA AND OTHER CONFIRMATORY TESTS
VASCULAR	
Microvascular:	UA may be normal or RBCs may be seen; mild proteinuria or, rarely, RBC casts or granular casts
Hemolytic-uremic syndrome (HUS)	
E coli O157:H7	In HUS/TTP: Anemia, thrombocytopenia, schistocytes on blood smear, $\uparrow$ LDH, $\uparrow$ bilirubin, $\downarrow$ haptoglobin, stool culture, renal failure
Thrombotic thrombocytopenic purpura (TTP):	
Signs/Symptoms: Neurological symptoms, fever, renal failure, petechiae, jaundice	In DIC: Anemia, schistocytes, $\uparrow$ D-dimer, $\uparrow$ fibrinogen, $\uparrow$ PT, PTT, $\downarrow$ platelets
Disseminated intravascular coagulation (DIC):	In preeclampsia: BP >140/90 mm Hg, proteinuria >300 mg, $\uparrow$ LFTs, low platelets
Sepsis, shock, malignancy, obstetric complications, placental abruption, amniotic fluid embolus, eclampsia	
Signs/Symptoms: Bleeding, petechiae	
Preeclampsia	
Signs/Symptoms: Headache, RUQ pain, pulmonary edema, scotomata	
Macrovascular:	Mild proteinuria and occasional RBCs; $\uparrow$ LDH
Renal artery thrombosis:	Renal arteriogram
History of atrial fibrillation, aortic dissection, recent MI; most often in elderly	$\downarrow$ antithrombin III
Signs/Symptoms: Flank or abdominal pain, sudden-onset hypertension	
Renal vein thrombosis:	Proteinuria and hematuria
Seen in patients with nephrotic syndrome; pulmonary embolism	IVC and renal vein imaging, ultrasound, or CT scan showing $\uparrow$ in renal size
Signs/Symptoms: Flank pain, anasarca	Eosinophilia, low complement levels, skin biopsy, renal biopsy
Atheroembolism:	
Age usually >50 years; often in ICU patients; recent surgery/procedure (angiography), administration of thrombolytics	
Signs/Symptoms: Acute arrhythmia, hypertension, edema, rash (livedo reticularis, subcutaneous nodules, palpable purpura)	

TABLE 9.5. **Clinical Presentation and Diagnosis of Postrenal AKI**

CAUSES/SUGGESTIVE CLINICAL FEATURES	UA/OTHER CONFIRMATORY TESTS
Urethral obstruction:	Frequently normal UA
Prostatic hypertrophy	Possible hematuria
Urethral stricture	Postvoid residual >100 mL
Bladder, pelvic or retroperitoneal neoplasm	Hydronephrosis on renal ultrasound, IVP, retrograde or anterograde pyelography, CT
Calculi	Other testing: PSA, SPEP, UPEP
Crystals, myeloma light chains	
Neurogenic bladder	
Anticholinergics, narcotics causing urinary retention	
Signs/Symptoms: Lower urinary tract symptoms, abdominal or flank pain, palpable bladder, enlarged prostate, oliguria/anuria	

QUESTION

A 30-year-old man presents for his yearly checkup. He reports no issues except a mild $\uparrow$ in urinary frequency. His physical exam is unremarkable. He is sent for blood work and a UA, which comes back positive for mild proteinuria. What is the next best step?

TABLE 9.6.   Nephrotoxic Drugs and Substances

DRUGS
Antimicrobials:
Aminoglycosides
Amphotericin B
Antivirals
Antiparasitics (pentamidine)
β-lactams
Cephalosporins
Fluoroquinolones
Rifampin
Sulfonamides
ACEIs
Anti-inflammatories:
NSAIDs
COX-2 inhibitors
Other:
Phenytoin
Allopurinol
Cimetidine
Furosemide
Thiazide diuretics
Lithium chemotherapeutics

SUBSTANCES
Ethylene glycol (oxalic acid)
Heavy metals (lead, arsenic)
Hemoglobin
Myeloma light chain deposition
Myoglobin (rhabdomyolysis)
Radiocontrast agents
Uric acid
Cocaine

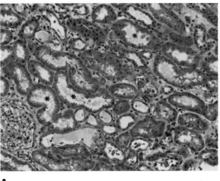

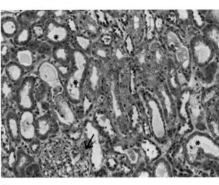

A   B

FIGURE 9.4.   Acute tubular necrosis. Renal biopsy shows tubular damage from drug toxicity. In both panels (**A**) and (**B**), there is a moderate degree of acute tubular necrosis (asterisks). Some tubules contain hyaline or epithelial casts in their lumina (green arrows), while several tubules show vacuolization of their cytoplasm (green arrowheads). One of the glomerular afferent arteriole shows swollen endothelia and occlusive change (black arrow). (Reproduced from Shah-Khan F, et al. Biopsy-proven acute tubular necrosis due to vancomycin toxicity. *Int J Nephrol.* 2011;2011:436856.)

Management

- Identify and treat the underlying cause.
- Ensure renal perfusion by maintaining adequate intravascular volume.
- Refer for dialysis in accordance with the **AEIOU** mnemonic.
- Eliminate further exposure to nephrotoxic drugs and substances (Table 9.6).
- Monitor and correct electrolyte abnormalities such as hyperkalemia, hypocalcemia, and hyperphosphatemia. Monitor urine output.
- Seek a urology consult for postrenal etiologies that cannot be managed by standard therapy. An example is renal stones >10 mm.

Chronic Kidney Disease

Clinically defined as the following:

- Urinary albumin excretion of >30 mg/day or GFR <60 mL/min/1.73m^2 for 3 months or more.

 ANSWER

Repeat the UA. The first step in any patient with proteinuria is to rule out transient proteinuria.

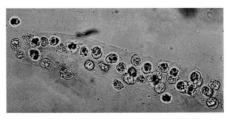

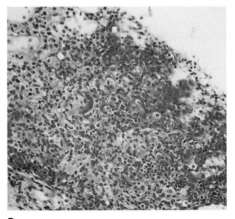

A   B

FIGURE 9.5.   Acute interstitial nephritis. (**A**) White blood cell cast. (**B**) Kidney biopsy highlighting the inflammatory interstitial infiltrate with prominent eosinophils. (Reproduced from Perazella MA. Diagnosing drug-induced AIN in the hospitalized patient: A challenge for the clinician. *Clin Nephrol.* 2014;81(6):381-388.)

- Divided into five stages for GFR and three stages for albumin levels. See Table 9.7.
- Kidney failure, or end-stage renal disease (ESRD), is defined as a GFR <15 mL/min and/or a requirement for renal replacement therapy in the form of dialysis or transplantation.
- Screening for CKD is recommended for high-risk patients (eg, those with diabetes, family history, hypertension, recurrent UTIs, urinary obstruction or vascular disease).
- Screening methods include the following:
  - Serum Cr to calculate GFR.
  - UA for proteinuria and microscopy.
  - For patients with type 2 DM, microalbumin to Cr ratio; a value of 30 to 300 mg/g of Cr suggests a moderate level of excretion, patients warrant further workup if the ratio of microalbumin to Cr is moderate or severe two times or more.
  - Renal imaging in patients with a history of urinary obstruction, recurrent UTIs, vesicoureteral reflux, family history of polycystic kidney disease.

Symptoms/Exam

Patients with stage 1 to 3 CKD are usually asymptomatic. Symptoms typically manifest in stages 4 to 5 when GFR ↓ to <30 mL/min. Signs and symptoms are those associated with complications of CKD: hyperkalemia (cardiac arrhythmia, muscle weakness), anemia (fatigue), bone disease (due to poor vitamin D formation), hypocalcemia (tetany, muscle spasms), volume overload (hypertension, pulmonary edema, extremity edema), uremia (pericarditis, restless leg syndrome, anorexia, nausea, vomiting, dry skin, pruritus, fatigue, and platelet dysfunction).

Diagnosis

To specify the cause of CKD, evaluate the following factors:

- Patient history, serum Cr, GFR, UA and microscopy, and renal ultrasound—useful to evaluate the presence of an obstruction.
- Spot urine protein-to-Cr ratio or 24-hour protein collection to quantify proteinuria. If etiology is not clear, further workup may be indicated to evaluate for causes of kidney disease, such as hepatitis B and C, syphilis, HIV, collagen vascular diseases, and multiple myeloma.
- Biopsy also indicated if the patient's serum Cr has remained unstable and imaging has not shown signs of chronicity.

KEY FACT

Diabetes and hypertension are the two main causes of chronic kidney disease.

TABLE 9.7.   **Stages of Chronic Kidney Disease Based on GFR and Albuminuria**

STAGE	Δ IN GFR	GFR (ML/MIN/1.73M²)	Δ IN ALBUMIN	ALBUMIN EXCRETION RATIO (MG/DAY)
1	Kidney damage with normal or ↑ GFR	≥90	Normal to mildly ↑	<30
2	Mild ↓ in GFR	60-89	Moderately ↑	30-300
3	Moderate ↓ in GFR	30-59	Severely ↑	>300
4	Severe ↓ in GFR	15-29		
5	Kidney failure	<15 or dialysis		

Q   QUESTION 1

A 57-year-old diabetic man in stage 3 CKD has undergone an emergency appendectomy. His postoperative pain persists despite treatment with acetaminophen. Which medication would you add to relieve his pain?

Q   QUESTION 2

A 67-year-old woman is hospitalized for suspected pneumonia. She has a history of CHF, CAD, CKD stage 2, and COPD. She takes several medications, including hydrochlorothiazide and lisinopril. The patient's diuretic use renders the Fe_{Na} of little value in monitoring renal function. What other calculation can you use?

Management

- The following measures have been proven to **slow the progression of CKD:**
  - **Reduction of proteinuria with ACEIs/ARBs:** Beneficial for both diabetic and nondiabetic nephropathy.
  - **Treatment of hypertension:** BP goal of <140/90 mm Hg, if normal urine protein; stricter control is warranted if patient has proteinuria.
  - Glycemic control in diabetic patients: HbA_{1c} goal <8%, especially in elderly patients.
  - Avoidance of nephrotoxins.
  - Statins may be used to lower lipids in patients with dyslipidemia.
  - Lowering protein intake to no more than 0.8 g/kg/day.
  - Smoking cessation.
- Patients with stage 3 to 4 CKD should be periodically monitored with the following lab studies:
  - Hemoglobin/hematocrit.
  - RBC indices.
  - Reticulocyte count.
  - Iron studies.
  - Fecal occult blood test.
  - Serum electrolytes.
  - Calcium, phosphorus, and PTH.
  - Serum albumin and total protein.
- Refer to surgeon for permanent vascular access or peritoneal dialysis catheter 6 months before anticipated date of dialysis.
- Refer to nephrologist when GFR <30 mL/min.
- Early nephrology referral has been shown to ↓ morbidity and mortality.

Complications

- **Anemia:** Erythropoietin (EPO) and repletion of iron stores.
- **Hyperkalemia:** Dietary restrictions, sodium polystyrene, and diuretics.
- **Acidosis:** Dialysis, sodium bicarbonate.
- **Renal osteodystrophy:** Phosphate binders, dietary restriction, calcium supplement, calcitriol.
- **Bleeding:** If patients are bleeding or require surgery, desmopressin, estrogen, or cryoprecipitate can be used.
- **Sexual dysfunction:** Treatment based on underlying cause.
- **Pericarditis:** Urgent dialysis is recommended.
- **Volume overload:** Diuretics, volume restriction, dialysis.
- Uremic neuropathy: Dialysis and trials of gabapentin can be used.
- **Uremia:** Dialysis.
- Dialysis-related complications:
  - **Vascular catheter–related infections** (*S aureus*, coagulase-negative *Staphylococcus*): Treat empirically with an IV first-generation cephalosporin and consider vancomycin coverage for MRSA. Tailor antibiotics to blood culture results from the catheter and a peripheral site. Consider removal of the catheter for fungal infections, sepsis, endocarditis, or persistent bacteremia.
  - **Peritoneal catheter–related infections** (*S aureus*, *S epidermidis*, enteric gram-negative rods): Often treated with infusion of antibiotics into the peritoneum. Add IV antibiotics in severe cases and consider catheter removal.
  - **AV fistula thrombosis:** Treatment options include intravascular clot removal and thrombolytics.

KEY FACT

Cardiovascular disease is still the most common cause of death in CKD, with risk and mortality ↑ in proportion to the ↓ in GFR.

ANSWER 1

A high-dose opioid such as fentanyl, hydromorphone, or tramadol would be beneficial for this patient as these drugs are metabolized in the liver.

ANSWER 2

Fe_{Urea}, which is not affected by diuretic use, calculated as $[(urine_{Urea} \times plasma_{Cr}) / (urine_{Cr} \times plasma_{Urea})] \times 100\%$.

Nephrotic Syndrome

Nephrotic syndrome is characterized by significant proteinuria (>3.5 g/24 hr) resulting from **noninflammatory** injury to the glomeruli, hypoalbuminemia (<3 g/dL), edema, and peripheral edema. Nephrotic syndrome may be 1°/idiopathic or 2° to a variety of disorders.

- **1° or idiopathic causes:**
  - **Minimal change disease:** Common in children, but can occur in adults. Usually preceded by an URI or in some cases by immunization. In adults, use of NSAIDs or Hodgkin lymphoma can also precipitate minimal change disease. Characterized by a sudden onset of heavy proteinuria. A fusion of foot processes of epithelial cells on electron microscopy is characteristic of minimal change disease; however, light microscopy will not reveal any abnormalities. Minimal change disease has an excellent response to steroids, and renal failure is uncommon.
  - **Focal segmental glomerulosclerosis (FSGS):** More common in African Americans and seen in sickle cell disease, hypertension, diabetes, IV drug use, and HIV. Can be primary or secondary with the former having an acute onset and the latter having a gradual onset of renal failure and proteinuria. Histologically, has many variants such as cellular, collapsing, and perihilar. When compared with minimal change disease, FSGS is associated with a higher frequency of renal failure. Generally treated with steroids, cyclosporin A, and cyclophosphamide.
  - **Membranous nephropathy (Figure 9.6):** Most common cause of nephrotic syndrome in adults and more common in whites, aged 30 to 50 years. Also seen in HBV, HCV, syphilis, malaria, gold and penicillamine use, and SLE. Approximately 25% of cases are associated with neoplasm. Membranous nephropathy presents with proteinuria, occasional microhematuria and hypercoagulability (renal vein thrombosis). Treated with steroids, cyclosporin, cyclophosphamide, and chlorambucil. Remission rate is 25%.
  - **Membranoproliferative glomerulonephritis (Figure 9.7):** Can present with nephritic or nephrotic features and is associated with infection, autoimmune disease, HCV, and cryoglobulins such as low C3. Treated with observation (nonnephrotic with stable renal function) or steroids, plasmapharesis, or interferon-α. Associated with a 50% mortality rate or progression to ESRD within 5 years of renal biopsy.
- **2° causes:**
  - **Diabetic nephropathy:** Leading cause of ESRD in the United States. Onset is 5 to 10 years after diagnosis for type 1 DM but is more variable in type 2 DM. Kidney biopsy will show Kimmelstiel-Wilson nodules. Mainstay of treatment

QUESTION 1

A 50-year-old man with a history of chronic lower back pain comes in with 1 week of ↑ lower extremity edema and ↓ urine output. He reports that over the last week, his urine has been dark and foamy. He denies shortness of breath or orthopnea. He has used ibuprofen 800 mg three times/day for the last year. He denies alcohol use. On exam, his BP is 135/80 mm Hg, and he has 3+ edema in his bilateral lower extremities up to his sacrum, but no rales, jugular venous distention, or ascites. What diagnosis will the blood and urine test results reveal?

QUESTION 2

A 25-year-old woman presents with 2 days of fatigue, ↓ appetite, swollen feet, and scant, cola-colored urine. She reports having sore throat and fever 2 weeks earlier that resolved without treatment. On exam, her BP is 165/102 mm Hg, she appears dehydrated, and has periorbital and 3+ lower extremity edema. UA shows blood and protein. RBC casts are seen on microscopic exam. What additional laboratory tests can confirm the diagnosis?

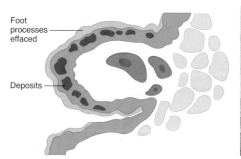
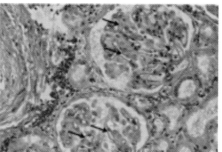

FIGURE 9.6. Membranous nephropathy. (A) Foot process effacement with subepithelial deposits. **(B)** Thickened capillary walls (arrows). (Reproduced with permission from USMLE-Rx.com; image B courtesy of Dr. Y. Chu.)

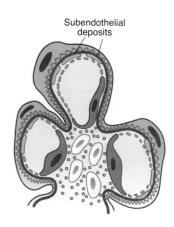

FIGURE 9.7. Membranoproliferative glomerulonephritis. (Reproduced with permission from USMLE-Rx.com.)

is tight glycemic control, BP control (ie, <140/90 mm Hg), and lipid control (ie, LDL <100 mg/dL). ACEIs are first-line agents in type 1 DM; ACEIs or ARBs are used in type 2.

- **Amyloidosis:** Most common in elderly patients. Two types are 1° amyloidosis in which amyloid light chain [AL] is deposited in the kidney and 2° amyloidosis in which amyloid acute phase reactant [AA] is deposited in the kidney. Diagnose via kidney biopsy and Congo red staining. Since majority of renal amyloidosis leads to ESRD, treatment consists of dialysis and kidney transplant.
- **Other etiologies:** Malignancy (classically, lymphoma or myeloma), infections (HIV, HBV, HCV, syphilis, leprosy, malaria), SLE, sickle cell disease, pre-eclampsia, drugs (gold, NSAIDs, penicillamine, IV drug use), insect bites, and poison ivy.

Symptoms/Exam

Loss of appetite, fatigue and malaise, edema, dyspnea from pleural effusions, ascites, weight gain, muscle wasting, frothy urine, opportunistic infections, and clotting disorders. Patients with nephrotic disease are also at ↑ risk for venous thrombosis and pulmonary embolism.

Differential/Diagnosis

See Table 9.8 for a comparison of nephrotic and nephritic syndromes. Relevant lab tests include the following:

- **UA and microscopy:** Reveals proteinuria. Oval fat bodies or Maltese cross may be seen under polarized light. Waxy and fatty casts.

ANSWER 1

Nephrotic syndrome from NSAID use, defined as proteinuria >3 g/day. Classically, microscopy shows oval fat bodies and fatty casts. Under polarized light microscopy, the oval fat bodies and fatty casts have a "Maltese cross" appearance. Additional laboratory findings include ↑ lipids and ↓ serum albumin.

ANSWER 2

Additional tests to confirm poststreptococcal glomerulonephritis (suggested by RBC casts on microscopy) include a rapid strep test and/or throat culture, which may be ⊖; ASO titer, which would be ⊕; and C3 complement level, which would be low. BUN and Cr will be elevated, demonstrating the AKI.

TABLE 9.8.   Comparison of Nephrotic and Nephritic Syndromes

	NEPHROTIC SYNDROME	NEPHRITIC SYNDROME
Findings	Proteinuria >3 g/day	Proteinuria <3 g/day
	Edema	Edema
	Hyperlipidemia and lipiduria	Hematuria
	Hypoalbuminemia (serum albumin <3 g/dL)	Hypertension
		AKI for days to weeks
	Hypercoagulability	Oliguria
	Fatty and waxy casts	RBC casts, WBC casts
	Oval fat bodies and Maltese crosses	Dysmorphic RBCs
1° or idiopathic	Minimal-change disease	PSGN (can present as nephrotic syndrome)
	FSGS	
	Membranous nephropathy	IgA nephropathy
	MPGN (can present as nephritic syndrome)	
2°	Diabetic nephropathy	SLE (can present as nephrotic syndrome)
	Malignancy (lymphoma or myeloma)	Goodpasture syndrome
	Infectious (eg, HIV, HBV/HCV, syphilis)	ANCA-related vasculitis:
	Amyloidosis	granulomatosis with polyangiitis (Wegener granulomatosis), microscopic polyarteritis nodosa, eosinophilic granulomatosis with polyangiitis (Churg-Strauss syndrome)

- **Twenty-four-hour urine collection:** Quantifies proteinuria. Spot urine sampling for protein-to-creatinine ratio can approximate 24-hour protein excretion.
- Serum albumin. Low in nephrotic syndrome.
- Additional labs to determine 2° causes: HbA_{1c}, SPEP/UPEP, complement levels, ASO titers, ANA, anti-dsDNA, and serologic tests for HBV, HCV, HIV, and syphilis.
- Consider renal biopsy if etiology is unclear.

Management

- Control peripheral edema with loop diuretics.
- Maintain good nutrition and limit salt intake for edema control.
- Administer ACEIs/ARBs to slow proteinuria.
- Institute lipid-lowering therapy with a target LDL generally <100 mg/dL.
- Heparin and warfarin therapy are used for thromboembolisms.
- Treat the underlying disease: Trial of steroid therapy for most nephrotic syndromes is warranted. 2° causes such as diabetes require strict glucose control while amyloidosis requires kidney transplant or dialysis.

Nephritic Disease

Typically consists of proteinuria (<3 g/day), hematuria, hypertension, renal insufficiency, and edema due to **inflammatory** changes in the glomeruli. May be primary/idiopathic or caused by a variety of disorders.

- 1° or idiopathic causes:
  - **Poststreptococcal glomerulonephritis (Figure 9.8):** Leading cause of acute nephritic syndrome and **classically seen 2 to 3 weeks after pharyngitis or skin infection.** Diagnosed via elevated ASO titers and anti-DNase B antibodies, along with low complement levels. Treatment is supportive, and renal failure typically resolves within 4 weeks, with only 5% of cases requiring acute renal replacement therapy.
  - **IgA nephropathy (Berger disease):** More common among Asians and Hispanics; with a higher prevalence in men than in women and patients in their teens to 20s. Patients present with episodic hematuria ± proteinuria, usually within 24 hours of a URI. The clinical picture is similar to PSGN but usually timing is a distinguishing factor between the two. Treat with ACEIs. Consider fish oil if proteinuria is <3 g/day or steroids if >3 g/day. Approximately 20% of cases progress to renal failure within 20 years.
  - **Hereditary (Alport syndrome):** The mode of inheritance is X-linked. Consider this diagnosis in patients with a family history of hematuria with sensorineural deafness and ocular abnormalities.
- 2° causes:
  - **SLE:** Lupus nephritis can be the presenting feature. Diagnosed by anti-dsDNA and anti-Smith antibodies, along with low complement levels. Eight to 15% of SLE patients progress to ESRD. Treatment is with steroids.
  - **Goodpasture syndrome:** A constellation of glomerulonephritis, pulmonary hemorrhage, and anti-GBM antibodies that can present with rapidly progressive glomerulonephritis (RPGN). Circulating antibodies to type IV collagen destroy basement membrane leading to sequela. Diagnosed via anti-GBM antibodies. Once recognized, treatment is urgent and includes plasmapheresis, steroids, and cyclophosphamide.
  - **ANCA-related vasculitis:** Includes granulomatosis with polyangitiis (Wegener granulomatosis), microscopic polyarteritis nodosa, and eosinophilic granulomatosis with polyangitiis (Churg-Strauss syndrome). These conditions are diagnosed via c-ANCA, p-ANCA, antimyeloperoxidase (MPO) antibodies,

KEY FACT

Complications of nephrotic syndrome include:
- Protein malnutrition
- Hypovolemia
- AKI
- Thromboembolism
- Infection
- Hyperlipidemia

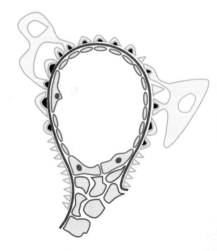

FIGURE 9.8. Acute (poststreptococcal) glomerulonephritis. Immune complex deposits below the podocyte foot processes creating subepithelial humps. (Reproduced from Wikipedia; courtesy of Michael Komorniczak.)

KEY FACT

PSGN can occur at any age but is most common in children 2 to 6 years of age. IgA nephropathy can present similarly to PSGN; however, it presents more in the second and third decades of life and occurs **usually a few days after a streptococcal infection.**

KEY FACT

Rheumatic fever from group A *Streptococcus* can be prevented with prompt administration of penicillin G and clindamycin; however, this treatment will not prevent PSGN.

anti-proteinase 3 (anti-PR3), and renal biopsy. Treatment is usually urgent and includes plasmapheresis, steroids, and cyclophosphamide.

■ Other causes: Henoch-Schönlein purpura, hypersensitivity vasculitis, cryoglobulinemia, drugs (gold, penicillamine).

Symptoms/Exam

Approximately 50% of cases are asymptomatic. Look for loss of appetite, fatigue and malaise, peripheral and periorbital edema, hypertension, oliguria, and dark urine (hematuria).

Differential

Table 9.8 distinguishes nephritic disease from nephrotic syndrome.

Diagnosis

■ **UA and microscopy:** RBC casts, dysmorphic RBCs, and WBCs. RBC casts are pathognomonic of glomerulonephritis.
■ **Twenty-four-hour protein collection or spot urine protein-to-creatinine ratio** determines proteinuria.
■ Obtain additional labs as indicated (complement levels, ASO titer, anti-DNase antibodies, anti-GBM antibodies, dsDNA, ANA, ESR, c-ANCA, p-ANCA).
■ Renal ultrasound.
■ Renal biopsy if diagnosis is unclear after workup.

Management

Treatment principles are the same as for nephrotic syndrome with emphasis on treating the underlying disease.

Hematuria

Can be classified as either microscopic or gross. Gross hematuria is defined as visible blood within the urine. Microscopic hematuria can be defined as ≥3 RBCs per high-power microscopic field in urinary sediment, from **two** of **three properly collected UA specimens.**

■ Remember that red urine is not always due to RBCs from the urinary tract. Other causes include the following:
  ■ Medications: Phenazopyridine, nitrofurantoin, cascara, methyldopa, phenacetin, phenindoine, phenolphthalein, phenothizine, senna.
  ■ Myoglobin in the urine.
  ■ Porphyria.
  ■ Beets, rhubarb, food coloring.
  ■ Contamination from vaginal or GI bleeding.
■ Causes of hematuria are characterized as glomerular or nonglomerular:
  ■ **Glomerular:**
    ■ Glomerulonephritis (see section on Nephritic Disease).
    ■ Alport syndrome (see section on Nephritic Disease).
    ■ Thin basement membrane nephropathy (benign familial hematuria).
  ■ **Nonglomerular** (categorized as renal or nonrenal):
    ■ **Renal:** Malignancy, vascular disease (malignant hypertension, AVM, nutcracker syndrome [left renal vein compression between the abdominal aorta and superior mesenteric artery], renal vein thrombosis, papillary necrosis), infection (pyelonephritis, TB, CMV, EBV), hereditary disease (polycystic kidney disease, medullary sponge kidney).

- **Nonrenal:** Malignancy (prostatic, ureteral, bladder), infection (prostatitis, cystitis), BPH, nephrolithiasis, endometriosis, coagulopathy (bleeding disorders or medication-induced disease), trauma (Foley catheter), vigorous exercise, *Schistosoma haematobium* (consider if from endemic areas of Africa, India, Middle East).

Symptoms/Exam

- **Gross hematuria:** Red or brown color change of urine.
- **Microscopic hematuria:** Often asymptomatic and discovered on urine dipstick or on UA obtained for other purposes.
- A focused history can help guide further evaluation and should include the following factors:
    - **Recent symptoms:** URIs may point toward PSGN or IgA nephropathy. Look for urinary tract symptoms that may suggest infectious or obstructive processes as well as flank pain radiating to the groin.
    - **Other:** Look for symptoms that predispose to glomerular disease, such as joint pain and rash in connective tissue disorder; edema in glomerular disease; and risk factors for endocarditis. Ask about recent vigorous exercise or traumas; ask about travel to areas where schistosomiasis is endemic and look at the eosinophil level. Determine if there is a family history of renal diseases or sickle cell trait/disease. Review medications, including use of NSAIDs and anticoagulants, although anticoagulants do not cause hematuria without trauma.

Diagnosis

Rule out benign causes of hematuria, such as menstruation, vigorous exercise, sexual activity, trauma, or infection.

Management

Benign causes of hematuria: If history suggests a benign cause, repeat UA 48 hours after cessation of activity. Treat patients with a UTI and repeat UA 6 weeks after treatment. Other causes of hematuria are discussed below.

GROSS HEMATURIA

Best initial step in evaluation: Centrifuge the urine and determine the urine sediment:
- **Red sediment:** Indicates hematuria. Patients with hematuria should have CT urography as the first initial step in diagnosis. In patients where a CT is contraindicated, an MRI without contrast or ultrasound is acceptable.

Cystoscopy should also be done for patients in the following three scenarios:
- If there is no evidence of infection or kidney stones.
- Patient >35 years and benign conditions have been ruled out.
- Patient has ↑ risk of malignancy. (See the Hematology/Oncology chapter for a discussion of RCC.)
- **Red supernatant:**
    - **Heme-positive dipstick:** Indicates myoglobinuria or hemoglobinuria.
    - **Heme-negative dipstick:** Phenazopyridine, beets, porphyria.

KEY FACT

Myoglobinuria can indicate rhabdomyolysis. Always suspect this in patients with "crush" injuries or if they are taking statins. Always anticipate that hyperkalemia could develop.

MICROSCOPIC HEMATURIA

Diagnosis

- UA and microscopy to determine the number and morphology of RBCs, crystals, and casts.
- Electrolytes, kidney function, blood counts, and coagulation.

- Smoking history
- Occupational exposure to benzenes, aromatic amines
- Age >40 years
- History of gross hematuria
- History of urologic disorder or disease
- History of irritative voiding symptoms
- History of UTI
- History of pelvic irradiation
- Analgesic abuse

- Differentiate between **glomerular and nonglomerular causes:**
    - **Glomerular causes:** See sections on AKI and Nephritic Disease.
    - **Nonglomerular causes:**
        - In low-risk patients without risk factors, workup includes urine cytology and renal ultrasound.
        - For patients with gross hematuria or associated risk factors (Table 9.9), obtain upper tract imaging (CT or IVP), lower tract imaging (cystoscopy), and urine cytology.
- If workup ⊖, UA, blood pressure, and urine cytology should be obtained at 6, 12, 24, and 36 months. If ⊖ for 3 years, further urologic testing is not needed.
- If during this 36-month interval, gross hematuria, abnormal cytology, or irritative voiding symptoms without infection are present, a complete evaluation should be repeated.

Management

- Directed at the underlying cause.
- Persistent, unexplained hematuria is most likely due to a mild glomerulopathy or nephrolithiasis.

Sodium and Water Disorders

Remember the following general principles when evaluating electrolyte abnormalities:

- Sodium levels must be determined by the patient's extracellular fluid (ECF) status. Recall that the serum sodium level tells us nothing about the total body sodium, only the patient's water control. A patient with an ↑ ECF such as with edema (volume expansion) has an ↑ total body sodium, which will in turn raise the ECF.
- Conversely, in situations with low total body sodium, such as in vomiting or volume depletion, the patient has a low total body sodium and exhibits symptoms of low ECF such as poor skin turgor and tachycardia.
- High serum sodium tells us that the patient has too much water loss. It tells us nothing about the total body sodium. In diabetes insipidus, for instance, the patient has free water loss and serum sodium will be high.
- Low serum sodium indicates that the patient has poor water excretion and has ↑ water intake (eg, SIADH).

HYPONATREMIA

Defined as a plasma sodium (Na^+) level <135 mEq/L. Recalling back to general principles, hyponatremia tells us that there is excess H_2O relative to sodium. Figure 9.9 outlines an algorithm for the differential diagnosis of hyponatremia.

Symptoms/Exam

- Symptoms and signs relate to the rate and severity of the decline in Na^+.
- Clinical presentation ranges from asymptomatic to nausea, vomiting, confusion, lethargy, seizures, or coma.

Diagnosis

- Obtain a thorough history to determine symptoms and identify potential causes of hyponatremia (see Figure 9.9).
- **Determine tonicity:** Plasma osmolality (P_{osm}) = $(2 \times Na^+)$ + (BUN / 2.8) + (glucose / 18). Normal tonicity of plasma is 280 to 300.
- There are three types of hyponatremia based on tonicity: hypotonic, hypertonic, and isotonic.

KEY FACT

Thiazide diuretics cause hyponatremia due to their effect on the distal collecting duct. Thiazides will not cause a proportional loss of both sodium and water when compared with loop diuretics, they cause more sodium loss and therefore can potentiate hyponatremia.

KEY FACT

An osmol gap of >10 can mean the presence of osmotically active substances such as alcohols (ethylene glycol, methanol), sugars (mannitol, sorbitol), ↑ lipids or proteins (MM, Waldenstrom macroglobulinemia).

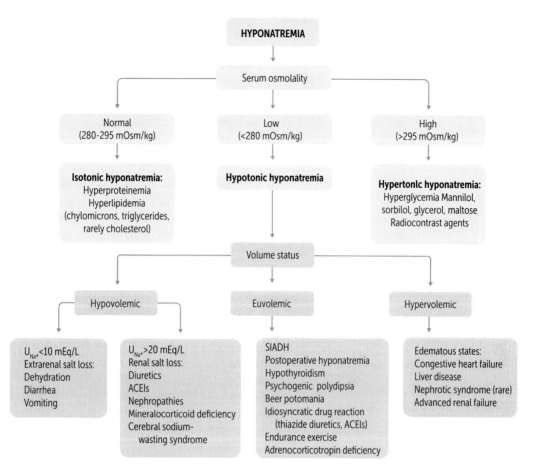

FIGURE 9.9. **Evaluation and differential diagnosis of hyponatremia.** (Reproduced with permission from USMLE-Rx.com.)

- Hypertonicity—seen in patients with hyperglycemia, recall that glucose is an effective osmol, therefore, it will cause a shift of water from intracellular to extracellular space, thereby diluting sodium concentration. IV mannitol infusion works through the same principle.
- Hypotonicity—most common type of hyponatremia. Seen in patients with renal failure. Caused by the inability to excrete water while still continuously taking in water. The ↑ water will dilute sodium concentrations and effective tonicity.
- Normotonicity—seen in patients with ↑ lipids or proteins. Note that the low sodium is an artifact.
- For hypotonic hyponatremia (P_{osm} <280), first determine volume status:
  - Perform a clinical exam to look for volume overload (elevated JVP, S3 gallop, ascites, edema), euvolemia, or volume depletion (dry mucous membranes, flat JVP).
  - A urine Na^+ <10 or a Fe_{Na} <1% (reliable only when the patient is oliguric and not taking diuretics) is found in hypovolemic hypotonic hyponatremia 2° to extrarenal fluid losses, such as from the GI tract, skin, or hemorrhage.
  - A urine Na^+ >20 suggests renal fluid loss as a cause of hypovolemic hypotonic hyponatremia, such as with diuretics, sodium wasting, and adrenal insufficiency.
  - Causes of euvolemic hypotonic hyponatremia (P_{osm} 280-300): hypothyroidism, adrenal insufficiency, SIADH (see next section), polydipsia, beer potomania, reset osmostat, thiazide diuretics.
  - Hypervolemic hypotonic hyponatremia is seen in CHF, nephrotic syndrome, cirrhosis, renal failure.

KEY FACT

Hypothyroidism and adrenal insufficiency both cause hyponatremia by mechanisms that are not completely understood.

 QUESTION

A 63-year-old woman with a history of hypertension has had fatigue of insidious onset, nausea, and vomiting for 1 week. Her medications include aspirin 81 mg, hydrochlorothiazide 25 mg, and a multivitamin. On exam, the patient is tired but in no acute distress. Her BP is 111/72 mm Hg supine, 90/62 mm Hg standing. Her mucous membranes are dry, and she has ↓ skin turgor. Lab tests reveal Na^+ 122 mEq/L, BUN 42 mg/dL, Cr 1.5 mg/dL, serum osmolality 265, and Fe_{Urea} <35%. What is the primary cause of the patient's hyponatremia?

- Normotonic hyponatremia (P_{osm} 280-300) is seen in pseudohyponatremia where hyperproteinemia and hyperlipidemia cause lab artifact.
- Hypertonic hyponatremia (P_{osm} >300) is seen in hyperglycemia and mannitol infusion.

Management

- Initiate fluid management per patient's volume status.
    - **Hypervolemia:** Fluid restriction and/or diuretics.
    - **Euvolemia:** Fluid restriction or hypertonic (3%) saline with caution. Demeclocycline if patient is unable to adhere to water restriction.
    - **Hypovolemia:** Isotonic or, rarely, hypertonic saline.
- Correct Na^+ by the patient's symptoms and rapidity of onset of the abnormality.
- **Acute symptomatic hyponatremia:**
    - ↑ Na^+ approximately 2 mEq/L/hr until symptoms resolve (for the first 2-3 hours), and then more slowly.
    - Consider careful use of hypertonic saline with a loop diuretic if volume overloaded.
- Acute asymptomatic hyponatremia:
    - Fluid restriction if Na^+ is >115 mEq/L.
    - If Na^+ is <114 mEq/L or >115 mEq/L (ie symptomatic), a bolus of 3% saline with a goal of an ↑ in Na^+ of 1.5 to 2 mEq/L/hr for 3 to 4 hours.
- **Chronic *symptomatic* hyponatremia:**
    - ↑ Na^+ more slowly (approximately 1 mEq/L/1-2 hr).
    - Again, consider careful use of hypertonic saline.
- **Chronic *asymptomatic* hyponatremia:**
    - Immediate correction is unnecessary.
    - Manage fluid per volume status as above.
    - Treat the underlying cause for long-term correction.

MNEMONIC

Causes of SIADH:

Surgery
Intracranial (infection, head injury, CVA)
Alveolar (malignancy, infection)
Drugs (opiates, antiepileptics, cytotoxics, antipsychotics)
Hormonal (hypothyroid, low corticosteroid level)

KEY FACT

Small cell lung cancer is the malignancy most commonly associated with SIADH.

ANSWER

Hyponatremia is a side effect of hydrochlorothiazide use and can come on insidiously. Periodic monitoring of electrolytes is recommended for patients taking thiazide diuretics. This patient's hyponatremia is worsened by both her acute renal failure and hypovolemia, which is evident from her orthostasis, dry mucous membranes, and poor skin turgor as well as her BUN:Cr ratio, which is >20.

SYNDROME OF INAPPROPRIATE SECRETION OF ADH

SIADH occurs when antidiuretic hormone (ADH) is secreted independent of the body's need to conserve water, leading to inappropriate water retention in the presence of Na^+ loss. May result from a variety of disorders.

- **CNS disorders:**
    - **Head trauma:** SAH, subdural hematoma.
    - **Infection:** Meningitis, encephalitis, brain abscess.
    - **Other:** Neoplasm, CVA, MS.
- **Pulmonary disorders:** Small cell lung cancer, pneumonia, lung abscess, TB, pneumothorax.
- **Medications:** SSRIs, TCAs, carbamazepine, haloperidol, chlorpromazine, chlorpropamide, theophylline, amiodarone.
- **Other:** Malignant neoplasia.

Diagnosis

- Euvolemic hyponatremia.
- P_{osm} <280 mOsm/kg.
- Urine osmolality >100 mOsm/kg; urine Na^+ >20 mEq/L.
- Low uric acid and BUN due to serum dilution and ↑ renal losses.
- SIADH is a diagnosis of exclusion.

Management

- As with other causes of hyponatermia, treatment of SIADH depends on the severity of the hyponatremia and the presence of symptoms.

- Asymptomatic patients can be treated with water restriction of 1 L/day.
- In patients with severe symptoms such as seizures or mental status changes, treat aggressively, but cautiously with hypertonic saline and loop diuretics.
- Correction of hyponatremia should not exceed a rate of 0.5 mEq/L/hr. Too rapid a rate of correction risks inducing central pontine myelinolysis.
- Demeclocycline for chronic SIADH.

HYPERNATREMIA

Defined as a plasma Na^+ level >145 mEq/L. Grouped into four broad categories by underlying mechanism:
- **Inadequate intake and ↑ water loss** (U_{osm} >600 mOsm/kg):
  - Most common cause.
  - ↑ insensible or GI losses (↑ sweating, burns, diarrhea).
  - Barriers to accessible fluids or inadequate replacement. Seen in elderly or institutionalized patients who lack access to free water.
- **↑ renal loss (polyuria):**
  - **Diabetes insipidus** (U_{osm} <600 mOsm/kg): A defect in the secretion or action of ADH. Can be central (due to ADH deficiency) or nephrogenic (due to the kidneys being unresponsive to ADH). Presents with hypernatremia with copious dilute urine (see the Endocrinology chapter).
  - **Postobstructive or post-ATN diuresis.**
  - Osmotic diuresis in diabetes.
  - Diuretic use.
- **1° hypodipsia:** Destruction of the hypothalamic thirst center due to neoplasm, vascular disease, granulomatous disease, or trauma.
- Iatrogenic causes: Due to accidental or intentional ingestion/infusion of hypertonic solution.

Symptoms/Exam

- Volume depletion: Dry mucous membranes, hypotension, and low urine output.
- CNS symptoms: Lethargy, weakness, irritability, confusion, seizures, and coma.

Diagnosis

- Review the patient's weight, BP, intake and output, and types of IV fluid.
- Think about the etiology of the hypernatremia: is the patient experiencing extra-renal loss, renal loss or was the cause iatrogenic.
- Check urine osmolality:
  - Low urine osmality (<250 mOsm/kg) with polyuria suggests diabetes insipidus.
  - High urine osmolality (>500 mOsm/kg) with low urine output suggests extra-renal loss.
  - High urine osmolality (>500 mOsm/kg) with high urine output suggests osmotic diuresis, post-ATN, postobstructive, or diuretic use.

Management

- As with hyponatremia, treatment depends on the presence of symptoms and the rapidity of onset of the abnormality.
- Acute hypernatremia that lasts <24 hours should be corrected within 24 hours.
- If the hypernatremia is chronic or of unknown duration, the correction should occur over 48 hours because too rapid a correction of hypernatremia can cause cerebral edema. Correct the serum sodium at a rate of 0.5 mEq/L/hr. Do not ↓ Na^+ >12 mEq/L per 24-hour period.
- Correction usually done with D5W or 0.45NS depending on the etiology and if the patient has ECF volume depletion.

KEY FACT

Postoperative patients generally have an ↑ amount of ADH secretion. this is important when calculating fluid dosing postoperatively.

KEY FACT

Hypernatremia in an elderly patient can be fatal as water shifts out of cells to compensate for the water loss causing cellular shrinking. This can drastically ↑ the risk of intracranial bleeding.

KEY FACT

Hypernatremia is usually due to free-water deficits.

QUESTION 1

A 58-year-old man reports feeling tired and weak for the last several weeks. He has a 60-pack-year smoking history and has had increasing shortness of breath and hemoptysis for the last month. On exam, vitals are significant for an O_2 saturation of 92% on room air. He has ↓ breath sounds on the left base. Lab results: Na^+ 119 mEq/L, K^+ 3.9 mEq/L, Cl 75 mEq/L, CO_2 22 mEq/L, BUN 28 mg/dL, Cr 1.2 mg/dL, osmolality 254 mOsm/L, urine Na^+ 48 mEq/L, urine osmolality 553 mOsm/kg. What is the cause of the patient's symptoms?

QUESTION 2

An 86-year-old female nursing home resident with baseline dementia presents with a seizure 2 days after being diagnosed with pneumonia and started on azithromycin. Her caregiver notes that her intake has ↓ over the last 2 days and she has become more somnolent. She is febrile at 38.9°C (102°F), BP 138/74 mm Hg, and pulse 104 bpm. On exam, she has dry mucous membranes and poor skin turgor; neurologic exam is nonfocal. Cardiac exam is notable for tachycardia. Lab results: Na^+ = 154 mEq/L, K^+ 3.2 mEq/L, Cl 107 mEq/L, CO_2 = 22 mEq/L, BUN 68 mg/dL, Cr 2 mg/dL, urine Na^+ 8 mEq/L, and urine osmolality 680 mOsm/kg. A CT scan of the head shows no acute intracranial process. What is the cause of her hypernatremia?

- Calculate the free-water deficit:

$$\text{Water deficit} = [(\text{plasma Na}^+ - 140) / 140] \times \text{TBW}$$

- Hypovolemic patients with unstable vital signs should be treated initially with isotonic normal saline. Once stabilization has occurred, the free-water deficit can be repleted by 5% dextrose in water or half isotonic normal saline.
- Correct 50% of the calculated free-water deficit in the first 12 to 24 hours, with the remainder corrected in the next 24 to 48 hours.
  - D5W @1.35 mL/hr × wt (kg) will ↓ [Na] by ~0.5 mEq/L/h in a 70-kg person.

Potassium Disorders

HYPERKALEMIA

Serum potassium >5.5 mEq/L. Causes of hyperkalemia include the following:
- **High K⁺ intake:** From supplements or diet (rarely occurs without baseline renal dysfunction).
- **Extracellular K⁺ shift** (↓ cellular entry or ↑ release):
  - Metabolic acidosis.
  - Insulin deficiency and hyperglycemia such as in diabetic ketoacidosis.
  - Tissue damage from rhabdomyolysis, trauma, or burns, or release during tumor lysis syndrome.
  - β-adrenergic blockade.
- **Impaired renal excretion:**
  - Renal failure.
  - ↓ renal perfusion, as seen with severe CHF or volume depletion.
  - Type IV renal tubular acidosis.
  - Hypoaldosteronism.
  - Adrenal insufficiency.
- **Medications:** ACE inhibitors, ARBs, NSAIDs, spironolactone, succinylcholine, β-blockers.

Symptoms/Exam

May be asymptomatic or may present with symptoms ranging from muscle weakness to ventricular fibrillation (VF).

Diagnosis

- Review the history, medications, and exam, focusing on chest pain, palpitations, muscle weakness, flaccid paralysis, and ileus.
- Obtain basic labs, including electrolytes, BUN, and creatinine.
- Consider additional labs as indicated by the history: CK for rhabdomyolysis; LDH, uric acid, phosphorus, and calcium for tumor lysis syndrome; U_{osm} and U_{K^+} to calculate the transtubular K⁺ gradient in hypoaldosteronism.
- ECG findings may be used as an indicator of severity. Figure 9.10 shows characteristically progressive changes that occur with increasing serum potassium levels.
  - **Mild:** Normal or peaked T waves.
  - **Moderate:** QRS prolongation or flattened P waves.
  - **Severe:** VF or asystole.

Management

- Check to see if the patient is receiving any potassium supplementation, if so, remove immediately.
- Obtain a stat ECG to evaluate for any changes.

- Look for any causes that might falsely elevate potassium such as hemolysis, elevated platelets, rhabdomyolysis.
- Repeat the blood draw to confirm elevated potassium.
- If potassium levels are still elevated, treat the underlying cause with the following:
  - IV calcium gluconate to stabilize the myocardium temporarily.
  - Insulin and glucose or β2-adrenergic agonists (such as albuterol) improve potassium entry into cells.
- Potassium exchange resins, such as sodium polystyrene sulfonate (Kayexalate), potassium-wasting diuretics such as furosemide, and dialysis are the only ways to permanently remove the potassium from the body.
- Hemodialysis is used for patients in renal failure when above treatments have failed.

HYPOKALEMIA

Defined as potassium (K^+) level <3.5 mEq/L. Causes include the following:
- Low K^+ intake.
- ↑ GI loss: diarrhea, vomiting.
- Intracellular K^+ shift, such as in metabolic alkalosis or use of β-agonists.
- Spurious hypokalemia can occur in cases of leukocytosis. In this case, large amounts of WBCs uptake K^+ in the blood tube, causing a falsely depressed K^+ level.
- Alkalosis can cause hypokalemia as it causes an intracellular K^+ shift.
- ↑ renal excretion, as with loop and thiazide diuretics, excess mineralocorticoids (hyperaldosteronism, Cushing, European black licorice ingestion), congenital (Bartter, Gitelman, Liddle, 17-α-hydroxylase deficiency), hyperglycemia (osmotic diuresis), hypomagnesemia, and renal tubular acidosis.

Symptoms/Exam

- Symptoms generally occur when serum K^+ is <2.5 to 3.0 mEq/L.
- Muscle weakness, fatigue, cramps, constipation, ileus. Severe symptoms include flaccid paralysis, hyporeflexia, tetany, rhabdomyolysis, and cardiac arrhythmias.

Diagnosis

- Twenty-four-hour urine collection for K^+:
  - **Extrarenal causes (GI losses, low intake, intracellular shifts):** <25 mEq/day.
  - **Renal causes:** >25 mEq/day.
- Spot urine for K^+ (more easily obtained, but less accurate):
  - **Extrarenal causes (GI losses, low intake, intracellular shifts):** <20 mEq/day.
  - **Renal excretion:** >40 mEq/day.
- ECG may show U waves, T-wave flattening, arrhythmias (PSVT, PVC, PAC, ventricular fibrillation, atrial fibrillation), ST depressions.
- See the Endocrinology chapter for evaluation of adrenal abnormalities.

Management

- Replete K^+, usually as KCl.
- Oral route preferred, taken with food to avoid abdominal pain and esophagitits associated with KCl.
- If repleting through a peripheral IV, rate should not exceed 10 mEq/L/hr. With a central line, rate can be up to 20 mEq/L/hr. IV site may burn.
- K^+-sparing diuretics in patients with chronic urinary K^+ loss.

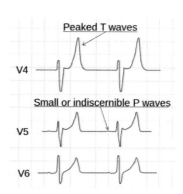

FIGURE 9.10. Electrocardiographic effects of hyperkalemia. (Reproduced from Wikimedia Commons; courtesy of Mikael Häggström.)

KEY FACT

Patients with hypokalemia are often also hypomagnesemic (commonly seen in alcoholics). The hypokalemia cannot be corrected unless the magnesium level is corrected. Treat both at the same time.

KEY FACT

Hypokalemia ↑ the risk of digoxin toxicity.

QUESTION 1

A 54-year-old man with a history of atrial fibrillation, currently on medications he cannot recall, presents to the ED with nausea, vomiting, and vision changes. He reports seeing "yellowish halos around objects." You order a CBC, CMP, and ECG. Based on the patient's presentation, what electrolyte abnormality is most likely to be seen?

QUESTION 2

A 60-year-old woman with a history of chronic renal failure on dialysis, hypertension, and diabetes presents with malaise, nausea, and ↓ appetite after missing her last dialysis appointment. Exam reveals rales halfway up both lung fields, jugular venous distention elevated at 15 cm, and an S3 gallop. She has 2+ edema of the knees bilaterally. Lab results show Na^+ 143 mEq/L, K^+ 7.6 mEq/L, Cl 107 mEq/L, CO_2 16 mEq/L, BUN 62 mg/dL, Cr 7.4 mg/dL. How would you treat this patient?

Acid-Base Disorders

Acid-base disorders are changes in serum pH that result from a change in either arterial P_{CO_2} or serum HCO_3^- (Figure 9.11). There are four types (see sections below): metabolic acidosis, metabolic alkalosis, respiratory acidosis, and respiratory alkalosis.

In a healthy person:
- pH = 7.40
- P_{CO_2} = 40 mm Hg
- P_{O_2} = 100 mm Hg
- HCO_3^- = 24 mEq/L

In a metabolic acid-base disorder, the primary change is in HCO_3^-. In a respiratory acid-base disorder, the primary change is in P_{CO_2}. In all acid-base disorders, the body compensates to return serum pH to 7.40. Remember that it will be close to 7.40 but never completely compensated in the disease state. In metabolic disorders, the compensation is respiratory. In respiratory disorders, the compensation is metabolic (Table 9.10). A good practice for identifying acid-base problems is to determine the following:
- Whether serum pH is acidemic or alkalemic.
- Presence of compensation (formulas will be discussed below).
- Anion gap.

METABOLIC ACIDOSIS

Metabolic acidosis is defined by a serum pH <7.35 due to a ↓ in extracellular HCO_3^-. It is caused by either a gain in acid or a loss of HCO_3^-. There are two categories of metabolic acidosis: anion gap (AG) metabolic acidosis and non-AG (hyperchloremic) metabolic acidosis.

ANSWER 1

The patient's history of atrial fibrillation, probably treated with digoxin, and vision disturbance point digoxin toxicity. Expect that the ECG will show peaked T-waves (Figure 9.10), as digoxin disrupts Na^+ K^+ ATPase and ↑ serum K^+ levels.

ANSWER 2

Hyperkalemia in the setting of chronic kidney disease means that the kidneys are unable to excrete potassium and that the patient requires dialysis to lower potassium to safe levels. Treatment may also include a stat ECG, a β2-adrenergic agonist or insulin, and calcium gluconate to prevent progression to arrhythmia.

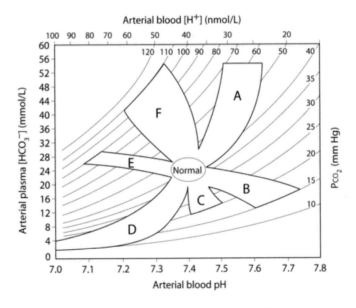

FIGURE 9.11. **Acid-base nomogram.** A = metabolic alkalosis; B = acute respiratory alkalosis; C = chronic respiratory alkalosis; D = metabolic acidosis; E = acute respiratory acidosis; F = chronic respiratory acidosis. (Reproduced with permission from USMLE-Rx.com.)

TABLE 9.10. Changes and Compensatory Mechanisms Seen in Acid-Base Disorders

DISORDER	PH	[H⁺]	[HCO₃⁻]	PCO₂	COMPENSATION
Metabolic acidosis	↓	↑	↓↓	↓	Respiratory alkalosis (ie, hyperventilation)
Metabolic alkalosis	↑	↓	↑↑	↑	Respiratory acidosis (ie, hypoventilation)
Respiratory acidosis	↓	↑	↑	↑↑	Metabolic alkalosis (renal HCO₃⁻ reabsorption)
Respiratory alkalosis	↑	↓	↓	↓↓	Metabolic acidosis (renal HCO₃⁻ excretion)

- **AG metabolic acidosis:** Production of endogenous or addition of exogenous acids.
  - Calculate the AG as follows:

$$AG = (Na^+) - [(Cl^-) + (HCO_3^-)]$$

- Normal AG is 6 to 10.
- Calculate the osmolar gap to assess for toxin ingestion.
- Osmolar gap = measured Osm – calculated Osm.
- Calculated serum osmoles = $(2 \times Na) + (BUN / 2.8) + (glucose / 18) + (ETOH / 4.6)$.
  - Osmolar gap >10 in ethanol, methanol, ethylene glycol ingestion.
  - Osmolar gap <10 in paraldehyde or salicylate ingestion.
- Causes of AG metabolic acidosis include (see Mnemonic MUDPILERS):
  - Lactic acidosis (tissue hypoxia, shock, hypovolemia, dehydration, sepsis).
  - Ketoacidosis (DM, ethanol, starvation).
  - Uremia.
  - Ingestion (paraldehyde, methanol, salicylate, ethylene glycol).
- **Non-AG (hyperchloremic) metabolic acidosis:** Loss of bicarbonate.
  - Calculate the urine AG to distinguish between renal and extrarenal losses of bicarbonate:

$$U_{AG} = U_{Na} + U_K - U_{Cl}$$

  - U_{AG} <0 suggests GI loss of bicarbonate, such as from diarrhea.
  - U_{AG} >0 suggests renal causes such as renal failure, renal tubular acidosis.

Approaching a patient with suspected metabolic acidosis:
- To determine whether a simple metabolic acidosis, whether there is adequate compensation, or whether a mixed problem, use **Winter's formula,** which provides the predicted P_{CO_2} to compare with the measured P_{CO_2}:

$$P_{CO_2} = 1.5 \times HCO_3^- + 8 \pm 2$$

- If measured and predicted P_{CO_2} are similar in value, then proper compensation has occurred.
- If measured P_{CO_2} is > predicted, then there must be concomitant respiratory acidosis.
- If measured P_{CO_2} is < predicted, then there must be respiratory alkalosis.
- After determining the compensation, calculate the AG: $(Na^+) - [(Cl^-) + (HCO_3^-)]$.
- If AG present, then calculate the **delta ratio,** $[AG - 12] / [24 - HCO_3^-]$, to determine whether there is a mixed acid-base disorder. Four delta ratios are usually seen:
  - <0.4: Indicates a hyperchloremic normal AG. Typically seen in patients with excessive diarrhea; a large quantity of HCO₃⁻ is lost, resulting in a lower the delta ratio.

KEY FACT

↑ AG suggests an AG metabolic acidosis, even if plasma HCO₃⁻ is normal.

KEY FACT

Hypoalbuminemia causes a ↓ in the AG. Remember to adjust for hypoalbuminemia. For every 1-g/dL decline in serum albumin, AG ↓ by 2.5 mEq/L.

QUESTION

A 17-year-old girl with a history of type 1 DM is admitted to the ED with persistent vomiting. She reports that she has not been taking her insulin regularly for the last few days. On exam, she is tachycardic and tachypneic; BP is stable. She is in mild respiratory distress, with dry mucous membranes and fruity breath. Lab results: Na 136 mEq/L, K 5.4 mEq/L, Cl 107 mEq/L, CO₂ 14 mEq/L, BUN 28 mg/dL, Cr 1.2 mg/dL, glucose 397 mg/dL; ABG shows pH of 7.1. UA shows 3+ glucose and is ⊕ for ketones. What is the underlying acid-base disorder?

- **>0.4-<1:** Indicates both a normal AG and high AG metabolic acidosis. Can be seen in patients with diarrhea and an underlying infection that progresses to shock, which causes elevated lactic acid.
- **1-2:** Indicates a high AG metabolic acidosis such as in DKA or lactic acidosis.
- **>2:** Indicates a high AG metabolic acidosis and a metabolic alkalosis. A good example is a patient with a preexisting metabolic acidosis who develops vomiting.

Symptoms/Exam

- Depend on the underlying cause:
  - Dehydration and fruity breath in diabetic ketoacidosis.
  - Tachypnea in salicylate intoxication.
  - Ataxia, confusion, seizures, coma in ethylene glycol intoxication.
- Patient can be asymptomatic or have nonspecific signs such as fatigue, anorexia, confusion, tachycardia, tachypnea, dehydration.

Diagnosis

- Calculate AG or urine AG as above.
- Labs: Evaluate via renal function, serum lactate, serum or urine ketones, salicylates.
- Calculate osmolar gap to rule out ingestion of alcohol (ethanol, methanol, ethylene glycol).

Management

- Treat the underlying cause.
- Bicarbonate therapy is controversial and, if used, is generally reserved for severe acidosis (arterial pH <7.10-7.15).

METABOLIC ALKALOSIS

Defined as an ↑ in plasma bicarbonate concentration: serum pH >7.45.

Diagnosis

- ↑ serum bicarbonate in chemistry panel.
- Measure urine chloride (U_{Cl^-}) concentration.
- Determine if there is proper compensation occurring via the following formula: $P_{CO_2} = 0.7[HCO_3^-] + 20 \pm 5$.
  - If predicted and measured P_{CO_2} are similar in value, then proper compensation has occurred.
  - If measured P_{CO_2} > predicted, then there must be respiratory acidosis as well.
  - If measured P_{CO_2} < predicted, then there must be respiratory alkalosis.

Management

- Treat chloride-responsive metabolic alkalosis with NaCl infusion.
- The presence of hypertension suggests 1° hyperaldosteronism, Cushing syndrome, exogenous mineralocorticoids or glucocorticoids, or Liddle syndrome.
- Treat the underlying cause (Table 9.11).

RESPIRATORY ACIDOSIS

Defined as an ↑ in P_{CO_2} (hypercapnia) due to ↓ alveolar ventilation. Serum pH <7.35. **Causes:**
- **Central:** Drugs (opiates, anesthetics, sedatives), stroke, infection.
- **Airway:** Obstruction (obstructive sleep apnea), asthma, COPD, obesity hypoventilation syndrome.

- **Parenchyma:** Pneumonia or bronchitis, pulmonary edema, pulmonary fibrosis, ARDS, pneumothorax, barotrauma.
- **Neuromuscular:** Spinal cord injury, kyphoscoliosis, poliomyelitis, Guillain-Barré syndrome, myasthenia gravis, MS, severe hypokalemia or hypophosphatemia.

Symptoms/Exam

- **CNS symptoms:** Headache, blurred vision, restlessness, anxiety.
- **CO_2 narcosis:** Tremors, asterixis, myoclonus, delirium, somnolence, seizures.

Diagnosis

- Arterial pH <7.40 and P_{CO_2} >40 mm Hg.
- Process can be acute or chronic. Compensation and therefore change in pH depends on chronicity:
  - Acute respiratory acidosis: HCO_3^- ↑ by 1 for every 10 mm Hg P_{CO_2} ↑.
  - Chronic respiratory acidosis: HCO_3^- ↑ by 3.5 for every 10 mm Hg the P_{CO_2} ↑.
- Distinguish intrinsic pulmonary disease from extrapulmonary disease using the alveolar-arterial (A-a) oxygen gradient:
  - A-a $(O_2) = (F_{IO_2}\% / 100) \times (P_{atm} - 47$ mm Hg$) - (P_{aCO_2} / 0.8) - P_{aO_2}$, where:
    - F_{IO_2} room air = 21%.
    - Atmospheric pressure = 760 mm Hg at sea level.
    - Water vapor pressure pH_2O (mm Hg) = 47 mm Hg at 37°C (98.6°F).
    - Respiratory quotient RQ $(V_{CO_2}/V_{O_2}) = 0.8$ (usual).
  - A normal A-a gradient is 10 to 20 mm Hg.
  - An A-a gradient >20 suggests intrinsic pulmonary disease causing impaired gas exchange.

Management

Initiate mechanical ventilation if necessary while correcting the underlying disorder.

RESPIRATORY ALKALOSIS

Defined as ↑ alveolar ventilation leading to a ↓ in P_{CO_2} (hypocapnia).

Symptoms/Exam

- Anxiety, tachypnea.
- **CNS symptoms:** Lightheadedness, altered mental status.
- Acute hypocapnea can cause intracellular shifts, leading to hypocalcemia, in turn leading to paresthesias, circumoral numbness, and carpopedal spasms.

Diagnosis

- Arterial pH >7.40 and P_{CO_2} <40 mm Hg.
- As with respiratory acidosis, respiratory alkalosis can be acute or chronic. Change in pH depends on chronicity:
  - Acute respiratory alkalosis: HCO_3^- ↓ by 2.2 for every 10 mm Hg P_{CO_2} ↓.
  - Chronic respiratory alkalosis: HCO_3^- ↓ by 5 for every 10 mm Hg P_{CO_2} ↓.
- Use the A-a oxygen gradient as above.

Management

Correct the underlying disorder (Table 9.12).

TABLE 9.11. Causes of Metabolic Alkalosis

Chloride Responsive

$(U_{Cl}^- <15$ mEq/L$)$

- Vomiting
- Diuretics (after discontinuation)
- Nasogastric suction
- Stool losses
- Posthypercapnic alkalosis
- Cystic fibrosis

Chloride Unresponsive

$(U_{Cl}^- >1°5$ mEq/L$)$

- Diuretics (current use)
- Hyperaldosteronism
- Cushing syndrome
- Exogenous mineralocorticoids or glucocorticoids
- Renovascular hypertension
- Hypomagnesemia, hypokalemia
- Liddle syndrome
- Bartter syndrome
- Gitelman syndrome

TABLE 9.12. Causes of Respiratory Alkalosis

- Hypoxemia
- Anxiety
- Salicylates
- Pain
- Sepsis
- Hepatic failure
- Congestive heart failure
- Pulmonary embolus
- Pneumonia
- Hyperthyroidism
- CNS lesions (stroke or neoplastic)
- Pregnancy (progesterone)

MIXED ACID-BASE DISORDERS

Defined as two or more independent acid-base disorders existing at the same time. Examples:

- A patient with DKA (metabolic acidosis) who develops pneumonia (respiratory acidosis).
- The "triple ripple": A patient overdoses on salicylates and has profuse vomiting caused by AG metabolic acidosis (salicylates) and metabolic alkalosis (vomiting) with respiratory alkalosis (salicylates directly stimulate the respiratory center).
- Identify the most prominent disorder by determining the greatest change in HCO_3^- or Pco_2.
- Apply the formula as shown above for expected compensation. If compensation is not appropriate, a coexisting disorder is present.

Other Urinary Tract Disorders

RHABDOMYOLYSIS

Defined as a breakdown of skeletal muscle fibers, leading to the release of muscle contents into the bloodstream. Causes include immobilization (eg, in elderly fall victims); crush injury; overexertion; infections; medical conditions such as hypothyroidism; and drugs such as statins, cocaine, and colchicine.

Symptoms

Myalgias, red to brown urine due to myoglobinuria.

Diagnosis

- ↑ in serum CK levels; may be >100,000 IU/L, serum myogoblin will also be elevated but this is nonspecific.
- Urine dipstick ⊕ for blood, but urine sediment with no RBCs (indicates that myoglobin is present and not hemoglobin).

Management

- Goal is to prevent renal failure.
- IV hydration to ensure renal perfusion (up to 12 L of fluid can be sequestered in necrotic muscle) and to flush out obstructing casts.
- Maintain urine output of 300 mL/hr until myoglobinuria is resolved.
- Alkalinize urine to pH >6.5 to ↓ toxicity of myoglobin to tubules.
- Use of mannitol and sodium bicarbonate is controversial.

Complications

- Hyperkalemia from muscle breakdown, causing cardiac arrhythmia or cardiac arrest. For any suspected rhabdomyolysis, do a stat ECG.
- Early hypocalcemia, but with hypercalcemia during the recovery phase.
- Hyperphosphatemia can also be seen.
- Metabolic acidosis.
- AKI from myoglobin precipitation, leading to tubular obstruction.

NEPHROLITHIASIS

Symptoms/Exam

- Presents with colicky flank pain ± radiation to the groin.
- Urinary frequency, urgency, and dysuria.
- Microscopic or gross hematuria.
- Male-to-female ratio is 3:1.

Diagnosis

- **Collect and analyze the stone!** Type of stone may change treatment.
- **Labs:**
  - UA: Hematuria.
  - BUN, Cr: Elevated only with bilateral obstruction.
  - Plasma calcium, phosphorus, and uric acid.
  - PTH for hyperparathyroidism if calcium is high-normal or elevated.
  - For recurrent nephrolithiasis, 24-hour urine collection (to assess volume, pH, Na^+, calcium, oxalate, phosphorus, citrate, uric acid, cysteine, and Cr).
- **Imaging:** CT scan is the gold standard for nephrolithiasis. Plain-film radiography can show radiopaque stones (calcium oxalate and calcium phosphate), but less radiopaque stones (uric acid, cysteine, and magnesium ammonium phosphate [struvite]) may go undetected (Figure 9.12).

Management

- Depends on stone size:
  - For stones <10 mm: Treat with pain control, hydration, α-blockers. The patient should also be instructed to strain their urine for stone evaluation. Analgesics are usually the "next best step."
  - Stones >10 mm and with uncontrolled pain, urosepsis, or acute renal failure require an urgent urology consult for immediate removal. Minimally invasive surgical techniques for stone removal include extracorporeal shock wave lithotripsy, percutaneous nephrostolithotomy, rigid and flexible ureterorenoscopy.
- After a first stone, bloodwork for electrolytes, calcium, phosphorus, uric acid, and parathyroid hormone is indicated.
- All patients should ↑ urine volume through daily ingestion of 2.5 to 3.0 L of fluid.
- Additional treatment depends on the type of stone:
  - **Calcium:** ↓ protein intake. Treat with thiazides in hypercalciuria and potassium citrate if normocalciuria. Calcium restriction has not been shown to reduce recurrences. May form more calcium oxalate stones and worsen osteoporosis (Figure 9.13).
  - **Uric acid:** Moderate protein intake. Consider potassium citrate. 2° to gout or ↑ cell turnover, as in leukemia or myeloproliferative disease. Stones are radiolucent. Urine alkalinization with potassium citrate or potassium bicarbonate. Allopurinol for patients with ↑ urinary uric acid levels.
  - **Cysteine:** Diagnostic of cysteinuria (a rare heritable disorder of cysteine transport in the proximal tubule). Urine alkalinization with potassium citrate or potassium bicarbonate.
  - **Magnesium ammonium phosphate (struvite):** Caused by UTI with urea-producing bacteria such as *Proteus* or *Klebsiella*. Can develop into a staghorn calculus involving the entire renal pelvis and calyces. Initiation of appropriate antimicrobial therapy can slow progress, but surgical intervention is generally required.

KEY FACT

Most kidney stones are calcium oxalate. The ureterovesical junction is the most common site of renal stone impaction.

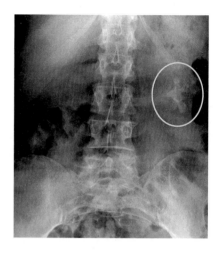

FIGURE 9.12. **Urinary calculi.** Prone abdominal radiograph showing left staghorn (oval) or struvite ($Mg-NH_4-PO_4$) stone filling the collecting system of the right kidney. (Reproduced with permission from USMLE-Rx.com.)

KEY FACT

Thiazide diuretics ↑ uric acid levels and should be avoided in patients with a history of uric acid stones and gout.

QUESTION

A 47-year-old man presents to the ED with acute onset of dysuria and severe left flank pain radiating to the groin. He is in discomfort, unable to find a comfortable position. On exam, you find exquisite left costovertebral angle tenderness with no peritoneal signs. UA shows 3+ blood with no nitrites and leukocyte esterase. A chemistry panel shows normal renal function. What imaging would you use for diagnosis?

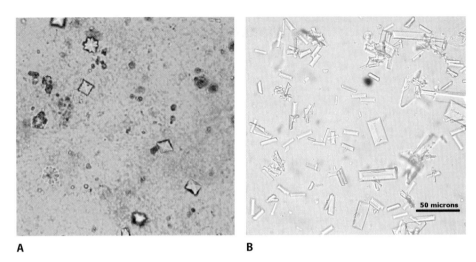

A   **B**

FIGURE 9.13.   **Kidney stones.** (**A**) Calcium oxalate "envelope-shaped" crystals on urine microscopy. (**B**) Struvite (magnesium ammonium phosphate) crystals. (Reproduced from Wikipedia; image A courtesy of NASA/JSC; image B courtesy of Joel Mills.)

POLYCYSTIC KIDNEY DISEASE

A hereditary disorder, most commonly of autosomal-dominant inheritance, involving renal cyst formation, with possible progression to renal failure. Hemorrhage into cysts may also occur, causing hematuria.

Symptoms

- Flank and abdominal pain, hematuria, hypertension.
- With advanced disease, kidneys can be enlarged and palpable.

Diagnosis

Imaging by CT (Figure 9.14) or ultrasound.

KEY FACT

Poor prognostic factors for decline in kidney function include hypertesion, male gender, early age of diagnosis, and early development of renal dysfunction.

ANSWER

A noncontrast helical CT scan. This presentation is consistent with nephrolithiasis, and noncontrast helical CT scan is the gold standard for detection of renal stones.

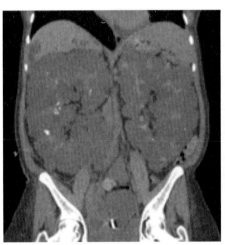
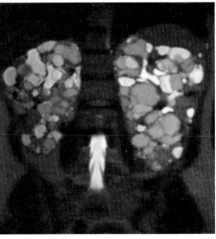

A   **B**

FIGURE 9.14.   **Polycystic kidney disease.** (**A**) Coronal noncontrast CT shows innumerable cysts within enlarged bilateral kidneys. (**B**) T2-weighted coronal MRI shows multiple cysts within bilateral kidneys. (Reproduced with permission from USMLE-Rx.com.)

Management

- BP control with a target of 130/80 mm Hg.
- Aspiration of cysts may help with pain from hemorrhage or compression. Remember that the most common extrarenal manifestation of ADPKD are hepatic cysts.
- Nephrectomy if severe pain from kidney enlargement or recurrent UTIs.
- Dialysis or kidney transplantation. If the patient elects to do a peritoneal dialysis, a colonscopy must be done to rule of diverticular disease as patients with ADPKD are more likely to get diverticulosis and this can cause complications in peritoneal dialysis.
- Screening family members is also important. Ultrasound is the screening tool of choice. The presence of three to five renal cysts is diagnostic of ADPKD.

NOTES

Dermatology

Jolie LeBlanc, MD

KEY FACT

Viral exanthams are often difficult to differentiate. The clinical history is key for diagnosis.

KEY FACT

Roseola's maculopapular rash appears only after 3-5 days of high fever, thus it is mainly diagnosed in retrospect.

Diagnosis of Dermatologic Disease

TERMINOLOGY

Skin lesions may be characterized as primary (ie, associated directly with a disease process; see Table 10.1) or as secondary (changes resulting from a variety of factors; see Table 10.2). They may also be distinguished by their configuration (see Table 10.3) and distribution (eg, localized or generalized).

DIAGNOSTIC TECHNIQUES

Key diagnostic techniques include the following:
- **Potassium hydroxide (KOH) prep:** Used to diagnose fungal infection. With a blade, scrape scale onto a glass slide, and add KOH (must be heated if not preserved with DMSO). KOH dissolves keratin but not hyphae walls. Look for branching structures (Figure 10.1).
- **Tzanck smear:** Used to test for HSV or VZV. Rupture the vesicle, scrape the base of the lesion, place fluid on a glass slide, and stain with Giemsa or Wright stain. Presence of multinucleated giant cells identifies HSV infection (Figure 10.2).
- **Wood's lamp:** Emits UV light ("black light"). Presence of fluorescence on skin is used to diagnose tinea capitis, pityriasis versicolor, erythrasma, vitiligo, melasma, and porphyria.

TABLE 10.1.   **Descriptions of Primary Dermatologic Lesions**

LESION	DESCRIPTION	EXAMPLES
Macule	Circumscribed, nonpalpable area of discoloration <1 cm	Flat nevi, café au lait
Papule	Circumscribed, elevated, solid area <1 cm. Top may be pointed, rounded, or flat	Acne, warts
Patch	Circumscribed, nonpalpable area of discoloration >1 cm	Sacral melanocytosis aka "Mongolian spot," vitiligo
Plaque	Circumscribed, elevated, solid area >1 cm, usually flat topped	Psoriasis
Vesicle	Circumscribed, elevated lesion <1 cm containing clear fluid	Blisters of herpes zoster, herpes simplex
Bulla	Circumscribed, elevated lesion >1 cm containing clear fluid	Bullous pemphigoid, second-degree burns
Pustule	Circumscribed, elevated lesion <1 cm containing purulent material	Acne, folliculitis
Nodule	Palpable, solid area >1 cm, deep-seated mass with indistinct borders that elevates the overlying epidermis, usually found in the dermal or subcutaneous tissue	Lipomas, tumors
Wheal	Transient circumscribed elevated area (papules or plaques) of erythema, resulting from tense edema of the papillary dermis	Urticaria

TABLE 10.2. Descriptions of Secondary Dermatological Lesions

2° CHANGE	DESCRIPTION	EXAMPLES
Scale	Dry, thin plates of keratinized epidermal cells (stratum corneum)	Psoriasis, ichthyosis
Lichenification	Thickening of skin, with exaggerated skin lines resulting from chronic rubbing or scratching	Atopic dermatitis, lichen planus
Erosion and oozing	Moist, circumscribed, depressed area due to loss of superficial layers of upper dermis, leaving denuded surface	Burns, bullous erythema multiforme
Crust	Dried exudate of plasma on the surface of the skin following trauma	Impetigo, contact dermatitis
Fissure	Sharply defined tear (linear or wedge-shaped) in the epidermis	Angular cheilitis
Scar	Flat, raised, or depressed area of fibrotic tissue as ulceration heals	Acne scars, burn scars
Atrophy	Thinning of one or more layers of skin, may have loss of skin markings or cause skin depression	Striae or "stretch marks"
Color	Red, pink, yellow, brown, tan, or blue; pay particular attention to blanching since failure to blanch suggests bleeding into the dermis (petechiae)	

Common Skin Disorders

COMMON PEDIATRIC SKIN DISORDERS

Table 10.4 outlines the presentation, diagnosis, and treatment of common viral and bacterial causes of rash in infants and children (Figure 10.3).

TABLE 10.3. Descriptions of Dermatologic Lesions by Configuration

CONFIGURATION	EXAMPLES
Annular (circular)	Granuloma annulare, urticaria, dermatophyte infections
Linear (straight lines)	Lichen striatus, incontinentia pigmenti, scabies
Grouped	Herpes simplex, herpes zoster
Discrete	Insect bites
Reticular (net-like)	Erythema infectiosum, telangiectasias of rosacea

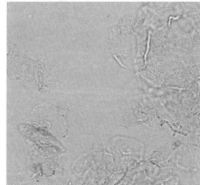

FIGURE 10.1. KOH preparation. Skin scrapings and preparation with potassium hydroxide demonstrates multiple septate hyphae of tinea capitis. (Reproduced with permission from USMLE-Rx.com.)

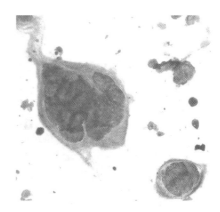

FIGURE 10.2. Tzanck smear. Multinucleated giant cells characteristic of HSV infection. (Reproduced with permission from Wolff K, Johnson RA. *Fitzpatrick's Color Atlas & Synopsis of Clinical Dermatology*, 6th ed. New York: McGraw-Hill, 2009, Fig. 27-7.)

TABLE 10.4.   Common Causes of Rash in the Pediatric Population

DISEASE	USUAL AGE	PRODROME	MORPHOLOGY/DISTRIBUTION
Measles (rubeola virus) *Figure 10.3A*	5-9 years	High fever, URI symptoms, conjunctivitis	Erythematous macules and papules become confluent (Figure 10-3Ai) Begins on the face and moves centrifugally
Rubella (rubella virus) *Figure 10.3B*	Teens and young adults	Absent or low-grade fever, malaise, upper respiratory symptoms	Rose-pink maculopapular; not confluent Begins on the face and moves downward rapidly
Erythema infectiosum or "fifth disease" (parvovirus B19) *Figure 10.3C*	3-12 years	Low-grade fever, malaise, sore throat, headache, nausea	Slapped cheeks followed by reticular erythema or maculopapular rash on extremities
Enteroviral exanthems (coxsackievirus, echovirus, other enteroviruses) *Figure 10.3D*	Young children	Fever (occasionally)	Extremely variable; may be maculopapular, petechial, purpuric, or vesicular Usually generalized, but may be acral
Hand-foot-mouth syndrome (coxsackievirus) *Figure 10.3E*	Young children	Fever (occasionally), sore mouth	Gray-white vesicles 3-7 mm in size on normal or erythematous base Hands and feet are most commonly affected, but may affect the diaper area and is occasionally generalized
Adenovirus exanthems (adenoviruses)	Young children	Fever; URI symptoms	Rubelliform, morbilliform, roseola-like rash Generalized
Chickenpox (VZV) *Figure 10.3F*	1-14 years	Fever, headache, and malaise 48 hours before exanthem	Macules and papules rapidly become vesicles on an erythematous base, followed by crusts Often begins on the scalp or face; more profuse on the trunk than on extremities
Roseola (HHV-6 linked)	<3 years	High fever for 3-5 days before exanthem	Maculopapular rash in rosettes appears **after** fever declines Affects trunk and neck but may be generalized. Lasts hours to days
Kawasaki disease *Figure 10.3G*	<5 years	High fever, irritability	Polymorphous—papular, vesicobullous, or morbilliform; erythema with desquamation Generalized, often with perineal accentuation and desquamation
Scarlet fever (group A streptococcus) *Figure 10.3H*	School age	Acute onset, with fever, sore throat	Diffuse erythema with sandpaper texture Facial flushing with circumoral pallor; linear erythema in skin folds
Staphylococcal scalded skin syndrome (*S aureus* epidermolytic toxin) *Figure 10.3I*	<5 years	None	Abrupt onset, with tender erythroderma Eruption with intensification in the neck, face, axillae, and groin
Henoch-Schönlein purpura *Figure 10.3J*	4-7 years	Possibly abdominal pain	Palpable purpuric or petechial rash Begins on the malleoli and extends to the buttocks

ASSOCIATED FINDINGS	DIAGNOSIS	SPECIAL MANAGEMENT
Koplik spots (Figure 10.3Aii), "toxic" appearance, photophobia, cough, adenopathy, high fever	Usually clinical; serologies	Report to public health; give immunoglobulin within 6 days of exposure
Postauricular and occipital adenopathy; headache, malaise, mild pruritus	Rubella IgM	Report to public health; check for exposure to pregnant women
Waxes/wanes for several weeks; occasionally presents with arthritis, headache, and malaise	Usually clinical; acute/ convalescent serologic test	May cause aplastic crisis
Low-grade fever, occasional myocarditis, aseptic meningitis, pleurodynia	Usually clinical; viral throat culture; rectal swabs in selected cases	In the presence of petechiae or purpura, meningococcemia must be considered
Oral ulcers, occasional fever, adenopathy	Same as for enteroviral exanthems	
Fever, URI symptoms, occasionally pneumonia	Viral isolation or acute/ convalescent seroconversion; rapid tests sometimes available	
Pruritus, fever, oral and genital lesions, occasional malaise	Usually clinical; serology, Tzanck smear, or direct immunofluorescence	Antihistamines for itching; **aspirin is contraindicated** (Reye syndrome); for severe symptoms, consider antiviral medication
Cervical and postauricular adenopathy	Clinical, mainly diagnosed in retrospect	
Conjunctivitis, cheilitis, glossitis, strawberry tongue (Figure 10.3Gi), peripheral edema (Figure 10.3Gii), adenopathy	Clinical; inflammatory markers can aid if atypical case	Admit to the hospital for IVIG and salicylates; echocardiography to look for coronary aneurysm
Exudative pharyngitis, palatal petechiae, abdominal pain	Throat cultures	IM penicillin or oral amoxicillin
Fever, conjunctivitis, rhinitis	Clinical; culture of *S aureus* from systemic site (not skin)	Neonate; if blistering is present, hospitalize for IV antibiotics and fluid/electrolyte therapy
Arthralgia, nausea, vomiting, diarrhea, GI bleeding	Clinical	Consider Rocky Mountain spotted fever or meningococcemia; steroids for severe cases

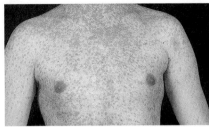

i

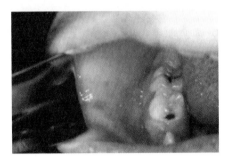

ii

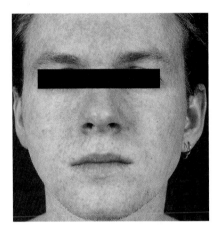

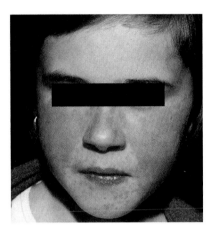

FIGURE 10.3A. Measles. Red blotchy rash seen in measles throughout the patient's trunk (i). (Reproduced with permission from Fauci AS, et al. *Harrison's Principles of Internal Medicine,* 17th ed. New York: McGraw-Hill, 2008, Fig. 185-3). Koplik spots (ii). Irregularly-shaped, bright red spots often with a bluish-white central dot within the buccal mucosa and tongue. (Source: CDC.)

FIGURE 10.3B. Rubella. Rash begins on face and spreads centrifugally. (Reproduced with permission from Wolff K, Johnson RA. *Fitzpatrick's Color Atlas & Synopsis of Clinical Dermatology,* 6th ed. New York: McGraw-Hill, 2009, Fig. 27-21.)

FIGURE 10.3C. Erythema infectiosum. (Reproduced with permission from Wolff K, Johnson RA. *Fitzpatrick's Color Atlas & Synopsis of Clinical Dermatology,* 6th ed. New York: McGraw-Hill, 2009, Fig. 27-24A.)

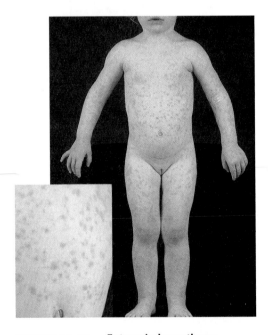

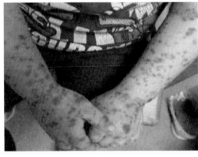

i

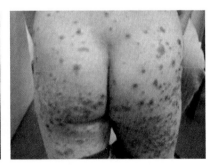

ii

FIGURE 10.3D. Enteroviral exanthems. (Reproduced with permission from Wolff K, Johnson RA. *Fitzpatrick's Color Atlas & Synopsis of Clinical Dermatology,* 6th ed. New York: McGraw-Hill, 2009, Fig. 27-19.)

FIGURE 10.3E. Hand-foot-mouth syndrome. Extensive involvement of the hands (i), legs and buttocks (ii) of a young boy infected with Coxsackievirus. (Reproduced from Biao D, et al. Circulation of Coxsackievirus A6 in hand-foot-mouth disease in Guangzhou, 2010-2012. *Virol J.* 2014;11:157.)

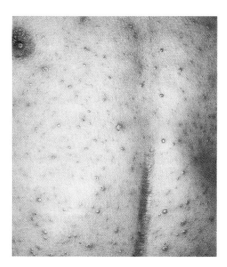

FIGURE 10.3F.   Chickenpox. (Reproduced with permission from Fauci AS, et al. *Harrison's Principles of Internal Medicine*, 17th ed. New York: McGraw-Hill, 2008, Fig. 173-1.)

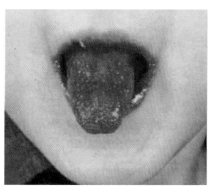
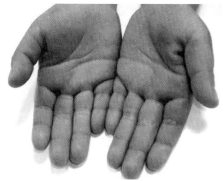

i   ii

FIGURE 10.3G.   Kawasaki disease. Strawberry tongue with bright red, swollen lips (i). Erythema of the palms accompanied by painful, brawny edema of the dorsum of the hands (ii). (Reproduced from Wikimedia Commons; courtesy of Dong Soo Kim.)

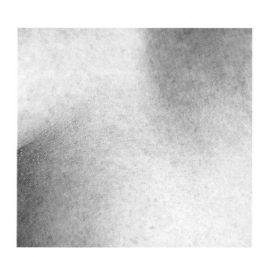

FIGURE 10.3H.   Scarlet fever. (Reproduced with permission from Fauci AS, et al. *Harrison's Principles of Internal Medicine*, 17th ed. New York: McGraw-Hill, 2008, Fig. 130-2.)

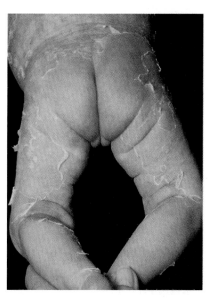

FIGURE 10.3I.   Staphylococcal scalded skin syndrome. (Reproduced with permission from Wolff K, et al. *Fitzpatrick's Dermatology in General Medicine,* 7th ed. New York: McGraw-Hill, 2008, Fig. 178-5.)

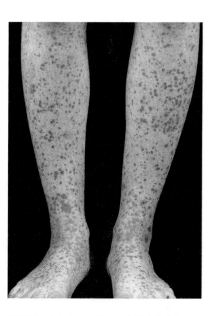

FIGURE 10.3J.   Henoch-Schönlein purpura. (Reproduced with permission from Wolff K, Johnson RA. *Fitzpatrick's Color Atlas & Synopsis of Clinical Dermatology,* 6th ed. New York: McGraw-Hill, 2009, Fig. 14-35.)

Q   **QUESTION**

A 6-year-old boy presents with purple macular rash on his bilateral lower extremities. Per his parents, 2 days ago he had a fever and stomach pain, but now is feeling better except for a mild limp. What is your next step?

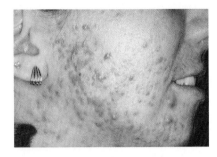

FIGURE 10.4. Severe inflammatory acne with pustules and comedones.

(Courtesy of Kalman Watsky, MD, as published in Kasper DL, et al. *Harrison's Principles of Internal Medicine,* 16th ed. New York: McGraw-Hill, 2005:295.)

KEY FACT

With recalcitrant acne in female patients, look for hirsutism and irregular menses, which may point to congenital adrenal hyperplasia, polycystic ovarian syndrome, or Cushing disease.

KEY FACT

Isotretinoin is teratogenic, so women must use a reliable method of birth control. Adverse effects include dry skin, cheilitis, hypertriglyceridemia, transaminitis (thus monitor LFTs), and depression.

KEY FACT

Steroid creams used on the face can cause dermatitis resembling rosacea.

ANSWER

This boy most likely has Henoch-Schönlein purpura. Perform urinalysis to evaluate for renal involvement and consider treating with prednisone.

ACNE

Defined as chronic inflammation and blockage of the pilosebaceous units with ↑ production of sebum and colonization of *Propionibacterium acnes.* Exacerbated by medications such as glucocorticoids; anabolic steroids; lithium; isoniazid (INH); some OCPs; cyclosporine; vitamins B_2, B_6, and B_{12}; and iodides.

- **Exam:** Will show noninflammatory open comedones ("blackheads") and closed comedones ("whiteheads") and/or inflammatory papules, pustules, and cysts (Figure 10.4).
- **First-line treatment:** Topical benzoyl peroxide; topical antibiotics (eg, clindamycin), topical retinoids.
- **Second-line treatment:** Oral antibiotics, typically doxycycline or erythromycin. Oral antibiotics may be first line in severe inflammatory acne with substantial cystic component. Also consider spironolactone if androgenic pattern in female (don't forget to check K^+!).
- **Third-line treatment:** Oral isotretinoin (Accutane), a retinoid that is anti-inflammatory.

ROSACEA

Chronic inflammatory facial dermatitis of adults characterized by papules and pustules on a background of telangiectasias and erythema.

Symptoms/Exam

- The earliest symptom is **flushing,** followed by erythema, telangiectasias, papules, pustules, and, rarely, lymphedema. Distribution is on the cheeks, nose, forehead, and chin.
- Triggered by **hot liquids, spicy food, alcohol, sun,** and **heat (the fun things!)**
- No comedones are seen (compare with acne vulgaris).

Differential

- Acne vulgaris, contact dermatitis, photosensitive eruptions, seborrheic dermatitis, SLE.
- Steroid creams used on the face can mimic rosacea.

Management

- Avoid exacerbating factors.
- **Topical treatment:**
  - First line: Metronidazole gel or cream.
  - Second line: Topical azelaic acid or topical ivermectin.
  - Third line: Sodium sulfacetamide lotion.
- **Oral treatment:** Low-dose doxycycline × 2 to 3 months. Appropriate in the presence of ocular involvement or if topical therapy is not effective.
- **Severe disease:** Isotretinoin.

Complications

Rhinophyma occurs primarily in middle-aged men with long-standing disease (Figure 10.5). Blepharitis and conjunctivitis are also potential complications.

ATOPIC DERMATITIS

A chronic, pruritic, inflammatory familial skin disease with allergic features. Characterized by recurrent flares of inflammatory rash, it often occurs in patients with other atopic disorders, such as **asthma** and **allergic rhinitis**. Typically begins in infancy; 50% incidence in the first year of life and an additional 30% between the ages of 1 and 5 years. Immune mediated, with roughly 85% of patients having ↑ IgE. Staphylococcal overgrowth is also thought to play a role in flares.

Symptoms/Exam

- Acute lesions can include vesicles on an erythematous base (see Figure 10.6). Skin lesions in older individuals with more chronic disease are characterized by **lichenification** as well as by excoriated and fibrotic papules.
- The **flexural** areas (neck, antecubital fossae, and popliteal fossae) are most commonly involved; other common sites include the face, wrists, and forearms.
- Infantile atopic dermatitis has a skin pattern opposite older children and adults, predominating on the face, truck, and neck.
- Other physical findings that support the diagnosis include xerosis (dry skin), infraorbital skin folds, periorbital darkening, hyperlinear palms (accentuation of fine palmar skin lines), keratosis pilaris, and anterior subcapsular cataracts and keratoconus.

Differential

Contact dermatitis, seborrheic dermatitis, drug reactions, psoriasis.

Diagnosis

Diagnosed visually. Pruritic recurrent flares, family history of atopy, and early age of onset are all suggestive of the diagnosis.

Management

- Ongoing treatment to prevent flares:
  - **Skin hydration with lotions and emollients.** Bleach in bath water may improve infected atopic eczema in children by decreasing bacterial colonization.
  - Eliminate exacerbating factors, including excessive bathing, low-humidity environments, emotional stress, xerosis, rapid temperature changes, and exposure to solvents and detergents.
- First line for flares: Topical corticosteroids, potency depending on severity and response.

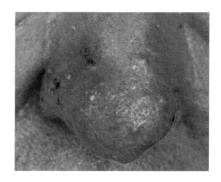

FIGURE 10.5. **Rhinophyma and pustules on a male with rosacea.** (Reproduced with permission from Wolff K, Johnson RA. *Fitzpatrick's Color Atlas & Synopsis of Clinical Dermatology,* 6th ed. Online Picture Gallery. New York: McGraw-Hill, 2009, Fig. 1e-R5.)

 KEY FACT

Examples of common topical steroids, ranked by potency:

Clobetasol 0.05%	*High potency*
Flucinonide (Lidex) 0.05%	
Betamethasone 0.05%	
Triamcinolone (TAC) 0.1%	
Triamcinolone (TAC) 0.025%	
Hydrocortisone 2.5%	*Low potency*

 KEY FACT

Extensor surface, axillary, gluteal, or groin lesions are more characteristic of psoriasis, while flexor surfaces, forearms, wrists and face are characteristic of atopic dermatitis.

 QUESTION 1

A 19-year-old man presents with acne minimally responsive to benzoyl peroxide and tretinoin. On exam he has multiple erythematous cystic lesions on chin, cheeks, and forehead, with healing scars. What's your next step?

 QUESTION 2

A 6-year-old girl with atopic dermatitis presents with her mother, who complains she is constantly slathering her daughter with hydrocortisone and lotion. You note dry, excoriated, erythematous patches with lichenification in her bilateral antecubital and popliteal fossa without signs of overlying infection. What's your next step?

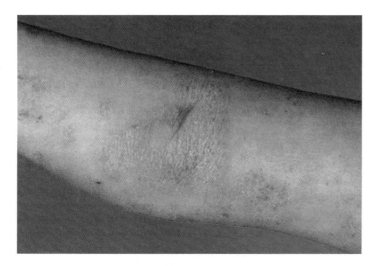

FIGURE 10.6. **Atopic dermatitis in the antecubital region of a child.** (Reproduced with permission from Wolff K, Johnson RA. *Fitzpatrick's Color Atlas & Synopsis of Clinical Dermatology,* 6th ed. Online Picture Gallery. New York: McGraw-Hill, 2009, Fig. 2e-Ad12.)

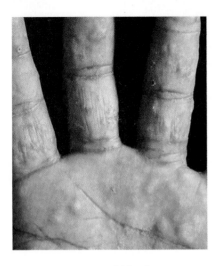

FIGURE 10.7.　Dyshidrotic eczema.
(Reproduced with permission from Fauci AS, et al. *Harrison's Principles of Internal Medicine*, 17th ed. New York: McGraw-Hill, 2008, Fig. 10-5.)

KEY FACT

Nummular eczema is often confused for tinea corporis and vice versa. If lesions worsen with steroid treatment, consider switching to an antifungal.

KEY FACT

Parkinson disease, stroke, and acute illness can present with seborrheic dermatitis. Severe and recalcitrant seborrheic dermatitis can also be a presenting symptom in patients with HIV.

A　ANSWER 1

Oral doxycycline (or tetracycline), as it has anti-inflammatory and antibacterial effects. If patient were female, consider OCPs.

A　ANSWER 2

This patient likely needs a stronger steroid ointment, ie, triamcinolone 0.1%. It's also important to review skin care and ensure use of unscented emollient without frequent baths or scrubbing.

- Second line:
  - Topical calcineurin inhibitors (tacrolimus/pimecrolimus) are appropriate for patients with inflamed skin.
  - Antihistamines can be given for pruritus.
- Third line:
  - Antibiotics for bacterial superinfection.
  - UVB or PUVA light therapy in difficult cases.

DYSHIDROTIC ECZEMA (POMPHOLYX)

An intensely pruritic, chronic recurrent dermatitis, typically involving the palms and soles (Figure 10.7).
- **Symptoms/exam:** Starts as an episode of **intense itching,** followed by the formation of small vesicles. Desquamation occurs over 1 to 2 weeks, leaving fissures and erosions. Recurrences may be seen.
- **Differential:** Tinea and contact dermatitis.
- **Management:** Treat with medium- to high-potency topical corticosteroids in mild cases and with a short course of systemic steroids in severe cases. Recalcitrant cases may respond to PUVA or UVA.

DISCOID (NUMMULAR) ECZEMA

Intensely pruritic dermatitis of unknown etiology.
- **Symptoms/exam:** Presents with nummular (coin-shaped) papules, scaling, crusting, and serous oozing. Lesions can be singular or multiple (up to 50) and are generally 2 to 10 cm in diameter and circular in shape. Distribution is over the trunk and lower extremities (the head is spared; see Figure 10.8).
- **Differential:** Tinea corporis; xerotic dermatitis, pityriasis rosea.
- **Management:** Treat with a short course of medium- to high-potency topical steroids. Systemic corticosteroids may be needed for more severe cases, but watch for rebound disease when using oral steroids. Avoid irritants (if identifiable).

SEBORRHEIC DERMATITIS

A chronic inflammatory eruption hypothesized to be caused by *Malassezia furfur* yeast (formerly *Pityrosporum ovale*) colonization. Known as "cradle cap" in infants.

Symptoms/Exam

- Presents with dry or **greasy,** salmon-colored scales on an erythematous base.
- Primarily affects the scalp, **postauricular region,** central facial area (especially the **eyebrows** and **nasolabial folds**), and flexural areas (Figure 10.9).
- Crust and fissures can develop and can become superinfected.

Differential

Atopic or contact dermatitis, psoriasis (seborrheic dermatitis is usually more "pinkish-red" compared with the deep red of psoriasis), impetigo, rosacea.

Management

- **Scalp:** First line: medicated shampoos (zinc pyrithione, selenium sulfide, or 2% ketoconazole); second line: coal tar shampoo.
- **Face, intertriginous areas:** First line: low-potency topical steroids; second line: topical antifungal cream. Use steroids on the face as short-term treatment only!
- **Infants:** Emollients ± 1% hydrocortisone ointment or an antifungal/hydrocortisone combination.

PSORIASIS

A chronic, noninfectious, immune-mediated inflammatory dermatosis. Roughly 2% of the population is affected, with a bimodal age distribution (peaks at 22 and 55 years). Early onset predicts a more serious disease course. Triggered by environmental factors such as infection, stress, trauma, and drugs (β-blockers, lithium).

Symptoms/Exam

- Presents with well-demarcated erythematous plaques covered by **waxy, silvery-white scales** (Figure 10.10). Characterized by bilateral involvement of the **extensor** surfaces, scalp, palms, and soles.
- Nail disease seen in most patients, including **nail pitting** and onycholysis (nail bed lifting).
- **Auspitz sign** is bleeding on removal of a scale.
- **Koebner** phenomenon is a form of the disease that occurs at sites of trauma.
- **Guttate psoriasis** generally follows a **streptococcal** infection (eg, strep throat) and presents with an acute symmetric eruption of "droplike" lesions on the trunk and limbs.
- More severe presentation is seen in **HIV**-infected patients.

Management

- **Mild to moderate disease:** First line: moderate-potency **topical corticosteroids**; second line: topical vitamin D analog or topical retinoids.
- **Moderate to severe disease:** First line: Phototherapy (UVB); second line: systemic agents (eg, oral retinoids, methotrexate, cyclosporine) or biologicals (eg, efalizumab, infliximab).
- **For guttate psoriasis**, treat strep throat given common association.

Complications

Psoriatic arthritis (affects 5% of patients, asymmetric oligoarthritis, classically "sausage digit" presentation); sacroiliitis.

PITYRIASIS ROSEA

An acute, self-limited disorder characterized by scaly oval papules and plaques. **Often seasonal** (peaking in the spring and fall). Generally found in adolescents and young adults in response to a viral infection (**HHV-6** and **HHV-7** have been implicated). **Affects females more often than males.**

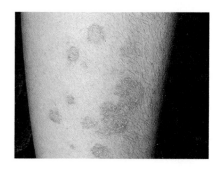

FIGURE 10.8. Nummular eczema. (Reproduced with permission from Wolff K, Johnson RA. *Fitzpatrick's Color Atlas & Synopsis of Clinical Dermatology,* 6th ed. New York: McGraw-Hill, 2009, Fig. 2-24.)

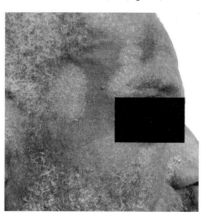

FIGURE 10.9. Seborrheic dermatitis. Extensive greasy scale-crust of the scalp, eyebrows, nasolabial folds and hair-bearing areas of the face. (Reproduced with permission from USMLE-Rx.com.)

 MNEMONIC

PSORIASIS:

Pink **P**apules / **P**laques / **P**inpoint bleeding (Auspitz sign) / **P**hysical injury (Koebner phenomenon) / **P**ain
Silver **S**cale / **S**harp margins
Onycholysis / **O**il spots
Rete **R**idges with **R**egular elongation
Itching
Arthritis / **A**bscess (Munro)
Stratum corneum with nuclei, neutrophils
Immunologic
Stratum granulosum absent / **S**tratum **S**pinosum thickening

 KEY FACT

Systemic corticosteroids are contraindicated in psoriasis because of severe rebound disease with medication withdrawal. However, potent topical steroids are sometimes needed to penetrate scale (eg, clobetasol).

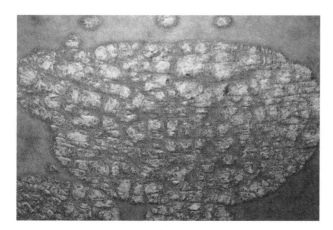

FIGURE 10.10. Psoriasis. (Reproduced with permission from Fauci AS, et al. *Harrison's Principles of Internal Medicine,* 17th ed. New York: McGraw-Hill, 2008, Fig. 52-7.)

Symptoms/Exam

- Presents as a generalized rash preceded by the appearance of a 2- to 5-cm **herald patch.** Days later, many smaller plaques appear on the trunk, arms, and thighs (Figure 10.11).
- Plaques are oval and pink, with a delicate peripheral **"collarette of scale,"** and are often distributed parallel to the lines of the ribs, creating the characteristic **"Christmas tree"** distribution.
- Sometimes accompanied by pruritus.

Differential

Guttate psoriasis, pityriasis versicolor, scabies, 2° syphilis.

Management

- Spontaneous resolution usually occurs in 1 to 2 months.
- **Moderate-potency steroids** may be given for itching.

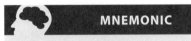

MNEMONIC

5 P's of Lichen Planus:

Purple
Polygonal
Papular
Pruritic
Planar (flat)

LICHEN PLANUS

An eruption characterized by flat, **purple, polygonal, pruritic papules** affecting the flexor surfaces, mucous membranes, and genitalia. Its cause is unknown but is thought to be immune related. Roughly two-thirds of cases occur in patients 30 to 60 years of age.

Symptoms/Exam

- The rash starts symmetrically on the limbs, especially the wrists. It may spread to become generalized within 4 weeks, but may also progress more slowly.
- Typical lesions are itchy, flat-topped polygonal papules a few millimeters in diameter (Figure 10.12). They classically show a surface network of delicate white lines (**Wickham striae**).
- Papules are initially red then violaceous, and can flatten or become hypertrophic. Although 50% of cases clear within 9 months, the condition often recurs.

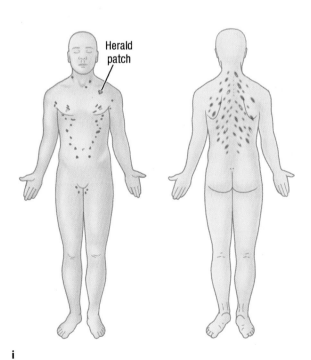

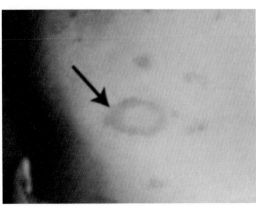

FIGURE 10.11. **Pityriasis rosea.** Distribution of pityriasis rosea (i). (Reproduced with permission from Wolff K, Johnson RA. *Fitzpatrick's Color Atlas & Synopsis of Clinical Dermatology*, 6th ed. New York: McGraw-Hill, 2009, Fig. 7-1.) Pink patches (ii, arrow) of pityriasis rosea. (Reproduced from the CDC.)

- Associated with chronic **HBV, HCV,** and **HIV.**
- Nail involvement in 10% to 15%.

Differential

Psoriasis, guttate psoriasis, pityriasis rosea, scabies.

Management

- The disease is usually self-limited.
- Moderate- to high-potency topical steroids are indicated for symptomatic treatment.
- Oral lesions are treated with steroid-containing paste.

CONTACT DERMATITIS

Any dermatitis that results from direct contact between skin and a substance. The two variants are allergen and irritant. **Irritants are responsible for 80% of cases.**

Irritant Contact Dermatitis

Trigger substance leads to breakdown of the normal epidermal barrier, causing the possibility of physical, chemical, or mechanical irritation. Reaction can be initiated by common irritants, such as daily-use products (eg, soap) or from one-time exposure to a chemical (eg, bleach, alkali). Patients with compromised skin barriers (eg, those with atopic dermatitis) are at higher risk.

- **Symptoms/Exam:** Erythema, fissures, and pruritus. In severe cases, bullae can develop. Often affects the hands, especially the web spaces, but location depends on exposure.
- **Diagnosis:** Usually clinical; patch testing can distinguish irritant from allergic dermatitis.
- **Management:** Involves avoiding triggers and restoring the normal epidermal barrier; emollients are useful. More severe cases can be treated with topical corticosteroids. Systemic steroids are generally not helpful without irritant removal.

Allergic Contact Dermatitis

In allergic dermatitis, a trigger substance induces a **delayed type IV immune response** in affected individuals. The first step takes 12 to 14 days to complete, and on re-exposure to an allergen, dermatitis occurs in 12 to 48 hours.

The most common plant allergen is oleoresin urushiol (found in poison ivy, poison oak, poison sumac, and mango skin). Other common allergens include nickel, formaldehyde, perfume, latex, and some medications.

Symptoms/Exam

- Presents with an intensely pruritic rash that is papular and erythematous, with indistinct margins.
- The rash can be linear (as in poison ivy) or can reflect the pattern of exposure to the allergen (eg, rings, clothing, footwear; see Figure 10.13).

Management

- **Avoid allergens.**
- **Mild cases** may be treated with medium- to high-potency topical steroids.
- With more severe oozing, wet-dry compresses may facilitate application of topical steroids by drying out the skin.
- **Severe cases,** involving >20% body surface area, can also be treated with a short course of oral corticosteroids.

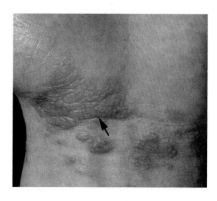

FIGURE 10.12. Lesions of lichen planus. Arrow showing Wickham striae. (Reproduced with permission from Wolff K, Johnson RA. *Fitzpatrick's Color Atlas & Synopsis of Clinical Dermatology,* 6th ed. New York: McGraw-Hill, 2009, Fig. 7-4A.)

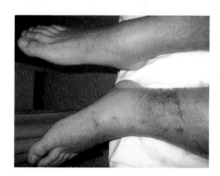

FIGURE 10.13. Contact dermatitis. Allergic contact dermatitis from exposure to poison ivy. (Reproduced with permission from USMLE-Rx.com.)

 QUESTION

A 22-year-old woman presents to urgent care complaining of ear drainage. On exam you note an erythematous lower earlobe with crusting and oozing, and a large, bronze stud piercing in place. What's the cause of her symptoms?

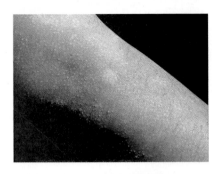

FIGURE 10.14. **Keratosis pilaris.** Keratosis pilaris in a patient with concurrent ichthyosis vulgaris. (Reproduced with permission from Wolff K, et al. *Fitzpatrick's Dermatology in General Medicine,* 7th ed. New York: McGraw-Hill, 2008, Fig. 85-1.)

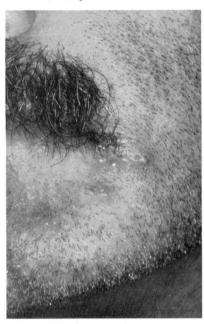

FIGURE 10.15. **Folliculitis in the beard area, with impetigo at the corner of the mouth.** (Reproduced with permission from Wolff K, et al. *Fitzpatrick's Color Atlas & Synopsis of Clinical Dermatology,* 5th ed. New York: McGraw-Hill, 2005:980.)

KEY FACT

Pseudomonal folliculitis is more common in people with recent hot tub exposure (aka "hot tub folliculitis") or on prolonged antibiotic therapy for acne treatment.

A **ANSWER**

This patient has allergic contact dermatitis, likely from a nickel allergy. She should remove the stud and wear hypoallergenic jewelry. Topical steroids would also provide symptomatic relief.

KERATOSIS PILARIS

Autosomal dominant condition caused by plugging of the follicle by keratin that has failed to exfoliate, leading to a red or skin-colored papule.

- Usually **asymptomatic**, but can cause pruritus. Typically found on the lateral face, trunk, upper and lower extremities, thighs, and buttocks (Figure 10.14).
- Conservative **treatment** (exfoliation, lactic acid preparations) is warranted. Try topical tretinoin for recalcitrant cases.

Bacterial Infections

FOLLICULITIS

An acute pustular infection of **hair follicles,** usually due to S *aureus.* Lesions are generally found in the hair-bearing areas. Sycosis barbae may develop in the beard area (Figure 10.15).

Diagnosis

Differential includes furuncles, carbuncles. If possible, **obtain a swab** to identify the causative organism.

Management

- For acute infections, use topical antibiotics if mild to moderate, and give systemic antibiotics with MRSA coverage if severe.
- For chronic infections: **First line:** Attempt to treat the underlying cause (occlusive clothing, poor shaving habits, underlying skin conditions). **Second line:** Systemic antibiotics with MRSA coverage. **Third line:** Consider evaluating for underlying fungal or parasitic etiology.
- **Hygiene** is key to treatment, along with weight loss and control of diabetes.

CELLULITIS

A bacterial infection of the skin, with extension into subcutaneous tissues. Seventy percent of patients are men. Additional risk factors include leg ulcers, trauma, intertrigo, tinea pedis, venous insufficiency, obesity, and a history of cellulitis.

Symptoms/Exam

- Presents with erythema, warmth, edema, and pain. May also have systemic symptoms such as fever, chills, and myalgias. Most commonly affects the extremities (73% of cases affect the lower extremities) but can involve any area of the body (Figure 10.16).
- **Margins** are generally **not well demarcated** (compare with erysipelas, which has distinct margins).
- Regional lymphadenopathy is common, and lymphangitis can be present.
- Abscess may be seen, as well as macular erythema that is largely confluent.

Differential

DVT, contact dermatitis, drug and foreign body reactions, insect stings, or venous stasis. Cellulitis is almost never bilateral.

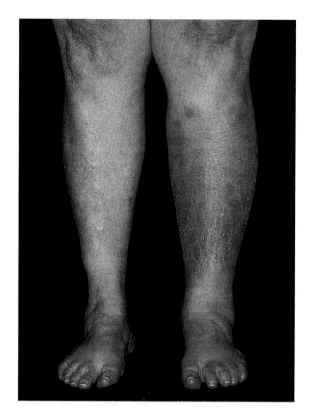

FIGURE 10.16. **Cellulitis of the lower extremity.** (Courtesy of Frank Birinyi, MD, as published in Knoop KJ, et al. *Atlas of Emergency Medicine,* 2nd ed. New York: McGraw-Hill, 2002:348.)

Diagnosis

- Cellulitis associated with furuncles, carbuncles, or abscesses is usually caused by S aureus. MRSA is very common and empiric treatment should always cover MRSA.
- Cellulitis that is diffuse or unassociated with a defined portal is most commonly caused by streptococcal species. β-hemolytic streptococci, including groups A, B, and, less often, C and G, are common causative agents.
- Facial cellulitis is associated with *Haemophilus influenzae* in children.
- Cellulitis following puncture wounds is most often caused by *Pseudomonas aeruginosa.*
- Exposure to fresh water or seawater is associated with *Aeromonas hydrophila* and *Vibrio* spp.
- Cellulitis after animal bites point to *Pasteurella multocida* and *Erysipelothrix.*
- Cultures are usually not helpful, establishing the diagnosis in only 50% of cases, and generally do not result in a change of antibiotic choice.

Management

- Per 2014 guidelines by the Infectious Diseases Society of America:
  - For cellulitis **without** signs of systemic infection, choose an antibiotic active against streptococci (ie, first-generation cephalosporin) and outpatient therapy.
  - For cellulitis **with** signs of systemic infection, choose IV antibiotic (ensure MRSA coverage, ie, vancomycin) and inpatient therapy.
- For **penicillin-allergic patients**, options include clindamycin or vancomycin.

Complications

Necrotizing fasciitis, gas gangrene.

Q QUESTION

A 45-year-old man with diabetes presents with an 8 × 7-cm warm, erythematous, painful, well-demarcated patch on his right lower extremity. A central oozing papule is noted. His vitals are notable for temperature of 39.1°C and heart rate of 113 beats/min. What is your next step in management?

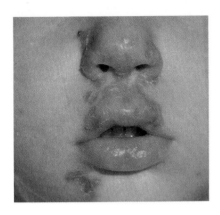

KEY FACT

Bullous impetigo is usually caused by *S aureus*, exfoliative toxins A and B.

KEY FACT

Recurrent impetigo suggests nasal carriage of *S aureus*. Treat with intranasal mupirocin.

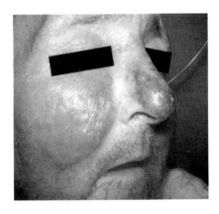

FIGURE 10.18.   Facial erysipelas.
Severe malar and nasal erythema and swelling with well demarcated borders.
(Reproduced from the CDC/Dr Thomas F. Sellers.)

  ANSWER

This man has cellulitis and his vitals show a systemic inflammatory response that warrant IV antibiotics covering MRSA (ie, vancomycin). The central papule likely represents a forming abscess and suggests staphylococcal infection.

IMPETIGO

A superficial skin infection due to **staphylococci** and/or **streptococci (group A)**. Affects men and women in all age groups. Lesions are classically found on the face.

- 1° lesions are thin-walled vesicles/pustules that easily rupture (Figure 10.17).
- Lesions spread rapidly and become crusted and are classically described as "**honey crusted.**"
- **Differential** includes HSV and fungal infection.
- **Remove crusts** via saline soaks and topical mupirocin.
- **Systemic antibiotics** (empirically directed against staph and strep) are appropriate for more severe cases.

ERYSIPELAS

An acute inflammation of the dermis by **group A β-hemolytic streptococci**. Elderly and immunocompromised patients are at higher risk.

- Presents with **well-demarcated erythema, edema, and tenderness** (a type of cellulitis), typically affecting the face and lower legs (Figure 10.18). Lesions can rapidly advance.
- Patients are generally systemically ill, presenting with fever, chills, and malaise.
- **Differential** includes staph cellulitis, angioedema, and allergic contact dermatitis.
- **Treat** with IV antibiotics directed against *Streptococcus*.
- **Complications:** Guttate psoriasis or acute glomerulonephritis can follow streptococcal infection.

HIDRADENITIS SUPPURATIVA

A chronic, suppurative cutaneous process that results from occlusion of follicles and 2° inflammation of the apocrine glands. Females are affected more often than males; it is more prevalent in obese women. Part of the **follicular occlusion triad** that consists of acne conglobata, hidradenitis suppurativa, and dissecting cellulitis of the scalp.

Symptoms/Exam

- Presents with recurrent deep boils for >6 months in flexural sites (Figure 10.19).
- Commonly affects the axillae, groin, vulva, and perineal or perianal areas, sparing the face (hence its proposed name, acne inversa). Lesions tend to recur.

Management

- Often challenging and should be approached stepwise.
- **For mild disease:** Start with topical clindamycin.
- **For moderate to severe disease:** A combination of oral antibiotics (first line: doxycycline, second line: clindamycin + rifampin) and surgical excision is used.

Mycotic Infections

TINEA (DERMATOPHYTES)

The most common type of fungal infection of the skin and nails. Often called "ringworm." The appearance of tinea is varied, depending on location, but commonly it

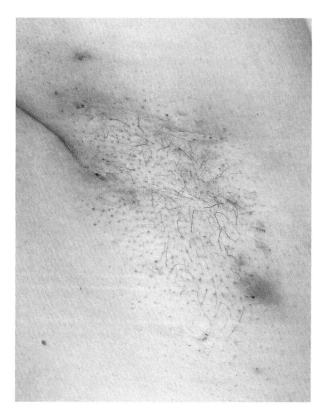

FIGURE 10.19.   **Hidradenitis suppurativa.** Note the bulging and depressed scars in the axilla. (Reproduced with permission from Wolff K, Johnson RA. *Fitzpatrick's Color Atlas & Synopsis of Clinical Dermatology*, 6th ed. New York: McGraw-Hill, 2009, Fig. 1-15.)

presents localized, erythematous, scaly lesions that form as pustules or vesicles with satellite lesions. Tinea is differentiated according to the site involved:

- **Tinea capitis:** Occurs primarily in children, typically causing patches of alopecia. Differentiate from seborrheic dermatitis (ie, "cradle cap"). First-line treatment is griseofulvin, second line is terbinafine.
- **Tinea pedis ("athlete's foot"):** Chronic cases usually require treatment with topical antifungal for 4 weeks. Interdigital tinea pedis, which is often macerated in appearance (Figure 10.20), require only 1 week of topical therapy. Resistant cases may require oral medication.
- **Tinea corporis ("ringworm"):** Lesions typically have sharply demarcated margins, with scaling (Figure 10.21). Treat with daily topical antifungal until clinical resolution (between 1 and 3 weeks). Resistant cases or extensive skin involvement may require oral medication.
- **Tinea cruris ("jock itch"):** Much more common in men. Obesity and sweaty physical activity are risk factors. Treat with topical antifungals. Use of talc or desiccant powders can help prevent recurrence.

Tinea Versicolor

A chronic fungal infection characterized by pigment changes. Caused by overgrowth of *Malassezia furfur*. More common in humid or tropical locations. Typically affects young adults.

KEY FACT

Amongst tinea, only tinea capitis is treated with oral antifungals as first line because of the need to penetrate the hair follicle. All other tineas are treated with topical antifungals.

KEY FACT

Tinea pedis is the most common underlying cause of cellulitis in otherwise healthy patients.

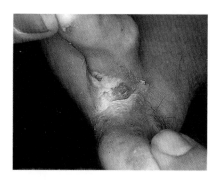

FIGURE 10.20.   **Interdigital tinea pedis.** (Reproduced with permission from Orkin M, et al. *Dermatology*. Originally published by Appleton & Lange. Copyright © 1991 by the McGraw-Hill Companies, Inc.)

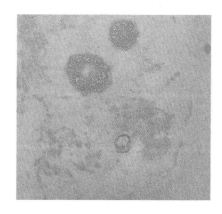

FIGURE 10.21.   **Tinea corporis.** Note the sharply demarcated margins with scale. (Reproduced with permission from Wolff K, et al. *Fitzpatrick's Color Atlas & Synopsis of Clinical Dermatology*, 5th ed. New York: McGraw-Hill, 2005:702.)

Symptoms/Exam

- In fair-skinned people, presents with brown or pinkish superficially scaly macules and patches that may be oval or round. Typically involves the trunk and proximal parts of the limbs.
- In darker-skinned people, hypopigmentation is seen (Figure 10.22).
- Wood's lamp ⊕ for pale yellow fluorescence.

Differential

Vitiligo, tinea corporis.

Diagnosis

Mostly clinical, can by aided by KOH scraping revealing hyphae and budding spores (**"spaghetti and meatballs"** appearance).

Management

- Topical antifungals; selenium sulfide 2.5% shampoo; zinc pyrithione shampoo.
- Systemic antifungals can be used for resistant cases.

Complications

Recurrence is common.

CANDIDIASIS/INTERTRIGO

A fungal infection that favors moist areas, with the intertriginous areas most commonly involved. Risk factors include diabetes mellitus, obesity, sweating, heat, maceration, and systemic/topical steroid use. Antibiotics and OCPs may also contribute.

Symptoms/Exam

- Plaques are very pruritic and occasionally painful with maceration.
- Brightly erythematous, sharply demarcated plaques with scalloped borders are seen, and often become macerated (Figure 10.23).

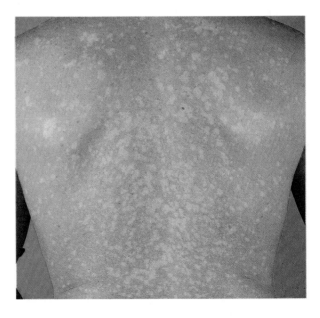

FIGURE 10.22. **Tinea versicolor.** Note the hypopigmented macules on the back of a tanned individual. (Reproduced with permission from Wolff K, Johnson RA. *Fitzpatrick's Color Atlas of Clinical Dermatology*, 6th ed. New York: McGraw-Hill, 2009, Fig. 13-13.)

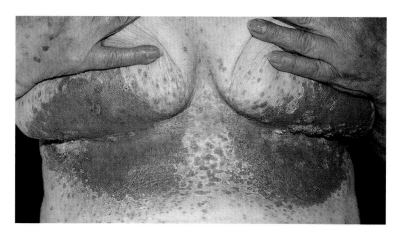

FIGURE 10.23.   **Cutaneous candidiasis/intertrigo.** Small peripheral satellite papules and pustules coalesce to create a large eroded area in the submammary region. (Reproduced with permission from Wolff K, Johnson RA. *Fitzpatrick's Color Atlas of Clinical Dermatology*, 6th ed. New York: McGraw-Hill, 2009, Fig. 25-23.)

- Satellite lesions (pustular lesions at the periphery) may coalesce and become part of a larger lesion.
- Clinical **diagnosis** is based on appearance and location, can be aided by KOH scraping showing pseudohyphae and yeast forms.
- Keep affected areas dry; **treat** with topical antifungals (powders or creams).

KEY FACT

Diaper rash may be candidal diaper dermatitis. Look for satellite lesions.

Viral Infections

MOLLUSCUM CONTAGIOSUM

Discrete, pearly pink, umbilical papules commonly involving the trunk, face, and neck, but may occur anywhere. Caused by a DNA poxvirus. Occurs mostly in children and young adults, and more common in immunocompromised patients. Spread by direct contact (eg, sexual contact, sharing towels).

Symptoms/Exam

- Presents with dome-shaped papules a few millimeters in size, with central umbilication or puncta (Figure 10.24).
- Lesions are usually multiple and grouped.
- Microscopic exam reveals intracytoplasmic inclusion bodies called Henderson-Paterson bodies.

Differential

Viral warts, skin tags.

Management

- The disease is self-limited, so often no therapy is necessary.
- In adults or older children, lesions can be removed via expression with forceps, with curettage under local anesthesia, or with cryosurgery.
- Topical imiquimod, cantharone, salicylic acid, or tea tree oil are also moderately effective.

Complications

Infection can be especially severe in immunocompromised patients.

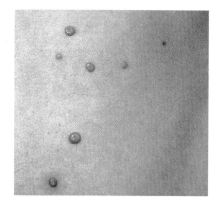

FIGURE 10.24.   Molluscum contagiosum on the chest of a female. Note the discrete, solid papules with central umbilication. (Reproduced with permission from Wolff K, et al. *Fitzpatrick's Dermatology in General Medicine*, 7th ed. New York: McGraw-Hill, 2008, Fig. 195-12A.)

 QUESTION

A 14-year-old boy presents to your office with a 2-week-long pruritic, crusting rash between his fingers and on his wrists and lateral feet. Topical corticosteroids have failed to improve his condition. How would you proceed?

VIRAL EXANTHEM

A rash associated with general features of a viral illness (myalgias, arthralgias, sore throat). Primarily seen in children and adolescents and can accompany many different viral infections.

- **Symptoms/Exam:** Erythematous and maculopapular rash, with a blotchy appearance, generally affecting the trunk and limbs. The viral cause is generally not identified.
- **Differential:** Chickenpox, measles, rubella, fifth disease, Coxsackievirus (hand-foot-mouth disease).
- **Management:** Emollients or cooling agents (calamine) for symptomatic relief.

Parasitic Infections

SCABIES

Caused by skin infection by the mite *Sarcoptes scabiei* (Figure 10.25). The female mite burrows into the skin to lay eggs. The infection is highly contagious and spreads through prolonged contact with an infected host.

Symptoms/Exam

- Presents with small pruritic papules, pustules, and burrows (Figure 10.26). Lesions are intensely pruritic, especially at night.
- Infection usually spares the face and scalp and is classically located in the web spaces of the hands. It is also common in the axillae, antecubital fossa, gluteal crease, feet, genitalia, nipples, and waistband (Figure 10.27).

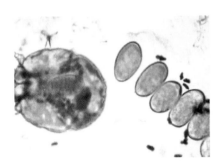

FIGURE 10.25. Microscopic appearance of scabies (*Sarcoptes scabiei*). (Reproduced with permission from Wolff K, et al. *Fitzpatrick's Dermatology in General Medicine*, 7th ed. New York: McGraw-Hill, 2008, Fig. 208-5.)

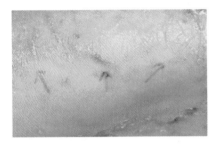

FIGURE 10.26. Linear burrows (arrows) of infection caused by scabies. (Reproduced with permission from Wolff K, Johnson RA. *Fitzpatrick's Color Atlas of Clinical Dermatology*, 6th ed. New York: McGraw-Hill, 2009, Fig. 28-18.)

 ANSWER

This is likely scabies. The skin should be scraped and examined under the microscope for characteristic mites. Treat with permethrin. Clothing and household contacts need to be treated as well.

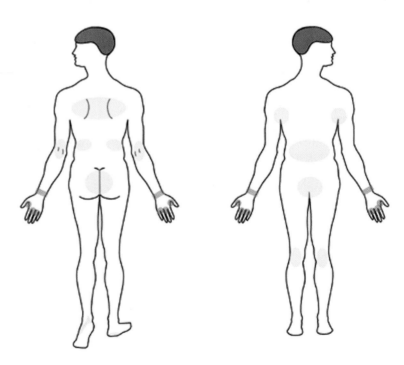

FIGURE 10.27. Common sites of scabies infection. Areas shaded red denote where mites are predominantly found. Areas shaded pink represent most common sites for the rashes to occur, but they can occur elsewhere. (Modified from the CDC/Alexander J. Da Silva, PhD/Melanie Moser.)

- Itching and rash are due to a type IV hypersensitivity reaction to the mite, eggs, and feces, and cause a delay of 2 to 4 weeks between infection and onset of symptoms.
- Excoriations and crusts develop due to scratching.

Diagnosis

- Often clinical based on location, exposure, characteristic rash, and intensity of itching.
- Confirm the diagnosis with skin scrapings and microscopy to identify mites, ova, and fecal pellets called scybala.

Management

- Apply permethrin 5% below the neck. Leave on for 8 hours and shower off. Repeat in 1 week.
- Wash clothes and linens in hot water.
- Consider empirically treating family members who sleep in the same room.

PEDICULOSIS

Skin infection by lice. The female louse lays eggs (nits) at the base of the hair that adhere to the hair shaft as it grows. Lice do not jump or fly and are not passed by pets. Head and body lice are interchangeable; genital lice ("crabs") are another species.
- Transmitted by direct contact or by fomites. May affect the head, body, or genital region.
- Patients may be asymptomatic or may present with pruritus resulting from allergy to lice saliva.
- Lice and nits are visible to the naked eye and are 2 to 4 mm in size.
- Diagnosed by direct visualization on exam.
- Permethrin 1% cream rinse is available OTC. Shampoo hair and towel dry. Apply permethrin cream and rinse in 10 minutes. Remove nits with comb. Repeat treatment in 7 to 10 days.

Immunologic and Autoimmune Disease

ERYTHEMA NODOSUM

A panniculitis (subcutaneous fat inflammation) usually on bilateral shins/lower extremities that is associated with a wide variety of disease processes (see mnemonic).
- **Symptoms/Exam:** Erythematous, tender nodules on anterior shins that spread to rest of lower extremities, usually associated with arthralgias, malaise, and fever on appearance. Turn purple/gray and resolve over 2 to 8 weeks (Figure 10.28).
- **Diagnosis:** Based on clinical exam and a search for the underlying cause. Must rule out TB/sarcoid, so a CXR is often warranted. Consider an ASO titer to rule out strep as it is the most common treatable cause.
- **Management:** Treat the underlying condition. If bothersome, can treat symptomatically with NSAIDs.

BLISTERING DISEASES

Pemphigus vulgaris and bullous pemphigoid are among the most common autoimmune blistering disorders. Table 10.5 outlines their presentation.

MNEMONIC

Underlying etiologies of erythema NODOSUM:

NO cause in 60% of cases (idiopathic)
Drugs (sulfas, iodide)
Oral contraceptives
Sarcoidosis
Ulcerative colitis/Crohn's
Micro (strep, TB, leprosy, any chronic infection)

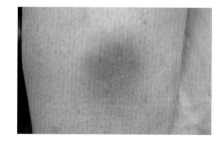

FIGURE 10.28. Erythema nodosum. 22-year-old woman with a history of sarcoidosis who developed painful non-ulcerated erythematous subcutaneous nodules on the extensor surfaces of the bilateral lower extremities. Skin biopsy demonstrated septal panniculitis consistent with erythema nodosum. (Reproduced with permission from USMLE-Rx.com.)

MNEMONIC

Bullous Pemphigoid is "**bullow**" (below) the epidermis

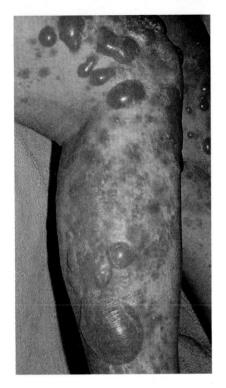

FIGURE 10.29.   Bullous pemphigoid.
(Reproduced with permission from Wolff K, et al. *Fitzpatrick's Dermatology in General Medicine,* 7th ed. New York: McGraw-Hill, 2008, Fig. 54-4.)

TABLE 10.5.   Bullous Pemphigoid Versus Pemphigus Vulgaris

	BULLOUS PEMPHIGOID	PEMPHIGUS VULGARIS
Site of blistering	Subepidermal	Intraepidermal
Epidemiology	Affects patients aged >60 years; the most common blistering disorder	Affects patients aged 40-60 years
Pruritus	Prominent	Not prominent
Nikolsky sign (superficial separation of skin with lateral pressure)	⊖	⊕
Frequency of oral mucosal lesions	Affect a minority of patients (<30%)	Affect > 50% of patients
Character of blisters and bullae	Intact, tense (Figure 10.29)	Rupture easily; flaccid (Figure 10.30)
Complications	Few complications	Superinfection; high mortality from sepsis if untreated; ocular involvement dictates a referral
Subtypes		Drug induced (penicillamine and ACEIs), paraneoplastic

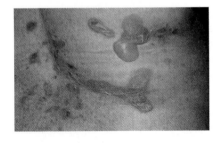

FIGURE 10.30.   Pemphigus vulgaris.
(Reproduced with permission from Wolff K, et al. *Fitzpatrick's Dermatology in General Medicine,* 7th ed. New York: McGraw-Hill, 2008, Fig. 52-3.)

KEY FACT

PPD testing for tuberculosis is a **type IV** hypersensitivity reaction.

Cutaneous Drug Reactions

Mechanisms of dermatologic drug reactions may be immunologic (Table 10.6) or nonimmunologic. Examples of nonimmunologic drug reactions include cutaneous phototoxicity with tetracycline or the itching and erythema caused by mast cell mediator release in response to NSAIDs or radiographic contrast. Table 10.7 outlines the etiologies and clinical presentation of severe cutaneous drug reactions.

TABLE 10.6.   Immunologic Mechanisms of Cutaneous Drug Reactions

MECHANISM	EXAMPLES
Type I: Classic immediate hypersensitivity	Urticaria, angioedema, anaphylaxis
Type III: Immune complex	Leukocytoclastic vasculitis, serum sickness, urticaria, angioedema
Type IV: Delayed hypersensitivity	Contact dermatitis, exanthematous reactions, photoallergic reactions
Systemic infection impairing immune response	Mononucleosis, ampicillin-induced rash, HIV, sulfonamide-induced toxic epidermal necrolysis
Unknown immunologic mechanisms	Lichenoid reactions, fixed drug eruptions

TABLE 10.7. **Differential Diagnosis of Severe Drug Reactions**

DIAGNOSIS	MUCOSAL LESION	TYPICAL SKIN LESION	FREQUENT SYMPTOMS AND SIGNS	OTHER UNRELATED CAUSES	DRUGS MOST OFTEN IMPLICATED
Stevens-Johnson syndrome	Erosions are usually at 2 or more sites	Small blisters on dusky purpuric macules or atypical targets (Figure 10.31) Rare areas of confluence may be seen Involves detachment of ≤10% of body surface area	Some 10%-30% present with fever	Postinfectious **erythema multiforme major** (acute dermatitis characterized by distinctive, fixed-target lesions [Figure 10.32]; caused by HSV or *Mycoplasma*)	Sulfa drugs, phenytoin, carbamazepine, lamotrigine, allopurinol
Toxic epidermal necrolysis	Same as above	Individual lesions like those of Stevens-Johnson syndrome (Figure 10.33) ⊕ Nikolsky sign; large sheet of necrotic epidermis Involves >30% of body surface area	Fever is nearly universal "Acute skin failure" and leukopenia are also seen	Viral infections, immunization, chemicals, *Mycoplasma* pneumonia	Same as above
Anticonvulsant hypersensitivity syndrome	Infrequent	Severe exanthems (may become purpuric); exfoliative dermatitis	Some 30%-50% of cases present with fever, lymphadenopathy, hepatitis, nephritis, carditis, eosinophilia, and atypical lymphocytes	Cutaneous lymphoma	Anticonvulsants
Serum sickness	Absent	Morbilliform lesions, sometimes with urticaria	Fever, arthralgias	Infection	
Anticoagulant-induced necrosis	Infrequent	Erythema, then purpura and necrosis, especially of fatty areas	Pain in affected areas	Digoxin	Warfarin
Angioedema	Often involved	Urticaria or swelling of the face	Respiratory distress or cardiovascular collapse	Insect stings, foods	NSAIDs, ACEIs, penicillin

Cutaneous Oncology

PRIMARY PREVENTION OF SKIN CANCER

UVA and UVB both lead to photoaging; UVB more commonly causes skin cancer. The following recommendations are for 1° prevention of skin damage and cancer:
 Minimize sun exposure during peak UV midday hours (10 AM-4 PM).

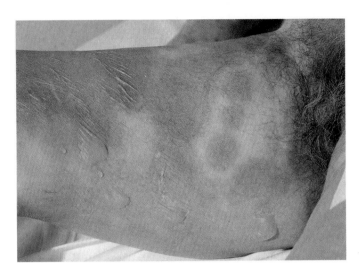

FIGURE 10.31. **Lesions of Stevens-Johnson syndrome.** (Reproduced with permission from Wolff K, et al. *Fitzpatrick's Color Atlas & Synopsis of Clinical Dermatology,* 5th ed. New York: McGraw-Hill, 2005:145.)

- Use sunscreen with at least SPF 15. Physical sunscreens (eg, titanium dioxide or zinc oxide) deflect or block the sun's rays. Chemical sunscreens absorb or filter UV rays. Broadband sunscreens may contain a combination of both.
- Use wide-brimmed hats, sunglasses, and protective clothing.

ATYPICAL NEVI

Nevi sharing features of melanoma. Typically large (>6 mm), hyperpigmented, and asymmetric, with irregular "fuzzy" borders ("fried egg" appearance).

- Lesions may occur anywhere on the body but are more common in sun-exposed areas (eg, the back). Appearance varies, but they usually show the **ABCDE** appearance (see mnemonic).
- **Rule out** melanoma.
- **Treat** with excisional biopsy only if melanoma is suspected.
- Increased incidence of melanoma in patients with atypical nevi.

MNEMONIC

The ABCDEs of Melanoma:

Asymmetric
Border irregularity
Color (multiple or black)
Diameter (>6mm)
Evolving (changing mole)

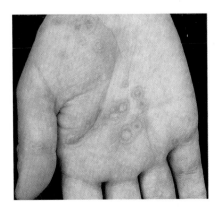

FIGURE 10.32. **Lesions of erythema multiforme.** (Reproduced with permission from Wolff K, et al. *Fitzpatrick's Dermatology in General Medicine,* 7th ed. New York: McGraw-Hill, 2008, Fig. 38-2.)

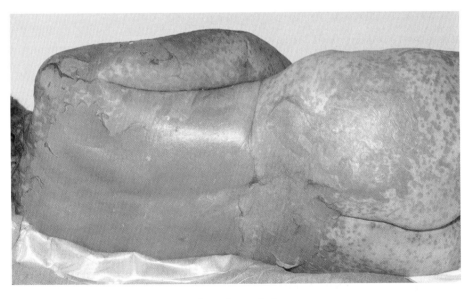

FIGURE 10.33. **Lesions of toxic epidermal necrolysis.** (Reproduced with permission from Wolff K, et al. *Fitzpatrick's Color Atlas & Synopsis of Clinical Dermatology,* 5th ed. New York: McGraw-Hill, 2005:147.)

MELANOMA

A malignancy of melanocytes that may occur on any skin or mucosal surface. It is the 7th most common cancer in the United States, with the incidence doubling every 10 years. Superficial spreading melanoma (which makes up 70% of cases) tends to stay "superficial" and has a better prognosis than nodular melanoma (15%), which tends to grow downward. *CDKN2A* is a gene associated with familiar melanoma. Risk factors are expressed in the mnemonic **MMRISK** (see below).

Symptoms/Exam

Presents with a changing mole (see Figure 10.34 and the mnemonic **ABCDE**) that may enlarge suddenly, begin to bleed, begin to itch, or become painful. May occur anywhere on the body, but more common in sun-exposed areas.

Differential

Atypical nevi; seborrheic keratosis.

Diagnosis

- Clinical exam and excisional biopsy.
- Tumor thickness (Breslow classification) and lymph node spread are the most important prognostic factors.
- No staging workup is necessary if the lesion is <1 mm in thickness, which is considered low risk.

Treatment

- Excision with appropriate borders.
- Sentinel lymph node dissection for melanomas >1 mm thick to determine if adjuvant therapy is needed.
- Close follow-up, depending on staging, at minimum with a skin exam yearly.

Complications

Metastasis. Five-year survival rates with lymph node involvement and distant metastasis are 30% and 10%, respectively.

BASAL CELL CARCINOMA

The most common skin cancer (80%); occurs in sun-exposed areas, especially the central face and ears.
- **Presents** with a shiny, "pearly" papule and telangiectasias (Figure 10.35), while more advanced disease can have an irregular appearance.
- **Differential** includes molluscum contagiosum and keratoses.
- **Diagnose** via shave biopsy.
- **Treat** with excision or destruction (electrodesiccation and curettage) of the lesion. Patient education for sun avoidance is key to further prevention. Mohs micrographic surgery is often indicated for BCC on the head and neck, and for large BCC or recurring BCC.
- **Complications** include metastatic spread, which occurs in <0.1% of patients.

ACTINIC KERATOSIS

A superficial keratotic lesion that is a precursor of SCC. Prevention by avoidance of sun exposure is key.

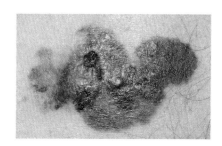

FIGURE 10.34. Superficial spreading melanoma. A highly characteristic lesion with an irregular pigmented pattern and scalloped borders. (Reproduced with permission from Wolff K, et al. *Fitzpatrick's Color Atlas & Synopsis of Clinical Dermatology*, 5th ed. New York: McGraw-Hill, 2005:318.)

MNEMONIC

Malignant melanoma risk:

MMRISK

Moles: atypical
Moles: total number >50
Red hair and freckling
Inability to tan
Severe sunburn, especially in childhood
Kindred: first-degree relative

KEY FACT

The central face and ears are high-risk areas of ↑ recurrence and metastatic potential for BCC.

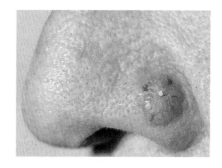

FIGURE 10.35. Nodular basal cell carcinoma. A smooth, pearly nodule with telangiectasias. (Reproduced with permission from Wolff K, et al. *Fitzpatrick's Color Atlas & Synopsis of Clinical Dermatology*, 5th ed. New York: McGraw-Hill, 2005:283.)

QUESTION

A 71-year-old man complains of a pruritic growth on his left ear that feels "rough." On exam you note an erythematous, hyperkeratotic, plaque with central crusting. What's your next step?

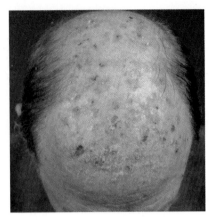

FIGURE 10.36. **Actinic keratosis.** Multiple premalignant keratotic lesions on the bald scalp of this individual. (Reproduced with permission from Wolff K, et al. *Fitzpatrick's Color Atlas & Synopsis of Clinical Dermatology,* 5th ed. New York: McGraw-Hill, 2005:263.)

KEY FACT

SCC is more common and more aggressive in immunosuppressed patients or transplant patients.

KEY FACT

In patients with psoriasis that is atypical or does not respond to steroids, consider cutaneous T-cell lymphoma and get a biopsy.

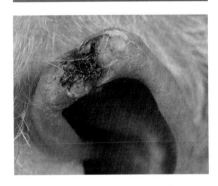

FIGURE 10.37. **Squamous cell carcinoma.** A hyperkeratotic nodule with ulceration. (Reproduced with permission from Wolff K, et al. *Fitzpatrick's Color Atlas & Synopsis of Clinical Dermatology,* 5th ed. New York: McGraw-Hill, 2005:279.)

 ANSWER

This is most likely an actinic keratosis given the rough, hyperkeratotic nature. However, the crusting may be a sign of SCC and warrants biopsy to further differentiate.

- **Presents** as a discrete, reddish-pink keratotic lesion, usually with a white scale, that feels "rough" (Figure 10.36). Found in sun-exposed areas, mostly on the face and dorsal hands.
- Biopsy is not indicated. **Diagnosed** by clinical presentation based on location and rough feel.
- **If single lesion or few lesions:** First-line treatment is cryotherapy, second line is shave biopsy, especially if suspicious.
- **If multiple or diffuse lesions:** Treat with topical 5-fluorouracil, topical imiquimod, photodynamic therapy (depending on availability and patient preference).

SQUAMOUS CELL CARCINOMA

Represents 20% of all skin cancers. May arise within actinic keratoses, within HPV-induced lesions, and within burn and radiation scars. SCC is more common than BCC in immunocompromised individuals.

- **Presents** with a hyperkeratotic lesion with crusting and ulceration (Figure 10.37). May occur anywhere, but most commonly seen in sun-exposed areas.
- **Treat** via surgical excision with clear margins.
- Has a higher rate of **metastasis** than BCC. The 5-year recurrence rate is 8%, and the metastatic rate is 5%.

CUTANEOUS T-CELL LYMPHOMA

A T-cell lymphoma that begins in the skin; the most common type is mycosis fungoides. Most often affects patients >50 years of age. Twice as common in men and more common in African Americans.

- Presents with pruritic, eczematous patches or plaques distributed over non–sun-exposed areas of skin. Tumors develop later in the disease course.
- May be misdiagnosed as psoriasis, eczema, or contact dermatitis. Chronicity, typical appearance, and failure to respond to steroids are all clues that a biopsy is indicated.
- **Sézary syndrome** is the leukemic form of T-cell lymphoma. Without treatment, patients succumb to opportunistic infections.

Miscellaneous Dermatologic Disorders

KELOID

A hypertrophic scar; more common in African Americans.

- Treatment involves intralesional corticosteroid injections.
- Surgical excision is **not** recommended, as lesions can recur larger than before.

DISORDERS AFFECTING THE HAIR

Table 10.8 outlines common dermatologic disorders of the hair.

TABLE 10.8. **Common Dermatologic Disorders Affecting the Hair**

DISORDER	HISTORY/EXAM	TREATMENT
Androgenic alopecia	Hereditary; affects individuals 12-70 years old; presents with gradual progression of hair loss over the temple and crown area	Topical minoxidil; finasteride
Alopecia areata	Nonscarring autoimmune alopecia characterized by well-demarcated patches of hair loss	Local steroid injection; topical steroids
Telogen effluvium	Diffuse loss of scalp, axillary, and pubic hair occurring 2-4 months after an inciting event (psychological stressors, major surgery, childbirth, crash diets, endocrine disorders)	Treat the underlying cause
Traction alopecia	Alopecia occurring in high-tension hair styles (tight braids, ponytails); may be permanent	Change in hair style

MELASMA

Splotchy hyperpigmented macules that affect sun-exposed areas of skin, most commonly on the face (Figure 10.38). Thought to be hormonally mediated. More common in women and darker-skinned persons (especially Hispanics). Often associated with pregnancy.

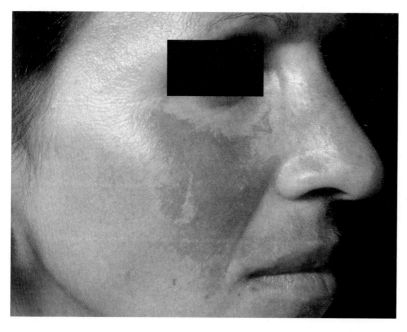

FIGURE 10.38. **Melasma.** Well-demarcated, hyperpigmented macules are seen on the cheek, nose, and upper lip. (Reproduced with permission from Wolff K, Johnson RA. *Fitzpatrick's Color Atlas & Synopsis of Clinical Dermatology*, 6th ed. New York: McGraw-Hill, 2009, Fig. 13-8.)

MNEMONIC

Don't confuse SKs (seborrheic keratosis) with AKs (actinic keratosis), which can become SCC. Think "**AK-47**" to remember which is more dangerous.

- Can be chronic, but if associated with pregnancy, it will usually regress within a year after delivery.
- Use **topical therapy** (hydroquinone cream) and strict **sunscreen** application. Hydroquinone must be used cautiously and for a maximal 3-month duration.
- If patients fail to respond, refer to a dermatologist for chemical peel or bleaching agents.

SEBORRHEIC KERATOSIS

The most common benign epidermal growth.
- Usually asymptomatic, hyperpigmented, hyperkeratotic papules and macules with a classic "stuck-on" appearance (Figure 10.39).
- No treatment is necessary, but growths can be frozen or curetted if bothersome.

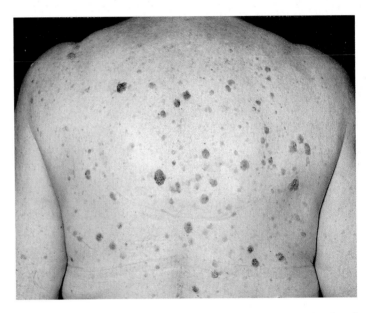

FIGURE 10.39.   **Seborrheic keratosis.** Multiple seborrheic keratoses with a "stuck-on" appearance are seen on the back. (Reproduced with permission from Wolff K, Johnson RA. *Fitzpatrick's Color Atlas & Synopsis of Clinical Dermatology,* 6th ed. New York: McGraw-Hill, 2009, Fig. 9-41.)

CHAPTER 11

Neurology

Lisa Moore, MD

MNEMONIC

Red flag symptoms in patients with headache:

SNOOP

Systemic symptoms or illness

Neurologic symptoms or signs (papilledema, asymmetric cranial nerve or motor function, abnormal cerebellar function)

Onset recently or suddenly

Onset after age 40 years

Prior headache history that is different or progressive

KEY FACT

Migraines are more common in women than in men, and typical age of onset is 10 to 30 years.

KEY FACT

Benign causes of headache can usually be diagnosed without imaging or labs based on the history and lack of focal neurologic deficits.

Headache

DIAGNOSIS OF DANGEROUS CAUSES OF HEADACHE

Consider imaging or further workup if the patient complains of one of these "red flag" symptoms. Table 11.1 summarizes key symptoms that may indicate a dangerous cause of headache.

MIGRAINE HEADACHE

Symptoms/Exam

- Recurrent headaches lasting 4 to 72 hours. To diagnose, at least two of the following characteristics must be present: **unilateral** distribution, **pulsatile** quality, severity limiting daily activities, and exacerbation by physical activity. One of the following characteristics must also be present: **nausea** or **vomiting, photosensitivity,** and sensitivity to noise or smell.
- **Migraine with aura** is preceded by a reversible symptom indicative of focal cerebral dysfunction. Examples of auras include gradual onset and spread of scotomas, scintillations, and/or hemianopic field defects; unilateral paresthesias or numbness; unilateral weakness; and speech disturbance. It is possible to have aura symptoms with gradual onset and no subsequent headache.
- Women who have migraine with aura should not use estrogen-containing contraceptives because of ↑ stroke risk.

Diagnosis

Based on symptoms, family history of migraines, and normal neurologic exam.

Management

- **Abortive therapy:** NSAIDs, acetaminophen, triptans, ergotamines, and antiemetics. Narcotic analgesics used as a last resort.
- **Prophylaxis:** β-blockers, calcium channel blockers, tricyclic antidepressants (TCAs), anticonvulsants. Avoidance or mitigation of triggers such as stress, missed meals, menses, and sleep deprivation.

TABLE 11.1. **Presentation of Dangerous Causes of Headaches**

SYMPTOM	POSSIBLE CAUSE
Sudden onset of "The worst headache of my life."	Subarachnoid hemorrhage
Neck stiffness with severe headache	Bacterial meningitis, subarachnoid hemorrhage
Sudden ↓ level of consciousness	Intracranial bleed, intracranial mass
Progressively worsening headache	Intracranial mass
Daily headaches that awaken the patient from sleep or are severe on arising in the morning	Intracranial mass with ↑ ICP
Onset of headache after 40 years of age	Intracranial mass
Progressive visual, motor, or balance disturbance, or cognitive changes	Intracranial mass, vascular lesion
Onset of headache after age 50 years of age	Temporal arteritis, intracranial mass

TENSION HEADACHE

Most common type of chronic recurring headache.
- **Symptoms/exam:** Presents as a bilateral headache with pain in the frontal and occipital regions in a **bandlike distribution that is triggered** by stress, glare, or noise.
- **Acute headache:** Treat with ASA, NSAIDs, ergotamines.
- **Prophylaxis:** TCAs, SSRIs, β-blockers, stretching and relaxation techniques.

CLUSTER HEADACHE

Occurs most often in middle-aged men.

Symptoms/Exam

- Recurrent, **unilateral**, excruciating **periorbital** headache that lasts 15 minutes to 3 hours.
- Cluster headaches classically take place in groups over days to weeks, occurring at the same time of day and in the same location.
- May be associated with Horner syndrome (miosis, ptosis, and anhidrosis), ipsilateral conjunctival injection, lacrimation, and nasal congestion (see section on Horner syndrome below).

Differential

Migraine, glaucoma, sinusitis, uveitis, trigeminal neuralgia.

Management

- **Acute attack:** 100% O_2, triptans, ergotamines, intranasal lidocaine, steroids, opiates. Treatment should start at the onset of symptoms and continue until headache-free for at least 2 weeks.
- **Prophylaxis:** Avoid triggers such as alcohol, stress, and medications causing vasodilation. To prevent acute recurrence, a prednisone burst and taper may be helpful. Medications for long-term prevention include calcium channel blockers, lithium, ergotamines, and anticonvulsants.

REBOUND HEADACHE

Presents as a chronic or nearly daily headache associated with **frequent use of medication for acute head pain,** with normal neurologic exam.
- **Management: Discontinue analgesics.** During withdrawal period, may also use triptans, prednisone, or ergotamines.
- **Complication:** One-third of patients **relapse** into analgesic overuse pattern.

POSTTRAUMATIC HEADACHE

Occurs following minor head injuries or hyperextension-flexion injuries ("whiplash"). Usually resolves in weeks to months.
- **Symptoms/exam:** Usually described as a generalized constant headache that is associated with changes in attention, concentration, and memory. May be associated with dizziness, nausea, irritability, insomnia, and ↓ light and sound tolerance. Onset within 2 weeks of trauma. Acute cases last <8 weeks. Chronic lasts >8 weeks.
- **Diagnosis:** Based on the history and a normal neurologic exam. Head CT may be indicated depending on timing and severity of head trauma.
- **Management:** Supportive care, NSAIDs, antiemetics, and TCAs.

MNEMONIC

Treatment of cluster headache:
STOLE (in no particular order)
Steroids
Triptans
Oxygen
Lidocaine, intranasal
Ergotamines

KEY FACT

The typical cluster headache patient is a middle-aged man.

QUESTION 1

A 16-year-old girl has had headaches for the last 2 years. They are associated with nausea and sensitivity to light and sound, and occur during her menses. She has some relief with OTC ibuprofen but would like to know if there is something stronger she can use. What test do you order before prescribing a triptan?

QUESTION 2

A 52-year-old woman is seen in the clinic because she is feeling "tired and achy all over." She has a headache by her right eye and blurred vision. She also complains of jaw ache when she chews. As you examine her, she reports pain when you palpate her scalp. How do you proceed?

TEMPORAL ARTERITIS (GIANT CELL ARTERITIS)

Temporal arteritis is a treatable neurologic emergency characterized by subacute inflammation of the external carotid arterial system and vertebral arteries. It is most common in **women >50 years of age.**

Symptoms/Exam

- Patients often describe a **new** temporal or diffuse headache that may be associated with **transient visual loss, scalp tenderness, jaw claudication.** Symptoms include fever, myalgia, malaise, anorexia, anemia, weight loss, tenderness, and stiffness in the shoulders and hips. About 40% of temporal arteritis patients have concurrent polymyalgia rheumatica.
- On exam, look for temporal arteries that may be dilated, tender, thickened, and nonpulsatile.

Differential

Glaucoma, uveitis, rheumatoid arthritis (RA), trigeminal neuralgia, retinal embolism, Takayasu arteritis.

Diagnosis

- Guided by the history and exam. If suspicious, check CBC, ESR, and CRP.
- ESR is usually >50 mm/hr, although rare cases may show a normal ESR. Normochromic, normocytic anemia with thrombocytosis is also common.
- Biopsy of the temporal artery shows vasculitis with mononuclear cell infiltration or granulomatous inflammation (Figure 11.1).

Management

Oral prednisone 40 to 60 mg daily for 1 to 2 months, with slow taper and monitoring of symptoms and ESR. ASA ↓ the risk of stroke or visual loss.

Complications

Visual loss affects about one in six patients. Associated with ↑ risk of cranial neuropathy, TIA, stroke, and thoracic aortic aneurysm.

KEY FACT

"A sed rate over 50 in a patient over 50" = temporal arteritis.

KEY FACT

Starting steroids is always the next best step when temporal arteritis is suspected. Temporal artery biopsy is the gold standard for diagnosis, with 100% specificity.

A ANSWER 1

Urine pregnancy test. Triptans have a pregnancy category C rating and may not be the best choice. They also ↑ the risk of serotonin syndrome in patients on SSRIs or MAO inhibitors.

A ANSWER 2

This patient needs to be started on prednisone immediately because her symptoms and exam are concerning for temporal arteritis. After starting prednisone, a temporal artery biopsy should be arranged.

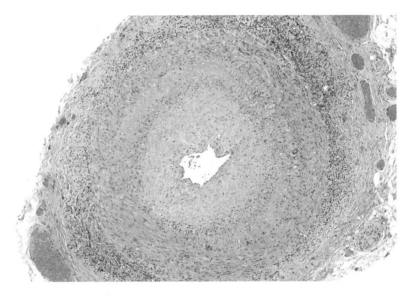

FIGURE 11.1.   **Temporal arteritis H&E stain.** (Reproduced from Wikimedia; courtesy of Nephron.)

IDIOPATHIC INTRACRANIAL HYPERTENSION (PSEUDOTUMOR CEREBRI)

A disorder characterized by **headache, ↑ ICP, and papilledema** unexplained by any other identifiable cause. Typically affects obese, hirsute-appearing young women. Associated causative factors include hypervitaminosis A, hypoparathyroidism, Addison disease, and medications (eg, corticosteroids, tetracycline, OCPs).

Symptoms/Exam

- Diffuse headaches that may worsen with straining. Often associated with visual loss or diplopia, transient visual obscurations, pulsatile tinnitus, or limited abduction of one or both eyes (abducens nerve palsy).
- A funduscopic exam shows papilledema (Figure 11.2). Visual function testing reveals a larger physiologic blind spot.

Differential

↑ ICP is caused by an intracranial tumor until proved otherwise. Also includes malignant hypertension, intracranial abscess or hemorrhage, hydrocephalus, dural venous thrombosis, and migraine.

Diagnosis

- **Imaging studies performed to rule out intracranial mass or dural sinus thrombosis.** Head CT or MRI may be normal or may show **small ventricles** or **empty sella.**
- LP shows elevated opening pressure with a normal CSF profile.

Management

- Start acetazolamide ± a diuretic.
- Discontinue contributing medications. Weight loss for obese patients.
- Repeated LPs or lumboperitoneal shunting may be necessary for refractory cases.

Complications

Optic atrophy and permanent visual loss.

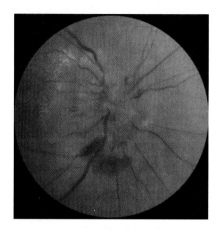

FIGURE 11.2. Papilledema. Color fundus photograph of the right optic nerve shows swelling of the optic nerve head with hemorrhage in a 26-year-old obese woman who presented with headaches, nausea, and vomiting. (Reproduced with permission from USMLE-Rx.com; courtesy of Dr. Nicholas Mahoney.)

QUESTION

An obese 37-year-old woman presents with headaches that worsen with lifting heavy objects and "ringing of the ears." She has also noted blurry vision. Exam shows limited abduction of her left eye, and funduscopy reveals optic disc swelling and hard exudates. How do you proceed?

KEY FACT

TIA is now differentiated from stroke by the absence of infarcted brain tissue, *not* the amount of time symptoms are present.

Cerebrovascular Disease

ISCHEMIC STROKE

- **Transient ischemic attack (TIA):** A transient episode of neurologic dysfunction caused by focal ischemia without acute infarction.
- **Ischemic stroke:** Sudden onset of focal neurologic symptoms that correlate with CNS infarction. Ischemic stroke may be due to embolism, thrombosis, or hypoperfusion. Accounts for about 80% of strokes.

Symptoms/Exam

Table 11.2 differentiates common symptoms that help to differentiate the location of the stroke.

Differential

Hemorrhagic stroke, seizure, complicated migraine, subdural hematoma, dural sinus thrombosis, Bell palsy, MS, intracranial mass, CNS infection, CNS inflammation, CNS arteritis.

KEY FACT

Lacunar infarct syndromes include clumsy hand, dysarthria, pure motor hemiparesis, pure hemisensory loss, and ataxic hemiparesis.

MNEMONIC

Stroke risk factors:
HEADS
Hypertension/**H**yperlipidemia
Elderly
Atrial fib
Diabetes mellitus/**D**rugs (cocaine)
Smoking/**S**ex (male)

TABLE 11.2.   **Key Stroke Syndromes**

LEFT (DOMINANT) HEMISPHERE	RIGHT (NONDOMINANT) HEMISPHERE	BRAIN STEM	CEREBELLUM
Left gaze preference	Right gaze preference	Hemiparesis or quadriparesis	Gait ataxia
Aphasia	Neglect (of the left side)	Sensory loss in hemibody or all limbs	Truncal ataxia
Right visual field deficit	Left visual field deficit	Ipsilateral face and contralateral body symptoms	Ipsilateral limb ataxia
Right hemiparesis	Left hemiparesis	Disconjugate gaze	
Right hemisensory loss	Left hemisensory loss	Dysphagia, ↓ consciousness	

MNEMONIC

Basic work up for stroke:

The 3 P's

Pipes—cerebral imaging
Pump—cardioembolic source
Plasma—hypercoagulable workup

A   **ANSWER**

To evaluate concern for ↑ ICP, a CT scan and LP must be done. These tests will confirm your suspicion of pseudotumor cerebri.

Diagnosis

- **Noncontrast CT:**
    - Must first rule out hemorrhage (Table 11.3).
    - Ischemic lesions do not usually appear during the first 24 to 48 hours after stroke. Lesions appear hypodense (dark) and ↑ in density with evolution.
- **MRI:** Shows ischemic changes within hours of the event as well as small infarcts missed by CT. MRI also offers better visualization of the posterior fossa (Figure 11.3).
- **Cerebral angiography:** The "gold standard" of cerebrovascular imaging. Shows the site and severity of occlusive disease, as well as intracranial artery dissection if present. However, CT and MRI are preferred because they are more readily available, less invasive, and angiography ↑ risk of stroke.
- **Workup for a cardioembolic source:** ECG and cardiac monitoring, carotid ultrasound or neck MRA, echocardiogram with bubble study.
- **Hypercoagulable workup:** Appropriate if the patient is <55 years of age or has associated symptoms or risk factors. Consider sickle cell disease in a child.

Management

- **Stabilize the patient** first. Assess the airway, avoid hypotension.
- **Permissive hypertension:** Do not treat unless SBP >220 mm Hg or DBP >120 mm Hg (SBP >185 mm Hg and DBP >110 mm Hg if undergoing thrombolytic therapy).
- **Thrombolysis** is indicated for ischemic stroke (not for TIA) in patients who meet the criteria listed in Table 11.3.
- If the patient is not an IV **recombinant tissue plasminogen activator** (tPA) candidate, cerebral intra-arterial thrombolysis or mechanical embolectomy may still be options.

TABLE 11.3.   **Criteria for IV Recombinant Tissue Plasminogen Activator**

INCLUSION CRITERIA	EXCLUSION CRITERIA
<3 hr from symptom onset	History of intracranial hemorrhage
Age ≥18 years	Prior stroke in previous 3 months
Head CT ⊖ for hemorrhagic stroke	Active bleeding
Extended window of 3-4.5 hr for age 18-80 years	Platelet count <100,000
	Current use of coumadin or direct thrombin inhibitors

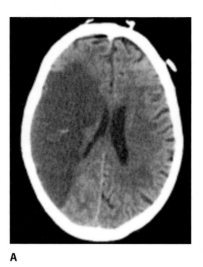
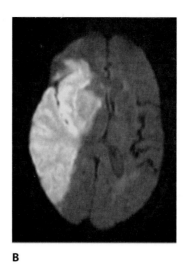
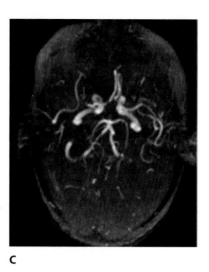

A   B   C

FIGURE 11.3.   **Acute ischemic stroke.** Acute left hemiparesis in a 62-year-old woman. (A) Noncontrast head CT with loss of gray and white matter differentiation and asymmetrically ↓ size of the right lateral ventricle in a right MCA distribution (indicating mass effect from associated edema). (B) Diffusion-weighted MRI with reduced diffusion (bright area) in the same distribution, consistent with an acute infarct. (C) Maximum-intensity projection of the intracranial vessels (time-of-flight MRA) shows the cause: an abrupt occlusion of the proximal right MCA (arrow). Compare with the normal left MCA (arrowhead). (Reproduced with permission from USMLE-Rx.com.)

- **Antiplatelet therapy**
  - Early antiplatelet therapy with ASA 160 to 325 mg, combination ASA-dipyrimidole, or clopidogrel.
  - Wait 24 hours to initiate if patient received tPA, otherwise give immediately.
  - Continue as long as benefits outweigh risks for secondary prevention.
- **Anticoagulation** is only indicated for patients with a cardioembolic source, eg, atrial fibrillation or cardiac thrombus.
- **Carotid endarterectomy:** For 2° prevention if ipsilateral carotid artery stenosis is >70%.

HEMORRHAGIC STROKE

The two etiologies of hemorrhagic stroke are intracerebral hemorrhage (ICH) and subarachnoid hemorrhage (SAH), compared in Table 11.4.

Symptoms/Exam

- Presents with sudden severe headache, nausea, vomiting, and ↓ level of consciousness.
- Papilledema.
- Rapid onset of focal neurologic symptoms is seen.

TABLE 11.4.   **Intracerebral Hemorrhage Versus Subarachnoid Hemorrhage**

	ICH (~ 90%)	SAH (~ 10%)
Causes	HTN, cerebral amyloid arthropathy, arteriovenous malformation (AVM), brain tumor, bleeding disorders, anticoagulation, thrombolytic therapy	Ruptured aneurysm, trauma, AVM
Other risk factors	Older age, high alcohol intake, smoking, black ethnicity	HTN, smoking, family history Hereditary syndromes: Ehlers-Danlos, Marfan, autosomal dominant polycystic kidney disease

- Meningeal irritation is possible and may lead to nuchal rigidity, more likely in SAH. One or both of the following signs may be present (Figure 11.4):
  - ⊕ Kernig sign: Passive extension of a flexed knee produces pain and resistance.
  - ⊕ Brudzinski sign: Passive flexion of the neck causes flexion of the hips and knees.

Differential

Ischemic stroke, seizure, subdural or epidural hematoma, dural sinus thrombosis, intracranial mass, meningitis, migraine, hypertensive emergency, temporal arteritis.

Diagnosis

- CT shows immediate **high-density (bright) lesions,** as in Figures 11.5 and 11.6.
- Check bleeding times, toxicology screen, CBC, and CMP.
- If the CT is normal but SAH is still suspected, obtain a **LP** to examine CSF for xanthochromia (yellowish color of CSF) or blood.

Management

- **Stabilize the patient:** Treat suspected herniation or ↑ ICP with mannitol, hyperventilation, and cooling blankets.
- **Consult neurosurgery:** Appropriate if treatable AVM, aneurysm, excisable tumor, or for decompression of superficial intracerebral hematomas. These measures can be lifesaving if the hemorrhage is large. Patients with small aneurysms may benefit from endovascular coiling.
- **Treat hypertension:** Gradually treat mean arterial pressure >130 mm Hg but maintain SBP >120 mm Hg.

Complications

Permanent disability, SIADH, seizure, rebleeding, death.

A ANSWER 1

When evaluating a TIA, studies and tests should be performed as if the patient has had a stroke because of its association with ↑ risk for having a stroke in the future.

A ANSWER 2

Concern for hemorrhagic stroke is high and a noncontrast CT of the head with CBC, chemistry panel, and coagulation studies are important first steps in evaluating this patient.

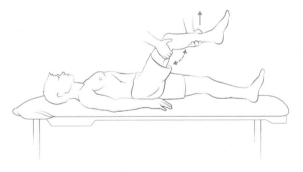

A

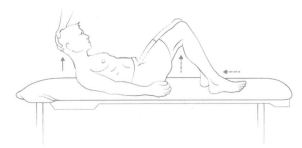

B

FIGURE 11.4. Kernig sign (**A**) and Brudzinski sign (**B**) in evaluation of subarachnoid hemorrhage. (Reproduced with permission from USMLE-Rx.com.)

Cerebral Lobe Dysfunctions

APHASIAS

Acquired language disorders, most often caused by cerebrovascular disease in dominant hemisphere.

- **Broca aphasia:** Speech that is **nonfluent, effortful,** sparse, and monotone, with impaired naming, repetition, and writing. **Comprehension is generally preserved,** and the patient is often aware of the deficit. Right hemiparesis and depression are common.
- **Wernicke aphasia: Fluent, possibly excessive** speech, with frequent paraphasias (substituting one word or phrase for another) and normal articulation. Patients may also have **impaired comprehension** of reading and speech as well as deficits in reading, writing, naming, and repetition. A right visual field cut may be present.
- **Global aphasia:** Involves impairment of all language functions, often accompanied by lethargy, right hemiparesis, hemisensory loss, apraxia, and visual field deficits.
- **Diagnosed** clinically and **treated** with speech therapy and supportive care.

Complications

Those with deficits of comprehension (eg, Wernicke aphasia) have a poorer prognosis for functional improvement or recovery than do those with deficits of expression.

AGNOSIA

Impaired recognition of familiar people or objects despite preservation of intelligence, attention, and perception. May involve visual, auditory, and/or tactile modalities.

- **Visual agnosia:** Inability to recognize familiar objects; often associated with right visual deficit. Impairment may be limited to identification or discrimination of **faces** of known people (prosopagnosia), **colors** (color agnosia), **objects** (object agnosia), or a whole item despite recognition of the parts (simultagnosia).
- **Auditory agnosia:** Inability to recognize familiar sounds despite intact hearing. Impairment may be limited to words, environmental sounds, or music.
- **Astereognosia:** Inability to identify objects through tactile stimulation despite intact sensation of touch. Patients may be able to describe and draw an object and name it from its image in the drawing yet not recognize it through touch.
- **Diagnosis:** Clinical. CT or MRI may be indicated to look for organic cause.
- **Management:** Supportive.

DYSARTHRIA

Poor articulation of appropriate words (slurred speech).

- **Symptoms/Exam:** May **present** with hoarseness and/or drooling. Reading comprehension and writing abilities remain intact.
- **Diagnosis:** Clinical, including testing for normal language functions to rule out aphasia; head **CT or MRI** to look for organic cause (eg, stroke).
- **Management:** Supportive with speech and language therapy.

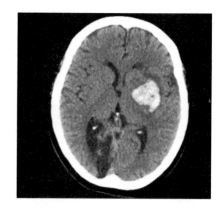

FIGURE 11.5. **Acute hemorrhagic stroke.** Unenhanced CT scan shows acute blood products with surrounding edema in the left basal ganglion with minimal mass effect on the left lateral ventricle in a 62-year-old woman with uncontrolled hypertension and acute onset of headache. (Reproduced with permission from USMLE-Rx.com.)

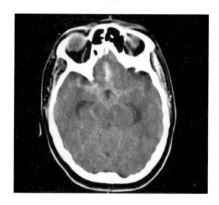

FIGURE 11.6. **Subarachnoid hemorrhage due to ruptured aneurysm.** Axial CT scan shows blood in the subarachnoid space that appears as hyperdense material collecting in the interhemispheric fissure and the cisterns near the skull base. The patient was a 50-year-old woman who collapsed suddenly in her bathroom. (Reproduced with permission from USMLE-Rx.com.)

 MNEMONIC

Wernicke aphasia is **W**ord salad.
Broca aphasia speech is **B**roken and effortful.

AMNESIAS

Severe disturbance of retained memory, with intact attention and language functions. Visuospatial functions are generally intact.

- **Transient global amnesia** is described as a paroxysmal, **transient loss of recent memory,** with preserved immediate recall and remote memory. Usually involves impaired ability to retain new information. Often caused by an emotional or physically stressful incident that occurred shortly before symptoms began. The patient may be confused and anxious, but **personal identity is retained.** Focal neurologic signs are absent. Typically lasts 30 minutes to 24 hours.
- **Korsakoff syndrome (KS)** is a permanent and significant impairment of short-term memory, with inability to form new memories and impaired remote memory that may result from **Wernicke encephalopathy (WE).** WE classically presents with the triad of **encephalopathy, oculomotor dysfunction, and gait ataxia,** but in reality confusion is the most common symptom. Caused by a deficiency in thiamine (vitamin B_1), and usually associated with heavy, long-term alcohol use. Patients who go on to develop KS have **apathy** and **lack of insight** into the disorder but are alert and responsive. Confabulation is common. Associated with peripheral neuropathy, hypothermia, nystagmus, and gait ataxia.

Diagnosis

- Based on the history and on the finding of anterograde amnesia with loss of recent memory. Otherwise neurologically normal in transient global amnesia. Peripheral neuropathy, nystagmus, and gait ataxia are present in Korsakoff syndrome.
- Head CT or MRI to examine for an underlying condition.

Management

- **Transient global amnesia:** Reassurance; neurology consult.
- **Korsakoff syndrome:** There is no treatment once a patient has progressed to have KS. Give thiamine before glucose to avoid precipitating WE in alcoholic patients or as soon as WE is recognized. Recommend a recovery program for alcoholic patients.

MNEMONIC

Korsakoff syndrome:

Alcoholics drink CANs of beer

Confusion
Ataxia
Nystagmus

KEY FACT

Transient global amnesia typically occurs in patients >40 years of age.

Seizure

Seizure is defined as a sudden change in neurologic function resulting from an abnormal, excessive, synchronous discharge of cortical neurons (Table 11.5).

TABLE 11.5. Types of Seizures

TYPE	PRESENTATION
Partial (restricted area; can become a generalized seizure)	Simple: intact consciousness; motor, sensory, autonomic, psychic Complex: impaired consciousness
Generalized (diffuse area)	Absence: petit mal; blank stare; no postictal state Myoclonic: quick, repetitive jerking Tonic: stiffening Tonic-clonic: grand mal; alternating stiffening and movement Atonic: commonly mistaken for fainting; "drop" seizures
Epileptic (recurrent seizures)	Any of the above Kindling, seizures beget seizures

FOCAL (PARTIAL) SEIZURE

Originate in one hemisphere. The terms simple, complex, and secondarily generalized have been replaced with descriptors such as without impairment of consciousness, with impairment of consciousness or awareness, and evolving to a bilateral convulsive seizure. Focal seizures are further categorized according to location:

- **Temporal lobe seizure:**
    - The seizure presents with unresponsive, quiet staring for 1 to 3 minutes and often is accompanied by an **aura** (eg, sensation of a particular smell, dizziness, nausea, or déjà vu).
    - Oral or ipsilateral manual automatisms may be present. Contralateral dystonic posturing of the arm and hand is common.
    - Postictal lethargy and confusion may last several minutes.
- **Frontal lobe seizure:**
    - Usually lasts 15 to 40 seconds without an aura or a postictal state.
    - Commonly occurs during sleep.
    - If the motor cortex is involved, rhythmic unilateral clonic activity may occur and spread across the body. Asymmetric tonic posturing is common with involvement of the supplemental motor area.
- **Occipital lobe seizure:**
    - Commonly begins with a visual aura that can range from spots or lights to formed visual hallucinations that are usually stereotyped from seizure to seizure.
    - May spread to the temporal lobe or the motor cortex.

Differential

Syncope, orthostatic hypotension, hypoglycemia, hypoxia, migraine, TIA, panic attack, psychogenic seizure, narcolepsy, tics.

Diagnosis

- Obtain a detailed history of the event, prodromal symptoms, witnessed seizures, and postictal state. Evaluate for risk factors—eg, head trauma, stroke, tumor, AVM, or a family history of seizures.
- Seizure threshold is lowered by many medications and triggers like sleep deprivation, stress, illness, or flickering lights. A few of the more common responsible medications include tramadol; diphenhydramine; and bupropion, venlafaxine, and other antidepressants.
- Check a CBC, CMP, and a toxicology screen as well as calcium, magnesium, alcohol, and ammonia levels.
- EEG and video EEG monitoring.
- **MRI** for new onset seizures to look for underlying brain lesion.

Management

Acute seizure: Stabilize patients and protect them from harm. Administer lorazepam IV or IM; diazepam IV or per rectum in gel form; or midazolam IV or sublingually. Give glucose if the patient is hypoglycemic. Treat severe hypertension. Correct any metabolic causes.

Complications

- May progress to a generalized seizure.
- Falls and injuries.
- Patients are at risk for depression, anxiety, and psychosis.
- Side effects and drug interactions associated with antiepileptic medications.

KEY FACT

Temporal lobe seizures are the most common seizures in adults.

KEY FACT

Do not start antiepileptics for a single isolated seizure.

QUESTION 1

A 78-year-old man with a history of CAD and type 2 DM presents to the ED because of difficulty speaking. The patient attempts to tell you his history but his speech is halting and he becomes frustrated. His wife explains that ever since they woke up this morning he cannot find the words he is looking for, and he is speaking in a very choppy manner. What is the next best step?

QUESTION 2

A mother brings her 8-year-old boy to the clinic because his teachers complain that he "daydreams too much" and has 20-second "staring spells" during which he stays still and does not react to anything that is said. He is doing well in school and has many friends. His exam is unremarkable. How do you proceed?

GENERALIZED SEIZURE

Generalized seizures involve the whole brain and are categorized as follows:

- **Tonic-clonic (grand mal):**
  - Tonic phase gradually progresses to a clonic phase, with each lasting about 30 seconds.
  - **Incontinence or tongue biting** may occur during the seizure.
  - The postictal state includes coarse breathing, with gradual awakening over several minutes. Postictal acidosis with ↓ HCO_3, ↑ CK, and ↑ prolactin may occur within 30 minutes after a seizure.
- **Absence (petit mal):**
  - Sudden-onset **staring spells**, usually **lasting about 10 seconds**, with immediate recovery. Those lasting 20 to 30 seconds may also have simple automatisms.
  - **Eye fluttering** or altered postural tone is common and may occur many times per day.
  - EEG shows **generalized spike-and-wave** discharges.
- **Myoclonic:**
  - Brief, **sharp muscle jerks** with no impairment of consciousness.
  - Movements may be symmetric, asymmetric, or multifocal.
  - EEG shows a **generalized polyspike-and-wave discharge.**
- **Tonic:**
  - Brief, sudden, bilateral, and symmetric tonic posturing, with brief impairment of consciousness and rapid recovery.
  - EEG shows **sudden, diffuse low-voltage β waves** or background attenuation.
- Diagnostic workup and management is the same as that for focal seizures.

FEBRILE SEIZURE

See the Child and Adolescent Medicine chapter.

STATUS EPILEPTICUS

A neurologic emergency consisting of continuous seizure activity lasting ≥5 minutes or repetitive seizures lasting >30 minutes, without a return to a baseline neurologic level between seizures. (Note: definitions of time for continuous seizure activity range from 5 to 30 minutes.)

Differential

Syncope, intracranial infection, migraine, hypoglycemia, psychogenic seizure.

Diagnosis

Made clinically in cases of sustained overt convulsions. An EEG may be needed for more subtle findings. In children <3 years of age, status epilepticus is more likely to have an underlying cause (such as CNS infection, vascular disorders, anoxia, trauma, intoxication, fever, or metabolic abnormalities). In older children, it is more often the result of a chronic seizure disorder.

Management

- Stabilize the patient, ABCs.
- **Lorazepam 4 mg IV** (0.1 mg/kg). Alternatives include diazepam and midazolam.
- If no response **after 1 minute, repeat** lorazepam 4 mg IV.
- If seizure persists start **fosphenytoin** or **phenytoin** bolus + infusion.
- Consider intubation.

A **ANSWER 1**

Perform a full neurologic exam and order a head CT without contrast to assess for stroke or intracranial lesion.

A **ANSWER 2**

The description of the child indicates appropriate development, so you suspect absence seizures. An EEG is the best diagnostic measure. Educational material is also important for the parents and school.

- If the patient continues seizing after 30 minutes, the seizure is considered refractory—begin continuous EEG monitoring.
- Next treatment steps are bolus + infusion of **phenobarbital,** sedation with **midazolam, pentobarbital,** or **propofol.**

Complications

Respiratory failure, rhabdomyolysis, hyperthermia, neuronal cell damage.

EPILEPSY

History of ≥2 unprovoked seizures greater than 24 hours apart.
- Medication choice depends on seizure type, patient response and comorbidities. Table 11.6 lists medication options.
- **Common side effects of antiseizure drugs:** GI symptoms, rash, somnolence, dizziness.
- **Rare but serious side effects:** Stevens-Johnson syndrome/toxic epidermal necrolysis, agranulocytosis, aplastic anemia, hepatic failure, serum sickness, multiorgan hypersensitivity, ↑ risk of suicidal ideation.
- Antiepileptics are teratogenic.
  - Perform a **pregnancy test** before starting any antiepileptic medication and offer **contraceptives** to all women of childbearing age.
  - Pregnant women with epilepsy may consider antiseizure drug withdrawal 6 months prior to planned conception if they have been seizure free for ≥2 years. All others should **continue the most effective seizure drug,** at the lowest possible dose. The exception to this rule is valproate, because of its association with **neural tube defects.** Women taking carbamazepine or valproate require **higher-dose folate supplementation** (4 mg/day).
- Surgery to remove seizure foci is possible in many patients.

KEY FACT

Most patients with >3 seizure-free years on medication will not have recurrences.

KEY FACT

Most cases of epilepsy start before 20 years of age.

Syncope

Episodic loss of consciousness and postural tone, with spontaneous recovery. Can occur with any global ↓ in cerebral perfusion. Incidence ↑ with age. Other types of syncope include orthostatic, neurogenic, and cardiac.

Symptoms
- Loss of consciousness, with loss of postural tone and spontaneous recovery.
- May be preceded by nausea, faintness, blurred vision, diaphoresis, vertigo, paresthesias, or pallor.
- No post-event confusion.

KEY FACT

The most common form of syncope is vasovagal/neurocardiogenic.

Possible causes (listed from most to least common): Neurocardiogenic, cardiovascular (eg, arrhythmia, myocardial dysfunction), orthostatic hypotension, and neurologic (eg, stroke, vertebrobasilar insufficiency).

TABLE 11.6. **Medications for Epilepsy**

	COMMON FIRST-LINE OPTIONS	COMMON ALTERNATIVES
Generalized and focal seizures	Phenytoin, carbamazepine, and valproic acid	Gabapentin, lamotrigine, levetiracetam, oxcarbazepine, and topiramate
Absence seizures	**Ethosuximide** or valproic acid	

QUESTION

A 75-year-old man comes to your clinic after falling when he got up at night to urinate. He denies any loss of consciousness and reports his vision going black before he fell to the ground. What will your next steps be?

Diagnosis

- Check medications, activities, and position at the time of the event.
- Check for orthostatic BP changes, consider tilt-table testing.
- ECG for arrhythmia; echocardiogram for cardiac outlet obstruction.

Management

Treat the underlying cause. Avoid precipitating factors and medications.

Vertigo

The perception of movement of the body or the environment when no movement occurs. May be central or peripheral.

CENTRAL VERTIGO

The illusion of movement of the body or environment in conjunction with nausea, vomiting, or gait ataxia.

- Associated with vertical, unidirectional, or multidirectional nystagmus that may be different in both eyes.
- **No extinguishing of symptoms or symptom latency occurs with provocative maneuvers** such as the Dix-Hallpike.
- Can distinguish from peripheral by presence of other neurologic deficits, which may include diplopia, dysarthria, facial motor or sensory asymmetry. Other motor or sensory deficits, hyperreflexia, extensor plantar responses, or limb ataxia may be present.
- **Possible causes:** Stroke, vertebrobasilar insufficiency, migraine-associated vertigo, multiple sclerosis.
- **Diagnosis:** By history and provocative maneuvers. Brain imaging with CT and/or MRI may be indicated to look for underlying etiology, MRI is best if ischemia of brain stem is suspected.
- **Management:** Treatment of the underlying disease. Supportive care with IV fluids if dehydrated from vomiting.

PERIPHERAL VERTIGO

Presents in the same manner as central vertigo, but symptoms are generally intermittent and more severe or distressing.

- **Hearing loss or tinnitus** is common.
- **Unidirectional or rotational nystagmus** (not vertical) may be present. Eyes drift toward the affected side.
- Provocative maneuvers such as the Dix-Hallpike (or Nylen-Bárány) maneuver elicit symptoms and nystagmus with symptom latency and extinguishment on repetition.
- **Possible causes:** Benign positional peripheral vertigo (BPPV), labyrinthitis, Ménière disease, acoustic neuroma, drug toxicity (aminoglycosides and some diuretics are known for ototoxicity).
- **Diagnosis:** Provocation of symptoms with the Dix-Hallpike (or Nylen-Bárány) maneuver. No imaging necessary unless there is question about central versus peripheral cause.

Management

- Meclizine for BPPV. Correct any underlying metabolic disorders.
- Discontinue or taper contributing medications.
- Offer education on desensitization exercises and otolith repositioning procedures.

Sleep Disorders

NARCOLEPSY

Sudden onset of irresistible sleep throughout the day; occurs during unusual circumstances such as talking, eating. Affects men and women equally. Usually has genetic association.

- **Symptoms/Exam:** Presents with cataplexy, the sudden loss of muscle tone with strong emotion, without loss of consciousness. Sleep paralysis and visual or auditory hallucinations may also be present. The age of onset tends to be 15 to 35 years of age.
- **Diagnosis of exclusion:** Narcolepsy should be high on your differential if there are two to six episodes of unintentional sleep a day. Order a sleep study to rule out other disorders, such as sleep apnea (see the Pulmonary chapter for more on sleep apnea).
- **Management:** Treat with timed naps around meals, stimulant medications, TCAs, and MAO inhibitors.

MNEMONIC

Symptoms of narcolepsy:
CHAP
Cataplexy
Hallucinations
Attacks of sleep
Paralysis on waking

NIGHT TERRORS

Non-REM sleep disorder characterized by a state of arousal with fear and anxiety, tachycardia, and diaphoresis during sleep. Individual is often difficult to arouse and will spontaneously go back to sleep. May be triggered by stressful events or certain medications.

- **Symptoms/Exam:** Usually occurs in children 2 to 7 years of age. Manifests as inconsolable screaming and thrashing. Episodes can last 30 minutes and may be associated with sleepwalking. The next day, the child has no recollection of events.
- **Management:** Supportive, focusing on parental reassurance and prevention of injury to the child. Waking the child several minutes before the usual time of occurrence for several days may break the cycle. Usually self-resolves by adolescence.

Movement Disorders

ATAXIAS

Incoordination and irregularity of voluntary movement. Categorized as follows:
- **Cerebellar ataxia:**
  - Presents with hypotonia and irregularities in the rate, amplitude, and force of voluntary movements. Terminal dysmetria, "overshooting," and terminal intention tremor are seen.
  - Complex movements are performed as a series of individual movements.
  - Nystagmus, gaze pareses, and defective saccadic and pursuit movement are possible.
- **Proprioceptive ataxia:**
  - Symmetrically affects the legs and gait, with limited or no arm involvement.
  - Involves impairment of vibratory sense, joint position sense, and proprioception.
  - Improved balance is achieved with use of a cane or other support or by watching one's own feet while walking. Symptoms worsen when the patient's eyes are closed.

Q QUESTION

A 16-year-old girl presents because of excessive sleepiness and unintentional nap-taking. Her mother has a history of narcolepsy treated with modafinil, and feels that her daughter has the same problem. She wants to know if you can start her on a medication. What is your response?

KEY FACT

Friedreich ataxia is the most prevalent inherited ataxia.

- Romberg sign is ⊕, and patients exhibit a wide-based, high-stepping gait, and poor heel-to-toe walking.
- **Vestibular ataxia:** Ataxia with unilateral nystagmus that ↑ with gaze away from the affected side. Romberg sign is ⊕, and patients fall *toward* the affected side.

Friedreich Ataxia

An idiopathic **progressive spinocerebellar disorder** typically presenting at 4 to 20 years of age. The most common hereditary ataxia. Typically **autosomal recessive,** with an expanded GAA trinucleotide repeat on chromosome 9 in the frataxin gene. Associated progressive **kyphoscoliosis** can lead to **restrictive lung disease** and **cardiomyopathy.**

Symptoms/Exam

- **Progressive mixed sensory and cerebellar gait ataxia** involves all limbs within 2 years of onset.
- Extensor plantar responses occur within 5 years.
- ↓ knee and ankle reflexes are seen, along with cerebellar dysarthria and impaired position and vibratory senses. Weakness of the legs and arms tends to be found late in the course of the disease.
- **Pes cavus** and kyphoscoliosis are common. Nystagmus, paresthesias, tremors, vertigo, spasticity, and ↓ vision and hearing are also seen.

Differential

Vitamin E deficiency, ataxia-telangiectasia, abetalipoproteinemia, spinocerebellar ataxia.

Diagnosis

- Sensory nerve action potentials are absent or ↓.
- MRI reveals cervical spinal cord atrophy and minimal cerebellar atrophy; chest and spine x-rays show kyphoscoliosis.
- Echocardiography reveals associated ventricular hypertrophy.

Management

Supportive care and treatment of associated cardiac and endocrine disorders. Orthopedic procedures can assist with foot deformities.

Complications

Disability with inability to walk unassisted may occur within 5 years of onset. Patients are typically bedridden 10 to 20 years after onset, though progression is variable. The average life span is 37 years.

Ataxia-Telangiectasia

An inherited **autosomal-recessive** disorder characterized by **cerebellar ataxia,** progressive pancerebellar degeneration, variable **immunodeficiency,** impaired organ maturation, predisposition to malignancy, and **ocular and cutaneous telangiectasia.** Onset is in infancy.

Symptoms/Exam

- Presents with nystagmus and cerebellar dysarthria, with gait, **limb, and trunk ataxia.** Loss of vibration and position sense, **choreoathetosis,** areflexia, and disorders of eye movement are seen.

ANSWER

First, the patient should undergo a basic workup, including a sleep log and overnight polysomnography to rule out other sleep disorders.

- **Telangiectasias** appear during the teen years, first on the eyes and then on sun-exposed areas of the skin (Figure 11.7).
- Mental deficiency typically appears in the second decade.
- Recurrent upper and lower respiratory tract infections are seen, hypogonadism, and insulin resistance.

Differential

Refsum disease, Niemann-Pick disease, Friedreich ataxia, cerebral palsy, familial spinocerebellar atrophies, cerebellar tumor.

Diagnosis

- Look for ↑ levels of AFP and CEA and/or chromosomal abnormalities such as inversions and translocations in chromosomes 7 and 14.
- Low lymphocyte count, ↓ IgA, IgG, and IgE; poor skin test response to common antigens.

Management

- Avoid all x-rays because of abnormal cellular sensitivity to ionizing radiation.
- Supportive care; antibiotics for any bacterial infections.

Complications

Death usually occurs in adolescence. Associated with ↑ risk of leukemia and lymphoma.

Acute Cerebellar Ataxia

Presents as sudden onset of truncal ataxia a few weeks after viral illness that may also be associated with dysmetria and nystagmus. Varicella, EBV, HSV-1, and coxsackievirus are the most commonly involved viruses.

- **Diagnosis:** Workup involves brain CT to rule out tumor; LP if patient is febrile or has meningitic signs; screen for toxins, including alcohol; consider urinary catecholamines if concerned for neuroblastoma, as all are also on the differential.
- **Management:** Supportive, and symptoms usually self-resolve within 2 to 3 weeks. Approximately 10% of patients have long-term neurologic deficits.

HUNTINGTON DISEASE

An **autosomal-dominant** disorder, with gradual onset and progression of **chorea** and **dementia**, usually starting at 35 to 50 years of age. Chromosome 4 shows excess **CAG trinucleotide repeats**.

Symptoms/Exam

- **Chorea:** Derived from the Latin word for dance (like choreography). Rapid, irregular, involuntary, and purposeless movement that goes from one body part to another.
- **Athetosis:** Slow, **sinuous, writhing movements** that may be generalized or restricted to one area of the body. Symptoms are ↑ by emotional stress and voluntary activity and are not present during sleep.
- Dystonia, tics, inhibitory pauses in voluntary movements, explosive speech, depression, and psychosis are common features.
- Also associated with irritability, moodiness, antisocial behavior, and later with dementia. Fidgetiness and restlessness may be seen early in the disease.

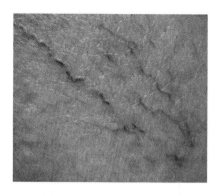

FIGURE 11.7. Blanching dilated superficial capillaries representing telangiectasia. (Reproduced with permission from Wolff K, et al. *Fitzpatrick's Dermatology in General Medicine*, 7th ed. New York: McGraw-Hill, 2008, Fig. 4-34.)

 MNEMONIC

Clinical features of cerebellar disease:

DANISH

Dysdiadochokinesia
Ataxia
Nystagmus
Intention tremor
Scanning dysarthria
Heel-shin test positive

 QUESTION 1

A 15-year-old boy with history of Friedreich ataxia presents to your office for an annual physical. He is still able to walk and gets regular physical and occupational therapy. He does report getting short of breath during his therapy sessions. What is this concerning for?

 QUESTION 2

A 65-year-old woman complains of worsening tremor. She reports that for the last 10 years she has noticed shaking of both hands whenever she reaches for things. Her mother and brother both have a similar tremor. She has noticed it goes away temporarily after a glass of wine, so she is wondering if there is a medication that might help. She has no other signs or symptoms concerning for Parkinson disease.

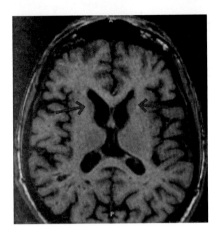

FIGURE 11.8. Huntington disease.
Axial T$_1$-weighted image demonstrates atrophy of the caudate nuclei, better seen on the right, resulting in slight expansion of the frontal horns of the lateral ventricles (right greater than left). (Reproduced with permission from USMLE-Rx.com.)

KEY FACT

Postural tremor is usually an exaggeration of normal physiologic tremor.

KEY FACT

The dementia of Creutzfeldt-Jakob disease has rapid onset and progression.

ANSWER 1

Heart failure or arrhythmia from cardio-myopathy. Patients with Friedreich ataxia should have annual echocardiographs, with additional workup as indicated if symptoms arise.

ANSWER 2

This case describes an essential tremor, which is a type of postural tremor. If it interferes with function, essential tremor can be treated with propranolol or primidone.

Differential

- Other hereditary causes of chorea: Wilson disease, spinocerebellar ataxias, ataxia-telangiectasia, Lesch-Nyhan syndrome.
- Acquired causes of chorea: Drug-induced (eg, levodopa), vascular, autoimmune disorders, Sydenham chorea.

Diagnosis

- Clinical suspicion is confirmed with genetic studies of the **huntingtin gene**.
- Head CT shows cerebral and caudate nucleus atrophy (Figure 11.8).

Management

- Supportive treatment. Dopamine receptor blockers for chorea symptoms; SSRIs to reduce aggression.
- Offer genetic counseling to family members.

Complications

Usually fatal 10 to 20 years after clinical onset. There is a high rate of suicide among patients with Huntington disease.

TREMOR

Rhythmic oscillatory movement, categorized as follows:
- **Postural tremor:** Tremor with sustained posture of an extremity. Symptoms ↑ with emotional stress or sleep deprivation and are not present during sleep. They also ↑ with use of TCAs, valproic acid, lithium, and bronchodilators.
- **Intention tremor:** Tremor during movement that ↑ as a target is approached. May be associated with cerebellar signs. No tremor at rest.
- **Resting tremor:** Tremor at rest. May affect the fingers, hands, forearms, or feet. Has a **frequency of 4 to 6 Hz.** Associated with hypokinesia or rigidity when due to parkinsonism (for more on Parkinson disease, see the Geriatric Medicine chapter).
- **Differential:** Along with differentiating between types of tremor, consider cerebellar disorders, Wilson disease, Parkinson disease, drug toxicity or withdrawal, and hyperthyroidism.
- **Diagnosis:** Guided by the history and exam. In intention tremor, MRI may show a lesion of the superior cerebellar peduncle.
- **Management:** Treat any underlying condition. β-blockers or anticonvulsants may reduce benign essential tremor. Severe intention tremor may be treated with thalamus stereotactic surgery or high-frequency stimulation via an implanted device.

CREUTZFELDT-JAKOB DISEASE

A **prion disease** characterized by **rapidly progressive dementia** in association with **diffuse myoclonic jerks.** Also known as subacute spongiform encephalopathy.

Symptoms/Exam

- Presents with rapidly progressive dementia, with late akinetic mutism and coma.
- Anxiety, **personality change,** depression, emotional lability, delusions, and hallucinations are also seen.
- Motor symptoms include myoclonus, cerebellar ataxia, rigidity, bradykinesia, tremor, chorea, and dystonia.

Differential

Alzheimer disease, Parkinson disease, progressive supranuclear palsy, intracerebral mass, hydrocephalus, multi-infarct dementia.

Diagnosis

- Definitive diagnosis is by immunodetection of the prion in brain tissue on biopsy.
- Brain MRI T_2-weighted and diffusion-weighted images show hyperintense signals in the basal ganglia.
- EEG may show periodic sharp waves or spikes. CSF protein may be ↑.

Management

Supportive. Disease is fatal within several months of diagnosis.

TICS

Repetitive, stereotyped movements or vocalizations. May be caused by transient tic disorder in children, or Tourette syndrome.

- **Symptoms/Exam:** Presents as blinking, sniffing, stretching of the neck or mouth, or touching something repetitively. Voluntary suppression may produce anxiety, whereas performing the tic may relieve tension. Symptoms ↑ with emotional stress and ↓ with voluntary activity. No symptoms occur during sleep.
- **Management:** Treatment with benzodiazepines or clonidine may be helpful. Antipsychotic medications such as haloperidol may be used for severe cases. Injected botulinum toxin can alleviate symptoms.

RESTLESS LEGS SYNDROME

- **Diagnosis:** Clinical. Check for **pregnancy, iron deficiency anemia**, uremia, or peripheral neuropathy. Family history is often ⊕.
- **Management:** Treated with levodopa, ropinirole, pramipexole, clonazepam, or gabapentin. Important to also treat underlying iron deficiency.

Demyelinating Diseases

MULTIPLE SCLEROSIS

A chronic **multifocal demyelinating** neurologic disorder that involves different parts of the CNS at various points in time. There is a female-to-male ratio of 2:1. The disease takes **four forms:** relapsing and remitting, 1° progressive, 2° progressive, and progressive relapsing (Table 11.7). Most cases are relapsing and remitting.

Symptoms/Exam

- Often nonspecific. Focal limb weakness, numbness, paresthesias, a bandlike sensation around the trunk or a limb, ataxia, diplopia, dysarthria, intention tremor, and bladder dysfunction. May also present as spastic paraparesis and sensory deficit.
- **Optic neuritis** (sudden loss or blurring of vision in one eye) is the presenting symptom in 25% of cases.
- Symptoms are transient, lasting days to weeks.
- A complete neurologic exam should be performed, looking for focal areas of sensory deficit and weakness or an afferent papillary defect. One specific finding is Lhermitte sign, an electric shock–like sensation down the spine with neck flexion.

Differential

ALS, acute disseminated encephalomyelitis, Bell palsy, brain or spinal cord infection, HIV, trauma, sarcoidosis, stroke, syphilis, SLE, Lyme disease, TIA, trigeminal neuralgia.

 MNEMONIC

Think Creutzfeldt-Jakob disease: 5 S's
Sporadic incidence
Startle myoclonus
Sharp waves on EEG
Signals hyperintense on MRI
Spongiform encephalopathy

 KEY FACT

Tourette syndrome is a neuropsychiatric disorder with onset in childhood, characterized by multiple motor tics and at least one vocal tic.

 MNEMONIC

Symptoms of restless legs syndrome:
URGE
Urge to move
Rest-induced
Gets better with activity
Evening and night accentuation

 KEY FACT

About 80% of patients with restless legs syndrome have periodic limb movement disorder, which is involuntary leg twitching during sleep.

 KEY FACT

The incidence of MS is highest among whites and increases farther away from the equator.

 QUESTION

A 29-year-old woman has fatigue and some right-sided clumsiness. These symptoms wane over weeks. Months later, she notices blurry vision and decides to get new glasses. However, new-onset left-hand numbness and a tingling sensation around her trunk prompt her to visit your clinic first, where she is found to have focal areas of ↓ sensation. What are your next steps?

TABLE 11.7.   **Types of Multiple Sclerosis**

TYPE	FEATURES
Relapsing and remitting	Relapses followed by incomplete remissions; during relapses, symptoms can grow more severe
1° progressive	Gradual, steady progression of symptoms from initial presentation
2° progressive	Gradual progression of symptoms and disability over time following a period of relapsing-remitting disease
Progressive relapsing	Gradual symptom progression over time accompanied by acute attacks of worse symptoms

KEY FACT

MS is the most common acquired neurologic disability in young adults.

MNEMONIC

To remember some of the classic characteristics of MS:

INSULAR

Intention tremor
Nystagmus
Slurred speech
Uthoff phenomenon (symptoms worsen with exposure to extremes of temperature)
Lhermitte sign
Ataxia
Relapsing

Diagnosis

- MRI is the most sensitive study and shows white matter lesions (Figure 11.9).
- Diagnosis requires evidence of CNS lesions disseminated in time and space—this is primarily based on clinical symptoms, MRI findings support the diagnosis.
- Visual evoked potentials show prolonged responses, and CSF is ⊕ for **oligoclonal bands.**

Management

- Relapsing-remitting MS: **Disease-modifying therapy** is first-line; agents include interferon-β, glatiramer acetate, dimethyl fumarate.
- Acute exacerbations: corticosteroids.
- Progressive: more difficult to treat. Azathioprine, cladribine, cyclophosphamide; interferons and glatiramer acetate are used but are less effective than in relapsing-remitting type.

A   **ANSWER**

New-onset neurologic symptoms in a young woman are concerning for intracranial or spinal cord lesions. An MRI is the best test to look for white matter lesions and diagnose MS.

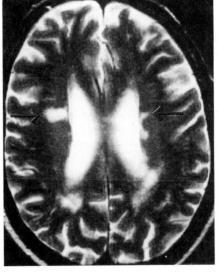

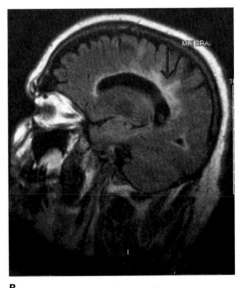

A   B

FIGURE 11.9.   **Multiple sclerosis.** Transaxial T_2-weighted MRI (**A**) and sagittal FLAIR image (**B**) show multiple MS plaques (arrows) in the periventricular matter oriented radially from the corpus callosum ("Dawson fingers"). (Reproduced with permission from Ropper AH, Samuels MA. *Adams & Victor's Principles of Neurology,* 9th ed. New York: McGraw-Hill, 2009, Fig. 36-1.)

Complications

Relapsing-remitting may progress to a chronic progressive form. Residual impairment of color vision and depth perception is common, as is chronic disability.

OPTIC NEURITIS

Partial or total vision loss, usually monocular, caused by optic nerve demyelination that presents with **eye pain**. Other symptoms include afferent pupillary defect and abnormal color vision.

- **Diagnosis:** Funduscopic exam may reveal papillitis and edema of the optic nerve, but most cases are **retrobulbar with a normal initial funduscopic exam.** CSF may show pleocytosis and ↑ IgG production.
- **Management:** IV methylprednisolone, followed by oral prednisone. Treatment does not affect long-term vision outcomes, but it does hasten recovery and reduce risk of conversion to MS temporarily.

TRANSVERSE MYELITIS

- **Symptoms/Exam:** Presents with rapidly evolving paraparesis or paraplegia with ascending paresthesias, sensory loss, sphincter dysfunction, and loss of deep sensation in the feet. History may include infectious illness in the preceding weeks. On exam, a sensory level on the trunk and bilateral extensor plantar signs are present.
- **Diagnosis:** Via CSF showing a moderate level of lymphocytes and an ↑ in total protein, although this may not be found early in the disease course. MRI shows focal demyelination in the expected level of the spinal cord.
- **Management:** Treat with IV glucocorticoids followed by oral steroids. Plasmapheresis is considered a second-line agent.

Eye Movement and Cranial Nerve Disorders

INTERNUCLEAR OPHTHALMOPLEGIA

Defined as a disconjugate gaze, with impaired adduction and nystagmus of the abducting eye, due to a lesion of the **medial longitudinal fasciculus.** Consider **MS** if the disease is bilateral or in a young adult. Vascular disease is likely in older patients or those with unilateral involvement.

- **Diagnosis:** On exam, the ipsilateral eye fails to adduct when the patient looks toward the opposite side (Figure 11.10). Nystagmus is present in the contralateral eye. Neuroimaging is required to look for possible etiologies.
- **Management:** Treat any underlying cause.

HORNER SYNDROME

Unilateral **miotic pupil** with **ipsilateral mild ptosis,** often associated with **ipsilateral anhidrosis,** caused by interruption of the sympathetic innervation of the eye (Figure 11.11).

- **Symptoms/Exam:** Reveals normal response to light and accommodation. The ipsilateral conjunctiva may be acutely injected, and the ipsilateral face may be warm and hyperemic. Slow pupillary dilation is seen on the affected side. Be sure to distinguish from Argyll Robertson pupil (associated with syphilis), in which the pupil accommodates but does not react. Common **causes** include cervical cord lesion, pulmonary apical or mediastinal tumor, neck trauma or mass, cluster headache, carotid artery thrombosis, and brain stem infarct.

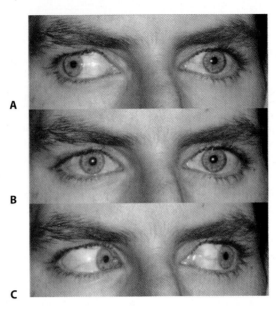

FIGURE 11.10. **Eye movements in internuclear ophthalmoplegia.** Right gaze (**A**) demonstrates impaired adduction of the left eye with normal abduction of the right eye, primary gaze (**B**), and left gaze (**C**). (Reproduced with permission from USMLE-Rx.com.)

- **Diagnosis:** Workup is based on the history and exam. MRI to look for intracranial lesion if there is numbness of the ipsilateral face and contralateral extremities or ipsilateral abducens palsy; chest x-ray for suspicion of chest tumor. Concomitant neck pain may be associated with carotid artery dissection and warrants an MRA.
- **Management:** Treat the underlying cause.

BELL PALSY

Abrupt onset of **LMN facial weakness** or paralysis that is usually **unilateral.** Caused by damage to the facial nerve CN VII (Figure 11.12).

Symptoms/Exam

- Symptoms progress over hours to 1 to 2 days. An **impaired sense of taste, hyperacusis,** and **lacrimation** are common.
- The ipsilateral eye may be difficult to close. Pain around the ipsilateral ear is possible.
- No abnormalities are found beyond the facial nerve territory.

Differential

Intracranial tumor, stroke, Ramsay Hunt syndrome, Lyme disease, sarcoidosis, AIDS, acoustic neuroma, Guillain-Barré syndrome.

KEY FACT

Bell palsy can be differentiated from a central lesion by involvement of the first branch of CN VII. In contrast, stroke leading to facial weakness spares the brow, as illustrated in Figure 11.12.

A   ANSWER

Chest x-ray. The physical exam is consistent with Horner syndrome, and the history of lung cancer is concerning for a new or mediastinal mass.

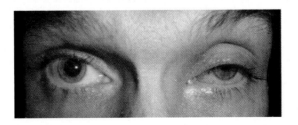

FIGURE 11.11. **Horner syndrome.** Anisocoria, ptosis of the left upper lid, and conjunctival hyperemia of the left eye are consistent with acute Horner syndrome. The patient was a 38-year-old male smoker with vague left eye pain and 40-lb weight loss. (Reproduced with permission from USMLE-Rx.com.)

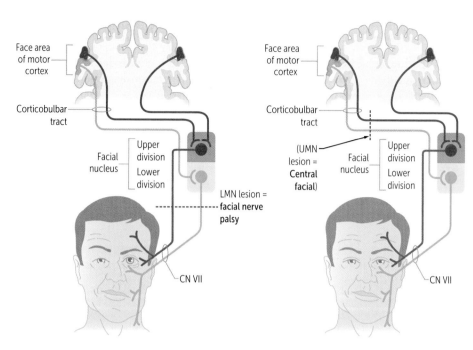

FIGURE 11.12.   Bell palsy versus stroke. Impact on normal motor nerve function in Bell palsy (**A**), a peripheral lesion affects all branches of the facial nerve, and in stroke (**B**), a central lesion affects only the lower branches of the facial nerve. (Reproduced with permission from USMLE-Rx.com.)

QUESTION 1

A 62-year-old woman presents with an intermittent dull ache on the lower right side of her face that is worsened by chewing and is not relieved by OTC analgesics. Her symptoms have been occurring for a month and are now "stabbing" and ↑ even with talking. Exam elicits pain on touching the lower right side of the patient's face. Head CT is negative. What is the diagnosis?

QUESTION 2

A 41-year-old has had ↓ feeling and strength in both legs after he became acutely ill following dinner a few days earlier. He also has "tingling" in his feet and some difficulty walking. Exam reveals ↓ lower extremity muscle strength with a lack of DTRs. The patient states that his arms now feel weaker as well. How do you proceed?

Diagnosis

- Based on the history and exam.
- Lab testing for Lyme disease, sarcoidosis, or HIV are not indicated unless there are other symptoms of these diseases.
- MRI should be considered if symptoms do not improve or worsen.

Management

- Oral corticosteroids ↓ duration of symptoms.
- Evidence now suggests that antivirals are *not* effective *alone*. There is conflicting evidence about whether or not there is benefit to adding an antiviral to steroids.
- Lubricating eye drops may be used, along with an ipsilateral eye patch or taping the eye shut during sleep, if the eye is difficult to close.

Complications

- Severe pain, older age, hyperacusis, and complete palsy at diagnosis are associated with a poorer prognosis, with disfigurement affecting about 10% of patients.
- Most patients have complete recovery within weeks to months without treatment.

RAMSAY HUNT SYNDROME

Ipsilateral facial weakness with herpetic eruption of the ear, palate, pharynx, or occipital scalp, caused by herpes zoster involvement of CN V, IX, and X. Additional symptoms may include deafness, tinnitus, or vertigo.

- **Management:** Treat acutely with **acyclovir** and **corticosteroids.**
- **Complications:** Postherpetic neuralgia in the affected areas or persistent facial weakness. Fewer than half of pativents achieve a complete recovery. For more on postherpetic neuralgia, see the Geriatric Medicine chapter.

MNEMONIC

Ramsay Hunt syndrome:
RH

Etiology: **R**eactivated **H**erpes virus
Complication: **R**educed **H**earing

TRIGEMINAL NEURALGIA

An **idiopathic facial pain syndrome** with onset often in the sixth decade. The male-to-female incidence ratio is 2:3. If the syndrome is bilateral or diagnosed in a young female patient, consider MS as a cause.

Symptoms/Exam

- Presents as **stabbing, brief unilateral pain** in the areas of the **2nd and 3rd branches of the trigeminal nerve (CN V)** (Figure 11.13). Touching the affected area, eating, or a draft of air over the face elicits the pain.
- Otherwise neurologically normal.

Differential

Temporal arteritis, TMJ dysfunction, atypical facial pain, glaucoma, brain stem tumor, MS, dental abscess, postherpetic neuralgia.

Diagnosis

Guided by the history and exam, often no imaging necessary. In a young patient, suspect MS and obtain evoked potential testing, an MRI, and CSF tests.

Management

Carbamazepine and **oxcarbazepine** are first-line agents but require monitoring of cell counts and LFTs. Baclofen and gabapentin can be considered as second-line therapies.

Complications

Spontaneous remissions can occur for months, but some patients have progression of the disorder, with more frequent symptoms and possibly persistent low-grade pain.

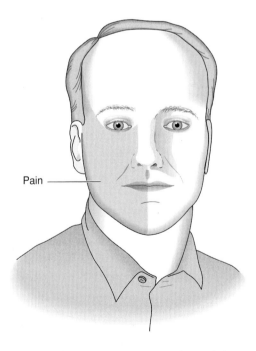

Pain

FIGURE 11.13. **Distribution of symptoms in trigeminal neuralgia.** (Reproduced with permission from Simon RP, et al. *Clinical Neurology*, 7th ed. New York: McGraw-Hill, 2009, Fig. 2-8.)

Spinal Cord Disorders

SPINAL ARTERIOVENOUS MALFORMATION

Symptoms/Exam

- Presents with weakness or paralysis of one or both legs, along with numbness or paresthesias in the same distribution. An upper, lower, or mixed motor deficit is seen in the legs.
- Associated with acute, **lancinating pain** in the back or legs, that **worsens when recumbent.** Hyperreflexia is seen caudal to the lesion. Sphincter function is compromised.
- Symptoms are also present in the arms with cervical lesions.
- A bruit, cutaneous angioma, or dermatomal nevus may be present over the affected area of the spine, but are rare findings.

Differential

Guillain-Barré syndrome, spinal cord infarction, transverse myelitis, MS, stroke, cauda equina syndrome.

Diagnosis

- MRI of the spine or CT myelography shows one or more enlarged and tortuous draining vessels in the subarachnoid space, usually at the lower spinal cord. The spinal cord may appear enlarged in the area of the lesion.
- CSF shows high protein but little or no cellular reaction.

Management

Embolization of the lesion or ligation of its feeding vessels and excision of the anomalous AVM nidus.

SUBACUTE COMBINED DEGENERATION OF THE SPINAL CORD

Degeneration of the dorsal and lateral white matter of the spinal cord caused by vitamin B_{12} deficiency.

- **Symptoms/Exam:** Presents with symmetric distal extremity weakness and paresthesias starting in the hands. Blood work may show macrocytic megaloblastic anemia and low serum vitamin B_{12} if not treated.
- **Management:** IM vitamin B_{12} injections. Progression without treatment can lead to ataxia, visual impairment, and psychosis.

Peripheral Neuropathies

GUILLAIN-BARRÉ SYNDROME

Acute inflammatory demyelinating polyneuropathy characterized by symmetric, progressive ascending muscle weakness that usually **starts in the legs** and may be **acute or subacute.** The condition is life-threatening if respiratory or swallowing muscles are involved. Can follow minor respiratory or GI illness, inoculation, or surgical procedures. It is unknown why the condition develops in certain people and not in others.

QUESTION

A 58-year-old right-handed man notices left calf "stiffness" that causes him to trip frequently. Over several months, right arm muscle cramping and twitching have led to difficulty buttoning his shirt. He presents with new difficulty swallowing and slurred speech. Exam reveals weakness and muscle atrophy in his extremities and hyperreflexia and fasciculations in the left lower extremity. An overactive gag reflex is present. What additional studies do you order?

KEY FACT

Guillain-Barré syndrome after a *C jejuni* infection is often severe.

MNEMONIC

Characteristics of Guillain-Barré syndrome:

4 A's

Acute inflammatory demyelinating polyneuropathy
Ascending paralysis
Autonomic neuropathy
Arrhythmias

KEY FACT

Corticosteroids can worsen Guillain-Barré symptoms.

Symptoms/Exam

- The hallmark is **lack of DTRs.** Progressive weakness of ≥2 limbs typically begins with the proximal lower extremities.
- Shortness of breath, constipation, facial weakness, dysphagia, ophthalmoplegia, dysarthria, and sensory disturbances are commonly seen.
- Also associated with disturbances in BP, heart rate, and pulmonary function.
- Symptom progression halts in <2 to 3 weeks.

Differential

Chronic inflammatory demyelinating polyneuropathy, HIV infection, transverse myelitis, intraspinal mass, porphyria, toxic neuropathy, poliomyelitis, botulism, tick paralysis, periodic paralysis syndrome.

Diagnosis

- Initial diagnosis based on clinical suspicion, but LP and electrophysiology studies should be performed in all patients for confirmation.
- CSF shows ↑ protein but a normal cell count, but may be normal in the first week.
- Electrophysiologic studies can show marked **slowing of motor and sensory conduction velocity,** consistent with denervation and axonal loss.

Management

- Plasmapheresis or IVIG may improve recovery time and ↓ residual neurologic effects.
- IVIG is preferable in children and in cases involving cardiovascular instability.
- Severe cases should be monitored in the ICU because of potential to require mechanical ventilation.

Complications

May have mild residual deficits. Relapse is possible years later. Fatal in 5% of cases.

DIABETIC NEUROPATHY

Polyneuropathy is the most common presentation. Patients experience numbness and tingling in a **stocking/glove distribution. Autonomic neuropathy** affects the internal organs and is associated with digestive, urinary, sexual, and visual changes.

- **Diagnosis:** May be made based on clinical symptoms, or screening monofilament exams. CBC, CMP, TSH and vitamin B_{12} levels should be tested to rule out other common causes of peripheral polyneuropathy. Consider EMG if diagnosis still unclear.
- **Management:** Involves improved glycemic control, foot care, TCAs, gabapentin, and capsaicin cream.

BRACHIAL PLEXUS DISORDERS

Usually a unilateral sensorimotor deficit traceable to one or more cords of the brachial plexus. May be due to trauma, radiation, infection, electrical injury, compression, or infiltration, but often there is no apparent cause.

- **Whole plexus lesion (C5-T1):** The entire arm is paralyzed, with sensory loss complete past a line drawn from the shoulder to the middle third of the upper arm.
- **Upper brachial plexus paralysis (C5, C6 ± C7):** Loss of shoulder abduction and elbow flexion. The affected arm is held internally rotated at the shoulder, with the elbow extended and the forearm pronated. Sensory loss occurs over a small area of the deltoid muscle. Also known as **Erb palsy** or "waiter's tip." Accounts for half of all neonatal brachial plexus injuries.

- **Lower brachial plexus paralysis (C8, T1):** Paralysis and wasting of the small muscles of the hand and of the long finger flexors and extensors, leading to **Klumpke palsy,** also known as "claw hand" deformity. Sensory loss is found on the ulnar border of the hand and the inner forearm. Horner syndrome is possible.
- **Brachial neuritis:** Acute onset of excruciating and generally unilateral shoulder pain followed days later by weakness of the shoulder and parascapular muscles. Numbness may also be seen.

Differential

Cervical radiculopathy, polymyalgia rheumatica, vertebral artery dissection.

Diagnosis

- Electrophysiologic testing of the affected muscles.
- AP and axillary lateral shoulder x-ray for concerns of related fracture.
- MRI may reveal infiltrative processes.

Management

- Physical/occupational therapy. Bracing prevents contractures.
- Possible surgery, with nerve grafting and muscle or tendon transfers.
- Corticosteroids for brachial neuritis.

Progressive Neurodegenerative Disease

AMYOTROPHIC LATERAL SCLEROSIS

A devastating neurodegenerative disease, with **degeneration of lower and corticospinal motor neurons.** Most cases are sporadic.

Symptoms/Exam

- Bulbar involvement: difficulty swallowing, chewing, coughing, breathing, and speaking.
- Vague sensory complaints and weight loss are common.
- **Upper and lower motor neuron (UMN/LMN) signs** in the bulbar region and upper and/or lower extremities include spasticity, hyperreflexia, atrophy, weakness or paralysis, fasciculations, hypotonia, and extensor plantar reflexes. Extraocular and sphincter muscles are generally spared. No sensory deficits.

Differential

Progressive bulbar palsy, pseudobulbar palsy (UMN bulbar symptoms), progressive spinal muscular atrophy (primarily LMN deficit in the limbs), 1° lateral sclerosis (purely an UMN deficit in the limbs), poliomyelitis, MS, cervical myelopathy.

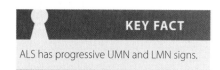

KEY FACT

ALS has progressive UMN and LMN signs.

Diagnosis

- Definitive diagnosis requires the **presence of UMN and LMN signs in three regions** as follows:
  - In the bulbar region and in at least two spinal regions (cervical, thoracic, or lumbosacral).
  - OR in three spinal regions.
- EMG findings of diffuse degenerative signs with normal or near-normal nerve conduction (except in severe atrophy) are highly suggestive. MRI and further lab workup are needed to eliminate other potential causes based on clinical situation.

Management

- Riluzole ↓ presynaptic glutamate release and may slow symptom progression.
- Symptomatic and supportive care. Anticholinergics ↓ drooling and saliva pooling.
- Spasticity may be improved with baclofen or diazepam.
- Physical therapy to ↓ contractures; braces or walker to promote mobility.

Complications

Progressive and fatal, usually within 3 to 5 years of onset.

Neuromuscular Disorders

MYASTHENIA GRAVIS VERSUS MYASTHENIC SYNDROME

The hallmark of myasthenia gravis is muscle weakness that worsens with activity and improves with rest. In contrast, myasthenic syndrome presents with proximal limb weakness that improves with activity. Different acetylcholinesterase inhibitors are used for diagnosis and treatment of myasthenia gravis (to help remember them, see the mnemonic). Table 11.8 distinguishes the clinical presentation, diagnosis, and treatment of myasthenia gravis from that of myasthenic syndrome.

MNEMONIC

Acetylcholinesterase inhibitors for myasthenia gravis:

E**d**rophonium is used to **d**iagnose
Py**rid**ostigmine is used to get **rid** of symptoms

TABLE 11.8. Myasthenia Gravis Versus Myasthenic Syndrome

DISEASE	MYASTHENIA GRAVIS	MYASTHENIC SYNDROME (LAMBERT-EATON SYNDROME)
General	An **autoimmune disease** Antibodies are usually against the postsynaptic muscle membrane acetylcholine receptors Associated with **thymoma,** thyrotoxicosis, SLE, and RA **Women are affected** more often than men	Generally **a paraneoplastic syndrome** Involves an immune-modulated defective release of acetylcholine in the neuromuscular junction Associated with **SLE, small cell lung cancer,** and **autoimmune diseases** such as pernicious anemia
Symptoms/Exam	**Muscle weakness that worsens with activity** and fluctuates during the day Involves slow progression of **ptosis, diplopia, altered tone of speech,** limb weakness, and difficulty with chewing, swallowing, or respiration Relapses and remissions for weeks Myasthenic **crisis** consists of absent gag reflex, limpness of the body, and ↑ respiratory muscle weakness	Presents with proximal limb **weakness that improves with activity,** extraocular muscles are generally spared May be associated with dry mouth, constipation, and impotence ↑ environmental or body temperatures worsen symptoms
Diagnosis	Electrophysiologic testing may show ↓ **response** of muscle to repetitive motor nerve stimulation High serum acetylcholine receptor antibody levels are found in 80%-90% of those with generalized disease **Edrophonium** (the Tensilon test) or neostigmine improves symptoms	Confirmed electrophysiologically by ↑ **response** to repetitive nerve stimulation Serum **autoantibodies to the P/Q subtype of voltage-gated calcium channels** are highly sensitive and specific to this syndrome
Treatment	Acetylcholinesterase inhibitors, eg, **pyridostigmine** Thymectomy for younger patients with weakness beyond the extraocular muscles Corticosteroids initially **worsen** weakness Azathioprine, plasmapheresis, IVIG, mycophenolate mofetil	Plasmapheresis, corticosteroids, azathioprine, or IVIG Guanidine hydrochloride may help severe cases but carries the risk of renal failure and bone marrow suppression Treat the underlying condition
Complications	Respiratory complications can be fatal	Worsens over time; respiratory compromise may result

Muscular Disorders

MUSCULAR DYSTROPHIES

Present with progressive muscle weakness and muscle wasting. Age at onset and distribution of symptoms depend on type (Table 11.9).

- **Diagnosis:** By muscle biopsy histology, which distinguishes different types of muscular dystrophy. If a physical developmental delay is observed, the level of serum creatinine kinase can distinguish peripheral from central disorders.

QUESTION

A 32-year-old woman experiences persistent double vision. She attributes it to stress, but a vacation yields minimal improvement. Weeks later, her problem worsens, and she becomes increasingly tired during the day, especially in the late afternoon to evening. She visits your office, where an exam reveals ptosis and hoarse voice. What further evaluation will confirm the diagnosis?

TABLE 11.9. **Presentation of Common Muscular Dystrophies**

TYPE	AGE AT ONSET	MODE OF INHERITANCE	DISTRIBUTION AND SYMPTOMS	PROGNOSIS	SERUM CK
Duchenne	1-5	X-linked recessive	The most common muscular dystrophy. Affects pelvic and shoulder girdle muscles, then extremities and respiratory muscles. Presents with muscular pseudohypertrophy; also associated with mental retardation, deformities, and contractures	Rapid progression. Fatal 15 years after onset	Markedly ↑
Becker	5-25	X-linked recessive	Affects pelvic muscles then shoulder girdle muscles	Slow progression	↑
Limb-girdle	10-30	Autosomal recessive; dominant, X linked or sporadic	Affects pelvic or shoulder girdle muscles, then other muscles. Presents with calf hypertrophy	Variable. May be severe in midlife	Mildly ↑
Facioscapulohumeral	Any	Autosomal dominant	Affects face and shoulder girdle muscles; then to pelvic muscles and lower extremities	Slow progression; minor disability	Can be normal
Myotonic	Any	Autosomal dominant	Weakness and myotonia (ie, "spasming") of facial, sternocleidomastoid, and distal extremity muscles; associated with baldness, cataracts, gonadal atrophy, cardiac abnormalities, mental retardation, and endocrinopathy	Variable	Normal or mildly ↑

ANSWER

A ⊕ Tensilon test and ↑ serum acetylcholine receptor antibodies confirm myasthenia gravis.

Management: Timely referral to early intervention and a pediatric neurologist are key. Physical therapy is the mainstay of treatment; glucocorticoids are beneficial for Duchenne and Becker muscular dystrophy.

INFLAMMATORY MYOPATHIES

Defined as muscle fiber destruction and inflammatory infiltration of muscles. Associated with some **autoimmune disorders,** including SLE, Sjögren syndrome, scleroderma, and RA. Peak incidence is in the **fifth and sixth decades. More women are affected** than men. Subtypes are as follows:

- Polymyositis:
  - Presents with muscle pain, weakness, and atrophy, especially of the proximal limb muscles. Begins with leg weakness that progresses to arm weakness. Dysphagia and respiratory difficulties are also seen.
  - Raynaud phenomenon, malaise, arthralgias, low-grade fever, and weight loss are common.
- Dermatomyositis:
  - Presentation similar to polymyositis, but with a **heliotrope rash,** which is an erythematous rash appearing over the eyelids, around the eyes, or on the extensor surfaces of the joints (Figure 11.14A).
  - Erythema over the face, neck, shoulders, and upper chest ("shawl sign").
  - **Gottron sign** consists of scaly patches over the dorsa of the proximal hand joints, periungual erythema, and nail bed capillary dilation (Figure 11.14B).
  - Skin or muscle **calcinosis** is common.
- **Inclusion body myositis:** Painless proximal weakness of the lower extremities and then the upper extremities, especially the quadriceps and finger flexors. Has a progressive course, with early loss of patellar reflexes.

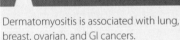

KEY FACT

Dermatomyositis is associated with lung, breast, ovarian, and GI cancers.

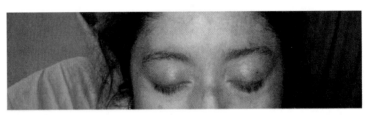

A

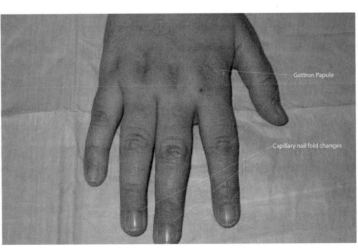

B

FIGURE 11.14. Dermatomyositis. (A) Heliotrope rash on the upper eyelids with associated eyelid swelling. **(B)** Gottron sign. Papules, nail fold telangiectasias, and dystrophic cuticles in dermatomyositis. (Reproduced from Dhoble A, et al. Dermatomyositis and supraventricular tachycardia. *Int Arch Med.* 2008;1:25.)

Differential

Myasthenic syndrome, myasthenia gravis, MS, ALS, polymyalgia rheumatica, trichinellosis, hypothyroidism, HIV myopathy.

Diagnosis

- Initial evaluation: Labs show ↑ serum CK and aldolase. An ANA panel should also be tested and may be positive. CXR for all patients to detect pulmonary involvement.
- Follow-up testing includes muscle biopsy (shows necrosis of muscle fibers and inflammatory cell infiltration), skin biopsy (if dermatologic findings), and EMG (reveals short, low-amplitude, polyphasic motor unit potentials, possibly with abnormal spontaneous activity).

KEY FACT

Muscle biopsy is the gold standard for diagnosis of polymyositis and dermatomyositis.

Management

- Glucocorticoids should be initiated and then lowered as serum muscle enzyme levels ↓. Consider a trial of methotrexate and azathioprine as second-line agents or in patients who are severely ill.
- Physical therapy to preserve function.
- For inclusion body myositis, immunosuppressive therapy with methotrexate or azathioprine is preferred, as response to glucocorticoids alone is limited.

Complications

Patients with dermatomyositis have an ↑ risk of malignancy. Those with respiratory muscle involvement can have hypercapnia and respiratory failure. Severe muscle inflammation can precipitate rhabdomyolysis, causing renal failure.

NOTES

Surgery

Sarah Stombaugh, MD

KEY FACT

The indications for coronary revascularization in the preoperative patient are no different from those in patients not facing surgery. Further evaluation or treatment should not be pursued unless it would be indicated in the absence of surgery.

KEY FACT

Check 12-lead ECG for patients undergoing vascular surgery who have at least one clinical risk factor and in patients undergoing intermediate-risk surgery who have CHD, peripheral arterial disease, or cerebrovascular disease.

KEY FACT

Poor glycemic control in both the chronic and acute setting is associated with a higher incidence of infection and delayed wound healing.

Preoperative Evaluation

Preoperative evaluation is required before all surgery. The goal of the preoperative evaluation is to assess risk of cardiovascular and other complications in the perioperative period. A thorough evaluation can help the physician and patient to weigh the risks and benefits of surgery, as well as to medically optimize a patient for surgery. The presence of comorbid conditions may necessitate additional lab, ECG, cardiac stress, PFT, or CXR testing. Nonselective imaging and lab screening tests have been shown to be of minimal value.

CARDIAC RISK EVALUATION

A preoperative cardiac risk assessment should address **three major components:**
- The patient's risk of a major **cardiac complication** (Table 12.1).
- The patient's current **functional status** (Table 12.2).
- The cardiac risk associated with the **planned procedure** (Table 12.3).

Guidelines for further cardiac evaluation and for the mitigation of cardiac risk are outlined in Figure 12.1.

PERIOPERATIVE β-BLOCKERS

Studies indicate that perioperative β-blockers ↓ cardiac complications in patients with known or suspected CAD. All studies used β_1-selective agents (eg, metoprolol, atenolol, bisoprolol). **Don't use β-blockers for patients with high-grade conduction system disease.** β-blockers are recommended for the following:
- Patients who are already taking β-blockers for angina, arrhythmia, and/or hypertension.
- Patients undergoing vascular surgery who have cardiac ischemia on preoperative evaluation.
- Intraoperatively and postoperatively to maintain a heart rate of 60 to 65 bpm.

TABLE 12.1.   Cardiac Risk Stratification

MAJOR	INTERMEDIATE	MINOR
MI within 6 months, with persistent ischemic symptoms	MI >6 months ago	Advanced age
	Stable/mild angina	Abnormal ECG
	Compensated or prior HF	Rhythm other than sinus (eg, atrial fibrillation)
Decompensated HF	DM	
Significant arrhythmias	Renal insufficiency	Poor functional capacity
Severe valvular disease		History of stroke
		Uncontrolled hypertension

TABLE 12.2. **Functional Status Assessment**

EXCELLENT (>7 METS)[a]	MODERATE (4-7 METS)	POOR (<4 METS)
Squash	Cycling	Vacuuming
Jogging (10-minute mile)	Climbing a flight of stairs	Activities of daily living (eg, eating, dressing, bathing)
	Golf (without cart)	
Scrubbing floors	Walking 4 mph	Walking 2 mph
Singles tennis	Yardwork (eg, raking leaves, weeding, pushing a power mower)	Writing

[a]MET = metabolic equivalent, a unit used to estimate the (energy) oxygen consumption during physical activity. 1 MET = oxygen consumption of a 70-kg, 40-year-old man in a resting state.

Perioperative Management

PERIOPERATIVE MANAGEMENT OF ANTICOAGULATION

- **Aspirin** can be continued for patients with a high risk of perioperative vascular complications. If discontinued, it should be stopped 7 days before surgery. Resume approximately 24 hours after surgery.
- **Warfarin** should be stopped 4 to 5 days before surgery and replaced with heparin or LMWH.
- **Unfractionated heparin** is stopped 5 hours before surgery, and **low-molecular-weight heparin (LMWH)** is stopped 12 to 24 hours before surgery. Unfractionated heparin or LMWH with warfarin therapy may be restarted postoperatively once hemostasis has been achieved.
- **Clopidogrel** should be stopped 7 to 10 days before surgery.
- **NSAIDs** should be stopped at least 3 days before surgery unless benefits exceed risks (eg, severe arthritis).

PERIOPERATIVE PROPHYLAXIS AND MANAGEMENT OF CHRONIC DISEASE

Table 12.4 outlines the indications for perioperative prophylaxis. Table 12.5 discusses the perioperative management of chronic diseases.

KEY FACT

Low-risk patients who are <40 years of age, have no additional risk factors for thromboembolic disease, and require general anesthesia for <30 minutes do not need DVT prophylaxis.

KEY FACT

LMWH should be avoided in patients with ↓ renal clearance because it is excreted by the kidneys. Unfractionated heparin is a better choice because it is metabolized by the liver and excreted in the urine.

KEY FACT

Sucralfate and H_2 receptor blockers both reduce the likelihood of GI bleeding by 50%, but they have known disadvantages such as ↓ absorption of medications and a possible ↑ risk of nosocomial pneumonia.

TABLE 12.3. **Degree of Cardiac Risk Associated With Surgical Procedures**[a]

LOW: "ABCDE-TURP"	INTERMEDIATE: "CHOPIN"	HIGH: "EVA"
Ambulatory procedures	**C**arotid endarterectomy	**E**mergency major procedures
Breast procedures	**H**ead procedures	**V**ascular procedures
Cataract procedures	**O**rthopedic procedures	**A**nticipated prolonged surgical procedures associated with large fluid shifts or blood loss
Dermatologic procedures	**P**rostatectomy	
Endoscopic procedures	**I**ntraperitoneal and intrathoracic procedures	
Trans**U**rethral **R**esection of the **P**rostate	**N**eck procedures	

[a]Cardiac risk is stratified as follows: low risk = <1%; intermediate risk = <5%; high risk = >5%.

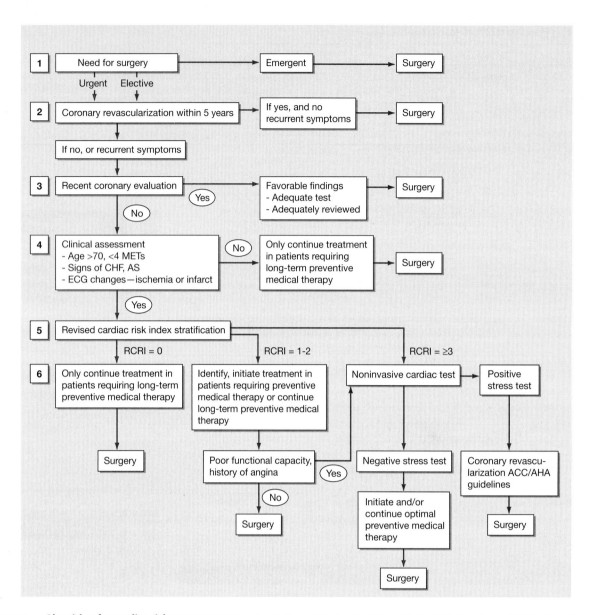

FIGURE 12.1. **Algorithm for cardiac risk assessment.** (Reproduced with permission from Fauci AS, et al. *Harrison's Principles of Internal Medicine*, 17th ed. New York: McGraw-Hill, 2008, Fig. 8-2.)

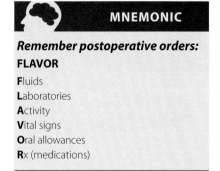

Postoperative Care

Recovery from surgery can be divided into three phases, as described below.

IMMEDIATE POSTOPERATIVE PERIOD

The principal causes of complications and death following major surgery are acute cardiac, pulmonary, and fluid derangements. Monitor postoperative patients until cardiopulmonary and neurologic function has returned to baseline.

INTERMEDIATE POSTOPERATIVE PERIOD

During the time from complete recovery from anesthesia until discharge from the hospital, the patient must recover basic bodily functions and become self-sufficient. Measures with which to achieve these goals are outlined in Table 12.6.

TABLE 12.4.   Indications for Perioperative Prophylaxis

CONDITION	AT-RISK GROUPS	RECOMMENDATIONS
Bacterial endocarditis	Patients with prosthetic valves, previous infective endocarditis, valvulopathy following heart transplantation, or complex CHD[a]	**Dental** (involving gingival tissue, dental periapical regions, or perforating the oral mucosa) **and respiratory tract procedures:** PO amoxicillin, IV ampicillin, PO cephalexin, or PO/IV clindamycin 30-60 minutes before the procedure Prophylaxis is **NOT** recommended for bronchoscopy, genitourinary/GI tract procedures
DVT	All surgical patients are at risk for DVT, especially those undergoing major surgery, those having orthopedic surgery, and those >40 years of age or with additional DVT risk factors	**"Minidose" heparin:** Usually 5000 U SQ BID-TID **LMWH:** Enoxaparin 30 mg BID or 40 mg QD Thromboembolic disease stockings Sequential compression devices **Warfarin:** Dose adjusted; for very-high-risk patients only
GI bleeding (due to stress-induced gastric mucosal disease)	At especially high risk for GI bleeding are patients with coagulopathy, those with respiratory failure requiring mechanical ventilation, and those with a history of GI ulcer/bleeding	H_2 receptor blockers, PPIs, sucralfate
Constipation	All postoperative patients on narcotic pain medications	Senna

[a]**Congenital heart disease (CHD)** only in the following conditions: unrepaired cyanotic CHD, completely repaired CHD with prosthetic material or device, and repaired CHD with residual defects to the site of a prosthetic patch or prosthetic device.

TABLE 12.5.   Perioperative Management of Chronic Diseases

CONDITION	POTENTIAL COMPLICATIONS	PREOPERATIVE MANAGEMENT	POSTOPERATIVE MANAGEMENT
DM, on insulin as outpatient	Hypo- and hyperglycemia; DKA; infection	Give 50% of usual long-acting insulin the morning of surgery (exception: glargine, which should be given at the usual dose the evening before surgery) with glucose drip	Strongly consider insulin drip titrating to normoglycemia; otherwise, restart long-acting insulin with supplemental short-acting insulin (with rapid titration of long-acting insulin)
DM, not on insulin	Hypo- and hyperglycemia; nonketotic hyperosmolar state	Omit oral hypoglycemic the day before surgery	Consider insulin drip; use regularly scheduled short-acting insulin if needed and restart oral agent when possible
Chronic steroid use (especially greater than the equivalent of prednisone 20 mg for 3 weeks)	Adrenal crisis (rare)	Continue usual dose	Can usually just give chronic dose; consider "stress-dose" steroids for longer/major surgeries—hydrocortisone 100 mg q 8 hr × 2-3 days
Liver disease	Mortality, hemorrhage, infection	Optimize treatment of underlying complications; high morbidity and mortality rates are seen in Child-Pugh Class C patients	Optimize treatment of underlying complications
Chronic kidney disease	Mortality, hemorrhage, electrolyte disturbance, infection	Monitor electrolytes; check bleeding time if uremia; assess for anemia/consider erythropoietin for elective surgery	Monitor electrolytes and fluid volume

TABLE 12.6.   Management of the Intermediate Postoperative Period

SYSTEM	MANAGEMENT
Fluid/electrolyte	Careful monitoring of volume status/electrolytes Postoperative fluid replacement includes maintenance fluid, losses from drains, third-space losses (eg, tissue edema, ileus), insensible losses (eg, burns, fever); postoperative rise in ADH may lead to hyponatremia
Pulmonary	Deep breathing exercises/incentive spirometry, adequate pain control, early mobilization, early recognition and treatment of cardiac failure
GI	Early feeding has been effective in most cases Patients receiving opioid pain medication may need stool softener and/or laxative Consider an NG tube if patients have marked ileus
NG tube	Low intermittent suction, frequent irrigation, addition of potassium to replace GI fluid loss
Infection	Routine postoperative antimicrobial use should be discouraged, as it is costly and is associated with ↑ rates of microbial drug resistance and incidence of *C difficile*

KEY FACT

Postoperative urinary retention should be suspected in patients who fail to pass urine after 3 hours of receiving anesthesia. An immediate bladder ultrasound should be done to assess how much urine volume is present. Urinary catheterization should follow to prevent hydronephrosis and renal injury.

KEY FACT

Incentive spirometry decreases the risk of postoperative complications secondary to atelectasis and should be taught to patients preoperatively.

KEY FACT

Two important infectious causes of fever in the first 36 hours after laparotomy are intraperitoneal leakage from injury to bowel and invasive soft tissue infection caused by either β-hemolytic streptococci or clostridial species (most commonly *Clostridium perfringens*).

Postoperative Fever

- Most early postoperative fever is caused by the inflammatory response to surgery and resolves spontaneously.
- The timing of fever after surgery is the key to generating differential diagnosis of postoperative fever (Table 12.7).

Pain Management

Postoperative pain serves no practical function and can give rise to a range of complications, including:
- Splinting of the diaphragm, which can lead to reluctance to breathe and can result in atelectasis and pneumonia.
- Limited mobility, which can lead to venous stasis and cause DVT.
- Release of catecholamines, leading to vasospasm and hypertension, causing stroke, MI, and bleeding.
- Table 12.8 outlines options for postoperative pain management.

TABLE 12.7.   The Five W's of Postoperative Fever

	POSTOPERATIVE DAYS	CONCERN	PREVENTION
Wind	1-2	Atelectasis, pneumonia	Incentive spirometry
Water	3-5	UTI	Early removal of Foley catheter
Walking	4-6	DVT, PE	Prophylactic anticoagulation; early mobilization
Wound	5-7	Surgical site infection	MRSA screening; preoperative skin cleansing with antiseptic; dressing changes
Wonder drugs	7+	Drug fever caused by medications, IV lines, blood production reaction	Change IV lines; type and screen blood products

TABLE 12.8.   **Postoperative Pain Medications**

ROUTE/MEDICATION CLASS	EXAMPLES	ADVANTAGES	SIDE EFFECTS
IV opioids	Morphine, hydromorphone, methadone	Potent analgesia	Respiratory depression, nausea, vomiting, altered sensorium
IV nonopioid analgesics	Ketorolac tromethamine (an NSAID), acetaminophen	Analgesic and anti-inflammatory	Potential for gastric ulcer; impaired coagulation; ↓ renal function with long-term use
PO analgesics	Acetaminophen with codeine (T#3); hydrocodone with acetaminophen (Vicodin)	Acetaminophen acts as an antipyretic and allows patients to be "transitioned" home with adequate pain relief	Tolerance with long-term use
Patient-controlled analgesia	Usually morphine	Controlled by the patient; the possibility of overdose is limited because the patient must be awake to self-administer. The maximum dose and timing are preset by the physician	Respiratory depression, nausea, vomiting, altered sensorium, inadequate analgesia if the patient is unable to depress the button
Continuous epidural analgesia	Morphine ± bupivacaine (topical to the epidural space)	Intense and prolonged segmental analgesia, ↓ respiratory depression, longer pain relief, ↓ alteration of sensorium than IV opioids	Pruritus, nausea, respiratory depression, hypotension, urinary retention (usually requires a bladder catheter)
Intercostal block	Bupivacaine	Useful for diminishing pain following thoracic and abdominal procedures	Risk of pneumothorax

CONVALESCENT PERIOD

The final postoperative phase begins when a patient is discharged from the hospital. The following support services should be considered to ensure a smooth transition home, minimize postoperative complications, and hasten the patient's recovery from surgery:

- Visiting/home nursing agencies.
- Physical/occupational therapy.
- Rehabilitation services.
- Wound care specialists.

Wound Management

Wound healing can be thought of as a **stepwise process** proceeding from coagulation and inflammation through fibroplasia, matrix deposition, angiogenesis, epithelialization, collagen maturation, and wound contraction.

LOCAL ANESTHESIA

- **Topical anesthesia** (eg, LET gel, EMLA cream): Used to ↓ the pain of infiltration.
- **Infiltrative anesthesia** (eg, lidocaine, lidocaine with epinephrine, bupivacaine).
- **Nerve block:** Good for fingers, toes, hands, feet, face, and mouth.

KEY FACT

Don't use lidocaine with epinephrine for digits, genitals, nose, earlobes, or skin flaps because of the risk of vasoconstriction and necrosis.

QUESTION

A 53-year-old woman becomes febrile (38.3°C [100.9°F]) 3 days after undergoing total colectomy, which was uneventful. The patient has been using incentive spirometry regularly. Vital signs are otherwise normal. Exam reveals normal heart sounds and clear lungs, surgical sites are clean, abdomen is soft with suprapubic tenderness, and Foley catheter is in place. What is the next best step?

WOUND PREPARATION

Thorough wound preparation facilitates wound healing and prevents wound infection.
- **Debridement.**
- **Foreign body removal:** Retained foreign bodies are at risk for developing infection. Wound exploration ± radiography or ultrasound (for radiolucent foreign bodies) is necessary.
- **Irrigation:** Copious irrigation is important to adequately clean wound.
- **Disinfection:** Povidone-iodine may be wound-toxic and should not be used in an open wound.

WOUND CLOSURE

The wound closure method is chosen, depending on the location, size, and mechanism of the wound as well as patient factors (eg, child).
- **Sutures:** In healthy patients, the ideal closure for small superficial wounds (eg, skin lacerations). Sutures are also used during surgery to close layers and ↓ tension.
- **Staples:** A quick and strong closure, cosmetically acceptable, used for scalp, torso, and extremities.
- **Skin adhesive** (eg, Dermabond): Works like glue. Minimal pain, used for low-tension wounds.

WOUND CARE

- **Antibiotic prophylaxis:** Consider antibiotics only in high-risk wounds such as heavily contaminated wounds, animal and human bites, or immunocompromised patients.
- **Tetanus prophylaxis:** Give tetanus vaccine to patients who have not had a three-dose 1° tetanus vaccine series or whose last tetanus vaccination was >10 years (>5 years if tetanus-prone wounds).
- **Suture removal:**
  - Face: 3 to 5 days.
  - Scalp: 5 to 7 days.
  - Trunk/arm/hand: 7 to 10 days.
  - Leg/foot: 10 to 14 days.

CAUSES OF WOUND DEHISCENCE

- **Dehiscence** is defined as undesired spontaneous separation of wound edges.
- The most common causes are **infection** and **excessively tight sutures.**
- Wound dehiscence can be caused by **host factors** and/or operator **factors** (Table 12.9).

TABLE 12.9. **Risk Factors for Wound Dehiscence**

HOST FACTORS
Smoking
Malnutrition, starvation
Steroids
Infection
Hypoxia and hypovolemia
Radiation
Trauma
Uremia
DM
Drugs (especially chemotherapeutic agents)
Advanced age

OPERATOR FACTORS
Tissue injury
Poor blood supply
Poor apposition of tissues (unclosed dead space, unreduced fracture)

Surgical Infections

MAJOR FACTORS

The three main determinants of surgical infection are:

- **Patient-related risk factors:** DM/perioperative hyperglycemia, tobacco use, remote infection at the time of surgery, obesity, malnutrition, low albumin, steroid use, prolonged preoperative hospital stay, prior site irradiation, and colonization with *Staphylococcus aureus.*
- **Procedure-related risk factors:** Presence of dead space, shaving of the site the night before procedure, improper preoperative skin preparation, improper antimicrobial prophylaxis, and implantation of foreign bodies.
- **Microbial factors:** Common pathogens are listed in Table 12.10.

TABLE 12.10. **Common Pathogens Causing Surgical Infections**

ORGANISM	CHARACTERISTICS
Staphylococci (*S aureus*)	The most common pathogen in wound infections; associated with foreign bodies
Streptococci	Can invade minor skin breaks and spread through connective tissue
Klebsiella	Often invades the inner ear, enteric tissues, and lung
Enteric organisms (Enterobacteriaceae and enterococci)	Often found with anaerobes such as peptostreptococci, *Bacteroides,* and *Clostridium*
Clostridium	Anaerobic; often found in ischemic tissue
Pseudomonas	Opportunistic in critically ill or immunosuppressed patients
Fungi, yeast, and parasites	Cause abscesses

QUESTION

A 62-year-old man presents to the ED with incisional pain and fever (38.0°C [100.4°F] at home) on postoperative day 9 after total cystectomy for bladder cancer. Exam reveals erythema surrounding the incision as well as serous drainage from the lateral edge. What is the next best step?

ANSWER

Open and debride the incision and start empiric antibiotics for possible wound infection and dehiscence.

MANAGEMENT OF INFECTION

- An infected surgical site **must be opened** either partially or entirely, depending on the extent of infection.
- Perform Gram stain and culture of purulent drainage.
- Administer empiric antibiotics.
- Switch to narrow-spectrum antibiotics once Gram stain and culture reveal a likely organism.

Acute Abdomen

Any sudden spontaneous nontraumatic disorder whose chief manifestation is in the abdominal area and for which urgent operation may be necessary.

Diagnosis

- **Abdominal exam** (Table 12.11).
- **Rectal exam must be performed** in all patients with an acute abdomen.
- **Pelvic exam** in female patients.
- **Imaging:**
  - **Abdominal radiograph (AXR)** may show signs of bowel obstruction or free air.
  - CT scan should be obtained routinely in adults.
  - In children, ultrasound is the best initial test, as it is not associated with any radiation exposure.

Management

Depends on the cause. Surgery is often required. In a patient with true acute abdomen, **urgent exploratory laparotomy** is sometimes necessary before the precise diagnosis can be made.

TABLE 12.11.   Abdominal Exam Findings Associated With Acute Abdomen

CONDITION	APPEARANCE	PALPATION	AUSCULTATION
Perforated viscus	Scaphoid abdomen	Tense; guarding and rigidity	Diminished bowel sounds; loss of liver dullness
Peritonitis	Motionless patient	Guarding and rebound tenderness	Absent bowel sounds (late)
Inflamed mass or abscess	Variable distention	Tender to palpation; special signs (Murphy, psoas, obturator)	Variable bowel sounds
Intestinal obstruction	Distention; visible peristalsis (late)	Diffusely tender to palpation; hernia or mass (some)	Hyperactive (early) or hypoactive (late) bowel sounds
Paralytic ileus	Distention	No localized tenderness	Hypoactive bowel sounds
Ischemic or strangulated bowel	No distention (until late)	Pain out of proportion to exam findings; rectal bleeding (some)	Variable bowel sounds
Bleeding	Pallor, shock; distention	Pulsatile (aneurysm) or tender (eg, ectopic pregnancy) mass; rectal bleeding	Variable bowel sounds

General Surgery

APPENDICITIS

A bacterial infection in the wall of the appendix that is due to obstruction of the proximal lumen, usually by fecolith. Can eventually lead to gangrene and perforation.

Symptoms/Exam

- Often begins with vague midabdominal pain, followed by **anorexia, nausea, vomiting,** and **low-grade fever.**
- Classically progresses to localized tenderness to palpation in the **RLQ.**
- Tenderness at the **McBurney point,** one-third the distance from the anterior superior iliac spine to the umbilicus.
- Patients may also have pain on flexion of the hip (**psoas sign**), pain on internal rotation of the hip (**obturator sign**), or pain on the right side when pressing on the left (**Rovsing sign**).
- **Appendicitis in pregnancy** can present with **RUQ tenderness** due to the gravid uterus.

Differential

- Women: PID, ectopic pregnancy, ovarian torsion.
- Men: Testicular torsion.
- All patients: Hernia, mesenteric adenitis.

Diagnosis

- Based on **exam findings.**
- **Labs:** Leukocytosis.
- **Imaging:**
  - **AXR: Not the imaging of choice** unless other conditions (eg, perforation, intestinal obstruction, ureteral calculus) are suspected.
  - **CT** scan is the most accurate imaging. Classic findings include an **enlarged appendix with wall thickening or enhancement or periappendiceal fat stranding** (Figure 12.2).
  - Ultrasound is less reliable than CT, but is a better initial test for children and pregnant women.

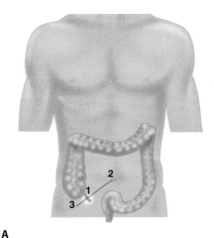

A

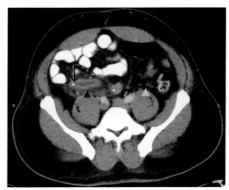

B

FIGURE 12.2.   Acute appendicitis. (A) McBurney point located two-thirds of the distance from the umbilicus. **(B)** CT scan shows an appendicolith in the proximal portion of an enlarged appendix with thickened, hyperenhancing wall. Note the inflammatory changes of the periappendiceal fat (red arrowhead), in distinction to the normal appearance of intra-abdominal fat shown by the yellow arrowhead. (Reproduced with permission from USMLE-Rx.com.)

 QUESTION

A 16-year-old boy with severe abdominal pain is brought to the ED. His mother states that he vomited after dinner last night; in the morning, he did not eat breakfast and complained of mild periumbilical pain. By 10 AM, he was curled up on his classroom floor, unable to move because of generalized abdominal pain. On presentation, he is febrile, tachycardic, and mildly hypotensive. Physical exam reveals abdominal guarding and tenderness at the McBurney point, with ↓ bowel sounds. CBC shows leukocytosis with left shift. CT reveals an inflamed mass in the RLQ. How should you manage this patient?

Management

- Appendectomy.
- Antibiotics ± percutaneous abscess drainage if surgery is contraindicated or unavailable.

Complications

- **Perforation:** Usually due to delay in seeking medical care. Occurs late (>12 hours after onset of symptoms) and associated with more severe pain and a higher fever.
- **Peritonitis:** Can be localized or generalized; results from microscopic perforation of a gangrenous appendix or gross perforation into the peritoneal cavity, respectively. These patients are taken for urgent surgery. Urgent laparotomy may be required if the diagnosis is unclear.
- **Appendiceal abscess:** Occurs when the infection is walled off by adjacent omentum or viscera. Patients with an abscess are better candidates for a nonoperative approach. Patients with abscess are usually treated with percutaneous drainage and IV antibiotics. Interval appendectomy (6-8 weeks later) is often done after inflammation has resolved.
- **Pylephlebitis:** A suppurative thrombophlebitis of the portal venous system.

GALLBLADDER DISEASE

Cholelithiasis With Biliary Colic

Intermittent RUQ pain caused by temporary obstruction of the cystic duct by a gallstone. Pain often increases after ingestion of fatty food.

Diagnosis

- **Labs:** Often normal, but elevated alkaline phosphatase and LFTs may be seen.
- **Imaging:** Initially, RUQ ultrasound is the best (Figure 12.3).

Management

- Dietary modifications, especially low-fat diet.
- Patient may be a candidate for elective cholecystectomy.

MNEMONIC

Think gallbladder disease in patients who are **F**emale, **F**orty, **F**at, and **F**ertile.

MNEMONIC

Remember Charcot triad with FEE:
Fever
Epigastric and RUQ pain
Emesis and nausea

A **ANSWER**

The patient has classic signs of acute appendicitis, including fever, leukocytosis, and periumbilical abdominal pain that progresses to the RLQ, and should be taken to the operating room for emergent appendectomy.

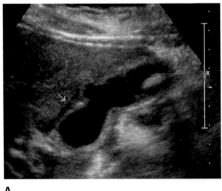
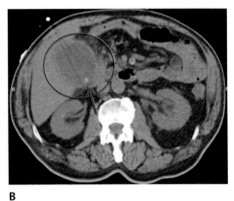

A   B

FIGURE 12.3. **Cholelithiasis. (A)** Gallbladder pericholecystic fluid (arrow) and wall thickening, with echogenic stone in fundus of 43-year-old woman with acute RUQ pain. **(B)** Noncontrast axial CT of the abdomen shows a distended, thick-walled gallbladder (circle) with surrounding stranding and evidence of a radiodense stone within the gallbladder (arrow). (Reproduced with permission from USMLE-Rx.com.)

SURGERY CHAPTER 12 383

Acute Cholecystitis

Inflammation of the gallbladder, most often secondary to cystic duct obstruction (Figure 12.4). Classically presents with **Charcot triad.**

Diagnosis

- **Murphy sign:** Present if the patient catches his or her breath upon deep palpation of the RUQ.
- **Labs:** Elevated WBC, alkaline phosphatase, and LFTs.
- **Imaging:**
  - RUQ ultrasound (Figure 12.3A): Best initial test ⊕ sonographic Murphy sign may be helpful in establishing the diagnosis.
  - CT scan is not the best diagnostic test for gallbladder disease, but if done for other reasons, may demonstrate gallstones (Figure 12.3B).
  - Hepatobiliary iminodiacetic acid scan or magnetic resonance cholangiopancreatography may be necessary if further imaging is required.

Management

- Urgent cholecystectomy: Often done for patients with early presentation.
- Interval cholecystectomy (6-8 weeks later): May be done if there is concern for significant inflammation.
- Endoscopic retrograde cholangiopancreatography: May be both diagnostic and therapeutic, especially in a patient with choledocholithiasis (see Figure 12.4).

ABDOMINAL WALL HERNIAS

An abnormal protrusion of intra-abdominal tissue through a fascial defect in the abdominal wall. Approximately 75% occur in the groin, most of these being inguinal hernias (Figure 12.5 and Table 12.12). Hernias can be completely reducible, incompletely reducible, or nonreducible (incarcerated), depending on the ability to manually push the herniated tissue back into the abdomen. Bowel strangulation is a dreaded complication that can occur in nonreducible (incarcerated) hernias.

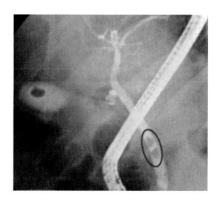

FIGURE 12.4. Endoscopic retrograde cholangiopancreatography image of acute cholecystitis. Three gallstones can be seen: one in the gallbladder and two partially obstructing stones in the distal common bile duct (circled). (Reproduced with permission from USMLE-Rx.com.)

KEY FACT

Choledocholithiasis is the presence of one or more gallstones in the common bile duct.

KEY FACT

Diastasis recti is a separation of the rectus abdominis muscles without a *fascial defect* and is often mistaken for an abdominal hernia. Most noticeable when patients strain or lift their head. This is common in women after pregnancy.

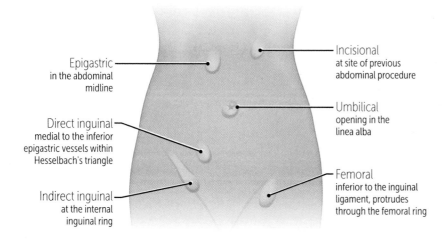

Epigastric — in the abdominal midline

Incisional — at site of previous abdominal procedure

Direct inguinal — medial to the inferior epigastric vessels within Hesselbach's triangle

Umbilical — opening in the linea alba

Indirect inguinal — at the internal inguinal ring

Femoral — inferior to the inguinal ligament, protrudes through the femoral ring

FIGURE 12.5. Hernia sites. (Reproduced with permission from USMLE-Rx.com.)

Q QUESTION

A 30-year-old woman who is otherwise healthy presents to you for the first time because she tested positive for the *BRCA1 mutation* and wants to know her options. Her 52-year-old mother was diagnosed with metastatic breast cancer at 38 years of age. How would you answer this patient?

TABLE 12.12.   Types of Hernias

TYPE	PATHOPHYSIOLOGY	LOCATION	CHARACTERISTICS
Indirect inguinal	A persistent processus vaginalis	The groin **lateral** to the inferior epigastric vessels	May present at birth Can descend into the scrotum
Direct inguinal	A defect of the transversalis fascia in Hesselbach triangle[a]	The groin **medial** to the inferior epigastric vessels	Most occur in middle-aged or elderly patients
Femoral	Occurs through the femoral canal	The upper thigh medial to the femoral vein	Less common; usually occurs in women Can easily become incarcerated or strangulated
Incisional/ventral	Breakdown of fascial closure from prior surgery	At the site of a previous surgical incision	Often asymptomatic May become larger on standing or with ↑ intra-abdominal pressure
Umbilical	Occurs through the fibromuscular umbilical ring	The umbilicus	Repair only if it persists beyond 5 years of age
Obturator	Occurs through the large obturator canal	Deep structures of the pelvis/thigh (not visualized externally)	Has a female-to-male ratio of 6:1 Can present as bowel obstruction
Epigastric	Occurs through defects in the aponeurosis of the rectus sheath	Midline between the umbilicus and the xiphoid process	Most commonly occurs in middle age but may also present in young children

[a]Hesselbach triangle is defined inferiorly by the inguinal ligament, laterally by the inferior epigastric arteries, and medially by the conjoined tendon.

MNEMONIC

Risk factors for breast cancer:
History ALONE

History of breast carcinoma, family history of *BRCA1* and *BRCA2*
Age
Late menopause
Obesity and lower social class
Nulliparity (or low/late parity) and lack of breastfeeding
Early menarche

ANSWER

You advise her that as a *BRCA* carrier she can undergo prophylactic bilateral mastectomy as well as bilateral salpingo-oophorectomy, if she has completed childbearing.

BREAST CANCER

Breast cancer is the most commonly diagnosed but second deadliest cancer in women. A mnemonic for remembering **risk factors for breast cancer** is History ALONE.
- OCP use is **not** a risk factor in average-risk women, but may be in those with a ⊕ family history.
- Screening methods include **mammography** and *BRCA1/BRCA2* mutation testing and are discussed in detail in the Community and Preventive Medicine chapter.

Differential
Fibrocystic disease, fibroadenoma, abscess, adenosis, scars, mastitis.

Diagnosis
- Breast cysts can be evaluated with ultrasound and then aspirated.
- Breast masses require either FNA or core needle biopsy, possibly followed by excisional biopsy.
- Any mass that is felt on exam **must** be further evaluated with biopsy, even if no abnormality is seen on mammography.
- **Algorithm:** If mass, then bilateral mammogram, then tissue sampling, then possible further workup, depending on tissue findings.

Management
Treatment for **early-stage breast cancer** is as follows:
- **Ductal carcinoma in situ (DCIS):** Excision (lumpectomy) with ⊖ margins and radiation therapy to the breast.

- **Lobular carcinoma in situ (LCIS):** A condition associated with ↑ risk of breast cancer arising elsewhere in the breast. Treatment with tamoxifen may be considered, but close follow-up and observation are usually indicated.
- **Invasive ductal or lobular carcinoma:** Lumpectomy followed by radiation therapy is equivalent to mastectomy. Mastectomy for large tumors or for patient preference.
- **Sentinel lymph node biopsy:** Indicated for invasive disease and may be indicated in certain cases of carcinoma in situ.
- **Adjuvant therapy:**
  - In general, any patient with an infiltrating ductal or lobular cancer >1 cm or with ⊕ lymph nodes should receive adjuvant therapy.
  - Hormone therapy with tamoxifen (for 5 years) is effective only in patients with breast cancer positive for estrogen receptor (ER) and/or progesterone receptor (PR). Where appropriate, tamoxifen ↓ the risk of recurrence by 40%.
  - Polychemotherapy ↓ the risk of recurrence by 25%.

The treatment approach for **advanced (metastatic) breast cancer** includes the following:
- **ER/PR-positive** masses:
  - **First-line therapy: Aromatase inhibitors** (eg, anastrozole, letrozole or exemestane) for postmenopausal women; prevent conversion of adrenal androgens into estrogens by aromatase enzymes in muscle and fat.
  - **Second-line hormonal therapy:** Megestrol acetate or tamoxifen.
- **ER/PR-negative masses (or progression of disease despite first-line treatment in hormone receptor-positive patients):**
  - Initial chemotherapy can be multiagent, but once patients progress after first-line treatment, single-agent treatment is commonly used.
  - Active chemotherapy drugs include paclitaxel, docetaxel, doxorubicin, methotrexate, vinorelbine, capecitabine, and 5-FU.
- **Patients with HER2 receptor overexpression:**
  - Overexpression of the HER2 receptor is associated with a poorer prognosis in breast cancer.
  - Trastuzumab is a humanized monoclonal antibody against the HER2 receptor found on breast cancer cells.
  - Patients with HER2 overexpression show responses to trastuzumab alone or in combination with chemotherapy.

BARIATRIC SURGERY

Bariatric surgery should be considered in patients with **BMI >40** or in patients with **BMI >35 with one or more obesity-related comorbidities** in whom traditional weight loss methods have failed. Obesity-related comorbidities include type 2 DM, hypertension, sleep apnea, nonalcoholic fatty liver disease, osteoarthritis, lipid abnormalities, gastrointestinal disorders, and heart disease.

Colorectal Surgery

SMALL BOWEL OBSTRUCTION

Small bowel obstruction (SBO) is the most common and surgically relevant disorder of the small intestine. Etiologies include postoperative **adhesions** (more than 50%), neoplasms, hernias, intussusception, foreign bodies, and gallstones.

MNEMONIC

Differential diagnosis of bowel obstruction:

HANG-IV

Hernia
Adhesions
Neoplasm
Gallstone Ileus

Intussusception
Volvulus

Symptoms

- **Proximal (high) obstruction:** Presents with abdominal pain and vomiting.
- **Mid- or distal obstruction:** Presents with periumbilical or poorly localized abdominal cramping, along with distention and constipation/obstipation. Feculent vomitus may also be seen.
- **Dehydration** and mild fever are seen.

Exam

- Vital signs are normal in the early stages.
- Peristalsis may be visible beneath the abdominal wall in thin patients.
- Exam reveals mild abdominal tenderness.
- Peristaltic rushes, gurgles, and **high-pitched tinkles** are sometimes audible.

Differential

- **Postoperative ileus:** Gas in the colon on AXR. Only mild dilation of small bowel.
- **Large bowel obstruction:** Obstipation and colonic dilation on AXR.
- **Intestinal pseudo-obstruction:** Symptoms and signs of obstruction without evidence of obstruction. Associated with SLE, drugs, and amyloidosis.
- **Other:** Acute gastroenteritis, acute appendicitis, acute pancreatitis.

Diagnosis

- **Labs:** Don't rely on labs, as these are often normal. Leukocytosis, evidence of dehydration, and/or electrolyte abnormalities may be seen. Creatine kinase and lactate are serum markers of intestinal compromise but are elevated only late in the course of disease.
- **Imaging:**
  - **Supine and upright AXRs:** Reveal a ladderlike pattern of dilated small bowel loops with air-fluid levels (Figure 12.6).
  - **CT:** Highly accurate in making the diagnosis and confirming the level of SBO. Also helpful in identifying the etiology.

Management

- **Partial obstruction** (gas seen in the colon on AXR): Can be managed expectantly with **NPO and an NG tube.**
- **Complete obstruction:**
  - Requires **operation**, in part to rule out **strangulation** (bowel dilation that impairs blood supply, which can eventually lead to necrosis, sepsis, perforation, and death).
  - Patients must be NPO and have an NG tube.
  - Treat dehydration and/or electrolyte abnormalities if present.
  - Antibiotics should be given if strangulation is suspected.

LARGE BOWEL OBSTRUCTION

Approximately 15% of intestinal obstructions in adults occur in the large intestine, most commonly in the **sigmoid colon.** The most common cause of large bowel obstruction (LBO) is **colorectal cancer;** other causes include diverticular disease, volvulus, inflammatory disorders, benign tumors, fecal impaction, and miscellaneous rare problems.

KEY FACT

Serial abdominal exams should be done in patients with partial SBO. Any acute change in exam should prompt repeat imaging and consideration of surgery.

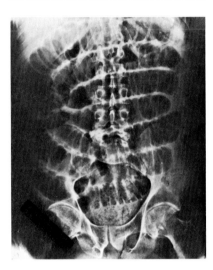

FIGURE 12.6. **Small bowel obstruction.** (Reproduced with permission from Doherty GM, Way LW. *Current Surgical Diagnosis & Treatment*, 12th ed. New York: McGraw-Hill, 2006:666.)

MNEMONIC

How do you know if a loop of bowel is dilated? Remember the 3-6-9 rule:

>**3** cm for the small intestine
>**6** cm for the large intestine
>**9** cm for the cecum

Symptoms/Exam

- Presents with abdominal cramping, constipation and/or obstipation, and vomiting. Onset can be rapid (volvulus) or insidious (cancer).
- Exam reveals abdominal distention, tympany, high-pitched "tinkles" on auscultation of bowel sounds, and tenderness to palpation ± signs of peritonitis (rebound tenderness).

Differential

SBO, paralytic ileus, pseudo-obstruction (Ogilvie syndrome).

Diagnosis

- **Labs:** May be normal. Leukocytosis and electrolyte abnormalities are seen with progression of disease.
- **Imaging:**
  - **AXR:** Demonstrates a dilated colon (distinguished from the small intestine by its haustral markings, which do not cross the entire lumen of the distended colon) with air-fluid levels.
  - **CT:** The best study for identifying the exact location and etiology of the bowel obstruction.
  - **Barium enema** if volvulus is suspected, as it can be therapeutic as well as diagnostic.

Management

- Surgery almost always required.
- The patient may require a **staged operation,** consisting of an initial colonic resection and diverting colostomy, followed by a later reanastomosis.

Diverticular Disorders

Approximately 65% of adults in the Western world develop diverticula by 80 years of age, most commonly in the sigmoid colon. Colonic diverticula are classified as false because they consist of mucosa and submucosa that have herniated through the muscular coats. True diverticula (containing all layers of bowel) are rare in the colon.

Diverticulosis

Defined as the presence of multiple false diverticula.

Symptoms/Exam

Usually asymptomatic. Exam reveals mild tenderness in the LLQ.

Differential

Diverticulitis, colon cancer.

Diagnosis

- **Labs:** Fever and leukocytosis are absent in patients with diverticula (and no diverticulitis).
- **Imaging:** Diverticuli can be visualized at colonoscopy and on CT and barium enema studies.

Management

High-fiber diet; bulking agents (psyllium); education and reassurance; surgical resection for massive hemorrhage or to rule out carcinoma.

Diverticulitis

A complication of diverticulosis that can range from mild inflammation to colonic perforation with peritonitis.

Symptoms/Exam

- Presents with acute onset of LLQ pain.
- Nausea, vomiting, or dysuria may be seen, depending on the location and extent of inflammation.
- Peritoneal signs are seen if the disease presents late (with perforation).
- Exam reveals low-grade fever, mild abdominal distention, LLQ tenderness, and a LLQ mass.

Differential

Appendicitis, mesenteric ischemia, bowel obstruction, Crohn's disease.

Diagnosis

- **Labs:** Leukocytosis; ⊖ fecal occult blood (if present, suggests malignancy).
- **Imaging:**
  - **AXR:** Reveals free air in the presence of a perforation. Shows ileus and partial obstruction ± LLQ mass.
  - **CT: The best initial study (preferably with IV contrast).** Reveals diverticuli, bowel wall thickening, and surrounding inflammation (Figure 12.7).
  - **Barium enema: Contraindicated** due to the possibility of barium leaking into the peritoneal cavity.

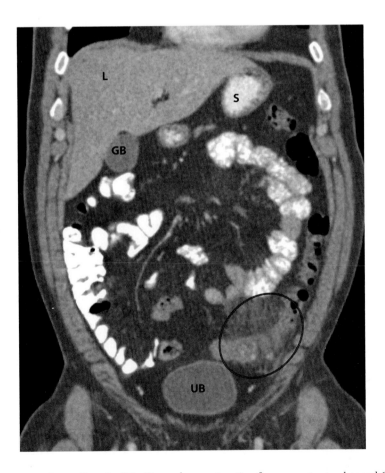

FIGURE 12.7.   Acute diverticulitis. Coronal reconstruction from a contrast-enhanced CT demonstrates sigmoid diverticula with perisigmoid inflammatory "fat stranding." The area of abnormality is circled in red. (L = liver; S = stomach; GB = gallbladder; UB = urinary bladder.)

Management

- **Expectant management:**
  - NPO, IV fluids.
  - Broad-spectrum antibiotics:
    - **Outpatient** (mild): Trimethoprim-sulfamethoxazole or metronidazole plus quinolone.
    - **Inpatient** (moderate to severe): IV piperacillin-tazobactam, ampicillin-sulbactam, quinolone to cover anaerobes and gram-negative rods.
  - Colonoscopy should be performed 4 to 6 weeks after the acute attack to exclude coexisting neoplastic disease. (Avoid colonoscopy during acute phase because of the risk of perforation.)
- **Surgical management:**
  - Indicated for abscess formation, **perforation, or failure of expectant management;** may sometimes be managed with percutaneous drainage of paracolic abscesses.
  - Severe cases usually require laparotomy and **possible colectomy** (often done as a **staged operation**). Laparoscopic operations are difficult in the setting of inflammation.

Sigmoid Volvulus

Rotation of a segment of the intestine on an axis formed by its mesentery that leads to obstruction of the lumen and circulatory impairment of the bowel. The sigmoid is the segment most commonly involved in colonic volvulus.

Symptoms/Exam

Presents with acute abdominal pain and obstipation. Exam reveals abdominal distention.

Differential

Cecal volvulus and other causes of LBO (carcinoma, benign tumors, fecal impaction, diverticular disease).

Diagnosis

- **AXR:** A single, greatly distended loop of bowel that has lost its haustral markings is usually seen rising up out of the pelvis (sometimes termed **megacolon**).
- **Barium enema:** The pathognomonic finding is the **"bird's beak"** or **"ace of spades"** deformity, named for the way the barium column tapers toward the volvulus (Figure 12.8). This procedure may be therapeutic.

Management

- **Endoscopic decompression** with a flexible colonoscope or sigmoidoscope.
- **Emergent operation (partial or total colectomy):** Performed if strangulation or perforation is present or if attempts at decompression are unsuccessful.

Fecal Impaction

May develop after excisional hemorrhoidectomy, in chronically debilitated patients, or from the use of constipating pain medications without stool softeners and fiber.

Symptoms/Exam

- Diarrhea (only passage of liquid stool due to obstructing inspissated fecal bolus).
- Pelvic pain and fullness.
- Digital rectal exam (DRE) reveals hard, dry stool that obstructs the rectum. Abdominal exam may reveal a pelvic or abdominal mass.

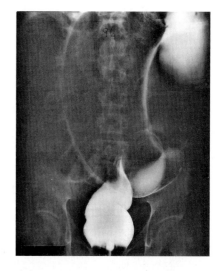

FIGURE 12.8. Sigmoid volvulus: greatly dilated sigmoid. Contrast barium enema shows stenosis known as "bird's beak" or "ace of spades" deformity.
(Reproduced with permission from Doherty GM. *Current Diagnosis & Treatment: Surgery,* 13th ed. New York: McGraw-Hill, 2010, Fig. 30-16.)

Differential

Other obstructing lesion or sigmoid malignancy.

Management

- Digital disimpaction at the bedside.
- Treatment in the operating room, with local or regional anesthesia, may be necessary to provide pelvic floor relaxation and pain control.

HEMORRHOIDS

Hemorrhoidal tissues that cause bleeding, pain, or mucus are pathologic, usually occurring in the setting of ↑ intra-abdominal pressure that can occur in pregnancy, in the presence of obesity, and with lifting or straining (ie, constipation).

Symptoms/Exam

- **Internal hemorrhoids:** Painless; present with bright red blood per rectum, mucous discharge, and rectal fullness or discomfort. Classification is based on the degree of prolapse:
    - **First degree:** Hemorrhoids do not protrude through the anus.
    - **Second degree:** Hemorrhoids prolapse but reduce spontaneously.
    - **Third degree:** Hemorrhoids prolapse and require manual reduction.
    - **Fourth degree:** Hemorrhoids cannot be reduced and may strangulate.
- **External hemorrhoids:** Present with severe perianal pain and perianal mass.
- Exam reveals vascular dilation, friable mucosa, and local perineal irritation.

Differential

Malignancy, diverticular disease, IBD, adenomatous polyps, procidentia.

Diagnosis

- **Labs:** CBC to rule out anemia if chronic bleeding is present.
- **Anoscopy.**

Management

- **Medical:** Best for first- and second-degree internal hemorrhoids. Consists of dietary changes (eliminating constipating foods and ↑ fiber), stool softener, exercise, and limiting toilet time.
- **Surgical:** Used when medical management fails and often indicated for third- and fourth-degree hemorrhoids. The three classic techniques are elastic band ligation, sclerosis, and excisional hemorrhoidectomy.

Complications

Bleeding, pain, necrosis, and, rarely, perianal sepsis.

Thrombosed External Hemorrhoid

Acute intravascular thrombosis that develops within an external hemorrhoid, causing severe perianal pain.

Symptoms/Exam

- Presents with sudden, severe perianal pain that peaks within 48 to 72 hours.
- Exam reveals a purplish-black, edematous, tense subcutaneous perianal mass (Figure 12.9).

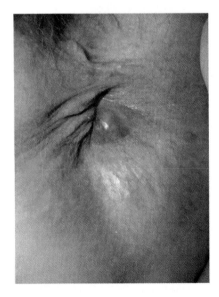

FIGURE 12.9. Thrombosed external hemorrhoid. External hemorrhoid with a small skin break that resulted in bleeding. (Reproduced with permission from LeBlond RF, et al. *DeGowin's Diagnostic Examination,* 9th ed. New York: McGraw-Hill, 2009, Plate 28.)

Differential

Nonthrombosed external hemorrhoid, internal hemorrhoid, skin tag.

Diagnosis

Physical exam.

Management

- **Less than 48 hours after onset of symptoms:** Excision of the entire thrombosis, simple incision with clot expression (higher recurrence rate).
- **Forty-eight to 72 hours after onset of symptoms:** Warm sitz baths, high-fiber diet, stool softeners, reassurance.

ANAL FISSURE

A split in the anoderm that results from forceful dilation of the anal canal, most commonly during defecation.

Symptoms/Exam

- Presents with pain with defecation, along with blood on the tissue and stool or dripping into the toilet water (but not mixed in the stool). Constipation is common.
- Exam reveals disruption of the anoderm in the anterior or posterior midline involving the epithelium immediately distal to the dentate line.

Differential

Crohn's disease, anal TB, anal malignancy, abscess or fistula disease, HSV.

Diagnosis

Anoscopy may reveal a proximal hypertrophied anal papilla above a fissure.

Management

- **Medical:** Stool softeners, bulking agents, sitz baths, topical anesthetic ointment, nitroglycerin ointment, nifedipine cream.
- **Surgical:** Consider surgery for chronic (>1 month) or chronic recurrent ulcers. Lateral internal anal sphincterectomy is the procedure of choice.

ANORECTAL ABSCESS AND FISTULA

When glands in the anorectum become infected, they can develop into an abscess and an associated fistula tract.

Symptoms/Exam

- Presents with severe, continuous throbbing anal pain.
- Anal swelling, fever, urinary retention, and sepsis may be seen.
- Exam reveals a tender perianal or rectal mass. A fistula tract may not be discovered until exam is performed under anesthesia.

Differential

Crohn's disease, pilonidal disease, hidradenitis suppurativa, diverticulitis, anal fissure.

KEY FACT

Anal fistula is a common complication of untreated anorectal abscess.

QUESTION

A 70-year-old man calls your answering service on Sunday night complaining of "bright red blood in my stool" for a few days. He had a normal colonoscopy 6 months ago and has no history of weight loss or anemia. When you see him in the office on Monday morning, he has stable vital signs and no abdominal pain, and anoscopy reveals a friable internal hemorrhoid. CBC reveals a stable hemoglobin/hematocrit. What is the next step in management?

Diagnosis
- No imaging is necessary in uncomplicated cases.
- Sinography, transrectal ultrasound, CT, and MRI can be useful in complex or recurrent cases.

Management
Surgical drainage under general anesthesia.

PILONIDAL DISEASE

An infection of natal cleft hair follicles, which, when obstructed, become distended and rupture into the subcutaneous tissue, forming an abscess. The highest incidence is in white males 15 to 40 years of age, with a peak incidence in those 16 to 20 years of age.

Symptoms/Exam
- Presents with pain, tenderness, purulent drainage, inspissated hair, and induration near the perianal region.
- Patients are typically overweight, hirsute males who perspire profusely.
- Exam of the coccyx or sacrum reveals small pits or abscesses on or close to the midline.

Differential
Abscess-fistula disease, hidradenitis suppurativa, furuncle, actinomycosis.

Diagnosis
Physical exam is adequate for diagnosis.

Management
- Surgical incision, drainage, and curettage of the abscess cavity to remove hair nests and skin debris.
- Meticulous skin care, hygiene, and shaving of the surrounding area for at least 3 months after the surgical procedure.
- May require more definitive surgery (eg, excision of pits, marsupialization).

Vascular Surgery

ABDOMINAL AORTIC ANEURYSM

A permanent local dilation of the abdominal aorta, defined as being >1.5 times the normal diameter. A diameter >3 cm is generally considered aneurysmal. Abdominal aortic aneurysm (AAA) is a relatively common condition and most patients are asymptomatic; however, it can be fatal when it ruptures. The risk of rupture increases with the size of the aneurysm. Risk factors for AAA include smoking, hypertension, a family history of AAA, and male gender.

Symptoms/Exam
- Usually **asymptomatic** until the aneurysm ruptures.
- Ruptured AAA presents with hypotension, abdominal or back pain, and **a pulsatile abdominal mass.** May also present with buttock, groin, testicular, or leg pain.

KEY FACT

Think pilonidal cyst in a young, hairy male patient with perianal abscess.

ANSWER

You prescribe a stool softener and advise your patient to ↑ his fluid intake, get regular exercise, and limit time spent on the commode.

KEY FACT

Larger AAAs can be felt as pulsatile masses.

Diagnosis

- **Ultrasound** is the standard imaging tool for screening/monitoring and is highly sensitive and specific (Figure 12.10A).
- CT scan should be obtained for symptomatic patients who are stable. CT scan is also recommended for preoperative aneurysm evaluation (Figure 12.10B).

Management

Asymptomatic patients: Management is based on **aortic diameter.**

- Aortic diameter **<3.0 cm:** No further testing.
- Aortic diameter **3.0 to 4.5 cm:** Annual ultrasound.
- Aortic diameter **>4.5 cm:** Refer to vascular surgeon.
- Aortic diameter **>5.5 cm:** Repair; the 1° methods of AAA repair are open and endovascular.
- Ruptured AAA: Emergent open repair or endovascular repair.

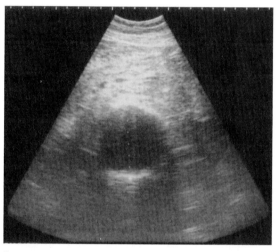

A

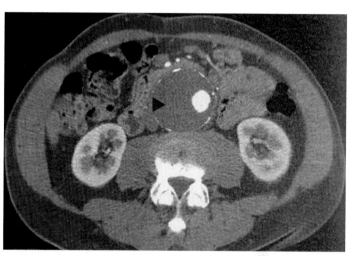

B

FIGURE 12.10. **Abdominal aortic aneurysm. (A)** Bedside ultrasound image of 6.5-cm abdominal aneurysm. **(B)** Transaxial image from contrast-enhanced CT showing 5.5-cm aneurysm with extensive mural thrombus (arrowhead). (Image A reproduced with permission from Tintinalli JE, et al. *Tintinalli's Emergency Medicine: A Comprehensive Study Guide*, 6th ed. New York: McGraw-Hill, 2004, Fig. 58-2; image B reproduced with permission from Doherty GM. *Current Diagnosis & Treatment: Surgery*, 13th ed. New York: McGraw-Hill, 2010, Fig. 34-16.)

NOTES

Child and Adolescent Medicine

Anna Jack, MD

The Newborn Exam

It is important to identify neonatal distress and become aware of congenital abnormalities and correctable defects:

- **History:** Maternal labs, maternal health during pregnancy and labor, outcomes of previous pregnancies, potential toxic exposures, and family history.
- **Apgar scores:** Performed at 1 and 5 minutes; may be repeated at 10 minutes if indicated (Table 13.1). Low 5-minute Apgar scores correlate with an ↑ risk of death in the first year as well as with cerebral palsy.

PHYSICAL FINDINGS

Skin

- **Acrocyanosis:** Blue hands and feet are often normal, but generalized cyanosis may be a sign of a congenital heart defect and warrants immediate evaluation.
- **Birthmarks:** Benign birthmarks include capillary hemangiomas and blue-grey spots (formerly called Mongolian spots). Birthmarks such as café-au-lait spots (Figure 13.1) and ash leaf spots can be a sign of an underlying disorder (eg, >6 café-au-lait spots may point to neurofibromatosis type 1 and ash leaf spots are associated with tuberous sclerosis).

Head

- **Scalp:**
  - **Caput succedaneum:** Swelling of the scalp caused by pressure on the head against the dilating cervix. Crosses suture lines (Figure 13.2).
  - **Cephalohematoma:** Bleeding between the skull and periosteum. Does not cross suture lines. Generally benign.
  - **Subgaleal hemorrhage:** Bleeding beneath the scalp; can result in extensive blood loss. Crosses suture lines.
- **Eyes:** An abnormal light reflex may be a sign of glaucoma, cataracts, or a tumor (ie, retinoblastoma).
- **Ears:** Low-set ears may be associated with congenital anomalies. Preauricular pits may be a sign of congenital hearing loss.

KEY FACT

Isolated cleft palate is more likely than cleft lip plus palate to be part of a syndrome. Complications include feeding difficulties, speech delay, and recurrent otitis media.

TABLE 13.1. Apgar Scores

SIGN	SCORE		
	0	1	2
Appearance	Blue or pale	Body pink; extremities blue	Completely pink
Pulse	Absent	60-100 bpm	>100 bpm
Grimace (reflex irritability)	No response	Grimace	Cry or cough
Activity (muscle tone)	Floppy	Some flexion	Flexion; active movement
Respirations	Absent	Slow, irregular	Good, crying

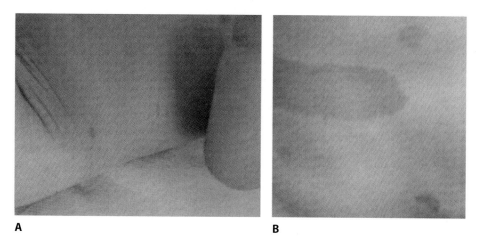

FIGURE 13.1. **Café-au-lait spots.** In an 8-month-old infant (**A**) and mother (**B**). (Reproduced from Benelli E, et al. Legius syndrome: case report and review of literature. *Ital J Pediatr.* 2015;41:8.)

- **Nose:** Check for the patency of both nares. Since infants are obligate nose breathers, blockage of the nasal passage by abnormal tissue (choanal atresia) may lead to respiratory distress.
- **Oropharynx:** Check for cleft lip or palate. Epstein pearls at the junction of the hard and soft palates are epithelial retention cysts and are considered normal.

Chest

Clavicular fractures may occur during delivery complicated by shoulder dystocia. Look for crepitus, step-offs, bruising, and tenderness.

Heart

Murmurs in the immediate newborn period are common and are usually benign (see the Cardiovascular Disease section below). Cyanosis, abnormal pulses, and signs of HF indicate heart disease.

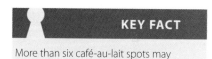
KEY FACT

More than six café-au-lait spots may indicate neurofibromatosis type 1.

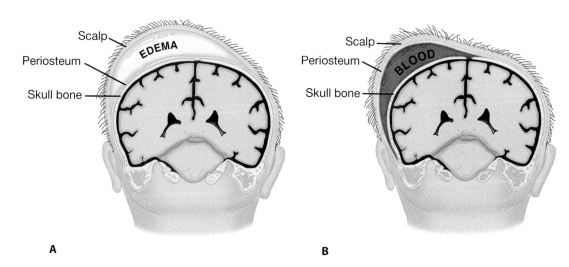

FIGURE 13.2. **Scalp swelling.** (**A**) Caput succedaneum—hematoma superficial to periosteum. (**B**) Cephalohematoma—hematoma is deep to the periosteum. (Reproduced with permission from Cunningham FG, et al. *Williams Obstetrics*, 23rd ed. New York: McGraw-Hill, 2010, Fig. 29-12.)

Abdomen

- An abnormal mass is most often associated with kidney disease (tumor, hydrone-phrosis, multicystic kidney disease).
- Consider diaphragmatic hernia in an infant with scaphoid abdomen and respiratory distress.
- Hepatosplenomegaly is associated with neonatal infection (cytomegalovirus [CMV]), metabolic disorders, and HF.

Genitalia

- Cryptorchidism may be present in up to 3% of term male infants and generally resolves by the first birthday.
- **Ambiguous genitalia:** The most common cause is congenital adrenal hyperplasia (CAH), which can lead to both XX virilization and XY feminization. Other causes include testicular regression syndrome, androgen insensitivity, testosterone biosynthesis disorders, and chromosomal abnormalities.
  - CAH is a group of autosomal-recessive enzyme deficiencies that lead to problems with adrenal hormone synthesis. Most forms include cortisol deficiency. Depending on the type of CAH, there may be symptoms of either mineralocorticoid deficiency or excess and androgen deficiency or excess.
  - Initial evaluation should include a history, physical exam, and karyotype. Measure gonadotropins (luteinizing hormone [LH], follicle-stimulating hormone [FSH]), adrenal steroids (cortisol, 17-OHP, adrenocorticotropic hormone [ACTH] stimulation test), testosterone precursors (DHEA, androstenedione), testosterone, dihydrotestosterone, and hCG (hCG stimulation test).
  - Management: Replace glucocorticoids, mineralocorticoids, and sodium as necessary in CAH. Provide hormone replacement as needed.
  - Surgical reassignment is controversial. In the past, early surgery was recommended, but as children reached adolescence, some rejected their gender assignment. This has raised the issue of waiting and allowing the child to express a preference.
  - A sensitive multidisciplinary team approach is crucial.

Musculoskeletal

- **Spine:** Pits or hair tufts at the base of the spine may suggest spina bifida occulta.
- **Upper extremities:** ↓ movement and asymmetric Moro reflex may indicate a brachial plexus injury.
- **Lower extremities:** Most flexible deformities result from intrauterine posture and usually resolve spontaneously.
- **Developmental dysplasia of the hip (DDH):** Defined as inadequate pressure of the femoral head against the acetabulum that leads to a shallow socket, with risk of future dislocation and gait abnormalities. Presents with asymmetric skin folds in the thighs. Provocative tests including Barlow and Ortolani maneuvers have low sensitivity, but a clunk felt may represent DDH. Risk factors include breech presentation, female gender, white race, and ⊕ family history. Ultrasound is used for diagnosis until 4 months of age, since radiographs do not detect the uncalcified femoral head before this time (Figure 13.3).
- **Metatarsus adductus (metatarsus varus):** Common congenital foot deformity characterized by **inward deviation of the forefoot.** Convexity along the lateral border of the foot. In advanced cases, a vertical crease in the arch may be seen. The angulation is at the level of the base of the fifth metatarsal, and this bone will be prominent. In most cases, the problem corrects itself with normal use of the foot or with stretching exercises. Rarely, casting or surgery may be needed. Approximately 10% to 15% of affected children also have hip dysplasia.

KEY FACT

Check for DDH with screening ultrasound in all breech female newborns. Also consider DDH in female newborns with ⊕ family history and in breech male newborns.

KEY FACT

Neural tube defects encompass a broad range of defects, including myelomeningocele, spina bifida, encephalocele, and anencephaly. Causes include genetic abnormalities, folate deficiency, maternal DM, and exposures (alcohol, anticonvulsants). Often idiopathic.

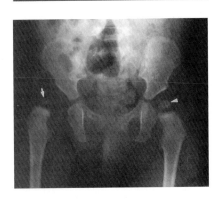

FIGURE 13.3. Developmental dysplasia of the right hip, severe. The right femoral epiphysis (arrow) is smaller than the left (arrowhead) and laterally displaced away from the acetabulum, and the right acetabular roof is shallow in comparison to the left. (Reproduced with permission from Chen MYM, et al. *Basic Radiology.* New York: McGraw-Hill, 2004, Fig. 7-11.)

- **Talipes equinovarus (clubfoot):** May be idiopathic, neurogenic, or syndromic (eg, arthrogryposis, Larsen syndrome). Idiopathic clubfeet may be hereditary. Presents with a **foot that turns inward and downward.** Plantar flexion of the foot at the ankle joint (equinus), inversion deformity of the heel (varus), and adduction of the forefoot and hindfoot (varus) are seen (Figure 13.4). Infants should be carefully examined for associated anomalies, especially of the spine. Corrected with manipulation of the foot to stretch the contracted tissues and with serial casting (the Ponseti technique).
- **Genu varum and genu valgum:** Varum (bowlegs) is normal until age 2 years, after which many children develop genu valgum (knock knees), which may persist until about age 8. Persistence of either condition beyond these ages requires referral and possible surgical repair or splinting.
- **Tibial torsion:** Internal rotation of the leg between the knee and the ankle is normal in the newborn, but justifies referral for splinting if it persists beyond 18 months.
- **Femoral anteversion:** Internal rotation at the hip causes the appearance of intoeing. Treatment is generally not necessary unless passive external rotation is not possible.

Neurologic

Look for normal newborn reflexes, including suck, rooting, grasp, tonic neck, and Moro. Several beats of ankle clonus and the Babinski reflex are normal in newborns.

- **Cerebral palsy:** Spectrum of disorders that are nonprogressive and originate from some type of cerebral insult or injury. The injury may occur before birth, during delivery, or in the perinatal period. The most common form involves spasticity of the limbs. The second most frequent presentation is ataxia. Associated neurologic deficits can include seizure, cognitive impairment, speech delay, and sensory loss. Physical, occupational, and speech therapy; orthopedic interventions as necessary.

NEWBORN SCREENING AND PROPHYLAXIS

Newborn Screening

Testing performed on all newborns to identify congenital disorders to prevent long-term sequelae.

- **Hearing:** Universal hearing screening helps identify most children with hearing loss. Risk factors for hearing loss include congenital infection, abnormal craniofacial anatomy, and ⊕ family history.

Newborn Prophylaxis

- **Hemorrhagic disease of the newborn** (bleeding disorder due to vitamin K deficiency): IM vitamin K is given for prevention.
- **Ophthalmia neonatorum:** Erythromycin or tetracycline ointment prevents gonococcal and chlamydial conjunctivitis.
- **Hepatitis B:**
  - Children born to mothers with ⊕ HbSAg should receive hepatitis B immune globulin (HBIG) and HBV vaccine in the first 12 hours of life.
  - In children ≤2000 g, HBIG should be given within 12 hours of delivery if the test result is still unknown or ⊕.
  - In children >2000 g, HBIG should be given as soon as the mother's test is ⊕ and should be given within 7 days.
  - **Prevention of perinatal HIV transmission:** See the Reproductive Health chapter.

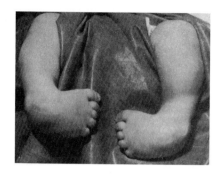

FIGURE 13.4. Talipes equinovarus (clubfoot). (Reproduced with permission from Brunicardi FC, et al. *Schwartz's Principles of Surgery*, 8th ed. New York: McGraw-Hill, 2005:1718.)

MNEMONIC

In genu val**GUM,** the knees are **GUM**med together.

KEY FACT

Newborn screening for genetic disease varies by state. All states test for PKU and congenital hypothyroidism, since early treatment will prevent cognitive and developmental impairment. Most states also check for galactosemia and sickle cell disease.

QUESTION

A 4-day-old boy, born at 37 weeks to a G1 now P1 mother via vacuum assisted delivery for prolonged variable decelerations presents for a weight check. He is being exclusively breastfed, but mother is worried that he is not "getting enough." He is down 10% from his birth weight and appears jaundiced. What should you do?

Circumcision

- **Benefits:** Slightly ↓ the risk of penile cancer, ↓ UTIs in the first year of life, and ↓ transmission of HIV infection.
- **Risks:** Bleeding, infection, injury to the urethra or other surrounding structures, removal of too much skin, unsatisfactory cosmetic outcome.
- **Contraindications:** Genital abnormalities (eg, hypospadias) or bleeding disorder.

PROBLEMS IN THE NEONATAL PERIOD

Birth Trauma

Complications associated with birth trauma include the following:
- **Intraventricular hemorrhage** (Figure 13.5): Risk factors include prematurity, birth trauma, and asphyxia.
- **Hypoxia:** Related to chronic intrauterine conditions such as placental insufficiency or to acute events such as cord prolapse or maternal hypoxia.
- **Fractures:** May occur with traumatic delivery. Clavicle fractures are most common.
- **Peripheral nerve injuries:** Often related to traumatic delivery but may be idiopathic. Shoulder dystocia is a risk factor for brachial plexus injury. Most brachial plexus injuries resolve spontaneously in the first year. Physical therapy may be beneficial.

Neonatal Jaundice

More than one-half of newborns develop clinical jaundice in the first week of life. Risk factors include maternal DM, male gender, prematurity, and Asian race. Etiologies are outlined in Table 13.2.

Symptoms/Exam

- Jaundice progresses from head to toe with ↑ bilirubin levels.
- **Physiologic jaundice:** Jaundice after first 24 hours, peaks at 3 to 5 days of life, lasts up to 1 week.

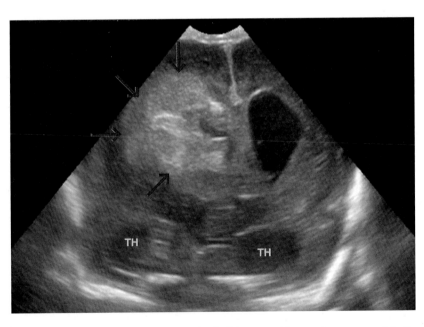

FIGURE 13.5. Neonatal hemorrhage. Grade IV neonatal hemorrhage centered in the right germinal matrix, extending into the right lateral ventricle and parenchyma (arrows) and associated with hydrocephalus (note the dilated temporal horns [TH] of the lateral ventricles). (Reproduced with permission from USMLE-Rx.com.)

TABLE 13.2. Etiologies of Unconjugated Hyperbilirubinemia

	CAUSE	DIAGNOSIS/COMMENTS
Hemolytic	Rh and ABO incompatibility	Maternal Coombs antibody for signs of isoimmunization
	Hereditary spherocytosis	Spherocytes on peripheral smear; confirm with a red cell osmotic fragility test
	G6PD deficiency	An X-linked disorder seen most commonly in African, Mediterranean, and Asian families
Nonhemolytic	Enclosed hemorrhage (cephalohematoma)	As blood is resorbed, bilirubin levels will ↑
	Inherited disorders of conjugation	Examples include Crigler-Najjar and Gilbert syndromes
	Physiologic (normal)	May be due to ↑ hematocrit (even in the absence of true polycythemia) and initial lack of gut flora
	Breast milk jaundice	Most likely related to free fatty acids in breast milk which can ↑ enterohepatic circulation of bilirubin; typically appears after the first week and may persist for many weeks
	Breastfeeding jaundice	Related to dehydration while the mother's milk supply is coming in; resolves when feeding is well established
	Infection	Congenital and acquired infections may cause jaundice

- **Pathologic jaundice:** Appears in first 24 hours, lasts >1 week, fast rate of rise (>5 mg/dL/day), higher bilirubin levels (>15 mg/dL), direct (conjugated) bilirubin >2 mg/dL.
- **Acute bilirubin encephalopathy:** Early signs include lethargy, hypotonia, and poor suck.

Differential

- Unconjugated bilirubinemia ("indirect").
- Conjugated bilirubinemia ("direct").
- Biliary tree disease.
- Hepatocellular disease.

Diagnosis

- Total and direct bilirubin levels.
- Hematocrit.
- Mother's hematocrit.
- Mother's and infant's blood type.
- DAT (Coombs test of infant).
- If conjugated bilirubinemia, consider LFTs and liver ultrasound.

Management

- **Unconjugated bilirubinemia:** Hydration, ↑ feeding, phototherapy, and exchange transfusion. A nomogram correlating safe bilirubin levels with age should be used to determine when to treat with phototherapy and exchange transfusion.
- **Conjugated bilirubinemia:** Treatment of underlying cause. Conjugated bilirubinemia is nontoxic (does not cause encephalopathy/kernicterus) and is not improved by phototherapy. Phototherapy causes bronzing of the skin.

Complications

The long-term complication of unconjugated hyperbilirubinemia is **kernicterus**, chronic bilirubin encephalopathy. Kernicterus presents with movement disorders and deafness.

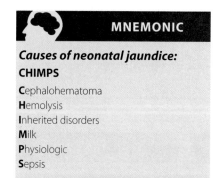

MNEMONIC

Causes of neonatal jaundice:
CHIMPS
Cephalohematoma
Hemolysis
Inherited disorders
Milk
Physiologic
Sepsis

KEY FACT

Screening and chemoprophylaxis for maternal GBS has ↓ the incidence of neonatal GBS sepsis. This benefit has been somewhat offset by a rise in non-GBS neonatal sepsis, especially in preterm and low-birth-weight infants.

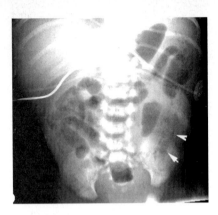

MNEMONIC

Congenital infections:

TORCHeS

Toxoplasmosis
Other (HBV, HIV, varicella, parvovirus, *Listeria*, TB, Zika)
Rubella
CMV
HSV
Syphilis

KEY FACT

CMV infection is the leading cause of sensorineural hearing loss in children.

KEY FACT

HSV is typically transmitted during vaginal delivery when the mother has active lesions or asymptomatic viral shedding. Prevent with antiviral therapy started at 36 weeks' gestation for pregnant women with recurrent genital herpes; cesarean delivery is indicated for women in labor with active genital lesions or prodromal symptoms.

Necrotizing Enterocolitis

The most common life-threatening GI illness in neonates. More common among premature infants. The etiology is unknown but may be related to ischemia and infection.

- Manifests as abdominal distention, feeding intolerance, and blood in the stools.
- **Diagnosis:** Radiographs may reveal pneumatosis intestinalis (intramural air; Figure 13.6).
- **Management:** NPO, broad-spectrum antibiotics; surgery may be necessary.

Neonatal Sepsis

May have **early** or **late** onset.

- **Early sepsis (first week of life):** Result of vertical transmission. Risk factors include prolonged rupture of membranes (>18 hours), maternal fever, chorioamnionitis, group B streptococcus (GBS) with inadequate treatment (<4 hours antibiotics), and prematurity.
  - Usually presents in the first 24 hours.
  - Characterized by temperature instability, respiratory distress, hypotension, and poor perfusion.
  - Common pathogens include GBS and *Escherichia coli*.
  - Pneumonia is a common cause.
- **Late sepsis (after the first week of life):** Risk factors include prematurity, indwelling lines, endotracheal intubation, prior antibiotics.
  - May present with poor feeding, temperature instability, lethargy, and apnea.
  - Causal organisms include *Staphylococcus aureus*, GBS, *Enterococcus*, *Pseudomonas*, and other gram-negative organisms.
  - Meningitis is more common in this period.
- **Diagnosis:** Laboratory abnormalities may include a low or high WBC count, thrombocytopenia, metabolic acidosis, hypoglycemia, and ↑ CRP.
- **Management:** Broad-spectrum antibiotics are appropriate while awaiting culture results (blood, urine, and CSF). Ampicillin with gentamicin is a common regimen.

Congenital Infections

See Table 13.3.

Meconium Aspiration Syndrome

Aspiration of meconium results in chemical pneumonitis, mucous plugging, and inactivation of surfactant. Risk factors include low amniotic fluid volume, postdates pregnancy, IUGR, and signs of fetal distress.

- Signs of respiratory distress, including tachypnea, grunting, nasal flaring, and retractions.
- **Diagnosis:** CXR shows patchy, coarse infiltrates and hyperexpansion.
- **Management:** Resuscitation should include suction of the hypopharynx under direct visualization **if the infant is depressed.** This does not prevent many cases of meconium aspiration, as aspiration also occurs in utero. Vigorous infants do not require suctioning.

Transient Tachypnea of the Newborn

Tachypnea due to retained fetal lung fluid. Risk factors include precipitous delivery, cesarean delivery, and maternal DM.

- Respiratory distress is generally present within several hours of birth. Respiratory rate typically exceeds 60 breaths/min.

TABLE 13.3. **Congenital Infections**

	TOXOPLASMOSIS	RUBELLA	CMV	HSV	SYPHILIS
TRANSMISSION	TRANSPLACENTAL	TRANSPLACENTAL	TRANSPLACENTAL	VAGINAL	TRANSPLACENTAL
Signs	Classic triad: Obstructive hydrocephalus, chorioretinitis, intracranial calcification Also presents with fever, hepatosplenomegaly, anemia, hyperbilirubinemia Maternal history of contact with cat feces or intake of undercooked meat or unpasteurized milk	Cataracts, cardiac involvement (especially patent ductus arteriosus [PDA]), "blueberry muffin rash," hearing loss	Sensorineural hearing loss Other manifestations include intrauterine growth retardation (IUGR), hepatosplenomegaly, thrombocytopenia, and CNS effects (microcephaly, chorioretinitis)	Mucocutaneous disease: Vesicular rash, keratoconjunctivitis CNS: Encephalitis, seizures Disseminated: Hepatitis, pneumonia, sepsis	**Early disease** (age <2 years): Typically presents in the first 6 weeks with jaundice, rash, rhinitis ("snuffles"), osteochondritis **Late disease** (age >2 years): Tooth and bone abnormalities, including Hutchinson teeth, hearing impairment, cognitive or developmental impairment
Diagnosis	Toxoplasma serology	Rubella serology	Urine culture for CMV	Viral culture	Serologic tests in mother and infant
Prevention/ Treatment	Pyrimethamine plus sulfadiazine	Maternal immunization before pregnancy	Ganciclovir may be beneficial	Antiviral therapy during pregnancy, cesarean delivery Acyclovir or valcyclovir	Treat mother during pregnancy Treat child with penicillin if mother is untreated or had an inadequate response to treatment, or if there are clinical signs of disease

- **Diagnosis:** CXR reveals streaky perihilar opacities and fluid in the fissures (Figure 13.7A and B).
- **Management:** Management is supportive; may require O_2. The syndrome typically resolves in 12 to 24 hours.

Respiratory Distress Syndrome (also Hyaline Membrane Disease)

Caused by surfactant deficiency. Greatest risk factor is prematurity. Other risk factors include maternal DM and cesarean delivery without labor.

- Poor lung compliance and atelectasis ↑ work of breathing and lead to eventual respiratory failure.
- **Diagnosis:** CXR shows ground-glass opacities (Figure 13.7C).
- **Management:** Prevent RDS with antenatal corticosteroids to improve lung maturity. Treat with exogenous surfactant and mechanical ventilation.

QUESTION

Shortly after the delivery of a term baby boy by cesarean section, you are called to the nursery to evaluate the infant. His respiratory rate is 55 breaths/min, and he is noted to be a bit dusky when he tries to breastfeed. His O_2 saturation is normal, but he has some mild retractions with respiratory effort. What is your management strategy?

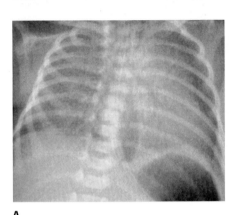
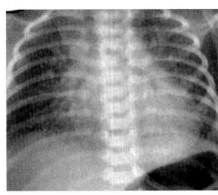
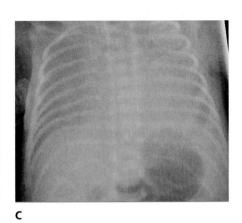

A   B   C

FIGURE 13.7. **Transient tachypnea of the newborn versus respiratory distress syndrome.** Frontal CXRs at 6 hours of life (**A**) and 2 days later (**B**) show initial findings of bilateral diffuse ground-glass appearance and fine granularity due to interstitial opacities (left) and resolution of the pulmonary parenchymal opacities, though perihilar streaky markings are still present (right). (**C**) Frontal CXR in a neonate with respiratory distress syndrome shows diffuse fine granular ("ground-glass") opacities and hypoaeration. (Images A and B reproduced from Alorainy IA, et al. Pictorial Essay: Infants of diabetic mothers. *Indian J Radiol Imaging.* 2010;20(3):174-181; image C reproduced with permission from USMLE-Rx.com.)

Cryptorchidism

Describes testes that have not descended into the scrotum. May be unilateral or bilateral. Approximately 3% of full-term male newborns have an undescended testis at birth.

- **Management:** By 1 year of age, 80% of all undescended testes are in the scrotum. Surgical orchidopexy is indicated if descent has not occurred by 1 year.
- **Complications:** Infertility and testicular malignancy. The risk of malignancy (although lower) persists even after placement into the scrotum.

GENETIC AND CONGENITAL DISORDERS

Chromosomal Abnormalities

- **Trisomy 21 (Down syndrome):**
  - Incidence: 1 in 600 live births; ↑ with ↑ maternal age.
  - Clinical features: Cognitive or developmental impairment, short stature, characteristic facies (epicanthal folds, midface hypoplasia), heart defects, and GI tract disorders.
  - Complications: ↑ risk of leukemia, hypothryoidism, congenital heart disease and Alzheimer dementia.
- **Trisomy 18 (Edwards syndrome):**
  - Incidence: 1 in 6000 to 8000 live births, with female newborns three times more likely to be affected than male newborns.
  - Clinical features: Severe cognitive or developmental impairment, IUGR, hypertonicity, abnormal facies, overlapping fingers, and "rocker-bottom" feet.
  - Prognosis: Most affected infants die within the first year of life.
- **Trisomy 13 (Patau syndrome):**
  - Incidence: 1 in 6000 live births. Affects slightly more girls than boys.
  - Clinical features: Cognitive or developmental impairment, midline facial defects, polydactyly, syndactyly, blindness, deafness, and heart defects. Complications include seizures.
  - Prognosis: Most patients die within the first 6 months.
- **Klinefelter syndrome (XXY):**
  - Incidence: 1 in 1000 live births.
  - Clinical features: Affected individuals are phenotypically male until puberty, when they may be noted to have small testicles (**micro-orchidism**), gyneco-

 ANSWER

Start a sepsis workup with CBC, cultures, CRP, and CXR. If the sepsis workup appears ⊖, the most likely diagnosis is transient tachypnea of the newborn. The infant should be closely monitored and supported with O_2 as needed. Always consider congenital cardiac anomalies in a newborn with respiratory distress.

mastia, and ↓ facial hair. Mild cognitive or developmental impairment is common.
- Management: Testosterone replacement.
- **Turner syndrome (XO):**
  - Incidence: 1 in 10,000 live births. Most fetuses conceived with this disorder are spontaneously miscarried.
  - Clinical features: Presents with short stature, absence of 2° sexual characteristics, the characteristic **"shield chest,"** **webbed neck**, edema of the hands and feet, and coarctation of the aorta. Complications include amenorrhea and learning disabilities.
  - Management: Estrogen replacement is needed for sexual maturation, and growth hormone is used for the treatment of short stature.

Autosomal Dominant Disorders

- **Neurofibromatosis type 1 (von Recklinghausen disease):** Neurofibromas are benign but have malignant potential and may compress nerves (Figure 13.8). Affected individuals are also at risk for CNS tumors, optic tumors, and pheochromocytomas.
- **Neurofibromatosis type 2:** Acoustic neuromas and other CNS neoplasms. Cutaneous manifestations are much less prevalent.
- **Tuberous sclerosis:** Presents with cutaneous lesions (**ash leaf spots** and shagreen patches). Associated with cognitive or developmental impairment; seizures; and CNS, pancreatic, renal, hepatic, and splenic involvement (Figure 13.9).
- **Marfan syndrome:** A triad of musculoskeletal changes (long limbs and ligamental laxity), lens dislocation, and aortic aneurysm. Penetrance is variable.

Autosomal-Recessive Disorders

- **Cystic fibrosis (CF):** Characterized by the triad of COPD, pancreatic exocrine insufficiency, and abnormal sweat chloride. See the Pulmonary chapter for the presentation, diagnosis, and management of CF.
- **Sickle cell disease:** Characterized by production of abnormal hemoglobin HbS. Deoxygenated HbS polymerizes, leading to distorted RBC morphology and ↑ blood viscosity. Associated with multiple complications (see the Mnemonic). Affected

MNEMONIC

Diagnostic criteria for neurofibromatosis type 1:
CAFÉ SPOT

Two or more of the following factors:
Café-au-lait spots (6 or more)
Axillary, inguinal freckling
Fibroma
Eye—Lisch nodules
Skeletal (eg, bowing leg)
Pedigree/**P**ositive family history
Optic **T**umor (glioma)

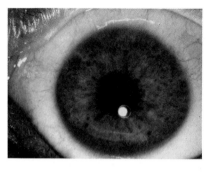

FIGURE 13.8. **Iris neurofibromas (Lisch nodules).** (Reproduced from the National Eye Institute.)

MNEMONIC

Complications of sickle cell anemia:
HbS PAIN CRISIS

Hemolysis, **H**and-foot syndrome
Bone marrow hyperplasia/infarction
Stroke (thrombotic or hemorrhagic)
Pain episodes, **P**riapism, **P**sychosocial issues
Anemia, **A**plastic crisis, **A**vascular necrosis
Infections (CNS, pulmonary, GU, bone, joint)
Nocturia, urinary frequency from hyposthenuria
Cholelithiasis, **C**ardiomegaly, **C**HF, **C**hest syndrome
Retinopathy, **R**enal failure or concentrating defects
Infarction (bone, spleen, CNS, muscle, bowel, renal)
Sequestration crisis involving the spleen or liver
Increased fetal loss during pregnancy
Sepsis

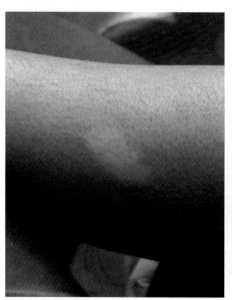

A

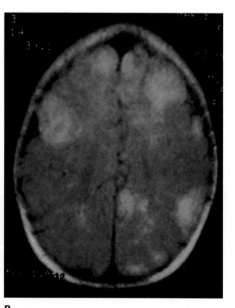

B

FIGURE 13.9. **Tuberous sclerosis.** Cutaneous ash leaf spots (**A**). CNS manifestation of tuberous sclerosis with cortical tubers (**B**). (Reproduced from Tonekaboni SH, et al. Clinical and para clinical manifestations of tuberous sclerosis: A cross sectional study on 81 pediatric patients. *Iran J Child Neurol.* 2012;6(3):25-31.)

children require routine screening for eye, liver, and kidney disease beginning at 5 years of age as well as stroke risk assessment beginning at 2 years of age. See the Hematology/Oncology chapter for a discussion of the presentation, diagnosis, and management of sickle cell disease.

- **Inborn errors of metabolism:** Absence of certain enzymes. The best-known type is phenylketonuria (PKU). Affected individuals are unable to convert phenylalanine to tyrosine, which leads to CNS damage and cognitive or developmental impairment. Treatment involves avoidance of phenylalanine in the diet.

X-Linked Disorders

- **Duchenne muscular dystrophy:**
  - Incidence: 1 in 3500 live births.
  - Clinical features: Proximal muscle wasting and distal muscle hypertrophy developing in the second and third years of life. Progressive, with almost all affected individuals requiring the use of a wheelchair by age 12.
  - Prognosis: Life expectancy is in the 20s. Respiratory failure and cardiomyopathy are the leading causes of death.
- **Hemophilia A and B:**
  - Incidence: 1 in 5000 live births. Hemophilia A (factor VIII deficiency) is much more common than hemophilia B (factor IX deficiency).
  - Management: Prevention of injury, factor replacement in the setting of active hemorrhage.
- **Fragile X syndrome:**
  - An example of genetic anticipation. Caused by a trinucleotide repeat on the long arm of the X chromosome that expands with each generation.
  - Clinical features: Female carriers may be mildly affected. Male offspring represent the full phenotype of cognitive and developmental impairment, macrocephaly, macro-orchidism, and behavioral disorders.

Exposure to Intrapartum Drugs

- **Fetal alcohol syndrome:** Presents with short palpebral fissures, epicanthal folds, a flat midface, absent philtrum, a thin upper lip, cognitive and developmental impairment, behavioral problems, and poor coordination (Figure 13.10). Heart defects and epilepsy are sometimes seen.
- **Opiates:** Opiate withdrawal (neonatal abstinence syndrome) presents with diarrhea, irritability, shrill cry, tremulousness, hypertonicity, and seizures. Onset of symptoms depends on the half-life of the opiate used and time of the last dose. Treatment is with opiates, weaned gradually.

Growth and Nutrition

Normal growth and nutrition in the first years of life are listed below. Plotting a child's growth on a standardized graph at all well-child visits is helpful in diagnosing FTT and growth abnormalities at a point when interventions may still be effective.

- **0 to 6 months of age:**
  - Weight loss in the first days is normal. Infants should be back to birth weight by the 10th day of life. Loss of >10% of birth weight raises concern for dehydration.
  - "Breast is best." Breastfeeding ↓ the incidence of obesity and DM, improves immune defenses, ↓ allergies later in life, and facilitates mother-infant bonding.

KEY FACT

Most families with hemophilia are aware that they carry the disease, but some remain unaware if the affected child has a new mutation or if the mutation has been passed from mother to daughter for several generations.

KEY FACT

Abnormal bleeding following circumcision or minor trauma in the early years may be the first clue to diagnosis of hemophilia.

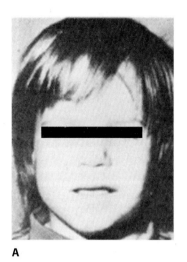
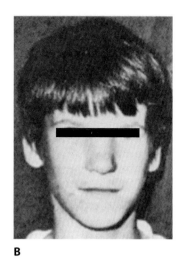
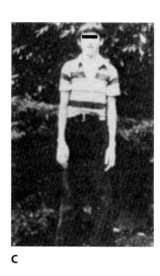

A   **B**   **C**

FIGURE 13.10.   Fetal alcohol syndrome. (A) At 2½ years. **(B, C)** At 12 years. Note the persistence of short palpebral fissures, epicanthal folds, flat midface, hypoplastic philtrum, and thin upper vermilion border. This child also has the short, lean prepubertal stature characteristic of young males with fetal alcohol syndrome. (Reproduced with permission from Cunningham FG, et al. *Williams Obstetrics*, 23rd ed. New York: McGraw-Hill, 2010, Fig. 14-2.)

- Exclusive breast or formula feeding should continue until 6 months of age to meet the infant's nutritional needs and ↓ the risk of developing allergies.
- Breastfed infants 0 to 12 months of age should receive 200 IU of vitamin D daily. Formula is fortified with vitamin D.
- Weight typically doubles by about 5 months of age.
- **6 to 12 months of age:**
  - Begin to add enriched cereals, fruits, vegetables, and meats to the diet. Add only one new item per week to ↓ the incidence of food aversions and to allow allergic reactions to be readily correlated with a new food.
  - To prevent infant botulism, honey should not be introduced until after 1 year of age.
  - Continue breastfeeding. Formula should be continued until 1 year of age and should then be switched to cow's milk.
  - Iron-rich foods should be introduced by 6 months of age.
  - Birth weight triples by 1 year.
- **12 months and older:**
  - Whole milk is best from age 1 to 2 years, at which time low-fat milk should be introduced.
  - Growth decelerates dramatically. Use the growth curve to assess adequacy.

> **KEY FACT**
>
> Absolute contraindications to breastfeeding are TB or HIV in the mother and galactosemia in the infant.

GROWTH DELAY

Although height and weight percentiles may adjust during the first 2 years of life, a persistent ↑ or ↓ in height percentiles between 2 years of age and the onset of puberty warrants further evaluation (Figure 13.11).

- Workup includes hand x-rays for bone age, CBC and ESR to evaluate for infection, kidney function and UA to assess for occult renal disease, stool studies to examine for malabsorption, karyotype for girls to assess for Turner syndrome, TSH to evaluate for hypothyroidism, and IGF-1 to look for growth hormone deficiency. Table 13.4 compares three common causes of growth delay.
- Long-term complications include vision loss, kidney failure, cardiovascular disease, peripheral neuropathy, and gastroparesis. Acute complications include diabetic ketoacidosis, hyperosmolar nonketotic state, and hypoglycemia.

> **KEY FACT**
>
> The anticipated height of a child can be determined by calculating the mean parental height and adding 6.5 cm for boys or subtracting 6.5 cm for girls.

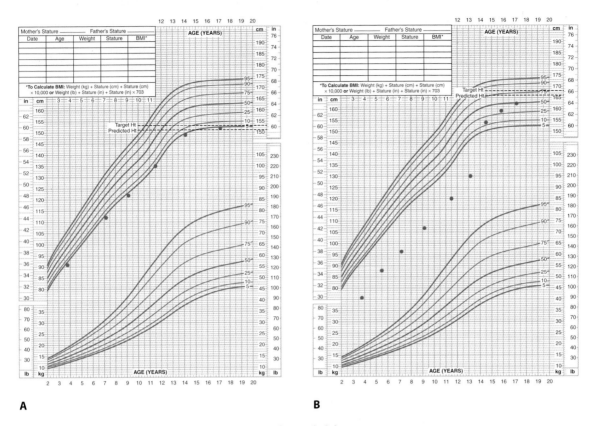

FIGURE 13.11. **(A) Familial short stature and (B) constitutional growth delay.** (Reproduced with permission from Hay Jr WW, et al. *Current Diagnosis & Treatment: Pediatrics,* 19th ed. New York: McGraw-Hill, 2009, Fig. 32-2 and 32-3.)

DISORDERS OF HEAD GROWTH

Microcephaly

Defined as a head circumference >2 SDs *below* the mean or a declining rate of head growth over time. The fontanelle may close early, and sutures may be prominent. Etiologies include trisomies, fragile X syndrome, TORCHeS infections, fetal alcohol syndrome, metabolic disorders, perinatal infections (GBS meningitis, herpes encephalitis), anoxic brain injury, and neurodegenerative disorders (eg, Tay-Sachs disease). Treatable causes include hypopituitarism, hypothyroidism, and severe protein-calorie undernutrition.

TABLE 13.4. **Common Causes of Growth Delay**

FAMILIAL SHORT STATURE	CONSTITUTIONAL GROWTH DELAY	GROWTH HORMONE DEFICIENCY
Parents are short	Parents are not necessarily short, but there may be a family history of late growth ("late bloomers")	Characterized by ↓ growth velocity and delay in skeletal maturation; growth delay may begin in infancy or later in childhood
Children are typically born with normal weight and length, but adjust to a lower percentile in the first 2 years of life; they will then have normal growth along that growth curve	Growth pattern is similar to that of familial short stature	May be isolated or occur with other pituitary hormone deficiencies
Skeletal maturation and the timing of puberty are consistent with chronologic age	Skeletal maturation and puberty are delayed, and linear growth continues beyond the typical age for reaching full height	Treatment is recombinant human growth hormone
No treatment is necessary	No treatment is necessary	

- **Diagnosis:** TORCHeS titers, metabolic workup, head CT, karyotype. Screen for maternal PKU.
- **Management:** Correct endocrine or metabolic disorders if present. Otherwise, treatment is largely supportive. Follow for possible cognitive or developmental impairment.

Macrocephaly

Defined as a head circumference >2 SDs *above* the mean. Etiologies include progressive hydrocephalus, subdural effusion, arachnoid cyst, porencephalic cyst, brain tumor, external hydrocephalus, benign enlargement of the subarachnoid spaces, neurofibromatosis, and tuberous sclerosis.

- **Symptoms/Exam:** An excessive rate of growth suggests ↑ ICP (hydrocephalus, extra-axial fluid collections, neoplasms). Macrocephaly with normal head growth rate suggests familial macrocephaly.
- **Diagnosis:** Imaging is not necessary if the infant is normal neurologically and head growth is consistent with catch-up or familial macrocephaly. Ultrasound may be used if the fontanelle is still open. Otherwise, CT or MRI is appropriate.

FAILURE TO THRIVE

Defined as persistent weight loss, a weight curve that declines across two major percentile lines, or weight persistently below the 3rd percentile (Table 13.5).

- Vitamin and nutrient deficiencies associated with FTT:
  - **Scurvy:** Vitamin C deficiency. Presents with bleeding gums, osteoid deficiency, and poor healing. Anorexia, irritability, and apathy may also be seen.
  - **Rickets:** Vitamin D deficiency (Figure 13.12). Presents with craniotabes (thinning of the skull), rachitic rosary (expansion of the anterior rib ends at the costochondral junctions), bowed legs, and tooth defects.
  - **Kwashiorkor:** Isolated protein deficiency presenting with edema and FTT.
  - **Marasmus:** Protein and calorie deficiency that presents with generalized wasting and FTT.
  - **Calcium deficiency:** Results in bone loss and failure to achieve maximal bone density. May contribute to later development of osteoporosis. Premature infants are at ↑ risk.

TABLE 13.5.   **Causes of Failure to Thrive by Metabolic Process**

INADEQUATE INTAKE	INADEQUATE ABSORPTION	EXCESSIVE LOSS	EXCESSIVE REQUIREMENT
Feeding mismanagement (eg, errors in formula feed, bizarre/ restricted diet, neglect, poverty)	Pancreatic insufficiency (eg, cystic fibrosis, Schwachman-Diamond syndrome)	Vomiting (eg, CNS abnormality, intestinal obstruction, metabolic abnormality, gastroesophageal reflux)	Chronic illness (eg, cystic fibrosis, congenital heart disease, inflammatory bowel disease)
Inability to feed optimally (eg, developmental delay, cleft palate, bulbar palsy, lip/tongue tie)	Small intestine disease (eg, dissacharidase deficiency, cow's milk protein intolerance, celiac)	Protein-losing enteropathy	Thyrotoxicosis
Anorexia (eg, chronic illness, anorexia nervosa)		Chronic diarrhea	Chronic infection (eg, TB, HIV)
Diencephalic syndrome			Malignancy
			Burns

Reproduced with permission from Guandalini S. *Essential Pediatric Gastroenterolgy, Hepatology, and Nutrition.* New York: McGraw-Hill, 2005, 57.

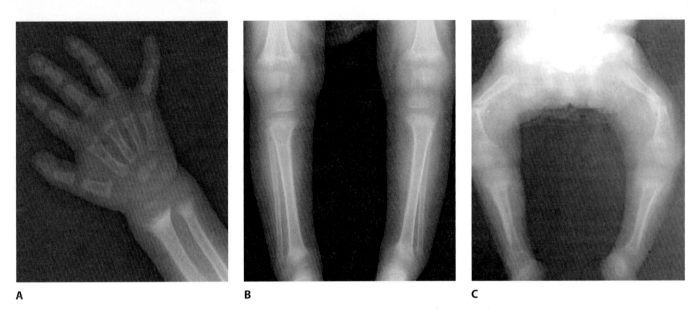

A   **B**   **C**

FIGURE 13.12. **Nutritional rickets.** Radiographs of the wrist (**A**) and knee (**B**) show cupping and flaring of the long bone metaphyses. Radiograph of the lower extremities (**C**) shows bowed legs with associated fractures and callus formation of bilateral mid-femurs. (Images A and B reproduced from Tamura M, et al. Detection of hereditary 1,25-hydroxyvitamin D-resistant rickets caused by uniparental disomy of chromosome 12 using genome-wide single nucleotide polymorphism array. *PLoS One.* 2015;10(7):e0131157; image C reproduced from Özkan B. Nutritional Rickets. *J Clin Res Pediatr Endocrinol.* 2010;2(4):137-143).

- **Diagnosis:** Testing guided by suspected etiology:
  - **Organic:** Consider GERD, problems with chewing/swallowing, malabsorption, protein-wasting nephropathy, genetic syndromes, tongue/lip tie and endocrine dysfunction.
  - **Nonorganic:** Assess for inappropriate or inadequate feeding by caregivers. May be related to lack of knowledge about feeding, bonding issues, socioeconomic issues, or abuse. Can have a mixed picture, with frustration or anxiety over organic illness leading to inadequate feeding.
- **Management:** Depends on underlying etiology. Institute a high-calorie diet, with particular attention to protein intake. Hospital admission to observe weight gain with adequate calories may be helpful.

OBESITY

Defined as a BMI >95th percentile for age and gender. At-risk children are between the 85th and 95th percentiles. Diagnosis is not made until age 2 years, although at-risk children may be identified earlier.

- **Management:** Lifestyle modification must involve the entire family. Limit sedentary activities like watching television. In most cases, the goal is to maintain current weight while linear growth catches up.
- **Complications:** Dyslipidemia, insulin resistance, **type 2 DM,** orthopedic problems, sleep apnea. See the Endocrinology chapter for a discussion of the presentation, diagnosis and treatment of DM (types 1 and 2).

Child Development and Behavior

DEVELOPMENTAL ISSUES

Colic

- Presents with the **rule of 3s** (see the Mnemonic).
- **Diagnosis:** If crying has developed suddenly, exogenous sources (eg, hair tourniquets, corneal abrasion, infection) should be ruled out.
- **Management:** Most cases are variations of normal behavior and resolve at about 4 months of age. Provide family support and close follow-up. Discuss methods to soothe colic (carrying, swinging, swaddling, changing formula or maternal diet in breastfeeding infants). Try H$_2$ blocker or PPI if GERD appears to be implicated. Screen for child abuse as risk is ↑.

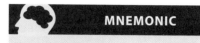

MNEMONIC

The colic rule of 3s:
3 hours a day
3 days a week
3 weeks or more

Elimination and Toilet Training

- Newborns typically have six to eight wet diapers per day; older infants will usually have four to six. Checking the number of diapers is a useful means of gauging hydration.
- Newborns often stool after every feed, but at 2 to 3 months stooling is much less frequent.
- Toilet training is generally initiated around 2 to 3 years of age but varies depending on the child's readiness and parental expectations.

Encopresis

Defined as repeated stooling in inappropriate locations after 4 years of age or after successful toilet training. More common in males. Often related to constipation and other causes of painful defecation (eg, anal fissures), leading to overflow incontinence of stool.

- Behavioral causes include control issues and fear of using public toilets.
- Physiologic causes include dehydration, lack of stool bulk, anal fissure, GI disorders, and metabolic disorders such as hypothyroidism.
- **Management:**
  - Treat underlying cause.
  - Treat constipation with stool softeners to make the passage of stool less painful.
  - May require disimpaction followed by regular use of a stool softener ± a stimulant laxative to establish a regular routine of one to two soft bowel movements a day.
  - Behavioral modifications include sitting on the toilet after each meal. Referral to pediatric behavioral health services may be necessary if significant behavioral problems persist.

Enuresis

- Defined as involuntary urination. Nocturnal enuresis (bedwetting) is seen in 15% of 5-year-olds and 1% to 2% of 15-year-olds. May be primary or secondary.
  - **1° enuresis:** Enuresis in a child who has never had an extended period of dryness. May be related to small bladder capacity, abnormal ADH secretion, sleep disorders, or psychological issues.
  - **2° enuresis:** Recurrence of bedwetting after a period of 6 months or more without bedwetting. 2° enuresis and daytime wetting are more often related to psychosocial issues.
- Consider UTI, neurologic disorders, structural abnormalities.

- **Management:**
  - **Behavioral modifications:** Reducing fluid intake in the evening and emptying the bladder before bedtime; bladder training to ↑ capacity; and bed alarms.
  - **Pharmacologic therapies:** Intranasal desmopressin (DDAVP) and imipramine. Enuresis often recurs after medication is stopped, but medical treatment may be helpful for sleepovers or camp.

Sleep Disorders

- Approximately 70% of infants sleep 8 hours at a time by 3 months of age, 80% by 6 months, and 90% by 12 months. Sleep disorders in children include the following:
  - **Nightmares:** Occur during REM sleep in 25% to 50% of children. Most common in children 3 to 5 years of age. The child can be awakened and consoled. Generally, **no intervention is required.**
  - **Night terrors:** See the Neurology chapter.

Strabismus

- Misalignment of the visual axes of the eyes. **Esotropia** is a form of strabismus characterized by convergent axes; **exotropia** refers to strabismus with divergent axes.
- **Diagnosis:** Intermittent esotropia may occur in normal infants up to 5 to 6 months of age. To confirm suspected strabismus, check the following:
  - **Light reflex:** The corneal light reflex from a penlight held along a toy that the child focuses on should appear symmetric.
  - **Cover test:** In an abnormal test, when the dominant eye is covered, the weaker eye will move to focus on an object.
- **Management:** Esotropia is more serious and often requires surgery. Exotropia may initially be treated with patching and exercises but may also need surgical correction.
- **Complications:**
  - Amblyopia (↓ visual acuity in the less dominant eye); diplopia (double vision); contracture of the extraocular muscles.
  - Acquired strabismus (occurring after the first year of life) is of more concern and may be the result of a significant visual deficit or CNS disease.

BEHAVIORAL ISSUES

- **Temper tantrums:** Common in children 1 to 4 years of age, as children learn to express desires and frustrations. Most episodes ↓ with age. Management focuses on protecting the child and others from harm and helping the child develop appropriate forms of expression.
- **Breath holding:** An involuntary response to minor injury or anger in which the child stops breathing after expiration. Loss of consciousness may occur. Occasionally associated with pica or iron deficiency anemia. Usually resolves by 6 years of age. If a child has frequent episodes, consider neurologic causes such as CNS tumor or seizure disorder. Manage with injury prevention.

DEVELOPMENTAL DELAY

Primary care physicians must screen for delays and refer children with suspected delays for further evaluation. Parents' concern about developmental delays is very sensitive and specific.

- The Denver Developmental Screening Test II, the most commonly used screening tool, is not sensitive for identifying language delays. Other tools such as Ages and Stages or Parents' Evaluation of Development Status are more sensitive.
- Children who fail to meet developmental milestones (Table 13.6) must be evaluated early to initiate appropriate therapies. Consider environmental causes (abuse/neglect), sensory causes (vision/hearing loss), motor delay (coordination defect leading to speech delay), psychiatric conditions.
- **Diagnosis:** Workup includes a careful physical exam for features of genetic syndromes (Down, fetal alcohol, and Turner syndromes), possible chromosome analysis and fragile X testing, lead levels, and testing of cognitive and adaptive skills. Loss of skills raises concern for a metabolic disorder or a neurodegenerative condition.
- **Management: Early intervention,** special education classes, appropriate occupational therapy.

Speech Delay

May be a result of hearing loss, isolated speech delay, autistic spectrum disorder. Be sure you consider parents' primary language or primary language spoken in home.

- Any child with delay in speech milestones should receive a hearing evaluation.
- **Red flags:**
  - No babbling by 12 months.
  - No words by 15 months.
  - Speech not intelligible to a noncaregiver by 2 years.
- **Management:** Speech therapy.

TABLE 13.6.   Developmental Milestones for Ages 1 Month to 5 Years

AGE	MOTOR	LANGUAGE/COGNITIVE	SOCIAL
1-2 months	Holds head up; rolls from side to back	Vocalizes	Spontaneous smile; recognizes parents
3-5 months	Reaches for objects; sits with support; rolls from back to side	Orients to voice	Laughs; responds to facial expressions
6-8 months	Sits alone briefly; rolls from back to stomach; passes objects between hands	Babbles	Sleeps through the night; stranger anxiety begins
9-11 months	Stands alone; pulls to stand; plays "pat-a-cake" and "peek-a-boo"; starts using pincer grasp	Follows 1-word commands; uses "mama" and "dada" nonspecifically; develops the concept of object permanence	Waves "bye-bye"
1 year	Walks independently; stacks 2 cubes	Uses "mama" and "dada" appropriately	Points to desired objects
18 months	Stacks 3-4 blocks; throws ball; walks up/down stairs with help	Uses 4-20 words; follows 2-step commands	Feeds self with hands; stranger anxiety peaks
2 years	Stacks 6-7 blocks; kicks ball; stands on 1 foot	Uses **2-word phrases;** uses pronouns; 50% of speech is comprehensible	Helps dress self; mimics parents; stranger anxiety subsides
3 years	Builds tower of 9-10 blocks; rides a **tricycle**	Uses **3-word phrases;** copies a circle; knows own name	Dresses self; feeds self with utensils
5 years	Runs and turns without losing balance; stands on 1 foot for 10 sec	Counts 10 or more things; answers questions appropriately	Magical thinking; plays with peers

Hearing Loss

Routine clinical hearing screening at well-child checks is essential. A child should turn toward a sound at 6 months and locate the source of a sound by 9 months. Speech delay can be a sign of hearing loss.

Symptoms/Exam: Distinguish conductive from sensorineural hearing loss.
- **Conductive hearing loss:**
  - Most often caused by otitis media and its sequelae (middle ear effusion). May also be caused by canal stenosis, impaction (cerumen or foreign body), and middle ear abnormalities (stapes fixation, ossicular malformation).
  - Hearing loss due to middle ear effusion is typically mild and temporary, but may affect language acquisition if it occurs during critical developmental periods.
- **Sensorineural hearing loss:**
  - A result of damage to or abnormal development of the inner ear or the auditory nerve (CN VIII). May be congenital or acquired (more often congenital). Etiologies include congenital or neonatal infections, ototoxic drugs, trauma, genetic syndromes (eg, Alport syndrome), and inner ear dysplasia.
  - Most cases are autosomal recessive and nonsyndromic. Inner ear dysplasia is the most common defect.
- **Diagnosis:** Hearing tests include otoacoustic emissions for screening. Auditory brain stem evoked response (ABER) is done if hearing loss is suspected.
- **Management:** Language acquisition programs (verbal and sign). For conductive hearing loss, correct the underlying cause (eg, tympanostomy tubes for middle ear effusion). For sensorineural hearing loss, treatment is hearing aids and possible surgical implants.

KEY FACT

The MMR vaccine and its components do not cause autism.

MNEMONIC

Signs of AUTISM:

Aloneness
Understanding (lack of)
Touch (hypersensitivity to)
Irrelevant and metaphorical language
Sameness (desire for)
Memory (rote)

AUTISM SPECTRUM DISORDER

Pervasive developmental disorder characterized by deficits in interpersonal relationships as well as speech and language delay. Uncommon condition (worldwide prevalence ~ 1%) with a male-to-female ratio of 3:1. Cause is unknown; there is likely a genetic component. It is **not** linked to vaccinations.
- Presents at 1 to 3 years of age. Early signs are poor eye contact, lack of stranger anxiety, and poor attachment to parents. Later signs include peculiar interests, stereotypic behaviors, and low IQ (generally <70).
- In Asperger syndrome, children have a lack of awareness of others and poor social functioning like those with autism, but cognitive impairment and language delay are generally absent.
- **Management:** Early intervention with behavioral education focused on sensory clues and appropriate interactions.

ATTENTION-DEFICIT HYPERACTIVITY DISORDER

Characterized by a **persistent pattern of inattention and/or hyperactivity-impulsivity** that interferes with functioning or development. Symptoms are present in ≥2 settings (eg, home and school), must have been present before 12 years of age, and have persisted for ≥6 months. Attention-deficit hyperactivity disorder (ADHD) may be classified as **inattentive, hyperactive/impulsive, or combined.**
- At least six symptoms in one or both of the following categories must be present for diagnosis:
  - **Inattentiveness:** Failure to pay close attention to detail, listen when spoken to directly, or follow instructions. Difficulty sustaining attention in tasks or or-

ganizing tasks and activities. Losing pencils, books. Reluctance to engage in tasks that require sustained attention. Easy distractibility. Forgetfulness in daily activities.
- **Impulsivity/hyperactivity:** Always "on the go." Fidgetiness (eg, difficulty remaining seated in class). Excessive running or climbing. Excessive talking. Difficulty engaging in quiet activities. Blurts out answers before questions have been completed. Interrupts and intrudes on others. Difficulty waiting for turn.
- **Management:**
  - Components of treatment include medication, behavior modification (often with a token economy that rewards good behavior), and environmental interventions such as preferential seating and ↓ stimuli.
  - The most commonly used medications are stimulants such as methylphenidate, which can cause growth delay and loss of appetite.
  - Intensive behavioral therapy may be helpful but is generally less effective than medication. Counseling is generally ineffective for ADHD but may be an important part of managing comorbid conditions such as depression and anxiety.
- **Complications:** Comorbid psychiatric problems are common and include mood and conduct disorders. All children should be evaluated for learning disabilities.

Preventive Medicine in Infants and Children

IMMUNIZATIONS

Vaccine schedules are updated annually. Current recommendations may be found on the Centers for Disease Control and Prevention Web site (www.cdc.gov/nip/ACIP). Contraindications to vaccines are outlined in Table 13.7.

DENTAL CARE

- Teething typically begins at 3 to 12 months. Parents should start cleaning teeth as soon as they appear.
- Encourage use of a cup by 1 year of age. Do not allow a bottle in bed (can lead to "baby bottle tooth decay").
- See the Community and Preventive Medicine chapter for recommendations on fluoride supplementation to prevent of dental caries in preschoolers.

T A B L E 1 3 . 7 .   Contraindications to Vaccines

VACCINE	CONTRAINDICATIONS
All vaccines	A previous anaphylactic reaction to a specific vaccine or any part of that vaccine
MMR and varicella	Pregnancy or known immunodeficiency
	Anaphylactic reaction to neomycin or gelatin
Influenza	Anaphylactic reaction to eggs
HBV	Anaphylactic reaction to baker's yeast
HAV	Anaphylactic reaction to aluminum or 2-phenoxyethanol

KEY FACT

Dental caries are the most common chronic disease of children aged 6 to 11 years and adolescents aged 12 to 19 years.

- Infants at higher risk for early dental caries should be referred to a dentist by 12 months of age. Risk factors include sleeping with a bottle, low socioeconomic status, mother with multiple caries, visible plaques/staining on teeth.

INJURY PREVENTION

Injuries are the leading cause of death in children and adolescents after the first year of life. The well-child check is an opportunity to counsel parents on injury prevention strategies such as keeping poisons locked and out of reach, drowning prevention, and "baby-proofing" to prevent falls and aspirations. Specific strategies include the following:

- **Car seats/seatbelts:**
  - Car seats and booster seats should be in the back seat of the car. Children should ride in the rear of the car until at least age 13 years.
  - Rear-facing car seats should be used until a child is older than 2 years of age and weighs more than the recommended weight limit allowed by the car seat manufacturer.
  - Booster seats should be used for children who have outgrown car seats.
  - A combination lap/shoulder belt should be used when a child has grown enough to fit the seat belts (usually 4 ft 9 in, or after age 8 years).
- **Bicycle helmets:**
  - Cycling is the leading cause of sports-related head injuries in children <14 years.
  - Use of properly fitting bicycle helmets when riding can prevent cycling-related injuries, but about half of children do not wear them.
  - Community interventions can greatly influence the rate of helmet use.

KEY FACT

Accidental injuries are the leading cause of death in children and adolescents after the first year of life.

SLEEP POSITION

Infants should sleep on their backs. This ↓ the risk of sudden infant death syndrome (SIDS) by approximately 50%. They should sleep on a flat surface with a tight-fitting sheet, without blankets, pillows, toys or crib bumpers. They should sleep in the same room as a parent, but not the same bed, for the first 6 months to a year.

TOBACCO EXPOSURE

- Exposure to secondhand smoke increases the risk of SIDS, asthma, pneumonia, bronchiolitis, otitis media, and hospitalizations in children.
- Children of smokers are more likely to become smokers.
- Primary care physicians should ask parents about smoking, advise them about the harmful effects, encourage them to quit, and provide resource connections.

LEAD SCREENING

The most common source of lead exposure is lead-based paint, which has been banned since 1977. Children may eat or inhale contaminated particles.

- High levels of lead are associated with seizures and coma. Moderate elevations are associated with behavioral problems and learning disabilities. Even low elevations are correlated with lower IQs.
- The CDC and the American Academy of Pediatrics recommend targeted screening of all Medicaid-enrolled and -eligible children, as well as those who were born outside of the United States.

- This recommendation also applies to all children deemed to be at risk (child lives or visits house built before 1978, child has a sibling or playmate who has or had lead poisoning). Screening of blood lead levels should be repeated at 2 years of age even if the level at 1 year is not elevated.

CHILD ABUSE

Physical Abuse

Physical indicators of abuse include the following:
- Injuries that do not correlate with the history.
- Specific pathognomonic injuries (eg, looped wire marks, cigarette burns, rib fractures, spiral fractures).
- Multiple injuries in varying stages of healing.
- Different types of injuries or disease (eg, burns and fractures).
- Overall evidence of poor care.
- Evidence of FTT.
- Infants who are severely shaken can present with sudden onset of seizure or coma with no signs of head trauma. They will typically have bilateral retinal hemorrhages and may have bilateral subdural hemorrhages on CT scan.
- When abuse is suspected, document all injuries, consider a skeletal survey, and report the case to Child Protective Services.

Sexual Abuse

- Behavioral changes may be an indicator of sexual abuse.
- Preschool children may present with fear states (eg, fear of adult males), nightmares, precocious sexual behavior, enuresis, encopresis, or behavior regression.
- School-aged children may exhibit sexual behavior, sexual aggression toward other children, school failure, truancy, running away, or depression.
- Adolescents may also develop problems with drugs, promiscuity, or prostitution.

KEY FACT

Abuse may be physical, sexual, emotional, or by neglect. In early childhood, FTT may be the first indicator.

Common Acute Conditions

RESPIRATORY DISTRESS

In all cases of respiratory distress, look for nasal flaring, grunting, and retractions. Listen for wheezing, crackles, and ↓ air movement. Cyanosis around the mucous membranes and nail beds is a sign of significant hypoxia.

Apnea

Defined as cessation of breathing for >20 seconds or for 10 to 20 seconds with signs of hypoxia. Subtypes are as follows:
- **Central:** Frequently identified early in infancy. May be related to infection, metabolic abnormalities, anemia, hypoxia, or CNS dysfunction.
- **Obstructive:** Occurs in later infancy and childhood. Obstruction causes cessation of airflow despite respiratory effort.
- **Mixed:** Both central and obstructive components are present.

Diagnosis

- In infants, check for metabolic imbalance with a basic metabolic panel and BUN/creatinine test. Look for signs of infection (CBC, UA, and CXR; consider CT and LP); check for respiratory syncytial virus (RSV) and pertussis; consider an ECG.

QUESTION

A panicked father presents with his 2-year-old daughter, who is coughing and wheezing. The child was entirely well and playing "tea party" with her older sister when the father started doing laundry, but looked ill when he returned. She has no significant medical history and no sick contacts. She is afebrile, slightly pale, and has an inspiratory wheeze. Her O_2 saturation is normal, and her CXR is significant only for mild hyperinflation of the right lung. What is your diagnosis?

- Consider an EEG if the patient has altered mental status or if a seizure focus is suspected. Admit for apnea monitoring.
- In older children, consider upper pharyngeal lesions such as tonsillitis and pharyngitis or laryngomalacia.

Apparent Life-Threatening Event

- Defined as an episode of apnea, change in muscle tone, and change in color (cyanosis or pallor).
- Differential includes infectious, cardiac, metabolic, and neurologic disorders. In 50% of cases, no diagnosis is found. GERD is often a diagnosis of exclusion.
- A single apparent life-threatening event is not associated with ↑ risk of SIDS.

Upper Airway Obstruction

May be caused by a foreign body, epiglottitis, or croup; distinguished as follows (see also Figure 13.13):

- **Foreign body:** Abrupt onset with no fever; not positional; presents with **inspiratory and expiratory stridor.**
  - **Diagnosis:** Expiratory CXR shows possible object and hyperinflation. Bilateral decubitus views may be necessary to demonstrate hyperinflation in children who cannot cooperate with instructions for expiratory CXR (Figure 13.14A).
  - **Management:** Removal via laryngoscopy or bronchoscopy.
- **Epiglottitis:** Most common in children 2 to 5 years of age. Most often caused by *Streptococcus pyogenes*, *Streptococcus pneumoniae*, and *Staphylococcus aureus*; on rare occasions, *Haemophilus influenzae* may be implicated (a significant ↓ in incidence has been seen 2° to routine vaccination).
  - **Symptoms/Exam:** Rapid onset with high fever; presents with drooling, and sore throat. Patients remain sitting or leaning forward ("tripod"). Primarily inspiratory stridor.
  - **Diagnosis:** A lateral neck x-ray reveals the characteristic "thumbprint sign" (Figure 13.14B).
  - **Management:** Secure the airway, send blood cultures, and start broad-spectrum antibiotics.
- **Croup:** Most common in children 6 months to 3 years of age, occurring during the fall and winter months. Caused by parainfluenza virus.
  - **Symptoms/Exam:** Barking (seal-like) cough, hoarseness, low-grade fever. Inspiratory and expiratory stridor may also be seen and may be provoked or worsened if the child is agitated or crying.
  - **Diagnosis:** CXR shows subglottic narrowing, the "steeple sign" (Figure 13.14C).
  - **Management:** Treat mild disease with humidified O_2. Moderate to severe disease should be treated with steroids and nebulized racemic epinephrine.

Lower Airway Obstruction

Causes in children include bronchiolitis, asthma, pneumonia, and foreign body obstruction. In infants, it can be associated with congenital anomalies of the airway (tracheal web, cysts, vascular rings, lobar emphysema).

- **Bronchiolitis:** An acute lower airway respiratory disease that causes small airway obstruction, typically occurring in the winter. It primarily affects infants <12 months of age and is caused by RSV.
  - **Symptoms/Exam:** Cough, coryza, and upper respiratory symptoms, usually with fever, precede wheezing and dyspnea. May present as apnea in younger children.
  - **Diagnosis:** CXR shows peribronchial cuffing, areas of hyperaeration, and atelectasis. Hypercapnia, hypoxemia, or both may be present. Obtain a nasal swab/wash for RSV.

KEY FACT

The key feature of a upper airway obstruction is inspiratory stridor.

ANSWER

This child almost certainly inhaled something radiolucent into her right bronchus while playing tea party. She needs urgent evaluation for removal of this object under direct visualization by ENT.

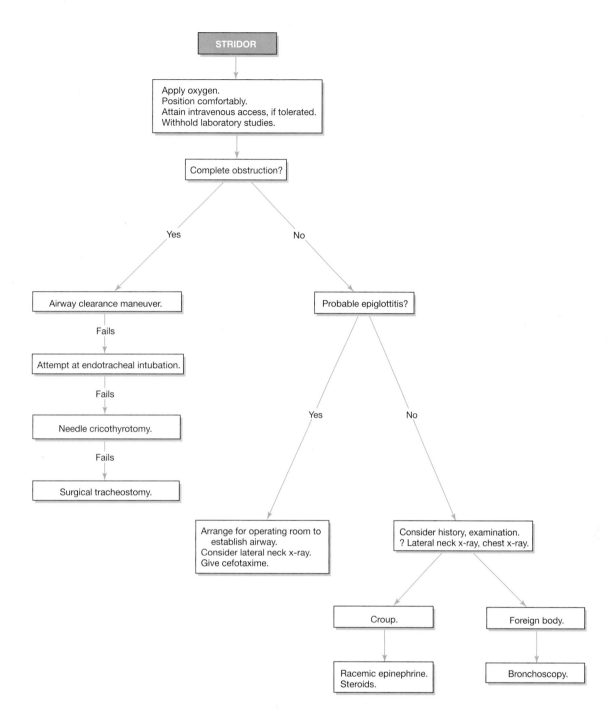

FIGURE 13.13.   Diagnosis and treatment of upper airway obstruction. (Reproduced with permission from Stone CK, Humphries RL. *Current Emergency Diagnosis & Treatment,* 5th ed. New York: McGraw-Hill, 2004:1054.)

■ **Management:** Primarily supportive. Give O_2 for hypoxia. Nebulized saline may be helpful. Limited evidence for nebulized albuterol and steroids but may be helpful in patients with a history of wheezing. Admit for low O_2 saturation, prematurity, age <3 months, or toxic appearance. High-risk infants (premature infants and those with preexisting lung or heart disease) should receive palivizumab, a monoclonal antibody, to ↓ the risk of contracting RSV.

■ **Complications:** Bacterial superinfection (pneumonia, otitis media). There is a possible correlation between bronchiolitis in infancy and the subsequent development of reactive airway disease.

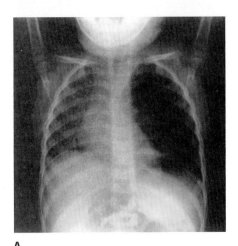
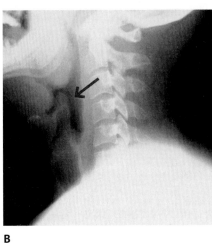
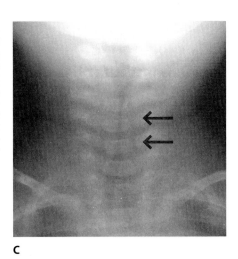

A   B   C

FIGURE 13.14. **Airway obstruction.** (A) Aspirated peanut (not visible) in the left mainstem bronchus, resulting in hyperinflated left lung with mediastinal shift. (B) Epiglottitis, known as the "thumbprint" sign (arrow). (C) Croup. Subglottic tracheal narrowing with an inverted "V" appearance below the larynx, the "steeple sign" (arrowheads). (Image A reproduced with permission from Lalwani AK. *Current Diagnosis & Treatment in Otolaryngology*, 2nd ed. New York: McGraw-Hill, 2008, Fig. 38-2; image B reproduced with permission from USMLE-Rx.com; image C reproduced with permission from Stone CK, Humphries RL. *Current Diagnosis & Treatment: Emergency Medicine*, 6th ed. New York: McGraw-Hill, 2008, Fig. 30-10.)

- **Asthma:** Expiratory wheezing and shortness of breath. Inability to speak, cyanosis, accessory muscle use, pulsus paradoxus, or signs of infection may indicate more serious disease.
  - **Management:** Exacerbations are treated with nebulized bronchodilators. Nebulized anticholinergics (ipratropium) ↓ hospitalizations. IV or PO steroids are required for moderate to severe exacerbations. For severe exacerbations, systemic bronchodilators (magnesium, terbutaline) may also help prevent intubation. Intubation is necessary in severe cases.
- **Pneumonia:** Common causative organisms are as follows:
  - **Newborns:** GBS, gram-negative enteric bacteria, CMV, *Listeria monocytogenes.*
  - **Infants:** *Chlamydia trachomatis*, RSV, *S pneumoniae*, *S aureus.*
  - **Toddlers:** Viruses, *S pneumoniae*, nontypable *H influenzae.*
  - **Children (4-14 years):** *Mycoplasma pneumoniae*, *Pneumococcus*, *Chlamydia pneumoniae.*
  - **Symptoms/Exam:** Presents with fever and respiratory findings (crackles, egophony, dullness to percussion).
  - **Diagnosis:** CXR shows evidence of parenchymal infiltrates.
  - **Management:** Antibiotics; hospitalize if the patient is unable to maintain an O_2 saturation >92% on room air. Some patients may respond to bronchodilators.

FEVER

Neonates (<30 days)

- Even well-appearing febrile children <1 month of age are at high risk for occult serious bacterial illness (SBI).
- Rectal temperature >38°C (100.4°F) is considered a fever in this age group.
- While viruses are the most likely source, consider late onset of congenitally acquired illnesses, such as rubella and CMV, or infections acquired at birth, such as GBS, *E coli*, and *Listeria.* Early infection may also be the first sign of a congenital abnormality (eg, in the GU system).

- **Diagnosis:** CBC with differential, blood culture, UA, urine culture, LP. Also consider CXR, stool culture, and viral culture.
- **Management:**
  - Admit and treat with broad-spectrum antibiotics while awaiting culture results.
  - Give ampicillin plus a third-generation cephalosporin or gentamicin.
  - Antibiotics may be discontinued at 48 hours if all cultures are ⊖ and the infant is clinically stable.

Infants (31-90 days)

- A positive viral test or a viral illness with a distinct phenotype may be considered the source of the fever.
- If no source is found, consider occult UTI, bacteremia, or meningitis.
- **Diagnosis:**
  - UA and urine culture in all infants.
  - CBC with differential and blood culture if UA is ⊖ or if the child is ill-appearing. Also consider LP if child is ill-appearing or if antibiotics are being started empirically. As indicated: CXR, stool culture, and viral culture.
- **Management:**
  - Start third-generation cephalosporin (eg, ceftriaxone) after collecting cultures if WBC >15 or <5, or if there are other concerns for infection.
  - Admit if the patient is ill-appearing or at risk for lack of follow-up.
  - Antibiotics may be discontinued at 48 hours if all cultures are ⊖ and the infant is clinically stable.

Infants and Toddlers (91 days-36 Months)

- Rectal temperature >39°C (102.2°F).
- Etiologies include viral infection, pneumonia, UTI, meningitis, and occult bacteremia. The source of the fever is more readily identifiable in this group than in younger children.
- **Diagnosis:** In the absence of an obvious source of infection (eg, otitis media, infectious diarrhea), diagnose as follows:
  - **Girls vaccinated against pneumococcus (two or more doses):** Check UA and urine culture if the child is <24 months of age.
  - **Boys vaccinated against pneumococcus (two or more doses):** Check UA and urine culture if the child is circumcised and <6 months of age or uncircumcised and <12 months.
  - If the child appears toxic or has not been adequately vaccinated against *Pneumococcus*, check CBC, blood cultures, UA, and urine culture. Also consider LP and CXR, based on clinical presentation.
- **Management:** All toxic-appearing children should receive empiric IV or IM antibiotics while awaiting cultures. Unvaccinated children with WBC >15,000 should also receive empiric antibiotics.

KEY FACT

Use of the pneumococcal conjugate vaccine and the Hib vaccine has dramatically ↓ the number of cases of invasive disease seen from *Pneumococcus* and *H influenzae* type B infections.

Children (>36 Months)

The risk of occult bacteremia is lower in this age group, and a source of fever is generally identifiable and treated as needed. In children <5 years of age with persistent fever, consider Kawasaki disease.

Febrile Seizure

- Usually presents as a brief (<15 minutes) tonic-clonic seizure associated with fever, in the absence of CNS infection or inflammation, no acute metabolic abnormalities peak age is 8 to 20 months, although febrile seizures may occur in children from approximately 6 months to 6 years of age. Underlying diseases are URIs or gastroenteritis. The seizure seems to be more the result of a rapid change in temperature than of absolute temperature. May be simple or complex.

- **Simple febrile seizure:** Typically occurs as a generalized, self-limited tonic-clonic seizure of several minutes' duration.
- **Complex febrile seizure:** Defined as a seizure that is focal, is associated with Todd paralysis, or lasts >15 minutes. Also includes >1 episode in 24 hours.
- **Differential:** Includes CNS infection and epileptic seizures.
- **Diagnosis:** Usually made clinically, but if the seizure has atypical features, a neurologic workup, including labs, MRI, and EEG, may be indicated. Consider LP in children <12 months old.
- **Management:** Simple febrile seizures are usually benign and treated with supportive care, airway management, and antipyretic given PO or rectally as needed. In rare cases, when children are prone to febrile seizure, diazepam can be used at seizure onset and repeated as necessary until the fever resolves.
- **Complications:** Children with a history of complex febrile seizures have a higher risk of developing epilepsy.

ACUTE OTITIS MEDIA

Commonly caused by *S pneumoniae*, *H influenzae*, and *Moraxella catarrhalis*.
- **Symptoms/Exam:** Presents with pain, fever, and hearing loss. May be preceded by a URI. Exam reveals a bulging tympanic membrane, with loss of visual landmarks (Figure 13.15). Loss of movement of the tympanic membrane, is both sensitive and specific.
- **Management:** First-line treatment is high-dose amoxicillin (80-90 mg/kg/day). If children are high risk, have severe disease or bilateral disease (associated with *H influenzae*), or have been treated in the last 30 days, treat with amoxicillin-clavulanate. Recurrent infections may be an indication for referral to ENT for placement of tympanotomy tubes. In patients >2 years of age without symptoms of systemic illness, acute otitis media may be treated supportively with pain control and close follow-up.
- **Complications:** Mastoiditis, hearing loss.

GI SYMPTOMS

Diarrhea

Rotavirus is the most common cause of acute diarrhea, particularly in the winter. Additional causes include other viruses, food poisoning, traveler's diarrhea, and diarrhea related to recent antibiotic use. Chronic diarrhea may be a sign of IBD, IBS, or celiac disease.
- **Diagnosis:**
  - The history and physical are important to identify signs of dehydration. Ask about the number of wet diapers and the presence of tears when crying.
  - Fecal leukocytes and stool cultures are not always necessary, but may be helpful when a child has bloody diarrhea or appears significantly ill. The serum WBC count is generally higher in bacterial than in viral infection.
  - A Chem 7 can help identify electrolyte abnormalities in patients with severe disease.
  - The combination of bloody diarrhea and acute renal failure should raise suspicion of hemolytic-uremic syndrome triggered by Shiga toxin–producing *E coli* O157:H7.
  - "Currant jelly" stools are the classic late sign of **intussusception.**
- **Management:** The most important intervention is rehydration. This can usually be done with oral intake, but significant dehydration should be treated with IV fluids

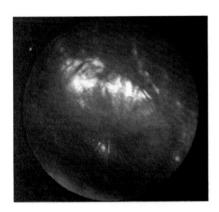

FIGURE 13.15. **Acute otitis media.**
(Reproduced from Wikimedia; courtesy of B. Welleschik.)

and occasionally with hospitalization. Most cases of infectious diarrhea will resolve without antibiotics. Even with bloody diarrhea, antibiotics should not be started empirically, as their role depends on the organism.

Vomiting

- In infants and children, common causes of vomiting include gastroenteritis (may precede diarrhea by a few days), intussusception, appendicitis, UTI/pyelonephritis, Reye syndrome, and hepatitis.
- **Diagnosis/Management:** Consider CBC, electrolytes, UA, urine culture, and LFTs, as indicated clinically. Evaluate for dehydration, and consider imaging for underlying causes.

Abdominal Pain

- The most likely etiologies of abdominal pain vary by age group:
    - **Infants:** Colic, constipation, gastroenteritis, intussusception, viral syndrome, volvulus.
    - **Preschool children:** Appendicitis, constipation, gastroenteritis, pneumonia, UTI, viral syndromes.
    - **School-aged children:** Appendicitis, pregnancy, gastroenteritis, pneumonia, peptic ulcer, PID.
- **Diagnosis:** Check CBC and electrolytes if the child appears ill. Obtain imaging as indicated by the clinical presentation:
    - **AXR** (flat and upright or lateral): Helps identify free air (an indication of perforation) and air-fluid levels (an indication of obstruction).
    - **CXR:** To identify lower lobe pneumonia.
    - **Ultrasound or abdominal CT with IV contrast:** Ultrasound to identify appendicitis, intussusception, or pyloric stenosis. If ultrasound is not available, CT with IV contrast can be performed.
    - **Testicular ultrasound:** To identify torsion.
    - **Upper GI series:** To identify midgut malrotation ± volvulus.
    - **Barium enema:** To diagnose intussusception or reduce intussusception identified by ultrasound.

HEAD TRAUMA IN CHILDREN

Types of head trauma in children include the following:
- **Concussion:** A brief loss or alteration of consciousness due to head trauma, followed by a return to normal. Brain tissue is not damaged, and there are no focal findings. Amnesia, vomiting, confusion, dizziness, and sleep disturbances may be seen. A postconcussive syndrome may last for weeks to months. Children should avoid activity that would put them at risk for another event (eg, competitive sports) until they have remained asymptomatic for at least 1 week.
- **Contusion:** A bruise of the brain matter. The child's level of consciousness diminishes, and focal findings correspond to the area of the brain that is injured. Obtain a head CT and admit for observation.
- **Diffuse axonal injury:** Characterized by coma without focal signs on neurologic exam. There may be no external signs of trauma. The initial CT scan is normal or may demonstrate only small, scattered areas of cerebral contusion and areas of low density. Prolonged disability may follow diffuse axonal injury.
- **↑ ICP ± herniation:** Etiologies include hemorrhage and generalized swelling in the setting of trauma. Symptoms include headache, vision changes, vomiting, gait difficulties, and a progressively ↓ level of consciousness. **Cushing triad (bradycardia, hypertension, and irregular respirations)** and papilledema are late findings.

KEY FACT

Use CT scans judiciously in children. CT scans are associated with ↑ lifetime cancer risk in children. This risk is greater in younger children.

QUESTION

A mother brings her 8-month-old son to the ED because he is having episodes of inconsolable crying during which he pulls his knees to his chest. Between episodes he is lethargic, and he has vomited twice. As you go in to examine him, the nurse tells you that he has just had an episode of bloody diarrhea. How do you proceed?

Evaluation and management: Goals are to promptly identify serious conditions and monitor for and treat sequelae. See the Emergency/Urgent Care chapter for more on diagnosis and treatment.

- For children of all ages, obtain a CT scan in patients who are at high risk for intracranial injury. High-risk patients are those who have severe mechanism of injury, abnormal mental status (GCS <14), or evidence of skull fracture.
- Children who are at moderate risk may be managed by observation for 4 to 6 hours or CT scan. Patients who are being observed may need a CT scan if symptoms persist or worsen.
- No further workup is needed in low-risk children.
  - **Age 0 to 2 years:** Neurologic exam may be normal. Children who are at moderate risk for intracranial injury include those with loss of consciousness for >5 seconds, nonfrontal scalp hematoma, or abnormal activity per parents.
  - **Age 2 to 18 years:** Patients in this age group are considered moderate risk if they have loss of consciousness, vomiting, or severe headaches.

Chronic Conditions in Children

CARDIOVASCULAR DISEASE

Heart Murmurs

Most common cardiovascular finding that leads to a cardiology referral. Innocent heart murmurs (also known as functional murmurs) are extremely common. Between 40% and 45% of children have an innocent murmur at some time during childhood.

Symptoms/Exam

- **Pathologic murmurs** may manifest as FTT, exercise intolerance, dyspnea with exertion/diaphoresis, syncope, dizziness, cyanosis, loss of consciousness, and tachypnea with feeds or activity.
- Assess the following factors: intensity, quality, timing in cycle, location, radiation, and variation with position (Table 13.8).

Diagnosis

Indications of pathologic murmurs include the following (see also Table 13.8):

- Cyanotic, symptomatic (FTT, tachypnea).
- Grade III or more.
- Diastolic murmur.
- Abnormal CXR or ECG.
- Comorbid syndrome with a high incidence of heart defects (eg, Down, Turner, Marfan, Williams, Noonan syndromes).

Management

Refer pathologic murmurs to a pediatric cardiologist; observe benign murmurs.

Ventricular Septal Defect

The most common congenital heart malformation, accounting for approximately 30% of all cases of congenital heart disease. Defects in the ventricular septum occur both in the membranous portion of the septum (most common) and in the muscular portion, permitting blood in the high-pressure left ventricle to shunt into the low-pressure right ventricle. Eisenmenger syndrome and shunt reversal occurs in approximately 25% of cases.

MNEMONIC

Features of innocent murmurs:
The 8 Ss
Soft
Systolic
Short
Sounds (S1 and S2) normal
Symptomless
Special tests (x-ray, ECG) normal
Standing/**S**itting (vary with position)
Sternal depression (pectus excavatum)

A **ANSWER**

This presentation raises concern for intussusception. If the child does not appear toxic, a barium enema may be both diagnostic and therapeutic. If there is suspicion of necrotic bowel or perforation, air insufflation may be attempted, but should only be done in a facility with surgical capabilities in case of failure as the child may need surgery.

TABLE 13.8.   **Types of Murmurs Based on Location of Loudest Intensity**

LOCATION/DIAGNOSIS	UNIQUE FEATURES
Right upper sternal border	
Venous hum	**Continuous;** disappears when the jugular vein is compressed, when the patient's head is turned, or when the patient is supine; benign
Aortic stenosis	Systolic ejection quality (with audible S1 and S2); radiates to the neck; presents with thrill in the suprasternal notch; often associated with a valve click
Left upper sternal border	Systolic ejection quality; usually seen in infants; often louder in the axillae than over the precordium; benign
Peripheral pulmonary stenosis	Systolic ejection quality; radiates to the back and axillae; may be associated with a valve click
Pulmonary stenosis	Continuous; **"machinery"** quality; bounding pulses
PDA	Systolic; fixed, split S2
ASD	Systolic; radiation to the back; weak, delayed femoral pulses
Coarctation of the aorta	
Left lower sternal border	**"Vibratory"** systolic ejection quality, no radiation, louder when the patient is supine; benign
Still murmur	Holosystolic; harsh quality; often radiates all over the precordium; often louder as the defect gets smaller
VSD	
Hypertrophic obstructive cardiomyopathy	Systolic ejection quality; louder when the patient is upright; often radiates to the apex; may be heard in patients who have chest pain with activity
Apex	Holosystolic, decrescendo, **"cooing dove"** quality
Mitral regurgitation	

Reproduced with permission from Le T, et al. *First Aid for the Pediatric Boards,* 1st ed. New York: McGraw-Hill, 2006:61.

Symptoms

- **Small to moderate shunts:** Often asymptomatic and acyanotic.
- **Moderate shunts:** May cause pulmonary vascular disease and right-sided failure.
- **Large left-to-right shunts:** Patients are ill early in infancy (with frequent upper and lower respiratory infections), growing and gaining weight slowly. Dyspnea, exercise intolerance, and fatigue are common. HF develops between 1 and 6 months of age. With severe pulmonary hypertension and shunt reversal, cyanosis is present.

Exam

- A systolic thrill is heard.
- **Small to moderate defects:** A loud, grade II to IV/VI holosystolic murmur is heard that is maximal along the lower left sternal border. Occasionally, a mid-diastolic flow murmur is heard. Small defects tend to have louder murmurs.
- **Large defects:** Right ventricular volume and pressure overload may lead to pulmonary hypertension, HF, and cyanosis. A grade II to IV/VI holosystolic murmur is maximal at the lower left sternal border. P2 is usually accentuated.

Differential

Mitral regurgitation; mitral valve prolapse.

Diagnosis

- **ECG:** LVH and/or RVH if the shunt is reversed.
- **CXR:** ↑ pulmonary vascularity.
- **Echocardiography:** Doppler is diagnostic and can assess the magnitude of the shunt as well as pulmonary arterial pressure.
- **Cardiac CT and MRI:** Can visualize the defect and other anatomic abnormalities.
- **Cardiac catheterization:** Reserved for those with at least moderate shunting; can measure pulmonary vascular resistance and the degree of pulmonary hypertension.

Q QUESTION

A 3-year-old girl presents for a routine well-child check. Her mother notes that she is now fully potty-trained and about to start preschool. Her height and weight have been stable at the 50th percentile and her developmental milestones are also appropriate for her age. On exam, you note that she has a quiet precordium, a regular rate, and normal S1 and S2, with a 2/6 systolic ejection murmur that is louder when she is supine. There is no radiation of the murmur to the neck, axillae, or back. What is your next step in management of this patient?

Management

- Small shunts do not require closure in asymptomatic patients.
- Symptomatic children should be managed with hypercaloric feeds, diuretics, and angiotesin-converting enzyme inhibitors.
- If symptoms persist despite maximal medical therapy or if there is ↑ pulmonary vascular resistance (affects approximately 50% of patients), the defect should be surgically or percutaneously repaired. The shunt should not be repaired if Eisenmenger syndrome has developed.
- Children who do not have surgery should be followed to assess for spontaneous closure of the defect or for the development of complications.
- Because infections can worsen HF, all children >6 months of age should receive the influenza vaccine, and all children <2 years of age should receive RSV prophylaxis.
- Endocarditis occurs more often with smaller shunts; antibiotic prophylaxis is mandatory for all patients.

Complications

Endocarditis; pulmonary hypertension/Eisenmenger syndrome. Surgical mortality is 2% to 3%, but ↑ to ≥50% if pulmonary hypertension is present.

Atrial Septal Defect

A communication between the right and left atria. The most common type is persistent ostium secundum, a defect of the mid-septum. Initially results in a left-to-right shunt as oxygenated blood from the higher-pressure left atrium passes into the right atrium. Over time, a large defect may lead to pulmonary over-circulation, pulmonary hypertension, Eisenmenger syndrome, right-to-left shunting, and cyanosis.

Symptoms/Exam

- Small defects are typically not hemodynamically significant and do not cause symptoms. Large defects may present with exertional dyspnea, arrhythmias, syncope, and heart failure.
- **A fixed, split S2** is heard.
- A systolic ejection murmur may be heard in the second and third interspaces. A right ventricular heave may also be present.

Diagnosis

- **Echocardiography:** Usually diagnostic. Saline bubble contrast and Doppler flow can demonstrate shunting.
- **ECG:** Shows incomplete or complete right bundle branch block, right axis deviation, and RVH.
- **CXR:** Demonstrates large pulmonary arteries, ↑ pulmonary vascularity, and an enlarged right atrium and ventricle.
- **Cardiac catheterization:** Can show an ↑ in O_2 saturation between the vena cava and the right ventricle; can also quantify the shunt and measure pulmonary vascular resistance.

Management

- Although there is no evidence of benefit from closure of small shunts, large shunts generally require closure. Percutaneous closure devices are now available.
- There is no ↑ risk of infective endocarditis unless mitral regurgitation is present as well, so antibiotic prophylaxis is recommended only in these cases.

ANSWER

Reassure the parents that the murmur is innocent, and observe the patient.

Complications

- Pulmonary hypertension, right-sided HF, **Eisenmenger syndrome,** and right-to-left shunting.
- Paradoxical emboli.
- ↑ risk of complications with scuba diving and at high altitudes.

Cyanotic Heart Disease

Cyanosis is seen when >5 g/dL of hemoglobin in the capillaries is deoxygenated. The most common causes of cyanotic heart disease in the newborn period are listed in Table 13.9. Infants with these disorders present with early cyanosis. The hallmark of many of these lesions is cyanosis in an infant without associated respiratory distress.

Symptoms/Exam

Table 13.9 outlines the common causes of cyanotic heart disease as well as its clinical presentation and treatment.

Diagnosis

Differentiate between cardiac and noncardiac causes:
- **Hyperoxia test:** Obtain an ABG; then place the patient on 100% O_2 for 10 minutes and perform a repeat ABG. If the cause of cyanosis is pulmonary, the PaO_2 should ↑ by 30 mm Hg. If the cause is cardiac, there should be minimal improvement in PaO_2.

MNEMONIC

Causes of cyanotic heart disease:
5 terrible Ts
Transposition of the great vessels
Total anomalous pulmonary venous return
Tetralogy of Fallot
Truncus arteriosus
Tricuspid atresia

QUESTION

A 2-year-old girl is brought to the ED after a spell of intractable crying and irritability. Her mother mentions that she has a heart problem and that whenever doctors examine her, they hear a loud murmur. Pulse oximetry reveals an O_2 saturation of 62%. On auscultation, you hear a 1/6 murmur in systole at the left upper sternal border. What is your therapeutic strategy?

TABLE 13.9. Causes, Presentation, and Treatment of Cyanotic Heart Disease

	DEFINITION	SYMPTOMS/EXAM	TREATMENT
Tetralogy of Fallot	Includes VSD, pulmonary stenosis, overriding aorta, and RVH	Cyanosis, dyspnea, loud pulmonary stenosis murmur; a VSD (holosystolic) murmur may also be heard; variable degree of cyanosis, depending on the amount of right-to-left shunting	Surgical repair through placement of a transannular patch across the pulmonary valve
Tricuspid atresia/ hypoplastic right heart	Complete or partial agenesis of the right ventricular cavity in which the left ventricle provides pulmonary blood flow through the ductus arteriosus	Tachypnea, dyspnea, anoxic spells, and evidence of right HF; cyanosis; a grade II–VI harsh blowing murmur heard best at the lower left sternal border	Anticongestive therapy; the Fontan procedure (connection of the systemic venous return to the pulmonary artery) is performed when ↑ cyanosis occurs
Transposition of the great vessels	Connection of the left ventricle to the pulmonary artery and the right ventricle to the aorta, causing the systemic and pulmonary circulations to operate in parallel	Cyanosis; a single S2 and no murmur	Early corrective surgery is recommended through an arterial switch operation of the great vessels
Total anomalous pulmonary venous return	All pulmonary veins terminate in a systemic vein or the right atrium	Tachypnea, feeding difficulties, and HF; widely fixed, split S2 and grade II–III/VI ejection-type systolic murmur	Surgery is always required
Truncus arteriosus	A single arterial trunk arises from the ventricles and divides into the aorta and pulmonary arteries	Mild or no cyanosis, early HF, systolic ejection click, wide pulse pressure	Anticongestive treatment and surgical repair

KEY FACT

Right axis deviation is normal for a neonate.

ANSWER

You recognize that this girl is likely having a hypercyanotic spell associated with tetralogy of Fallot. You bring her knees up to her chest and administer a single dose of IV morphine, and her O$_2$ saturation rapidly improves to 92%.

MNEMONIC

Tetralogy of Fallot

Pulmonary stenosis
Right ventricular hypertrophy
Overriding aorta
Ventricular septal defect

MNEMONIC

Diagnosis of Kawasaki disease:
CRASH and Burn

Conjunctivitis—perilimbic sparing
Rash
Adenopathy—usually cervical
Strawberry tongue
Hand and foot changes
Burn—fever for >5 days

- **CXR:** Vasculature on CXR provides information about pulmonary blood flow.
- **ECG:** Provides information about rhythm and, grossly, ventricular size. Examine both the axis and the magnitude of the deflections. Remember that right axis deviation is normal for a neonate.
- **Echocardiography:** The gold standard of diagnosis, as well as a noninvasive means of assessing the cardiac anatomy.

Management

For cyanotic heart disease in which circulation is ductus dependent (requiring a patent ductus arteriosus), immediate treatment with prostaglandins, which delay closing of the ductus, may be lifesaving while the child is transported to a facility for cardiac surgery.

Kawasaki Disease

Previously called mucocutaneous lymph node syndrome, Kawasaki disease is an acute febrile vasculitis of childhood involving small and medium-size arteries, with characteristic involvement of the coronary arteries. The cause is unclear, and no specific diagnostic test is available. Approximately 80% of affected patients are younger than 5 years of age, and the male-to-female ratio is 1.5:1.

Symptoms/Exam

The condition is defined by the presence of fever for at least 5 days and at least four of the following features (Figures 13.16 and 13.17).
- Bilateral, painless, nonexudative conjunctivitis.
- Lip or oral cavity changes (eg, lip cracking and fissuring, strawberry tongue, inflammation of the oral mucosa).
- Cervical lymphadenopathy (≥1.5 cm in diameter and usually unilateral).
- Polymorphous exanthema.
- Extremity changes (redness and swelling of the hands and feet, with subsequent desquamation).

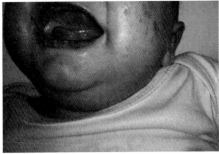

A

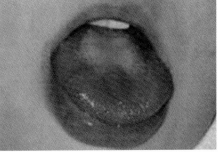

B

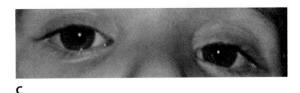

C

FIGURE 13.16.   **Kawasaki disease.** (**A**) Cherry-red lips and hemorrhagic fissures in a boy with prolonged high fever, (**B**) strawberry tongue, and (**C**) infected conjunctivae. (Image A reproduced from Leonardi S, et al. Severe Kawasaki disease in a 3-month-old patient: a case report. *BMC Res Notes.* 2013;6:500; images B and C reproduced from Stagi S, et al. Kawasaki disease in a girl with Turner syndrome: a remarkable association. *Ital J Pediatr.* 2014;40:24.)

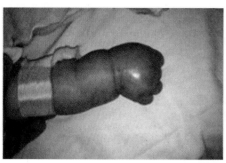
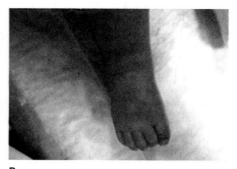

A   **B**

FIGURE 13.17.   **Manifestation of Kawasaki disease in distal limbs.** Erythema and edema of the distal limbs are an early manifestation of Kawasaki disease (**A** and **B**). Later the skin on the fingers may become cracked. (Reproduced from Leonardi S, et al. Severe Kawasaki disease in a 3-month-old patient: a case report. *BMC Res Notes.* 2013;6:500.)

Differential

Juvenile rheumatoid arthritis, infectious mononucleosis, scarlet fever, viral exanthems, leptospirosis, Rocky Mountain spotted fever, toxic shock syndrome, staphylococcal scalded-skin syndrome, erythema multiforme, serum sickness, SLE, Reiter syndrome.

Diagnosis

- Patients often have pyuria, transaminitis, normocytic anemia, and reactive thrombocytosis.
- Hyponatremia can be associated with an ↑ risk of cardiac complications.
- Screen with echocardiography or angiography for coronary artery aneurysms.

Management

- High-dose ASA and IVIG in the acute phase, followed by low-dose ASA for 6 to 8 weeks or until the coronary aneurysm resolves.
- Corticosteroids are not recommended, as they may be associated with an ↑ incidence of aneurysms.
- Serial echocardiograms at the time of diagnosis, at 2 to 4 weeks, and at 6 to 8 weeks. More frequent imaging may be required if abnormalities are present.

Complications

- **Coronary artery lesions:** Range from mild transient dilation of a coronary artery to large aneurysm formation. Untreated patients have a 25% risk of developing an aneurysm of the coronary arteries. Those at greatest risk for aneurysm formation are males, young children (<6 months), and those not treated with IVIG.
- **Other:** Also associated with myocarditis, pericarditis, and valvular heart disease (usually mitral or aortic regurgitation).

PULMONARY DISEASE

For pediatric asthma and asthma-associated conditions, see the Pulmonary chapter.

Bronchopulmonary Dysplasia

A chronic lung disorder that can develop in children who received prolonged mechanical ventilation to treat RDS. Risk factors include preterm delivery, low birth weight, and RDS, with an incidence of approximately 30% for infants with a birth weight of <1000 g. Although neonates with bronchopulmonary dysplasia (BPD) have an ↑ risk of mortality, lung function is normalized in early childhood in most survivors.

QUESTION

A 5-year-old boy presents with a 5- to 6-day history of persistent high fever and irritability. Three days ago, he was given antibiotics for presumed acute otitis media, but his fever did not resolve. On exam, he is found to have an erythematous rash, cracked lips, and a "strawberry tongue." He refuses to stand on both feet and cries every time he attempts to walk. Both ear canals appear red, which you attribute to the child's excessive crying. Do you continue the course of antibiotics?

Symptoms/Exam

- Patients present with dyspnea, tachypnea, cyanosis, and hypoxia.
- Exam reveals hypoxia with ↑ O_2 requirement.

Differential

Meconium aspiration syndrome, persistent pulmonary hypertension, congenital infection (eg, CMV), cystic adenomatoid malformation, recurrent aspiration, congenital heart disease, overhydration, idiopathic pulmonary fibrosis.

Management

- Inhaled corticosteroids with occasional use of β-adrenergic agonists.
- Chest physiotherapy is used for the thick secretions that may contribute to airway obstruction or recurrent atelectasis.
- RSV prophylaxis.
- Comprehensive interdisciplinary planning on discharge to ensure adequate follow-up.

Complications

Pulmonary hypertension, recurrent respiratory infections, cor pulmonale, exercise intolerance, ↑ risk of COPD, neurodevelopmental problems.

GASTROINTESTINAL DISEASE

Pyloric Stenosis

Most common in firstborn sons.
- **Symptoms/Exam:** Usually presents at 2 weeks to 2 months of life with projectile, nonbilious vomiting. An olive-sized mass may be felt in the epigastrium.
- **Diagnosis:** Ultrasound is diagnostic (Figure 13.18). Check electrolytes; hypochloremia and hypokalemia may be severe. Must confirm not false positive due to pyloric spasm.
- **Management:** Pylorotomy is curative. Correct electrolyte abnormalities before surgery.

A ▶ **ANSWER**

Recognizing that this child has Kawasaki disease, you discontinue antibiotics and admit the boy to the hospital for appropriate therapy.

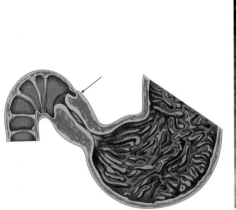

A

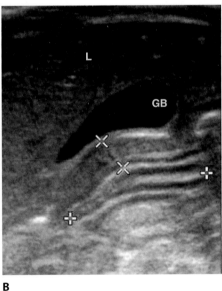

B

FIGURE 13.18.   **Hypertrophic pyloric stenosis. (A)** Schematic representation of a hypertrophied pylorus. The arrow denotes protrusion of the pylorus into the duodenum. **(B)** Longitudinal ultrasound of the pylorus showing a thickened pyloric musculature (X's) over a long pyloric channel length (plus signs). GB = gallbladder; L = liver. (Image A reproduced with permission from Doherty GM. *Current Diagnosis & Treatment: Surgery*, 13th ed. New York: McGraw-Hill, 2010, Fig. 43-9; image B reproduced with permission from USMLE-Rx.com.)

Intestinal Obstruction

Forms of intestinal obstruction in infants can be distinguished by clinical and radiographic findings, as described in Table 13.10, see also Figures 13.19 to 13.21. Surgical resection of the affected area is required in most cases.

Meckel Diverticulum

An ileal diverticulum that may contain ectopic gastric tissue. Male infants are affected more often than female infants.
- **Symptoms/Exam:** Painless rectal bleeding. Intussusception leading to intestinal obstruction.
- **Diagnosis:** A technetium scan can identify ectopic gastric tissue.
- **Management:** Surgical resection of symptomatic lesions (asymptomatic diverticula do not need to be removed).

Gastroesophageal Reflux Disease

Reflux of stomach contents into the esophagus caused by inappropriate relaxation of the LES. Children with neurologic deficits have a higher incidence of this condition.
- **Symptoms/Exam:** Spitting up, vomiting, apnea, colic, FTT.
- **Diagnosis:** Usually clinical. pH testing may be useful if symptoms are atypical. EGD is helpful in identifying esophagitis.

> **KEY FACT**
>
> Approximately 90% of cases of meconium ileus occur in patients with **CF.**

> **MNEMONIC**
>
> **Meckel diverticulum rule of 2s:**
> **2** inches long
> **2** feet from the ileocecal valve
> **2** types of tissue
> Presentation before age **2** years

TABLE 13.10.   Intestinal Obstruction in Infants

SITE OF OBSTRUCTION	CLINICAL FINDINGS	PLAIN RADIOGRAPHS	CONTRAST STUDY
Duodenal atresia	Down syndrome (30%); early vomiting that is sometimes bilious	Dilated stomach and proximal duodenum; no air distal ("double bubble" sign; Figure 13.19)	Not needed
Malrotation and volvulus	Associated congenital anomalies (>25%); bilious vomiting with onset at any time in the first few weeks; later signs include blood in stool, malabsorption, protein-losing enteropathy, diarrhea	Dilated stomach and proximal duodenum; paucity of air distally (may be a normal gas pattern)	UGI study shows a displaced duodenojejunal junction with a "corkscrew" deformity of twisted bowel (Figure 13.20)
Jejunoileal atresia, meconium ileus	Bilious gastric contents of >25 mL at birth; progressive distention and bilious vomiting	Multiple dilated loops of bowel; intra-abdominal calcifications if in utero perforation occurred (meconium peritonitis)	Barium or osmotic contrast enema shows microcolon; contrast refluxed into the distal ileum may demonstrate and relieve meconium obstruction (successful in about 50% of cases)
Meconium plug syndrome	Distention; delayed stooling (>24 hr)	Diffuse bowel distention	Barium or osmotic contrast enema outlines and relieves plug
Hirschsprung disease	Down syndrome (10%-15%) Early signs include delay or failure to pass meconium, vomiting, abdominal distention, reluctance to feed; later, fever, explosive diarrhea may develop; stool may be palpable in colon, not rectum on digital exam	May reveal a dilated proximal colon and absence of gas in the pelvic colon	Barium enema shows a narrowed segment distally, with a sharp transition to a dilated proximal colon (Figure 13.21)

Data from Hay WW, et al. *Current Diagnosis & Treatment in Pediatrics,* 18th ed. New York: McGraw-Hill, 2007:47.

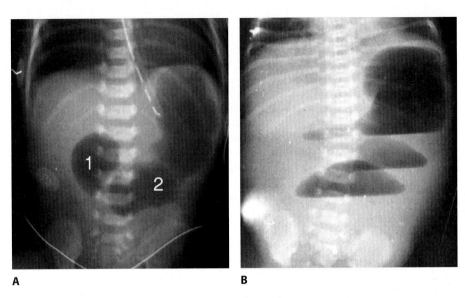

A   **B**

FIGURE 13.19.   **Bowel atresia. (A)** Characteristic "double bubble" sign (1 and 2) of duodenal atresia in an infant with bilious emesis. **(B)** Multiple dilated loops of small bowel with air-fluid levels in an infant with jejunal atresia. (Image A reproduced with permission from Brunicardi FC, et al. *Schwartz's Principles of Surgery,* 9th ed. New York: McGraw-Hill, 2010, Fig. 39-13; image B reproduced with permission from Brunicardi FC, et al. *Schwartz's Principles of Surgery,* 9th ed. New York: McGraw-Hill, 2010, Fig. 19-14.)

 Management:
  - Conservative treatment includes small feeds at shorter intervals. Medical options include H_2 receptor antagonists and proton pump inhibitors.
  - Indications for surgery include persistent vomiting with FTT, esophagitis, and apnea or pulmonary symptoms that persist after several months of medical treatment.
- **Complications:** Prolonged symptoms may lead to esophagitis, occult blood loss, anemia, esophageal stricture, and inflammatory esophageal polyps. Aspiration pneumonia, coughing, and wheezing may result if gastric secretions reflux into the airways.

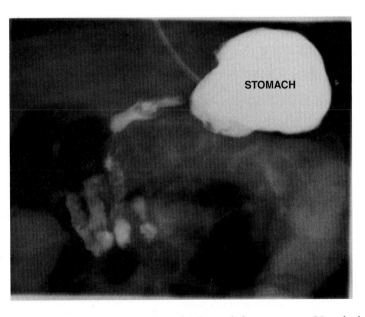

STOMACH

FIGURE 13.20.   **Midgut malrotation.** Frontal radiograph from an upper GI study shows a spiral pattern of duodenal and proximal jejunal loops in the right abdomen, consistent with midgut malrotation. The duodenojejunal junction should normally be to the left of the patient's spine. (Reproduced with permission from USMLE-Rx.com.)

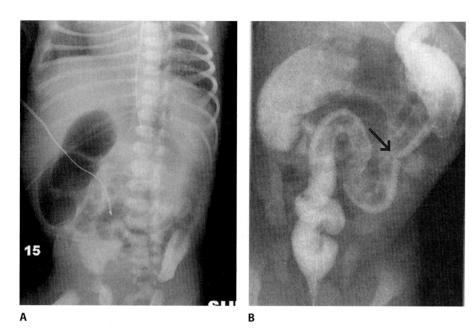

A **B**

FIGURE 13.21. **Hirschsprung disease.** (**A**) AXR showing dilated, air-filled right colon in an infant with infrequent stools. (**B**) Barium enema showing relatively large transverse colon caliber, with transition to small-caliber colon at the splenic flexure. Note the stool (arrow) in the aganglionic sigmoid colon and rectum. (Reproduced with permission from USMLE-Rx.com.)

Cow's Milk Allergy

Most common food allergy in infancy. More likely in patients with a family history of atopy.

Symptoms/Exam

Usually presents by the first month after introduction of cow's milk, but may take several months to develop. Presents with colic, GERD, hematochezia, or rash. May also present in breastfed infants whose mothers consume dairy.

Diagnosis

Food challenge.

Management

Dietary changes that avoid cow's milk protein should lead to improvement within 3 weeks. Do not change to soy protein, as there is a 50% likelihood that patients who are allergic to cow's milk will also be allergic to soy. Usually outgrow by 2 to 3 years of age.

CHILDHOOD CANCER

Leukemia

Acute lymphoblastic leukemia (ALL) is the most common malignancy in children. Incidence peaks at 2 to 5 years of age and is higher in children with Down syndrome.

Symptoms/Exam

Presents with bruising, purpura, pallor, bone pain, fever. Exam may show lymphadenopathy, petechial rash, and hepatosplenomegaly.

Q **QUESTION**

You are preparing to discharge a 2-day-old boy delivered by the normal spontaneous vaginal route when the nurse tells you that he has not yet passed any stool. The baby is breastfeeding, but seems to spit up most of what goes down, and his mother is becoming discouraged. You examine the infant and note that his belly is somewhat distended. You are not sure if you can feel a mass in the left side of the abdomen. What is the next step in evaluation?

Diagnosis

- Labs reveal abnormal WBC count (low or high), anemia, thrombocytopenia, and elevated LDH and uric acid.
- Bone marrow biopsy shows at least 25% blasts.

Management

Chemotherapy. Prognosis is good, with most ALL patients entering complete remission after induction chemotherapy.

Brain Tumor

The most common solid tumor in childhood. Children who have tuberous sclerosis or neurofibromatosis or have received brain radiation are at greatest risk.

Symptoms/Exam

- **Before 2 years of age: Typically infratentorial.** Vomiting, unsteady gait, and cranial nerve palsies may be seen.
- **After 2 years of age: Typically supratentorial.** Headache, vomiting, seizures, motor deficits, and changes in behavior. Headaches are classically daily, severe headaches that are worse with lying down and awakening from sleep.

Diagnosis

- CT or MRI of the brain with contrast; MRI is more sensitive.
- Biopsy of the lesion is sometimes indicated.

Management

Depends on tumor type. Most require surgical resection and/or radiation. Chemotherapy is also helpful in certain tumors.

Osteosarcoma

The most common malignant bone tumor in children. Peak incidence is in adolescence.

Symptoms/Exam

Presents with pain and swelling at the site of the tumor. Typically involves **ends** of the bone (distal femur, proximal humerus). **No systemic symptoms.**

Diagnosis

- X-ray: Aggressive lytic bone lesion with **"sunburst"** pattern of periosteal reaction, typically in the metaphysis of a long bone (Figure 13.22).
- Bone biopsy.

Management

Surgical resection and chemotherapy.

Ewing Sarcoma

The second most common malignant bone tumor in children. Peak incidence is at 10 to 20 years of age. Older age is a poor prognostic feature.

Symptoms/Exam

Presents with pain and swelling at the site of the tumor. Typical locations are **midshaft** of long bones, pelvic bones, and ribs. **Systemic symptoms** often seen.

ANSWER

This scenario raises concern for Hirschsprung disease or an atresia. An AXR would be a good starting point, although a contrast enema may also be needed to make a definitive diagnosis.

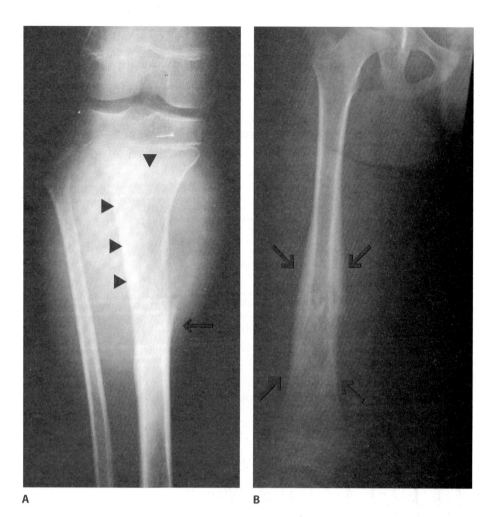

A   B

FIGURE 13.22.   Osteosarcoma versus Ewing sarcoma. (A) Lytic lesion of the proximal tibial
metaphysis (arrowheads) with sunburst appearance (arrow) compatible with osteosarcoma.
(B) Moth-eaten destructive lytic lesion in the mid-diaphysis of the femur with associated onion
skin periostitis (arrows). (Image A reproduced with permission from Doherty GM. *Current Diagnosis & Treatment: Surgery,*
13th ed. New York: McGraw-Hill, 2010, Fig. 40-38; image B reproduced from Monument MJ, et al. Microsatellites with macro-
influence in Ewing sarcoma. *Genes (Basel).* 2012;3(3):444-460.)

Diagnosis

- X-ray demonstrates an aggressive lytic bone lesion, most commonly in the diaphysis
  of a long bone. Often associated with **"onion-skinning"** periosteal reaction.
- Bone biopsy reveals a small, round blue cell.

Management

Surgical resection, chemotherapy, and radiation.

Rhabdomyosarcoma

The most common soft tissue sarcoma occurring in childhood. It can occur anywhere
in the body and accounts for 10% of solid tumors in childhood. The peak incidence
is at 2 to 5 years of age; 70% of children are diagnosed before age 10 years. A second,
smaller peak is seen in adolescents with extremity tumors. Males are affected more
often than females.

Symptoms/Exam

- Presenting symptoms and signs of rhabdomyosarcoma result from disturbances of normal body function due to tumor growth.
- Presents with a painless, progressively enlarging mass.
- Orbital invasion may cause proptosis; mucosal invasion may cause chronic drainage (nasal, aural, sinus, vaginal). Cranial nerve palsies are also seen.
- Bowel or bladder invasion may cause urinary obstruction, constipation, and hematuria.

Diagnosis

- Biopsy of the mass.
- When rhabdomyosarcoma imitates striated muscle and cross-striations are seen on light microscopy, the diagnosis is straightforward. Immunohistochemistry, electron microscopy, or chromosomal analysis is sometimes necessary to make the diagnosis.
- CT or MRI can determine the extent of the 1° tumor and assess regional lymph nodes.
- A lung CT can rule out pulmonary metastasis, the most common site of metastatic disease at diagnosis.
- A skeletal survey and a bone scan are obtained to rule out bony metastases.

Management

- Tumors should be excised if possible.
- Chemotherapy and radiation are appropriate for all patients and can shrink large tumors before surgery is attempted.

Neuroblastoma

KEY FACT

Neuroblastoma is an extremely malignant neoplasm. Most patients do not present with symptoms of the 1° lesion, but with complications of metastatic disease.

The third most common pediatric malignancy after ALL and AML. Accounts for approximately 10% of all childhood cancers. More than 80% of cases present before 4 years of age, and the peak incidence is at 2 years of age. Neuroblastomas arise from the neural crest cells of the adrenal medulla or sympathetic ganglia. The tumor most frequently originates in the adrenal glands, neck, chest, or pelvis. Prognosis is generally poor, with overall survival <30%.

Symptoms/Exam

- Systemic symptoms.
- Can present with an asymptomatic or painful abdominal mass. The tumor/abdominal mass may cross the midline.
- Bone pain results from metastases.
- Tumor can invade the spinal cord, leading to muscle weakness or sensory changes.
- The majority of patients already show signs of metastatic disease at presentation.

Diagnosis

- ↑ levels of serum catecholamines or urinary catecholamine metabolites (VMA and HVA).
- Biopsy of the mass.
- CT or MRI can determine the local extent of disease, and nuclear medicine MIBG imaging can assess for distant metastases (Figure 13.23).

Management

Depends on staging. Often includes chemotherapy and surgical resection of tumor. If bone marrow is involved, may require autologous bone marrow transplantation.

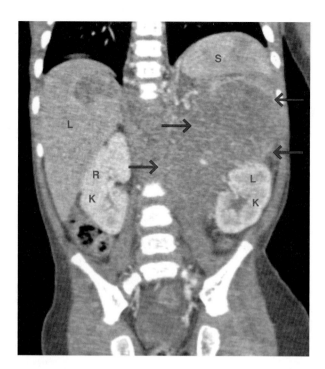

FIGURE 13.23. **Neuroblastoma.** Coronal reformat from contrast-enhanced CT shows a massive left suprarenal mass displacing the left kidney inferiorly. L = liver; LK = left kidney; RK = right kidney; S = spleen. (Reproduced with permission from USMLE-Rx.com.)

Wilms Tumor

Second most common abdominal malignancy after neuroblastoma. A tumor of the kidney consisting of a variety of embryonic tissues. Approximately 75% of children affected are <5 years of age; the peak incidence is at 2 to 3 years of age. The constellation of Wilms tumor, aniridia, GU anomalies, and cognitive impairment (WAGR syndrome) is associated with deletion of chromosome 11p13.

Symptoms/Exam

- Presents with abdominal enlargement ± pain, hematuria, malaise, weakness, anorexia, weight loss, and fever.
- Hypertension is noted in more than one-half of patients.
- An abdominal mass is felt that does not cross the midline.

Differential

Abdominal masses, including hydronephrosis, multicystic or duplicated kidneys, neuroblastoma, teratoma, hepatoma, and rhabdomyosarcoma.

Diagnosis

CT is required to determine the extent of the mass as well as to assess for bilateral disease, venous invasion, and metastases (Figure 13.24).

Management

- Surgical excision (nephrectomy) to completely remove the tumor and ureter.
- Very large tumors may be treated preoperatively with radiation therapy and chemotherapy to ↓ their size.
- Metastatic foci in the lung or liver may be resected or treated with radiation therapy.
- Overall survival is 85%.

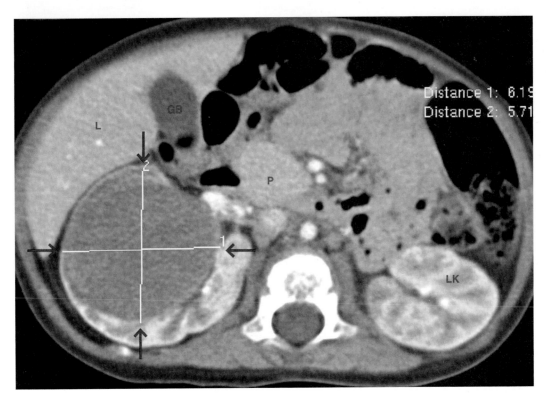

FIGURE 13.24.   **Wilms tumor.** Centered in the right kidney (arrows) on transaxial image from contrast enhanced CT. GB = gallbladder; L = liver; LK = left kidney; P = pancreas. (Reproduced with permission from USMLE-Rx.com.)

MUSCULOSKELETAL AND RHEUMATOLOGICAL DISORDERS

Legg-Calvé-Perthes Disease

Avascular necrosis of the proximal femur. Most frequently occurs in boys ages 4 to 8 years.

- **Symptoms/Exam:** Presents with persistent pain, limp, and limited ROM. Can be painless.
- **Diagnosis:** X-ray changes occur over several weeks. At several weeks, ↓ bone density, a necrotic center, and femoral head sclerosis are apparent (Figure 13.25).
- **Management:** Goal is to keep the femoral head in the acetabulum and preserve ROM. In most cases, observation is adequate with ↓ weight bearing. In children >6 years of age, a brace is recommended. Some patients require surgery.

Osgood-Schlatter Syndrome

Overuse injury that leads to inflammation at the tibial tuberosity at the insertion site of the patellar tendon. Seen in girls 11 to 13 and boys 12 to 15 years of age.

- **Symptoms/Exam:** Presents with pain at the tibial tubercle, especially with activities that involve climbing and jumping.
- **Diagnosis:** X-rays typically normal but may reveal fragmentation at the tibial tubercle.
- **Management:** Rest, ice, anti-inflammatories.

Slipped Capital Femoral Epiphysis

Disruption at the growth plate that leads to displacement of the proximal femoral head. Most common in **overweight adolescent boys.** Generally, presents with vague progressive pain and limp, but may occur suddenly with trauma.

KEY FACT

Hip pathology can present with knee pain. Always evaluate the hip in a child presenting with knee pain or limp.

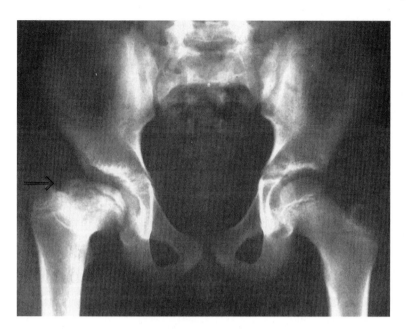

FIGURE 13.25.   Legg-Calvé-Perthes disease. Note the sclerosis, fragmentation, and collapse of the right femoral epiphysis (arrow) in comparison with the left femur. (Reproduced with permission from Chen MYM, et al. *Basic Radiology.* New York: McGraw-Hill, 2004, Fig. 7-48.)

- **Diagnosis:** Bilateral AP and frog-lateral x-rays reveal the classic appearance of an ice-cream scoop slipping off its cone. Approximately 30% of affected patients have asymptomatic slipped capital femoral epiphysis on the other side (Figure 13.26).
- **Management:** Surgical pinning.
- **Complications:** Avascular necrosis may occur in up to one-third of cases.

Septic Arthritis

- Causative organisms vary with age:
    - **Younger than 4 months:** *S aureus* and GBS.
    - **Four months to 4 years:** *H influenzae* and *S aureus.*
    - **Four years and older:** *S aureus* and *S pyogenes.*
    - **Adolescence:** Consider *Gonococcus.*

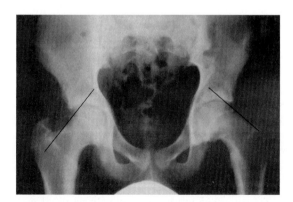

FIGURE 13.26.   Slipped capital femoral epiphysis, left. Frontal radiograph demonstrates medial displacement of the left femoral epiphysis. The "Klein line" is drawn in red. Note that the abnormal left femoral epiphysis does not protrude lateral to this line, whereas the right epiphysis does intersect this line. (Reproduced with permission from Skinner HB. *Current Diagnosis & Treatment in Orthopedics,* 4th ed. New York: McGraw-Hill, 2006, Fig. 11-14.)

 QUESTION

An 18-month-old boy is brought to your office for fussiness and fever. He demands to be held and will not stand on his own. The child will not allow you to bend his leg at the knee or hip. What should you include in your workup?

- **Symptoms/Exam:** Presents with pain, fever, malaise, swelling, and ↓ ROM of the joint. Early changes may not be seen on radiographs; late changes include destruction of the joint space.
- **Management:** Drainage is key. The knee may be aspirated or washed arthroscopically, but the hip generally requires surgical drainage. Use broad-spectrum IV antibiotics while awaiting cultures.

Osteomyelitis

Infection occurring in the bone resulting from either direct or hematogenous spread of bacteria. The metaphyses of long bones, especially the femur and tibia, are the most common locations in children.

- *Staphylococcus* infection is most common, but *Streptococcus* and *Haemophilus* are also seen. In patients with sickle cell, think *Salmonella.* In patients with a puncture wound, consider *Pseudomonas.*
- **Symptoms/Exam:** Infants may present with fussiness and pseudoparalysis of a limb. Older children will generally have fever and acute tenderness and will refuse to bear weight on the affected limb.
- **Diagnosis:** ↑ WBC, CRP, and ESR. ⊕ blood culture in 40% to 50%. X-ray findings lag behind clinical findings. MRI and bone scan are more sensitive. Aspiration of the bone for culture can help identify an organism and narrow the antibiotic spectrum.
- **Management:** IV antibiotics with surgical debridement as indicated.

Scoliosis

Defined as lateral curvature of the spine >10 degrees. Idiopathic disease is most common and usually presents at 8 to 10 years of age. There is an association with Marfan syndrome, cerebral palsy, muscular dystrophy, and neurofibromatosis. The disease is seen four times more often in girls and frequently runs in families.

- **Diagnosis:** First noted by the family or on exam. Forward bending test may show elevation of the rib cage on one side. To assess severity, check x-rays to calculate the angle of defect (Figure 13.27). There is no evidence to support universal screening.
- **Management:** Based on symptoms, obviousness of the deformity, and the likelihood of progression. Refer to orthopedics for a curve >20 degrees. Mild disease may be followed with serial exams and bracing; more severe disease may require surgery to correct the deformity and preserve respiratory capacity.

Juvenile Idiopathic Arthritis

The majority of cases of juvenile idiopathic arthritis (JIA) improve with age, and many patients become asymptomatic after puberty. However, joint damage acquired during active disease may contribute to later disability, even in the absence of an ongoing disease process. JIA is defined by age **<16 years,** arthritis, and symptoms persisting **>6 weeks.** Subtypes are as follows:

- **Systemic JIA** (also known as Still disease): Presents with fever, rash, arthritis, hepatosplenomegaly, and leukocytosis. Systemic symptoms generally regress within 1 year. Arthritis may regress, but may also continue and become extremely destructive. Differential includes reactive or postinfectious arthritis; other connective tissue disease (eg, SLE); malignancy (eg, leukemia). ANA and rheumatoid factor (RF) are usually ⊖. Treated with NSAIDs, corticosteroids, methotrexate, other immune-modifying agents.
- **Polyarticular JIA:** Involves ≥5 joints. Presents with **symmetric** chronic arthritis that may wax and wane. Systemic symptoms may be present but are generally mild. Iridocyclitis rarely occurs. Labs reveal ↑ ESR; mildly ⊕ ANA. Treated with NSAIDs; disease-modifying medications (eg, methotrexate, TNF-α blockers).

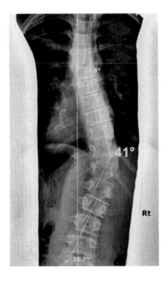

FIGURE 13.27. Idiopathic scoliosis. Standing radiograph shows S-shaped thoracolumbar scoliosis with right thoracic curvature centered at T11-T12 with Cobb angle of 41 degrees. (Reproduced from Wood G. Brace modifications that can result in improved curve correction in idiopathic scoliosis. *Scoliosis.* 2014;9:2.)

KEY FACT

Unlike adults, children with RA generally have a ⊖ RF.

ANSWER

CBC, radiographs, and ESR. Suspicion is high for osteomyelitis or septic joint (knee or hip), with pain in the other joint being an example of referred pain. It is often necessary to proceed with MRI (sensitive for osteomyelitis) and/or joint aspiration (for septic joint), even with a ⊖ x-ray. Start broad-spectrum antibiotics while awaiting blood culture results. *S aureus* or *H influenzae* is the most likely culprit in toddlers.

Pauciarticular JIA: Asymmetric chronic arthritis in **one to four joints** (typically weight bearing). Iridocyclitis is a significant risk, and children require frequent ophthalmologic exams. ESR and WBC are normal; RF is $\ominus$ but ANA is $\oplus$. Other causes of arthritis (eg, reactive) must be ruled out. Management is the same as that for polyarticular JIA.

Adolescent Growth and Development

Stages of normal growth and development are as follows (see also Table 13.11):
- **Early adolescence:**
  - Occurs at 11 to 13 years of age and merges with mid-adolescence at 14 to 15 years.
  - Characterized by **concrete thinking** and **body image disruption.**
- **Mid-adolescence:**
  - Begins around 14 to 15 years of age and blends into late adolescence at about 17 years.
  - Issues involve **autonomy;** may lead to parental conflict.
- **Late adolescence:**
  - Begins at approximately 17 to 21 years of age. The upper end is particularly variable and depends on cultural, economic, and educational factors.
  - Adolescents begin to think about the future and form stable, intimate relationships.
  - Executive function and self-regulation skills solidify.

TABLE 13.11. Stages of Development in Adolescence

STAGE	CHARACTERISTICS	GROWTH
Preadolescence	Low investment in sexuality Information about sexuality comes from friends, school, and family Physical appearance is prepubertal	2° sexual characteristics have begun to appear
Early to mid-adolescence	Physical maturation begins Curiosity about one's own body persists Sexual fantasies are common Masturbation begins Sexual activities are often nonphysical (eg, phone calls, e-mail)	Growth rapidly accelerates, reaches peak velocity, and begins decelerating; stature reaches 95% of adult height 2° sexual characteristics are well advanced
Late adolescence	Full physical maturation Sexual behavior and thoughts are more expressive Intimate physical and sharing relationships may develop Sexual behavior can include masturbation, petting, oral, anal, and vaginal intercourse	Physically mature; statural and reproductive growth are virtually complete

TANNER STAGING

Describes the development of pubic hair and breasts for girls and pubic hair and genitalia for boys (see Figures 13.28 and 13.29). Progression through the five stages is predictable. Lack of this predictable progression can indicate a pubertal disorder and may require further examination and possible referral to an endocrinologist.

Adolescent Consent and Confidentiality

Adolescents may fail to seek or delay seeking health care for a number of reasons. In addition to lack of access, finances, and awareness of clinical services, they may have concerns about confidentiality. Adolescents are more likely to seek care about sensitive issues if they feel that the health provider will not disclose that information to their parents. Laws about confidentiality vary from state to state.

- Minors have the right to consent for reproductive health care, treatment of STIs, treatment of rape or incest, and emergency health care. **No parental consent is required in these cases.**
- Minors who are considered "emancipated" do not require parental consent for medical decisions. Emancipation may be based on whether a minor is pregnant or a parent, is or has been married, is financially independent, or is in the armed forces.
- **The age of consent is 18 years,** although it varies by state.

> **KEY FACT**
>
> Teens should be aware of the physician's legal responsibility to report situations in which patients are at risk for suicide or homicide or are victims of sexual or physical abuse.

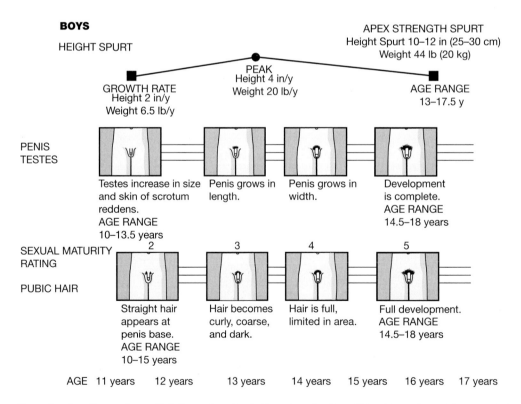

FIGURE 13.28. Sexual maturation and growth in boys. (Reproduced with permission from Hay Jr WW, et al. *Current Diagnosis & Treatment: Pediatrics,* 19th ed. New York: McGraw-Hill, 2009, Fig. 3-3.)

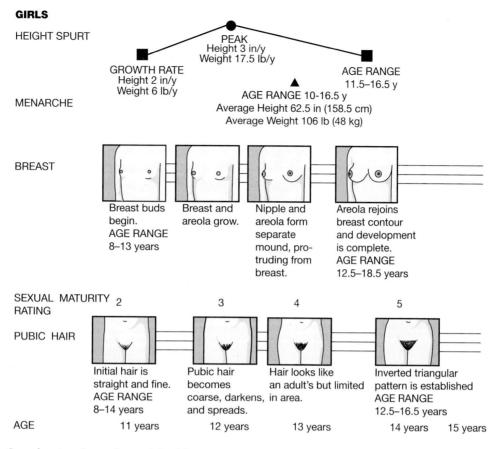

GIRLS

HEIGHT SPURT

PEAK
Height 3 in/y
Weight 17.5 lb/y

GROWTH RATE
Height 2 in/y
Weight 6 lb/y

AGE RANGE
11.5–16.5 y

MENARCHE

AGE RANGE 10-16.5 y
Average Height 62.5 in (158.5 cm)
Average Weight 106 lb (48 kg)

BREAST

Breast buds begin. AGE RANGE 8–13 years

Breast and areola grow.

Nipple and areola form separate mound, protruding from breast.

Areola rejoins breast contour and development is complete. AGE RANGE 12.5–18.5 years

SEXUAL MATURITY RATING   2   3   4   5

PUBIC HAIR

Initial hair is straight and fine. AGE RANGE 8–14 years

Pubic hair becomes coarse, darkens, and spreads.

Hair looks like an adult's but limited in area.

Inverted triangular pattern is established AGE RANGE 12.5–16.5 years

AGE   11 years   12 years   13 years   14 years   15 years

FIGURE 13.29. **Sexual maturation and growth in girls.** (Reproduced with permission from Hay Jr WW, et al. *Current Diagnosis & Treatment: Pediatrics,* 19th ed. New York: McGraw-Hill, 2009, Fig. 3-4.)

Preventive Medicine in Adolescence

ROUTINE SCREENING IN ADOLESCENTS

Guidelines for routine screening of adolescents are as follows:
- **Exam:**
  - Measure BP.
  - Conduct subjective hearing tests at every well-child visit.
  - Conduct a Snellen test for visual acuity.
  - Calculate BMI.
  - Screen for depression and anxiety.
  - Screen for alcohol and substance abuse.
  - Confirm dental home.
- **Labs:** Often **not necessary in the asymptomatic teenager,** screening laboratory tests should be kept to a minimum. General guidelines are as follows:
  - **Hemoglobin or hematocrit:** Anemia screening is recommended at the first encounter or at the end of puberty.
  - **Sickle cell screening:** Obtain at the first visit with African American adolescents.
  - **Cholesterol and fasting triglyceride testing:** Indicated in teens with obesity, heart disease, hypertension, and DM (or a strong family history of hyperlipidemia).

- **High-risk or symptomatic adolescents:** TB, anemia.
- **STI testing:**
  - **Sexually active female adolescents:** Patients should receive a Pap smear starting at age 21 years regardless of coitarche. Frequent gonorrhea/chlamydia testing (every 6-12 months) is recommended in high-risk youth, as is testing for syphilis, hepatitis B and C, HIV, and trichomoniasis.
  - **Sexually active male adolescents:** Do not routinely screen unless history of STI, or men who have sex with men.
  - **Men who have sex with men:** Annual syphilis, gonorrhea, chlamydia (genital and rectal), and hepatitis A/B/C screening.
    - HIV screening is recommended for all adolescents at least once, may ↑ frequency if at high risk.

ADOLESCENT IMMUNIZATIONS

- **Diphtheria, tetanus:** A booster of tetanus toxoid, reduced diphtheria toxoid, and acellular pertussis (Tdap) is recommended at age 11 to 12 years.
- **Meningococcal conjugate vaccine:** Administer to all 11- to 12-year-olds. A booster vaccine is recommended at age 16 years.
- **Influenza vaccine:** Recommended annually.
- **Hepatitis A and B:** Administer if vaccines were not received during childhood.
- **Pneumococcal vaccine:** Indicated in adolescents with chronic illnesses (sickle cell disease, HIV, asplenia, B-cell immune deficiency) and, in particular, in those with cardiovascular or pulmonary disease.
- **HPV vaccine:** Three doses of HPV vaccine are recommended for boys and girls starting at age 9 years.
- **Rubella:** Administer if vaccine was not received during childhood.

HEADSS ASSESSMENT

Adolescence is generally a period of extremely good physiologic health and well-being. Underlying psychosocial issues may thus have more significance than physical ones during this period. The **HEADSS** assessment is a systematic approach to these issues.

ANTICIPATORY GUIDANCE

Adolescents should receive health guidance annually, but information shared should be kept confidential. Recommendations for health guidance are designed to help adolescents approach development with greater knowledge and understanding, particularly as they develop cognitively and psychologically. The goals of anticipatory guidance are as follows (see also the mnemonic **SAFE TEENS**):

- **Promote a better understanding of physical growth, psychosocial and psychosexual development,** and the importance of becoming actively involved in health care decisions.
- **Provide information regarding dietary habits,** the benefits of a healthy diet, and ways to achieve a healthy diet and manage weight safely.
- **Reduce injuries by encouraging the use of helmets, seat belts, and sunscreen.**
  - **Motor vehicle safety,** eg, the roles of driver, passenger, and pedestrian as well as on the influence of substance abuse and the importance of using seat belts.
- **Educate adolescents about responsible sexual behaviors.**
  - Provide information to parents and adolescents, both together and separately. Emphasize the healthy expression of sexuality.

MNEMONIC

Adolescent psychosocial screening:
HEADSS

Home
Education/employment
Activities
Drugs
Sexuality
Suicide/depression screen

MNEMONIC

Anticipatory guidance:
SAFE TEENS

Sexuality
Accident
Firearms/homicide
Emotions/suicide
Toxins
Environment (school, home, friends)
Eating (**N**utrition)
Shots/immunizations

- Issues to discuss include timing of the initiation of sexual activity, sexual orientation and gender identity, abstinence resources (sex education, family planning clinics, professional education), and information on consent and violence prevention.
- Discuss the use of contraception and latex condoms to prevent STIs, including HIV infection.
- **Provide information about the benefits of fitness and physical activity:** Counsel regarding the use of adequate equipment, protective gear and clothing, helmets, safe facilities, proper rules of safe play, and rational approaches toward activities requiring advanced skill levels.
- **Discourage use of addictive and/or toxic substances:** Instruct patients in the potential dangers (including sudden death) that may occur not only with regular substance abuse but also with experimental use of drugs and alcohol. Include a discussion of nicotine, opioids, and steroids.
- **Ask about firearms:** Adolescents with firearms in the home need to learn proper use, safety, and legal issues associated with guns.

KEY FACT

Injuries are the most significant health problem of adolescents. A strong need for peer approval and lack of ability to appreciate consequences may lead youths to participate in a variety of risk-taking behaviors. Providing safety guidelines for teens is crucial in ↓ mortality from high-risk behavior and in reducing teen pregnancy, STIs, and unwanted sexual experiences such as sexual abuse or exploitation.

KEY FACT

Differing family values, cultural values, and personal experiences may give rise to varying sex education needs, which may include understanding body functions, exploring personal values, and setting sexual limits with partners.

NOTES

CHAPTER 14

Psychiatry and Behavioral Science

Amber Robins, MD, MBA

Mood Disorders

MAJOR DEPRESSIVE DISORDER

Defined as **severe depression** that has a significant effect on a patient's ability to function. Variable age of onset. Those aged 18 to 29 years are three times more likely to have major depressive disorder (MDD) than those who are 60 years or older. There is a two- to four-fold ↑ risk in first-degree family members. Variable course for MDD with patients experiencing remission (depression resolving completely or nearly completely). Recovery (extended remission of symptoms) can begin as early as 3 months of onset. Relapse is common.

Symptoms

Defined as one or more episodes of **depressed mood** or **anhedonia** (loss of interest or pleasure) for **at least 2 consecutive weeks,** as well as by at least five of the symptoms of depression, summarized by the mnemonic **SIG E CAPS.**

Differential

- **Adjustment disorder with depressed mood:** A reaction to a specific incident or psychosocial stressor, leading to depressed mood. Symptoms begin within 3 months of the stressor and lessen within 6 months (after removal of stress, behavior change and adaptation).
- **Grief:** Feelings of emptiness and loss that occur in waves, which mostly occur after death of a love one or major loss of functioning due to illness/accident or with a parent or significant other's loss of functioning such as with progressive dementia. Differentiated from MDD due to MDD being persistent depressed mood.
- **Mood disorder due to a medical condition:** A variety of disorders (eg, anemia, hypothyroidism, pancreatic cancer, Parkinson disease, SLE, infection, organic CNS disorders-tumors, vascular lesions) can lead to MDD.
- **Substance/medication-induced depressive disorder:** Depressive symptoms that start after use of a medication or after substance use or withdrawal, and that reappear after subsequent use of the substance/medication.
- **Bipolar disorder:** Episodes of major depressive symptoms alternating with manic periods.
- **Schizoaffective disorder:** Predominantly a psychotic disorder with accompanying mood symptoms.

Management

- **Behavioral:** Many forms of individual, couple, family, and group psychotherapy are appropriate and are as effective or more effective than medication in mild and moderate depression. Couples therapy is particularly effective for adults with depressive symptoms. If utilizing either psychotherapy alone or medication alone does not work, using both in combination has a significantly improved response rate over either modality separately.
- **Pharmacologic:** Select the medication with the most tolerable side effect profile while maximizing efficacy (see Table 14.1). The latest data indicate that sertraline is favored for efficacy and acceptability. Allow at least 4 to 6 weeks to assess the efficacy of a medication and continue antidepressants for at least 6 months after remission in moderate and severe depression. A change in treatment should be considered if there has been no response in 4 to 12 weeks.
  - Selective serotonin reuptake inhibitor (SSRI) (eg, paroxetine, fluoxetine, sertraline): Generally, first-line medication owing to its **lower side effect profile.** Serotonin-norepinephrine reuptake inhibitors (SNRIs), tricyclic antidepressants (TCAs), and monoamine oxidase inhibitors (MAOIs) have all demon-

TABLE 14.1. **Common Antidepressants and Side Effects**

CLASS	EXAMPLES	COMMON SIDE EFFECTS	MEDICALLY SERIOUS SIDE EFFECTS
SSRIs	Paroxetine (Paxil), fluoxetine (Prozac), sertraline (Zoloft), citalopram (Celexa), escitalopram (Lexapro), fluvoxamine (Luvox), others	Headache, sedation or activation, weight gain, GI discomfort, orgasmic or ejaculatory delay	Serotonin syndrome (tachycardia, hypertension, fever, hyperthermia, myoclonus, convulsions, coma)
SNRIs	Duloxetine (Cymbalta), venlafaxine (Effexor)	Same as SSRIs, and constipation, dizziness	Lowered seizure threshold, hypertension
TCAs[a]	Amitriptyline (Elavil), nortriptyline (Norpramin), clomipramine (Anafranil)	Dry mouth, constipation, bladder problems, sexual problems, blurry vision, drowsiness, orthostatic hypotension	Tachycardia, arrhythmias, rhabdomyolysis; in overdose, cardiotoxicity
MAOIs	Isocarboxazid (Marplan), phenelzine (Nardil), tranylcypromine (Parnate)	Orthostatic hypotension, edema, weight gain, GI distress, dizziness, headache, sedation	Hypertensive crisis: Avoid tyramine-containing foods and medicines: cheese, wine, pickles, decongestants, OTC cold meds. Never combine with SSRI because of the risk of hyperserotonemia
Other	Bupropion (Wellbutrin)	Insomnia, "jitteriness"	Lowered seizure threshold
	Mirtazapine (Remeron)	↑ appetite, sedation, dry mouth, constipation	Lowered seizure threshold
	Trazodone (Desyrel)[a]	Sedation (often used for sleep), GI distress, headache	Prolonged QT, dysrhythmias, priapism, serotonin syndrome

[a]Consider a baseline ECG before prescribing a TCA or trazodone, particularly in the elderly, to evaluate for congenital prolonged QT. Consider interactions when prescribing another QT prolonging medication!

strated a level of efficacy similar to that of SSRIs. Table 14.2 compares SSRIs and other pharmacologic treatments.

- **Adjunct therapies** for refractory depression: Atypical antipsychotics, mood stabilizers, and levothyroxine may be added, although this is usually done under the care of a psychiatrist.

TABLE 14.2. **Considerations for Treatment Choice in Major Depressive Disorder**

CONSIDERATION	CHOICE OF SSRI
Depression with low energy level	An activating SSRI (like fluoxetine) or bupropion
Depression with anxiety symptoms	A calming SSRI like paroxetine or a TCA like imipramine; avoid bupropion
Obsessive compulsive features	Any SSRI or clomipramine
Trouble sleeping	Trazodone or mirtazapine
Comorbid chronic pain	Consider duloxetine (however, evidence that this is more effective than any other SSRI is slim)
Sexual side effects are problematic	Bupropion
Need to quit smoking or lose weight	Bupropion (do not use for those with anorexia or bulimia!)
Seizure disorder	Do **not** use bupropion, mirtazapine, or SNRIs
Did it work for a close relative?	Give that medication a try

KEY FACT

FOR CHILDREN AND ADOLESCENTS:
- The FDA recommends that paroxetine **not** be used for treatment of MDD in children and adolescents.
- In 2004, the FDA issued a black-box warning regarding the risk of ↑ suicidality in children and adolescents prescribed antidepressant medications. However, this warning must be balanced with the risk of suicidality related to the depression.

KEY FACT

Don't forget to ask about manic symptoms before prescribing an antidepressant. Initiating an antidepressant can launch a clinically important manic episode.

KEY FACT

ALERT! Many questions on the Family Medicine Boards have addressed choosing appropriate antidepressants, especially within a specific class (eg, "Which SSRI would be the most appropriate for . . . ?").

KEY FACT

Always assess suicide risk! Ask directly about suicidal thoughts and plans!

- **Antidepressant discontinuation syndrome** can occur within days after abrupt medication cessation if a patient has been taking a medication for >6 weeks. Supervised tapering over 6 to 8 weeks may be required to minimize symptoms of antidepressant discontinuation syndrome, which include symptoms from the mnemonic **FINISH**.
- **Electroconvulsive therapy (ECT):** Primarily used for patients who show a lack of response to several antidepressants or have **severe depression** with psychosis, a high risk of suicide, or prior response to ECT. More effective than antidepressants in those who are severely depressed. ECT is not only effective but also very safe for both pregnant women and the elderly. Primary side effect is temporary retrograde amnesia as well as posttreatment confusion that lasts for minutes to hours. Permanent memory loss for events prior to the ECT is rare.
- **Treatment phases of MDD:**
  - **Acute phase:** About 12 weeks.
  - **Continuation phase:** Full remission of symptoms, but at high risk for relapsing within the next 4 to 6 months. Continue antidepressant treatment at acute-phase doses and eventually taper down.
  - **Maintenance phase:** Continue antidepressant treatment at acute-phase doses for prevention.

Complications

- **Psychosis:** Patients with severe MDD can develop psychotic symptoms such as auditory hallucinations, paranoia, and delusions. In such cases, the response rate is 40% with antidepressants alone, 20% with antipsychotics alone, and 70% with both taken together.
- **Suicidality:** Severe untreated MDD can lead to suicidality. Women tend to attempt more suicides, whereas men tend to succeed more often. Risk factors for suicide include:
  - Prior attempts.
  - Family history of completed suicide.
  - Degree of premeditation or plan.
  - Access to a weapon or proposed plan.
  - Active substance abuse.
  - Impulsivity.
  - Recent psychiatric inpatient discharge.
  - Protective factors include social support and family connectedness, parenthood, religiosity.
  - If a high risk of suicidality is present, the clinician must hospitalize the patient to ensure his or her safety.
  - Safety contracts are not effective in preventing suicide. Do a thorough suicide assessment including risks and protective factors. Include involved family or significant others in safety planning.

DYSTHYMIA

Defined as **depressed mood** occurring on most days and lasting **at least 2 years.** Although **less severe** than MDD, dysthymia significantly impairs work and social functioning because of its chronicity. Dysthymia is a risk factor for developing MDD.

Symptoms

Diagnostic criteria for dysthymia are as follows:
- **Two** of the following symptoms must be present, most of the day, more days than not, for at least 2 years:
  - Poor appetite or overeating.
  - Insomnia or hypersomnia.

- Low energy, fatigue.
- Poor concentration.
- Low self-esteem.
- Hopelessness.
- During a 2-year period, affected patients must **not have had a symptom-free period for >2 months.**
- Symptoms must lead to significant impairment in daily functioning.

Differential

- **Major depression:** A more severe form of depression.
- **Depression due to a medical condition:** Depressive symptoms may be similar to those of dysthymia, but are caused by a medical condition (eg, hypothyroidism, anemia).
- **Bipolar disorder:** Characterized by periods of mania or hypomania in addition to the depressive symptoms.
- **Substance abuse disorders:** Presentation is often similar to that of dysthymia, but symptoms are precipitated by the use of or withdrawal from alcohol or an illicit substance.

Management

- **Behavioral:** Various forms of individual, couple, family, and group psychotherapy may be of benefit.
- **Pharmacologic:** SSRIs; other classes of antidepressants.

BIPOLAR DISORDER

Characterized by **manic or hypomanic behaviors** that are sometimes accompanied by a depressive disorder. Male-to-female ratio is 1:1. Individuals are at higher risk if family members are affected. The mean age of onset is around 18 years.

Symptoms

- The symptoms of a manic episode of bipolar disorder are expressed in the mnemonic **DIG FAST.**
- To qualify as mania, symptoms **must last 4 to 7 days** and must produce social or occupational dysfunction. If there is no social or occupational dysfunction, the symptoms qualify as **hypomania.**

Differential

- **MDD:** Characterized by depressive symptoms without manic or hypomanic episodes.
- **Schizophrenia:** Although bipolar patients may exhibit signs of psychosis during a manic phase, schizophrenics do not experience mania.
- **Attention deficit/hyperactivity disorder (ADHD):** Distractibility and impulsivity are components of bipolar disorder, but ADHD patients do not exhibit other manic symptoms.
- **Cyclothymia:** Consists of mood swings between dysthymia and hypomania. However, depressive symptoms are not of sufficient severity to warrant a diagnosis of MDD, and manic symptoms do not reach the threshold sufficient for a manic episode.
- **Medical conditions leading to manic symptoms:** Include use of illicit substances (methamphetamines, cocaine), thyroid disorders, Cushing syndrome, HIV or HSV encephalitis, antidepressant treatment, steroid treatment, and neurologic disorders such as MS, frontal lobe syndromes, and temporal lobe epilepsy.

KEY FACT

Types of bipolar disorder:
Type I: At least one manic episode with or without major depression lasting at least 1 week.
Type II: At least one hypomanic episode with a major depressive episode lasting at least 1 week.

MNEMONIC

DIG FAST
- **D**istractibility
- **I**njudiciousness or **I**mpulsivity (poor judgment—eg, spending sprees, sudden travel, sexual indiscretion, reckless driving)
- **G**randiosity (↑ self-esteem)
- **F**light of ideas (racing thoughts)
- **A**ctivities—psychomotor agitation; ↑ goal-directed activities (eg, socializing, hypersexuality, ↑ productivity)
- **S**leep—↓ need for sleep
- **T**alkativeness—pressured speech

QUESTION

A 24-year-old white female college student presents to your office complaining, "I never have any energy, even though I sleep all the time. And I seem to inhale all the food around me—I don't want to be this way! I don't know why I stay in school; I'll never finish. I'm not worth the money my parents are spending on this! I have friends, and I like my classes, but I bring down anyone who's around me. I can't remember more than a day here and there in the last 2 years that I haven't felt this way. Will it ever get any better than this?" How do you respond?

Management

- **Pharmacologic:** Mood stabilizers (lithium, valproic acid, carbamazepine, lamotrigine, atypical antipsychotics; Table 14.3) **treat at least one phase** of bipolar disorder (mania or depression) **without worsening the other phase.** Antidepressants are **not** mood stabilizers, as they are known to precipitate mania.
- **Behavioral:** Individual therapy, cognitive behavioral therapy (CBT), interpersonal therapy, and family therapy have been shown to be effective in the treatment of bipolar patients. Establishing a therapeutic alliance is key.

Complications

Associated with a high rate of **completed suicides** (up to 15%). Although bipolar disorder is not associated with a downward drift of socioeconomic status, patients have high divorce rates, multiple jobs, and a high incidence of achievement followed by decline. Bipolar disorder is associated with several **comorbid conditions;** 60% have **substance abuse,** and 50% have **anxiety disorders.**

PREMENSTRUAL DYSPHORIC DISORDER

A severe form of premenstrual syndrome (PMS) defined by nonspecific psychological, behavioral, and somatic symptoms occurring during the final week prior to the onset of menses, starts to improve with menses, and becomes minimal/absent in the week after menses. Affects 1.8% of menstruating women. Onset of premenstrual dysphoric disorder (PMDD) can occur any time after menarche. Symptoms stop after menopause.

Symptoms

- Presents with depressed mood, feelings of hopelessness, self-deprecating thoughts, anxiety, tension, ↑ emotional lability, persistent and significant anger or irritability, anhedonia, lethargy, appetite changes, poor concentration, sleep disturbances, and a sense of being overwhelmed.
- Physical symptoms include bloating, breast tenderness, hot flashes, headache, and joint pain.

Differential

- **PMS:** Characterized by milder physical or behavioral symptoms prior to menses that do not interfere with performance or interpersonal relationships.
- **Mood disorders:** Symptoms do not resolve with menses.
- **Medical conditions:** Include dysmenorrhea, migraine, IBS, fibrocystic breast disease, and hypothyroidism.

TABLE 14.3. **Mood-Stabilizing Medications and Side Effects**

DRUG CLASS	DRUG	SIDE EFFECTS	MEDICALLY SERIOUS SIDE EFFECTS
Mood stabilizer	Lithium	Cognitive dulling, tremor, sedation, nausea, diarrhea, T-wave flattening	Lithium toxicity, **hypo**thyroidism (in long-term use), nephrogenic diabetes insipidus
Mood stabilizer/ anticonvulsant	Valproic acid (Depakote) Carbamazepine (Tegretol)	Weight gain, sedation, cognitive dulling	Thrombocytopenia SIADH, agranulocytosis, Stevens-Johnson rash

Diagnosis

- Specified symptoms must be present and limited to the luteal phase.
- Must lead to significant impairment in one or more areas of daily life.
- Rule out medical etiologies or other psychiatric conditions.

Management

- Recommend lifestyle changes such as aerobic exercise, ↓ caffeine, ↓ sodium intake, smaller and more frequent meals, and a diet rich in complex carbohydrates.
- Stress reduction, anger management, and individual, couple, and group therapy may be of benefit.
- Nutritional supplementation, with a daily multivitamin, vitamins D and E, calcium, and magnesium. Vitamin B_6 is also thought to be helpful, but data suggest that there may be harm from too much B_6—safe intake is 100 mg daily.
- Pharmacologic treatment with antidepressants or anxiolytics. NSAIDs can be used before or at onset to relieve physical symptoms. Spironolactone may be useful for significant bloating. OCPs or medroxyprogesterone acetate may stabilize hormonal swings.
- Ovulation suppression with GnRH agonists; danazol for severe symptoms refractory to other treatments.
- Bilateral oophorectomy should be used only in the most severe and refractory cases.

KEY FACT

PMDD is distinguished from PMS by the severity of its symptoms and by its disruption of performance and interference with interpersonal relationships.

POSTPARTUM MAJOR DEPRESSION

A major depressive episode with onset within 6 months of childbirth. Affects 1 in 10 childbearing women. Onset can begin prior to delivery to several months after delivery, lasting several months to the second year postpartum. ↑ risk of postpartum major depression (PMD) with prior history of depression, bipolar disorder, and/or family history of bipolar disorders.

Symptoms

Presents with depressed mood, anhedonia, sleep disturbance, ↓ energy, weight loss, a sense of hopelessness or guilt, ↓ concentration, thoughts of suicide or death, and thoughts of harming the infant.

KEY FACT

The mainstay of treatment for severe PMD consists of SSRIs in combination with supportive psychotherapy.

Differential

- Normal physiologic response to childbirth.
- "Baby blues": Mild symptoms that usually peak after postpartum day 4 or 5 and resolve by postpartum day 10. Affects 30% to 80% of childbearing women.
- Preexisting psychiatric disorders.
- Medical conditions such as thyroid dysfunction and anemia.
- **Puerperal psychosis:** Constitutes a psychiatric emergency. Most often associated with infanticide.

KEY FACT

"Baby blues" typically peak 4 or 5 days after delivery and resolve after 10 days.

Management

- **Behavioral:** Individual or group therapy; couples therapy often helpful.
- **Pharmacologic:** Used in patients with moderate to severe PMD; treatment is the same as that for major depression (SSRIs, TCAs). There is no evidence of morbidity in breastfed infants with SSRIs or TCAs, but the drugs and their metabolites have been found in breast milk. Weigh the risks and benefits, and discuss options with the patient.
- **Referral:** For any woman with suicidal/infanticidal ideation, no response to antidepressant therapy, or psychotic symptoms, immediate referral to psychiatry should be initiated and inpatient treatment considered.

KEY FACT

Postpartum psychosis is a psychiatric emergency.

Prevention

Identify at-risk women before delivery (eg, those with poor family support, stressful life events, a history of a mood disorder, or previous PMD).

Complications

Untreated PMD can have serious adverse effects on the mother and can also adversely affect the emotional and psychological development of the child.

PSYCHOTROPIC MEDICATIONS DURING PREGNANCY AND BREASTFEEDING

Women and their physicians tend to **overestimate the teratogenic risk** of psychotropic medications during pregnancy and to **underestimate the risk of untreated maternal mental illness.**

- Antidepressants:
  - **TCAs: Not associated with major congenital malformations.** Some reports link TCA use to postpartum irritability, shakiness, and urinary and bowel obstruction.
  - **SSRIs:** Extensive research has shown **no association between major congenital malformations and fluoxetine,** but preliminary studies show a possible ↑ in persistent pulmonary hypertension in the newborn when SSRIs are given **after 20 weeks' gestation. Paroxetine is contraindicated in pregnancy** in the wake of studies showing an association with cardiac malformations. Case reports link SSRIs with perinatal irritability, hypoglycemia, and shakiness.
  - Both SSRIs and TCAs have also been shown **not to have neurobehavioral toxicity,** and children exposed in utero have been found to develop normally. In contrast, studies have shown that untreated depression does have a negative effect on children's development.
- Mood stabilizers:
  - **Carbamazepine and valproic acid:** Both have a **well-established risk** of neural tube defects (1% and 5%, respectively). Carbamazepine may also ↑ the risk of neonatal hemorrhage.
  - **Lithium:** Use during the first trimester is associated with a **10% to 20% higher risk of Ebstein anomaly** (tricuspid valve malformation). However, the **overall risk is still low (0.1%),** as the incidence of this anomaly is low to begin with.
    - Lithium remains the preferred medication for the treatment of pregnant patients with severe bipolar disease, as benefit outweighs the risks.
    - In other patients, it may be safer to discontinue the medication in the first trimester and resume it in the second or third trimester.
    - In the perinatal period, hypotonia, cyanosis, and diabetes insipidus have generally been reported to be rare and self-limited.
- Antipsychotics:
  - **High-potency neuroleptics** are considered **safe** in pregnancy. By contrast, study data are limited regarding the atypical antipsychotics (olanzapine, risperidone, quetiapine).
  - **Perinatal toxicities** (tremor, restlessness, dystonia) have been reported, but tend to resolve within weeks. Limited data exist regarding the neurobehavioral effects of these agents.
  - Again, the **benefits** (such as ↓ substance abuse and continuity with prenatal care) must be **weighed against the above risks.**
- ECT: Considered safe and effective during pregnancy.
- Medication use and breastfeeding:
  - All psychotropic medications are **secreted in breast milk.** Therefore, infants of mothers taking such medications must be **monitored for behavioral changes.** Check drug levels in infants with symptoms.
  - **Carbamazepine** and **valproic acid** are **not contraindicated** in breastfeeding but are associated with infant **thrombocytopenia** and **anemia.**

Anxiety Disorders

GENERALIZED ANXIETY DISORDER

Defined as excessive worrying that is out of proportion to the situation and lasts **at least 6 months.** There is a 2:1 female predominance, usually beginning in childhood or adolescence. The condition is generally **chronic,** but has flares of worsening severity.

Symptoms

Presents with **excessive worrying and anxiety** about a variety of subjects, more days than not, with difficulty controlling the worry. Three of the following symptoms—at a functionally impairing level—must be present:

- Restlessness.
- Easy fatigability.
- Poor concentration.
- Muscle tension.
- Insomnia.
- Irritability.

Differential

- **Posttraumatic stress disorder (PTSD):** Must have a precipitating traumatic event.
- **Major depression:** Accompanied by depressive symptoms.
- **Panic disorder:** Consists of discrete, short-lived panic attacks.
- **Obsessive compulsive disorder (OCD):** Anxiety that is due to obsessions and is relieved by compulsions.

Diagnosis

Rule out medical causes (eg, hyperthyroidism, substance abuse).

Management

- **Behavioral:** CBT, mindfulness-based stress reduction.
- **Pharmacologic:** Antidepressants, buspirone, and long-acting benzodiazepines (eg, clonazepam).

PANIC DISORDER

Characterized by **recurrent unexpected** panic attacks, with fear of additional ones occurring. Onset is from late adolescence through the third decade of life.

Symptoms

- Characterized by episodes of **abrupt anxiety** that peak after 10 minutes and are associated with several features of **autonomic arousal.**
- Must include at least four of the following features of autonomic arousal: **palpitations,** tachycardia, chest discomfort, **shortness of breath,** nausea, a choking sensation, trembling, dizziness, **paresthesias,** sweating, chills, hot flashes, dissociation, and **fear of losing control or dying.**

Differential

- **Psychiatric:**
    - **PTSD:** Must have a precipitating traumatic event.
    - **Generalized anxiety disorder:** Characterized by continuous anxiety, but no discrete attacks.

KEY FACT

Agoraphobia, which is sometimes a complication of panic disorder, is fear of being in a place from which escape would be difficult, or where it might be difficult to get help if a panic attack were to occur.

QUESTION 1

A 60-year-old woman presents to your office, saying, "Everyone knows I have a PhD in worry! If I know you're supposed to arrive at 3 PM, I start worrying at 1 PM that you've had a crash. You could have fallen asleep while driving. You could have forgotten to pick up the groceries; it could start snowing any minute! Sometimes I get so worried that I can't sleep. I can't even go to work! I don't know what is going to happen next with the world—it's all so out of control!" What counseling could you provide in the office?

QUESTION 2

A 25-year-old man discloses to you, "I don't know what it is. Nothing happened. I was just sitting there watching TV. All of a sudden, I had a terrible feeling, my heart was racing, and I couldn't breathe. Both hands started tingling and I was sweaty all over. I knew I was having a heart attack and was going to die." What is the best nonpharmacologic treatment for this patient?

- **Phobia:** A specific trigger for panic is present (eg, fear of flying, fear of heights, fear of bridges, fear of spiders).
- **Medical:**
  - **Endocrine:** Hypoglycemia, hyperthyroidism, pheochromocytoma.
  - **Cardiac:** Arrhythmia, MI.
  - **Pulmonary:** COPD, asthma, pulmonary embolus.
  - **Pharmacologic:** Side effects of medications (eg, SSRIs, albuterol); acute intoxication with a stimulant.

Diagnosis

Rule out medical causes first (eg, ECG, CXR, metabolic panel).

Management

- **Behavioral:** CBT.
- **Pharmacologic:** SSRIs (fluoxetine, sertraline, paroxetine), benzodiazepines.

OBSESSIVE COMPULSIVE DISORDER

Chronic syndrome of intrusive, recurrent, undesired thoughts (**obsessions**) and/or uncontrollable repetitive behaviors or rituals (**compulsions**) that lead to significant distress in a patient's daily life. Prevalence of OCD is 1.2%, with a mean onset in the second decade. Rarely presents after 35 years of age.

Symptoms

- **Obsessions: Recurrent** and persistent ideas, impulses, thoughts, or images that are perceived to be intrusive and meaningless and cause anxiety or grief. Not anxieties about real-life problems.
- **Compulsions: Uncontrollable** repetitive behaviors or rituals. May temporarily relieve anxiety.

Differential

- **Obsessive-compulsive personality disorder:** Generally lacks the obsessions and compulsive behaviors and rituals common to OCD. Patients are perfectionists, with inflexibility and obsessive attention paid to detail. Patients typically are not disturbed by their symptoms, whereas in OCD, they often are.
- **Generalized anxiety disorder:** Anxiety tends to be generalized to all areas of the patient's life, and the patient does not present with ritual behaviors to relieve anxiety.
- **Schizophrenia:** The patient is typically unaware that the obsessions are a product of his or her own mind and will have other symptoms characteristic of schizophrenia, such as psychotic and negative symptoms.

Diagnosis

The following criteria must be met to characterize a disorder as OCD:

- The presence of obsessions or compulsions.
- The patient recognizes that the obsessions or compulsions are to the **point of excess or unreasonable.**
- The obsessions or compulsions **interfere with daily living,** cause anguish, or are significantly time consuming (>1 hour in 1 day).

Management

- **Behavioral:** Begin with CBT, with the goal of stopping intrusive thoughts and behaviors. Effective for 70% of patients who agree to the process.

- **Pharmacologic:** Generally, medications should be started if behavioral treatment alone is unsuccessful. SSRIs are indicated and may need to be titrated to higher doses than those used to treat depression or other anxiety disorders. Clomipramine (a TCA) is also indicated in the treatment of OCD.

Complications

Can cause depression if untreated. Can also lead to significant impairment in one's life, such as loss of income, family stressors, and substance abuse.

POSTTRAUMATIC STRESS DISORDER

Avoidance, hyperarousal, and **reexperiencing** of a traumatic, life-threatening event that overwhelms the person's coping mechanisms. Onset most commonly occurs within 3 months following trauma. Risk factors include young age, a history of prior trauma, a history of mental illness, low IQ, and minimal social support. Experiences as a refugee and domestic and street violence are important to consider.

Symptoms

- **Reexperiencing:** Frequent intrusive memories and sensations of the experience of the event (flashbacks, hallucinations, and nightmares).
- **Avoidance/numbing:** The patient avoids any reminder of the event, such as conversations, people, and places. For example, a patient who has experienced combat may avoid all films about war. He or she may also feel detached from others or emotionally restricted and have little hope for the future.
- **Hypervigilance:** The patient may be easily startled and has a persistently ↑ autonomic response, characterized by difficulty sleeping, irritability, anger, and difficulty concentrating.

Differential

- **Acute stress disorder:** Similar to PTSD, but lasts 3 days to <1 month.
- **Adjustment disorder:** May have symptoms similar to those of PTSD, but they are not caused by a life-threatening, severely traumatic event.
- **OCD:** The patient experiences recurrent intrusive thoughts, but they are not the result of a severe trauma.

Diagnosis

- Patients must have witnessed or **experienced a life-threatening or severe injury-threatening event** that elicited a response of intense horror, hopelessness, and fear.
- All three symptoms of **avoidance, reexperiencing, and ↑ arousal** must be present.
- Symptoms must last >1 month.
- Symptoms must lead to severe impairment and significant distress in the patient's life.

Management

- **Behavioral:**
  - **CBT:** Effective, as is psychotherapy geared toward reducing survivor guilt, hopelessness, and anger. Goal of CBT is fear extinction and improved coping through conditioning and modifying thoughts.
  - **Couple or family therapy:** May be helpful in reducing the negative effects of PTSD on family members who may not understand or be aware of the trauma inflicted on the patient.
- **Pharmacologic:**
  - SSRIs (fluoxetine) are effective in treating all three clusters of PTSD (ie, reexperiencing, avoidance/numbing, and hyperarousal).

KEY FACT

Acute stress disorder is diagnosed when symptoms occur within 3 days to 1 month of the event, but do not last >1 month. In PTSD, symptoms last >1 month.

Q   QUESTION

A 32-year-old woman says, "I can't stop cleaning my house! I spent 4 hours yesterday cleaning the kitchen sink. This is crazy!" For which complications of this illness should you monitor?

- TCAs (desipramine, amitriptyline) are most helpful in treating reexperiencing symptoms.
- For mood swings, mood stabilizers such as carbamazepine or valproic acid are effective. β-blockers such as propranolol can help ↓ hypervigilance, and benzodiazepines (alprazolam, clonazepam) can be used for anxiety.

Complications

Comorbid conditions associated with PTSD include alcohol and substance abuse, MDD, somatoform disorders, dissociative disorders, other anxiety disorders, and ongoing trauma.

SPECIFIC PHOBIAS

Persistent and marked **fear of a specific object or situation** that leads to marked anxiety and avoidance that impair the patient's life. Fear of animals or natural environments (eg, snakes, heights, water) and fear of blood and injections usually start in childhood, whereas fear of situations (eg, flying, small spaces) may start in the second decade of life.

- **Notable symptoms:** Fear experienced is **excessive** in relation to the object and situation. The patient recognizes that the fear is unreasonable. Exposure to the feared object or situation causes **extreme** anxiety and panic. The object or situation is avoided or dreaded.
- Differential includes:
    - **Panic disorder:** Panic attacks are not related to fear of a specific object or situation.
    - **PTSD:** Panic symptoms are triggered by severe trauma.
    - **Generalized anxiety disorder:** Anxiety is generalized and is not related to a specific situation or object.
- **Behavioral therapy:** CBT is geared toward extinguishing the anxiety response to the specific situation. This is done through **desensitization** or repeated exposures to the inciting agent.
- **Pharmacologic treatment:** Antianxiety medications such as benzodiazepines can help ↓ anxiety and ↑ exposure to the offending object or situation. These medications are best used in the short term before or during triggering situations, and can be combined with behavior therapy when needed.

KEY FACT

Fear is a normal reaction to an actual threat or danger. A phobia is an excessive and unreasonable reaction to a certain situation or object.

Psychotic Disorders

DELUSIONAL DISORDER

Chronic disorder of delusions (**fixed false beliefs may be bizarre or nonbizarre in nature**) that occur ≥1 month. An uncommon disorder, with a prevalence of 0.2%. More prevalent in older age groups.

Symptoms

- Presents with highly specific delusions not attributable to physiologic changes from substance use or another medical condition. Some patients with delusional disorder develop schizophrenia. Prognosis is good in most cases.
- Patients are otherwise normal and maintain a high level of functioning.

ANSWER

Depression and substance abuse.

Differential

- **Schizophrenia:** Associated with more functional impairment, auditory hallucinations, and thought disorders.
- **Substance-induced delusions:** Seen primarily with CNS stimulants such as cannabis and amphetamines.
- **Medical conditions:** Include thyroid disorders, Huntington disease, Parkinson disease, Alzheimer disease, Lewy body dementia, CVAs, metabolic causes (uremia, hepatic encephalopathy, hypercalcemia), alcohol withdrawal, and other causes of delirium.

Management

- Patients are often resistant to treatment or medications.
- The first goal is to create a strong physician-patient alliance. Avoid directly challenging the patient's beliefs, but do not pretend to be in full acceptance of the delusions.
- Low-dose **antipsychotics** are indicated (atypicals such as olanzapine or risperidone are preferred). **Antidepressants,** especially clomipramine, may be helpful.
- The goal of medications is to help the patient avoid acting on the delusion.

SCHIZOPHRENIA

A **chronic** disorder characterized by **delusions, hallucinations, disorganized speech, behavioral disturbances,** and **impaired social function** (without any mental status changes). Lifetime prevalence is 0.3 to 0.7%, manifesting earlier (18-25 years of age) and more severely in men and later (26-45 years of age) in women, with an equal male-to-female ratio (1:1). **Prevalence is higher** in the presence of a ⊕ **family history** (10% if there is a sibling or parent with schizophrenia). Earlier age of onset is predictor of worse prognosis. Suicide risk is high.

Symptoms

Patients must have at least a **6-month period** of continuous symptoms of:
- **Hallucinations,** mostly auditory.
- **Delusions** characterized as fixed false beliefs that are not shared by others in the same culture and that persist despite evidence to the contrary.
- **Disorganized speech, described as** "word salad."
- **Catatonic** or bizarre behavior.
- **Negativity,** flat affect, alogia (poverty of speech), avolition, lack of purposeful action.

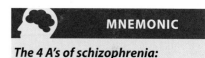

MNEMONIC

The 4 A's of schizophrenia:
Affective flattening
Asocial
Auditory hallucinations
Alogia (poverty of speech)

Differential

- **Mood disorders:**
  - **Bipolar disorder:** Psychotic symptoms can occur during manic or depressive episodes.
  - **Schizoaffective disorder:** Predominantly a mood disorder (mania or depression), with psychotic symptoms (lasting at least 2 weeks) during normal mood.
  - **Depression with psychotic features:** Depression predominates, with superimposed psychotic features. Patients are not psychotic when depression improves or resolves.
- **Delusional disorder:** Delusions tend not to be bizarre, and there are no associated symptoms such as hallucinations, thought disorders, or negative symptoms.
- **Drug-induced psychosis:** Amphetamines or cocaine can lead to paranoia and hallucinations. LSD, PCP, ketamine, and MDMA (ecstasy) can all lead to psychosis. Typically accompanied by other signs of substance abuse.
- **Organic causes:** Include medical conditions such as neurosyphilis, dementia, delirium, complex partial seizures, Huntington disease, heavy metal exposure, neoplasms, and medications (eg, prednisone).

KEY FACT

Schizophrenia often starts with negative symptoms without the delusions or hallucinations (positive symptoms). This is called the **prodromal** or **residual** phase.

- **Negative symptoms:** If the patient has negative symptoms only, other disorders should be ruled out, including Parkinson disease, depression, hypothyroidism, frontal lobe injury, PTSD, and substance abuse.

Diagnosis

Diagnosis is made by the history. Patients must have either bizarre delusions or hallucinations or two or more of the above symptoms (thought disorder, disorganized speech, catatonia, negative symptoms). Initially, **medical causes must be ruled out.** Consider BMP, calcium, CBC, TFTs, LFTs, VDRL, vitamin B_{12}, folate, HIV, a toxicology screen, brain imaging (CT or MRI), and EEG (if clinically indicated).

Management

- Antipsychotics are the treatment of choice. **Atypical neuroleptics,** or second-generation antipsychotics (SGAs), are **often first-line agents** (eg, olanzapine, quetiapine, risperidone), but typical or first-generation antipsychotics (eg, haloperidol, fluphenazine, chlorpromazine) are often just as effective, though with some intolerable side effects.
- Acutely, the goal of therapy is to **minimize symptoms and side effects** and, once the patient is stable, to titrate to the lowest effective dose that will maintain maximal functioning and prevent recurrence.
- Since 25% to 50% of schizophrenics continue to have residual symptoms and impaired functioning, psychosocial treatment is a component of therapy and includes **CBT, individual therapy, group therapy, family therapy,** and **social skills training.** In more severe cases, a **multidisciplinary team** (case manager, nurse, and physician) is often needed to prevent hospitalization.
- "Potency" in typical antipsychotics refers to their potency in binding to the D_2 dopamine receptor—the higher the potency, the greater the likelihood of extrapyramidal symptoms. Atypical antipsychotics (also called SGAs) have fewer extrapyramidal symptoms. There is no fundamental difference in efficacy. Table 14.4 compares typical and atypical antipsychotics by side effects and toxicity.
- All antipsychotic medications have risk of sedation, sexual dysfunction, postural hypotension, cardiac arrhythmias, and sudden cardiac death. Avoid combining with other medications that prolong the QT interval.
- Aripiprazole and ziprasidone have the least effect on weight gain of all the atypical antipsychotics. Weight gain is the worst with clozapine and olanzapine.
- Clozapine is most effective for treatment-resistant psychosis.

Complications

- Without treatment, patients with schizophrenia may experience "**downward drift**" in socioeconomic class and deterioration in family and peer relationships.
- **Tardive dyskinesia** (involuntary movements of the tongue, lips, face, trunk, and extremities) can be caused by long-term treatment with typical antipsychotics such as haloperidol. This complication can be minimized through use of atypical antipsychotics or by adding benztropine concurrently with typical antipsychotic medication.

PSYCHOSIS IN CHILDREN

Prepubertal onset of schizophrenia is extremely rare. Psychosis can occur among children with major depression or mania.

- **Differential diagnoses to consider:** Substance intoxication, medical conditions such as SLE, thyrotoxicosis, and temporal lobe epilepsy, as well as auditory and visual hallucinations can occur in nonpsychotic children under extreme stress.

TABLE 14.4.   **Typical and Atypical Antipsychotics and Side Effects**

CLASS/POTENCY	DRUG	SIDE EFFECTS	MEDICALLY SERIOUS SIDE EFFECTS
Typical, high-potency antipsychotics	Haloperidol (Haldol), fluphenazine (Prolixin)	Sedation, akathisia	Acute dystonic reactions, neuroleptic malignant syndrome, tardive dyskinesia (in long-term use)
Typical, midpotency antipsychotics	Thioridazine (Mellaril), chlorpromazine (Thorazine)	Sedation, anticholinergic side effects (dry mouth, constipation, urinary retention, tachycardia)	Acute dystonic reactions, neuroleptic malignant syndrome, tardive dyskinesia (in long-term use), prolonged QT interval
Typical, low-potency antipsychotics	Thiothixene (Navane), perphenazine (Trilafon), trifluoperazine (Stelazine)	Orthostatic hypotension and other anticholinergic effects, sedation, hyperlipidemia	Acute dystonic reactions, neuroleptic malignant syndrome, tardive dyskinesia (in long-term use)
Atypical antipsychotics (SGAs)	Olanzapine (Zyprexa) Risperidone (Risperdal) Quetiapine (Seroquel) Clozapine (Clozaril) Aripiprazole (Abilify) Ziprasidone (Geodon)	Weight gain, sedation, anticholinergic at high doses, hyperlipidemia / Weight gain, hyperprolactinemia / Weight gain, sedation, anticholinergic at high doses, hyperlipidemia / Drooling, sedation, anticholinergic effects, hyperlipidemia / Fewest side effects, though has the typical ones. / Hyperprolactinemia	Diabetes mellitus Side effects of typical antipsychotics (when used in high doses) Cataracts Agranulocytosis Prolonged QT interval

- **Treatment** should be under the care of a child psychiatrist, as antipsychotics are indicated. Children seem to have a weaker response to antipsychotics than adolescents and adults. Family support and education, as well as the proper educational setting for a child, is crucial to treatment success.

PSYCHOTROPIC MEDICATIONS IN CHILDREN AND ADOLESCENTS

Pharmacokinetics in children and adolescents are different from pharmacokinetics in adults. Children have greater hepatic capacity, ↑ glomerular filtration rate, and less fatty tissue. Half-lives may be shorter.

- **Mood disorders:** SSRIs have generally been found to be safe in children and adolescents, with the precaution of black-box warnings regarding ↑ risk of suicide. Fluoxetine has been shown to have the most favorable risk-to-benefit ratio in children and adolescents. The risks and benefits of both treating and not treating psychiatric disorders must be fully explained to children/teens and their caregivers. Manic episodes are treated as they are among adults.
- **OCD and anxiety disorders:** SSRIs are first-line treatments; buspirone and long-acting benzodiazepines can also be used.
- **Psychosis and schizophrenia:** The best-studied medications are chlorpromazine and haloperidol; however, overall, atypical antipsychotics are preferred in children. Risperidone is used for psychosis as well as behavior disorders. Be sure to check BMI, lipids, and fasting blood glucose, and monitor for weight gain.

Substance Abuse Disorders

Substance abuse is the compulsion to use substances despite adverse consequences. **Substance dependence** is physiologic and/or emotional reliance on the substance.

- **Abuse can be present without dependence:** For example, a person who expends significant energy acquiring and using cocaine, with adverse legal, financial, work, and interpersonal consequences, but only uses cocaine sporadically, has substance abuse, but not dependence. Commonly abused substances include the following:
  - **Alcohol:** The prevalence of alcoholism is 4.6% in women and 9.2% in men. Alcohol-related deaths are the **fourth leading cause of preventable deaths** in the United States (with higher prevalence in certain cultures such as Native Americans). While there is no direct genetic link, it is clear that alcoholism tends to run in families and is likely the product of a complex and poorly understood gene-environment interaction. In **men**, "safe" levels of alcohol consumption equal **two drinks per day**; in **women**, "safe" levels of alcohol consumption equal **one drink per day**.
  - **Opiates:** Prescription opioid and heroin abuse has ↑ to epidemic proportions over the last 25 years. **Data from the CDC suggest that rising rates of opioid prescriptions are a driving factor in the 15-year ↑ in opioid overdose deaths.** Results from the 2010 national survey on drug use and health found an estimated 2.1 million Americans had substance use disorders related to prescription opioid pain relievers and an estimated 467,000 were addicted to heroin. The age of onset is generally in the teens, with the death rate among opioid abusers 20 times greater than that in the nonusing population. Improving the way opioids are prescribed is now more emphasized in the United States, with some states having drug prescription monitoring programs.
  - **Stimulants:** There are an estimated 1.5 million people in the United States who are current cocaine users. A higher rate of adults aged 18 to 25 years use cocaine.

Symptoms/Exam

Table 14.5 outlines the presentation and treatment of common substance abuse disorders.
- All patients should be screened for substance abuse disorders. Questions should be asked in a **nonjudgmental** manner and in a **confidential** environment to ensure the most open responses. The **CAGE questionnaire** is an example of a tool used to screen for alcohol abuse disorders.

Diagnosis

- **Substance abuse** requires at least **one** of the following criteria:
  - Continued use in **physically dangerous** situations (eg, drinking and driving).
  - **Legal problems** due to use.
  - Continual **failure to complete important obligations.**
  - Persistent use despite detrimental social or interpersonal impact.
- **Substance dependence** requires **three or more** of the following criteria:
  - Physiologic **tolerance** or **withdrawal.**
  - Persistent desire or unsuccessful **attempts to cut down** or stop using.
  - Use for a **longer amount of time** or in larger amounts than was originally intended.
- **Substance use disorder** includes four main categories of behavior:
  - Impaired control.
  - Social impairment.
  - Risky use.
  - Pharmacologic indicators of tolerance or withdrawal.

KEY FACT

DSM-5 no longer separates "substance abuse" versus "substance dependence" as these disorders occur on a continuum of substance use disorders.

KEY FACT

Substance abuse can be characterized either by brief episodes or by more chronic patterns.

MNEMONIC

CAGE questionnaire for alcohol abuse:

C: Have you ever felt the need to **C**ut down on your drinking?
A: Do you get **A**nnoyed when people talk to you about your drinking?
G: Do you feel **G**uilty or bad about your drinking?
E: Do you ever have an **E**ye opener (a drink first thing in the morning)?

A score of 2 or greater is clinically significant for alcohol abuse.

KEY FACT

The majority of people who abuse alcohol have a comorbid psychiatric disorder.

TABLE 14.5.   **Presentation and Treatment of Substance Abuse Disorders**

DRUG	MEDICAL COMPLICATIONS	WITHDRAWAL SYMPTOMS	TREATMENT

Alcohol	**General:** Cirrhosis, pancreatitis, ataxia, delirium, GI bleed, hepatitis, hypertension, cardiomyopathy, anemia, sexual dysfunction, depression, peripheral neuropathy, memory loss, depression, ↑ risk of cancer (esophageal, stomach, lung, colon)
	In pregnancy: Fetal alcohol syndrome
		Early (8 hours after last drink): Sweating, flushing, sleep disturbances, hallucinations, seizures, mild mental status changes
		Late (48 hours after last drink): DTs (tremor, hallucinations, delirium, ↑ autonomic tone)
			Withdrawal: Benzodiazepines (long-acting, eg, chlordiazepoxide, diazepam)
			Long-term treatment:
			  Naltrexone: ↓ cravings and relapse.
			  Disulfiram: Causes flushing, nausea, and vomiting when mixed with alcohol
			  SSRIs: ↓ cravings

Cocaine	**General:** Hypertension, tachycardia, arrhythmias, vasospasm of coronary arteries (MI) and cerebral arteries (CVA), hemoptysis, chest pain, nasal septum necrosis, dehydration, malnutrition, weight loss **In pregnancy:** Fetal hypoxia and placental abruption	Depressed mood, fatigue, disturbing dreams, ↑ appetite, insomnia or hypersomnia, agitation, or retardation	No specific treatment for withdrawal; no pharmacologic treatments for dependence
Opiates	**IV use:** Endocarditis, HIV, HBV/HCV, cellulitis, abscesses, septic arthritis, osteomyelitis, pneumonia, meningitis, pulmonary emboli, nephrotic syndrome **In pregnancy:** Infant withdrawal	Depressed mood, nausea, vomiting, diarrhea, yawning, insomnia, myalgias, runny nose, watering eyes, dilated pupils, sweating, fever	**Overdose antidote: Naloxone/ Naltrexone** **Withdrawal:** Methadone, clonidine, buprenorphine, clonidine-naltrexone **Long-term treatment:** Methadone maintenance, buprenorphine, naltrexone

- Main activities are **centered on the substance** (eg, intoxication or obtaining drugs).
- **Giving up important activities** for drugs (eg, work).
- **Persistent use,** regardless of the knowledge that continued use can lead to physical or psychological problems.

Management
Before formulating an approach toward substance abuse, it is important for the clinician to use motivational interviewing techniques and understand what **phase of behavioral change** the patient is in. It is also crucial to recognize that substance abuse has a **relapsing and remitting pattern.**
- Pharmacologic treatments: See Table 14.5.
- Nonpharmacologic treatments: **Psychotherapy,** methods include the following:
  - **Therapeutic communities:** Residential treatment centers. Treatment duration is generally 6 to 18 months; communities tend to have strict limits and are highly structured. Associated with high dropout rates, but successful for highly motivated individuals.
  - **Group therapy.**
  - **Individual therapy:** Includes CBT, harm reduction (minimizing negative effects of behaviors), and psychoeducation.

KEY FACT

The stages of behavioral change are precontemplation, contemplation, preparation, action, maintenance, and relapse.

QUESTION

A 55-year-old man has nausea, vomiting, and diarrhea 2 days after he was admitted to your service for cellulitis. He appears feverish and diaphoretic and is yawning repeatedly. Exam reveals no abdominal tenderness, rebound, or guarding. You note that his eyes and nose are watering, and his pupils are unusually dilated. On further questioning, you find that the patient takes oxycodone, which he buys from a friend. What treatment do you give him to relieve his symptoms?

- **Family support/education:** Essential in the treatment of abusers, as family members are strongly affected by negative behaviors. Education (eg, Al-Anon) helps families recognize what to expect and how best to be supportive.
- **Peer support groups:** Self-help organizations such as Alcoholics and Narcotic Anonymous. Such groups tend to focus on relapse prevention and maintenance of sobriety. Users are supported by peer mentors who have maintained abstinence. They may then graduate to peer lead the groups.

SUBSTANCE USE AND ABUSE IN ADOLESCENTS

Use of substances during adolescence may compromise physical, cognitive, and psychosocial aspects of adolescent development and can be a risk factor for substance abuse later in life. Commonly used substances include alcohol, marijuana, opioids, cocaine, amphetamines, sedative-hypnotics, hallucinogens, inhalants, nicotine, anabolic steroids, γ-hydroxybutyrate (GHB), and 3,4-methylenedioxymethamphetamine (ecstasy). When discussing substance use with adolescents, physicians must be aware of state confidentiality laws.

Diagnosis

Clinical history, specific physical examination findings (see Tables 14.6 and 14.7), and a drug screen if drug abuse is suspected.

Management

- Counsel about the dangers of substance use and abuse.
- Family therapy.
- **Smoking:** Nicotine patches, gum.
- **Alcohol:** Recommend participation in Alcoholics Anonymous or Alateen.
- **Illicit drug use:** Recommend drug rehabilitation programs.

Complications

Death and injury (from motor vehicle accidents, other unintentional injuries, homicide, and suicide); physical and sexual abuse; ↑ sexual activity (teen pregnancy, STIs); alterations in mood, sleep, and appetite; frank psychosis indistinguishable from schizophrenia; irreversible cardiomyopathy; noncardiogenic pulmonary edema; pulmonary hypertension; drug overdose with multiorgan system failure.

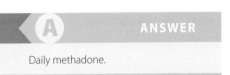

A ANSWER

Daily methadone.

TABLE 14.6.   **Presentation of Substance Use and Abuse**

VARIABLE	PRESENTATION
Physical	Fatigue, insomnia or hypersomnia, runny nose, shortness of breath, injected eyes, pinpoint pupils
Emotional	Personality change, sudden mood changes, irritability, irresponsible behavior, low self-esteem, poor judgment, depression, withdrawal, general lack of interest
Family	Breaking rules or withdrawing from the family, high family conflict, lack of bonding
School	Truancy, academic failure, lack of commitment to school and education, early persistent behavioral problems
Social/behavioral	Peer group involvement with drugs and alcohol, problems with the law

TABLE 14.7.   Physiologic Effects of Common Illicit Substances

SYMPTOM	SUBSTANCE
Eyes/pupils	
Mydriasis	Amphetamines, MDMA or other stimulants, cocaine, jimsonweed, LSD; withdrawal from alcohol or opioids
Miosis	Alcohol, barbiturates, benzodiazepines, opioids, PCP
Nystagmus	Alcohol, barbiturates, benzodiazepines, inhalants, PCP
Conjunctival injection	LSD, marijuana
Lacrimation	Inhalants, LSD; withdrawal from opioids
Cardiovascular	
Tachycardia/hypertension	Amphetamines, MDMA, cocaine, LSD, marijuana, PCP; withdrawal from alcohol, barbiturates, or benzodiazepines
Hypotension	Barbiturates, opioids; withdrawal from depressants. Orthostatic hypotension—marijuana
Arrhythmia	Amphetamines, MDMA, cocaine, inhalants, opioids, PCP
Respiratory	
Depression	Opioids, depressants, GHB
Pulmonary edema	Opioids, stimulants
Core body temperature	
↑	Amphetamines, MDMA, cocaine, PCP; withdrawal from alcohol, barbiturates, benzodiazepines, or opioids
↓	Alcohol, barbiturates, benzodiazepines, opioids, GHB
PNS response	
Hyperreflexia	Amphetamines, MDMA, cocaine, LSD, marijuana, PCP; withdrawal from alcohol or benzodiazepines
Hyporeflexia	Alcohol, benzodiazepines, inhalants, opioids
Tremor	Amphetamines, cocaine, LSD; withdrawal from alcohol, benzodiazepines, or cocaine
Ataxia	Alcohol, amphetamines, MDMA, benzodiazepines, inhalants, LSD, PCP, GHB
CNS response	
Hyperalertness	Amphetamines, MDMA, cocaine
Sedation/somnolence	Alcohol, benzodiazepines, inhalants, marijuana, opioids, GHB
Seizures	Alcohol, amphetamines, MDMA, cocaine, inhalants, opioids; withdrawal from alcohol or benzodiazepines
Hallucinations	Amphetamines, MDMA, cocaine, inhalants, LSD, marijuana, PCP; withdrawal from alcohol or benzodiazepines
Gastrointestinal	
Nausea/vomiting	Alcohol, amphetamines or other stimulants, cocaine, inhalants, LSD, opioids, peyote, GHB; withdrawal from alcohol, benzodiazepines, cocaine, or opioids

SUICIDALITY

Suicide is the third leading cause of mortality among adolescents and the tenth leading cause for the United States. The suicide rate of adolescent boys is four times higher than that of adolescent girls, and white adolescent boys have the highest rate. The incidence of unsuccessful suicide attempts is 10 times higher in adolescent girls than in adolescent boys. Firearms account for the majority of suicide deaths in both sexes. The suicide rate ↑ in the seventh decade of life.

With the normal mood swings of adolescence, short periods of depression are common, and a teenager may have thoughts of suicide. Teens with a same-sex or transgender orientation are at significant risk for suicidal thoughts and suicide attempts. Those who have not "come out" (have not claimed a nonheterosexual identity) are at highest risk. LGBT teens are at higher risk for victimization and bullying, which is also thought to contribute to an ↑ risk of suicidality. Accompanied by an ↑ risk of depression and substance abuse.

Symptoms/Exam

Social withdrawal; symptoms of depression; anger; a history of a previous suicide attempt. For child/adolescents, inability to keep up with schoolwork.

Diagnosis

Determine the extent of the patient's depression and assess the risk of inflicting self-harm. The history should include medical, social, emotional, and academic background. Inquire about the following:

- Common signs of depression.
- Recent stressful events.
- Evidence of long-standing problems in the home, or with peers. For children/adolescents, assess for problems at school.
- Drug or substance use and abuse.
- Signs of psychotic thinking, such as delusions or hallucinations.
- Evidence of marked depression.

Management

- Medical therapy should be aimed at treating medical complications of the suicide attempt.
- Physical protection is needed to avoid harm to self if a plan is in place.
- Provide emergency psychological consultation for any patient who is severely depressed, psychotic, or acutely suicidal.
- Safety contracts are not effective in preventing suicide. Do a thorough suicide assessment for risks and protective factors, as with adults. Remove firearms and potentially lethal medications from the home. Involve family in safety planning.

MNEMONIC

STOPS FIRE for evaluating risk in self-injury:

Suicidal ideation during or before self-injury
Types of self-injury in which the patient engages
Onset of self-injury
Place on the body of injury
Severity of damage caused by self-injury
Functions of the self-injury for the patient
Intensity or frequency of urges to self-harm
Repetition of behavior
Episodic frequency of injury

SELF-INJURIOUS BEHAVIOR

Only 1% to 4% of adults participate in self-injurious behavior; however, approximately 15% of adolescents report some form of self-injury. Behavior includes cutting, skin carving, burning, severe abrading/scratching, or punching/hitting as well as more severe forms of self-injury. Typical age of onset is between 14 and 24 years.

- **Comorbid conditions:** Borderline personality disorder, dissociative disorders, eating disorder, MDD, alcohol dependence.
- **The relationship with suicidality is complex.** Many who self-injure are not suicidal, but as the severity of self-injury increases, the risk of suicide increases. Therefore, it is critical to evaluate self-injury severity.

Management

- Therapeutic alliance is key. Work to develop an understanding of the behavior, including recognition that the self-injurious behavior is serving a function for the patient.
- Motivational interviewing techniques may be helpful. Reflectively listen and validate emotions with a nonjudgmental attitude. It is also important not to be overly concerned, as this may be a reinforcing behavior.
- Pharmacological treatments: Topiramate, clozapine, naltrexone.
- Psychotherapeutic treatments: DBT (most evidence available, though with mixed results), CBT, other therapy techniques with a focus on addressing underlying psychological dysfunction and skill building.

EATING DISORDERS

Teenagers and younger children continue to develop eating disorders at an alarming rate. The spectrum of eating disorders includes **anorexia nervosa, bulimia nervosa, eating disorders not otherwise specified, and binge-eating disorder.** The relationship between biology and environment in the development of eating disorders is complex. Contributing factors appear to include the influence of the media (television, magazines, movies, videos), in which thin young women are often depicted as the norm. Anorexia and bulimia are distinguished as follows:

- **Anorexia nervosa:** Diagnosis requires the following four diagnostic criteria, as defined in the DSM-IV:
  - Refusal to maintain weight within a normal range for height and age (>15% below ideal body weight).
  - Fear of weight gain.
  - Severe body image disturbance (body image is the predominant measure of self-worth, along with denial of the seriousness of the illness).
  - In postmenarchal girls, absence of the menstrual cycle, or amenorrhea (>3 cycles).
- **Bulimia:** Defined as episodic and uncontrolled ingestion of large quantities of food, followed by recurrent inappropriate compensatory behavior to prevent weight gain, such as self-induced vomiting, diuretic or cathartic use, strict dieting, or vigorous exercise.

Symptoms

- **Anorexia:** Amenorrhea, depression, fatigue, weakness, hair loss, bone pain, constipation, abdominal pain.
- **Bulimia:** Normal or near-normal body weight, mouth sores, dental caries, heartburn, muscle cramps and fainting, hair loss, easy bruising, intolerance to cold, menstrual irregularity, abuse of diuretics and laxatives, misuse of diet pills (leading to palpitations and anxiety), frequent vomiting (resulting in throat irritation and pharyngeal trauma).

Exam

- Assess vitals to evaluate for bradycardia, hypotension, or orthostatic hypotension.
- Perform a detailed physical and dental exam, including height, weight, and BMI.
- **Anorexia:** Signs include brittle hair and nails; dry, scaly skin; loss of subcutaneous fat; fine facial and body hair (lanugo hair); and breast and vaginal atrophy.
- **Bulimia:** Signs include a callused finger (Russell sign; results when the finger is used to induce vomiting); dry skin; periodontal disease; and sialadenosis (swelling of the parotid glands).
- Obtain a psychiatric history to assess for substance abuse and mood/anxiety/personality disorders.
- Ask about suicidal ideation.

Diagnosis

- Explore body image, exercise regimen, eating habits, sexual history, current and past medication use, diuretic and laxative use, binging and purging behavior, and substance use.
- Obtain electrolytes, CBC, LFTs, and ECG to evaluate for arrhythmias and electrolyte disturbance.

Management

- The goal of treatment is restoration of normal body weight and eating habits, along with resolution of psychological difficulties.
- **Behavioral therapy:** Intensive psychotherapy and family therapy.

KEY FACT

The commonalities among the eating disorders include disturbance in body image and a drive for thinness.

QUESTION 1

A 17-year-old high school senior is brought by her mother, who is concerned about her daughter's abnormal eating habits. The girl denies that she has a problem, stating that she is just picky with her food and is attempting to become a vegetarian. She has lost 18 pounds over the last 6 months, and her periods have stopped. What is your advice for her anxious mother?

QUESTION 2

A 16-year-old girl comes to your clinic for 2° amenorrhea. She tells you that she feels better than ever after joining her neighborhood gym. The girl is sexually active and uses condoms for contraception. You obtain a urine pregnancy test, which is ⊖. What is the next step in your workup?

- **Pharmacotherapy:** TCAs, SSRIs, lithium carbonate.
- Enteral or parenteral feeding in patients with severe malnutrition.
- Hospitalization as indicated in cases of severe malnutrition or failed outpatient therapy.

Complications

Severe malnutrition, cardiac arrhythmias, suicide attempt, osteopenia, heart failure, dental disease.

FEMALE ATHLETE TRIAD

Many young women engage in exercise to control body weight and improve exercise capacity. The consequences of excessive exercise can include amenorrhea, infertility, and delay of puberty and menarche. The likelihood of amenorrhea varies with the type and amount of exercise as well as with the rapidity of ↑ in exercise. Activities that are associated with low body weight and amenorrhea include running, ballet dancing, and figure skating. Gradual ↑ in exercise is less likely to lead to amenorrhea than acute ↑. Amenorrhea occurs only when there is relative caloric deficiency due to inadequate nutritional intake for the amount of energy expended.

- **Management:** Educate patients on the need for adequate caloric intake to match energy expenditure. Take an interdisciplinary approach with sports coaches, family, school, and school counselors. Estrogen replacement for women with amenorrhea (OCPs). Patients should be encouraged to take 1200 to 1500 mg of calcium daily, along with supplemental vitamin D (400 IU daily).
- **Complications:** Exercise-induced amenorrhea; loss of bone density.

Behavioral Disorders

PERSONALITY DISORDERS

Distinguished by **persistently inadequate adaptive capacities** and patterns of behavior, leading to significant impairment in areas such as social relationships and occupational performance. Disorders start in **early childhood** and persist through adulthood. They are **coded on Axis II.**

Symptoms

Personality disorders are classified into three clusters that share characteristics:
- **Cluster A** (odd and eccentric):
  - Paranoid
  - Schizoid
  - Schizotypal
- **Cluster B** (dramatic, emotional, and erratic):
  - Antisocial
  - Borderline
  - Histrionic
  - Narcissistic
- **Cluster C** (anxious and fearful):
  - Avoidant
  - Dependent
  - Obsessive compulsive

KEY FACT

The "female athlete triad" consists of an eating disorder, amenorrhea, and osteoporosis.

KEY FACT

Personality disorders are classified into three clusters: cluster A ("weird"—odd and eccentric); cluster B ("wild"—dramatic, emotional, and erratic); and cluster C ("wimpy"—anxious and fearful).

A **ANSWER 1**

Interview the girl alone, and look for signs and symptoms of an eating disorder and sexual abuse.

A **ANSWER 2**

Obtain a better history about the type and amount of exercise to determine the cause of amenorrhea.

Differential

- Distinguish from personality changes caused by a medical condition, intellectual disability, and Axis I disorders.
- Personality disorders have an early-childhood onset and possess characteristics not found in Axis I disorders, such as intact reality testing, normal abstracting ability, and the absence of formal thought disorders. They may occur in concert with an Axis I disorder.

Diagnosis

The diagnosis is made after several visits, when the persistent patterns of behavior become apparent.

Management

- Because personality disorders are developed across an individual's life span, patients are often **resistant to treatment** and require a multidisciplinary approach for effective management as opposed to cure.
- **Dialectical behavior therapy,** in group and individual treatment, has the best evidence of efficacy among psychotherapeutic treatments and focuses on learning to manage emotions and reactions. **Psychoanalysis** and psychodynamic psychotherapy may help the patient recognize and change maladaptive behavior patterns.
- Although of limited utility, **pharmacologic treatments** are used in some cases. In **antisocial** and **borderline** personality disorder, mood stabilizers such as lithium and carbamazepine are sometimes used; in **paranoid** and **schizotypal personality disorder,** low-dose **antipsychotics** have been given.

Somatoform Disorders

A group of psychiatric disorders that share the common feature of **overimportance of physical symptoms (with no clear medical etiology)** in a patient's life. This often leads to a feeling of being misunderstood by health providers. Somatization frequently leads to inappropriate workups, hospitalizations, and procedures (up to $30 billion per year) and may cause the patient harm, hence the importance of any appropriate diagnosis and treatment plan.

Symptoms

Generally categorized as follows:

- **Somatization disorder:** A **chronic** disorder characterized by **multiple clinically significant symptoms** (a completely ⊕ ROS: especially GI, sexual, musculoskeletal, and neurological symptoms) that vary over time and are **not explained by medical findings.** Patients usually have an extensive treatment history, with age of onset <30 years of age. Higher prevalence in women.
- **Conversion disorder:** Usually characterized by self-limited symptoms that affect voluntary motor or sensory systems and **suggest a neurologic disorder,** but are **not consistent with anatomic structures.** Age of onset is 10 to 40 years of age. **Preceded by stress or trauma.**
- **Hypochondriasis:** A chronic preoccupation with or **fear of having a serious medical disease** that is not relieved by appropriate evaluation or reassurance. Usually begins in early adulthood.
- **Body dysmorphic disorder:** Chronic preoccupation with **an imagined defect in physical appearance;** usually begins in adolescence. Is **not** the same as an eating disorder.
- **Chronic pain syndrome:** Long-standing **pain without an identified organic cause** is the central feature.

QUESTION 1

A 35-year-old woman presents for an initial visit. Her chart is lengthy, showing multiple primary care providers, numerous ED visits for self-mutilation, and history of alcohol abuse. The woman says she was referred to you by a friend, and throughout the visit she continually praises you, saying that you are not like the other doctors, who were just interested in prescribing pills and making a cut from the drug companies. On further questioning, she reveals that she hasn't had any stable partners because they all were shallow, empty users who didn't care about her. As she talks about herself, you begin to remember complaints about this patient and her inappropriate aggressive behavior in the waiting room. What is the most likely diagnosis?

QUESTION 2

A 22-year-old woman is brought to the office by her mother. She complains of sudden onset of bilateral blindness. She denies any trauma. Her mother states, "I can't believe this is happening. First, her father is dying of cancer, and now this." As the patient moves toward the exam table, you are struck by how easily she avoids all obstacles that lie between her and the table. On exam, you note normal bilateral pupillary responses, and you are surprised that she has none of the expected bruises or scrapes. You order a visual evoked potential, and it comes back normal. What is the most likely explanation for the patient's symptoms?

KEY FACT

Somatoform disorders are motivated by inner psychic gain; symptoms are unintentional or involuntary and are precipitated by stress.

Differential

- **Malingering:** Motivated by external gain (eg, drug seeking, insurance fraud); symptoms are intentional, with poor cooperation in evaluation.
- **Factitious disorder (Munchausen syndrome):** Motivated by assumption of the sick role, in which symptoms are fabricated or self-inflicted. Histories are often vague, and patients go from hospital to hospital seeking care.

Diagnosis

A careful assessment and evaluation should be performed using standard medical workups, with an emphasis on avoiding exhaustive and unnecessary testing.

Management

- Stress empathy, along with the importance of establishing and maintaining a strong primary care relationship. Schedule routine, frequent visits to ↓ "emergency" visits and calls.
- Avoid categorizing the diagnosis as mental or physical; address in "stress" terms or emphasize the mind-body connection.
- Comorbid psychiatric disorders should be addressed and treated.
- Consider a psychiatry/behavioral health referral to provide a framework for treatment (not to take the place of the primary care provider).
- Individual, couple or group therapy may be of benefit, as may stress identification and reduction.
- Prevent iatrogenesis by limiting workup and treatments to objective findings (not complaints).

ANSWER 1

Borderline personality disorder.

Mind-Body Syndromes

CHRONIC FATIGUE SYNDROME

Etiology is unknown, although an infectious source is suspected. Many report sudden onset of symptoms after a severe flulike illness or infectious mononucleosis. All potential endocrine, neurological, infectious, and psychiatric disorders must be ruled out. Childhood trauma or physical inactivity ↑ risk for CFS in adults.

Diagnosis

Diagnosis is made by observation of severe unexplained fatigue for at least 6 months that is not resolved by rest and is functionally impairing, plus four or more of the following criteria:

- Impaired memory or concentration.
- Sore throat.
- Tender or enlarged lymph nodes.
- Muscle pain and arthralgias.
- Headache.
- Sleep disturbance.
- Postexertional malaise.
- Causes at least a 50% reduction in activities.

Management

Similar to somatoform disorders as well as other supportive treatments. Do not continue treatment indefinitely without evidence of clinical response. The only beneficial interventions in CFS are CBT and graded exercise therapy (ie, home exercise program).

KEY FACT

While mind-body syndromes like chronic fatigue and fibromyalgia don't have a clearly agreed-upon etiology or pathology, they require a multidisciplinary approach and are clearly exacerbated by stress and emotional pain.

ANSWER 2

Conversion disorder.

Therapeutic Drugs in Psychiatry

DRUG-DRUG INTERACTIONS

Table 14.8 shows psychotropic drugs that can potentially interact with other medications.

Abuse and Violence

FAMILY AND INTIMATE PARTNER VIOLENCE

Affects individuals from all socioeconomic and cultural backgrounds and all family structures, including same-sex relationships, and is vastly underreported by victims and overlooked by physicians. Victims are more commonly women. Children of abused parents are at ↑ risk for abuse or neglect. Additional risk factors include marital/couple stress or instability, alcohol or drug abuse, social stressors (eg, unemployment, poverty), and a family history of violence. **The highest risk of injury or death occurs during the time and after the victim leaves the perpetrator.**

Symptoms

- Although there is insufficient evidence of the benefit of **universal screening**, experts recommend screening all women during prenatal and routine well-care visits. The incidence of domestic violence increases during pregnancy and postpartum.
- In the outpatient setting, abuse may present as vague, recurrent somatic complaints, depressive symptoms, or ↑ use of medical services.
- Physical abuse is often preceded or accompanied by psychological abuse (insulting, controlling financial and social life, denying of basic needs) and/or sexual abuse.
- Use the patient's own words when documenting symptoms. Document name of abuser, type of violence (emotional, physical, verbal, or sexual), and if weapons are used.

KEY FACT

Serotonin syndrome is a rare but sometimes fatal syndrome that presents as nausea, hyperthermia, hyperreflexia, agitation, autonomic dysfunction, muscle rigidity, delirium, and coma.

MNEMONIC

Questions for detecting domestic violence:

SAFE

Stress/**S**afety?
Afraid/**A**bused?
Friends/**F**amily aware?
Emergency plan?

TABLE 14.8. **Psychotropic Drug Interactions**

DRUG	LEVEL RAISED BY	LEVEL LOWERED BY	OTHER INTERACTIONS
Lithium	Thiazides, ACEI, NSAIDs, metronidazole	Theophylline, anything causing urinary alkalinization (NaHCO₃)	Can cause neurotoxicity (rare): Antipsychotics, carbamazepine, methyldopa, calcium channel blockers Can cause serotonin syndrome (rare): SSRIs, TCAs
Valproic acid	ASA, erythromycin, ibuprofen	Phenobarbital, phenytoin, carbamazepine	↓ efficacy of AZT, warfarin, benzodiazepines
Carbamazepine	Valproic acid, antifungals, calcium channel blockers, INH, protease inhibitors, grapefruit juice	Phenytoin, phenobarbital	↓ efficacy of warfarin, benzodiazepines, many AEDs, antidepressants, OCPs
SSRIs	↑ risk of serotonin syndrome with MAOIs, lithium, other serotonergic agents		

Exam

- Look for patterns of injuries, such as bruises in various stages of healing.
- If physical signs of abuse are present, document them in detail and take identifying photographs.

Differential

Bleeding disorder; affective, anxiety, and somatoform disorders.

Management

- Validate the patient's right to be free from abuse (eg, "You don't deserve to be hurt like this") and offer support.
- Recognize that abuse often occurs in repeated cycles: escalating tension leads to violence leading to remorse and reconciliation (honeymoon period). Do not expect victims to leave right away, and avoid blaming or giving up on them if they return to the abuser.
- Help the patient establish a safety plan.
- If you suspect that children are being harmed or neglected, report to Child Protective Services.
- Psychotherapy.
- Know your state's laws with respect to reporting requirements for suspected abuse.

Complications

Learned helplessness, low self-esteem, depression, anxiety, substance use disorders, and PTSD; physical injury and disability; exacerbation of chronic medical conditions; death by suicide or homicide.

KEY FACT

Pregnancy and attempted separation are especially high-risk times for abuse victims.

SEXUAL VIOLENCE

Any actual or attempted sexual contact that is against the victim's will or that occurs when the victim is unable to consent because of age, disability, or impairment. At least 1 in 3 women and 1 in 33 men have been victims of rape or attempted rape. More than half of lifetime rapes occur before age 18. Certain groups are more vulnerable, including adolescents, survivors of childhood sexual or physical abuse, disabled persons, persons with risky alcohol and substance use, and sex workers.

Symptoms

- Patients who present acutely after sexual assault may have symptoms of trauma that are physical (**bruises, broken bones**), sexual (**genital lacerations, abrasions, bruises**), and/or psychological (**feeling fearful, withdrawn, angry**).
- Patients with a past or ongoing history of sexual violence may have symptoms of psychological sequelae such as **depression** or **PTSD**, or they may present with chronic somatic complaints such as **headache, nausea,** or **fatigue.**

Exam

- After an acute sexual assault, care should be taken to conduct the exam in a way that allows for adequate collection of forensic evidence and avoids retraumatizing the victim. If available, call on a certified sexual assault nurse examiner or a rape victim's advocate.
- Document all signs of trauma and abuse.
- Patients with a past or ongoing history of sexual violence may experience added fear and anxiety with the routine physical (especially pelvic) exam. Limit invasive exams to those absolutely necessary, and offer to have a support person present.

KEY FACT

Emergency contraception is the standard of care for young women capable of becoming pregnant at the time they are raped. The sooner they get it, the more effective it will be at preventing pregnancy.

Diagnosis

- All patients with suggestive signs or symptoms (physical or psychological) should be asked about their exposure to sexual violence.
- All victims of sexual assault should be offered testing for STIs (including oropharyngeal and anal sites if applicable) and pregnancy.

Management

- In the setting of acute assault, if clinically applicable, make sure to offer **emergency contraception** to prevent pregnancy, **postexposure HIV prophylaxis and HBV vaccination,** and **empiric STI treatment.**
- Compassion and advocacy throughout the clinical encounter tell victims that you are there to help. An independent victim's advocate, if available, should be provided.
- Work with law enforcement when applicable.
- Offer acute and ongoing psychological counseling.

Complications

Undesired pregnancy; STIs; depression, anxiety, eating disorders, PTSD, and substance abuse; chronic headaches, sleep disturbance, and GI complaints; suicidal behavior.

MANDATORY REPORTING OF ABUSE

It is essential that physicians understand the role they play in recognizing and reporting abuse of any kind. Guidelines are as follows:
- **Child abuse:** Mandatory reporting laws exist for all suspected cases of child abuse or neglect, and physicians are required to report all such cases.
- **Domestic violence:** Reporting laws regarding domestic violence vary from state to state, with few states requiring reporting. Nonetheless, domestic violence should by no means be considered a "private matter," and physicians must screen for it in primary care visits. In this context, physicians should not judge their success on the basis of whether a patient leaves his or her partner, but they should let victims know that the abuse is not their fault; that they do not merit such treatment; and that the violence they are confronting is unacceptable.
- Pregnancy is a known period of heightened risk for domestic violence.
- **Who and when to screen:** As part of a routine health history; with every new intimate relationship; all young women >14 years of age; with each pregnancy. Some questions to ask on the topic of abuse, suggested by the Family Violence Prevention Fund: Do you feel controlled or isolated by your partner? Do you ever feel afraid of your partner?
- **Elder abuse:** Approximately 1 to 2 million older Americans are victims of abuse or neglect by their primary caregivers. Physicians are **mandatory reporters** of elder abuse and neglect.
- Don't forget to ask your adolescent patients about gang violence or bullying and their sense of safety in school and in their neighborhoods.

The Patient-Physician Relationship

COMMUNICATION

Good communication is key to strong patient-physician relationships. A good relationship with your patients leads to **higher adherence** and **greater patient satisfaction**

KEY FACT

Sexual abuse in any age female patient has a lifelong association with functional GI disorder.

KEY FACT

One in seven women is a victim of domestic violence.

MNEMONIC

Guidelines for domestic violence surveillance:

RADAR

Remember to ask about partner violence
Ask directly about violence
Document information in the patient's chart
Assess the patient's safety
Refer the patient to outside resources (eg, legal services, support groups, shelters)

(not to mention ↓ **likelihood of litigation!**). Components of effective communication:

- **Make eye contact** and a brief personal connection at the beginning.
- **Avoid interrupting the patient** while keeping patients on track.
- Do not appear rushed. Sit down with the patient.
- **Manage expectations** by asking patients about their expectations.
- **Empower patients** to ask questions and make decisions about their own medical care.
- **Respect confidentiality:** Do not disclose information to family members who may also be under your care (especially important to remember with adolescent patients).
- **Provide information:** Summarize the plan, review medication dosages, use patient handouts. **Assess literacy level** before providing written materials.
- Don't talk excessively (or at all) about yourself—the encounter is about the patient!
- Be attentive to nonverbal forms of communication.

CULTURAL COMPETENCE

It may not be realistic for physicians to be familiar with all of their patients' cultural backgrounds; however, it is important for clinicians to understand how culture affects the patient-physician relationship and hence treatment outcomes. Above all, you must take care **not to apply stereotypes** or prejudices to patients whose gender, race, ethnicity, sexual orientation, or culture may differ from your own. It is important to be knowledgeable about cultural issues prevalent in populations in your community. Be aware of your own feelings, biases, and prejudices as you interact with patients.

Techniques to **minimize cultural misunderstandings** include the following:

- Be respectful (address all patients as Ms. or Mr.).
- Where feasible, use competent interpreters who are not only bilingual but also bicultural.
- Spend more time with the patient if needed.
- Ask patients to explain what the symptom or illness means to them and how it might be treated in their culture.
- Anticipate that patients may have had negative interactions with the medical system in the past.
- Review treatment plans carefully and have patients demonstrate an understanding of these plans.
- Be nonjudgmental and accepting of patients' cultural differences.
- Work to create a culture of safety for transgender patients by respecting the pronoun and name they choose to use. When possible, use patient forms that have options for "partnered" as well as married or single. Do not make assumptions about the gender of a patient's sexual partner(s).

KEY FACT

An exception to the requirement for confidentiality occurs when physicians feel that patients may be at risk of hurting themselves or others.

KEY FACT

Harm reduction is a method by which physicians seek a middle ground between what they feel is best and what the patient wants. This method helps the patients modify behaviors to ↓ self-harm (eg, ↓ smoking vs smoking cessation; using clean needles vs quitting heroin). The physician must **understand and respect** the patient's wishes, as such understanding will foster a stronger relationship and ↑ the likelihood of adherence.

Geriatric Medicine

Mary Bonnet, MD

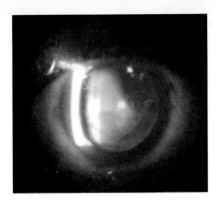

FIGURE 15.1. **Cortical cataract.** Slit-lamp photograph of a 69-year-old man's left eye shows nuclear and cortical changes to the lens consistent with a cataract. The patient had a 2-year history of ↓ visual acuity. (Reproduced with permission from USMLE-Rx.com.)

Sensory Disorders

CATARACTS

Opacity of the lens that ↓ visual acuity. Caused by oxidative damage to the lens, leading to ↑ deposition of insoluble proteins in otherwise transparent tissue (Figure 15.1). Risk factors include smoking, diabetes, and corticosteroid therapy.

- **Symptoms/Exam:** Presents with painless blurred vision (Figure 15.2). Symptoms are progressive, developing over months or years. Lens opacities can be grossly visible or seen as a diminished red reflex.
- **Diagnosis:** Slit-lamp biomicroscopy during ophthalmologic exam (see Figure 15.1).
- **Management:** Decision to treat is based on the degree of functional impairment imposed by the cataracts. Surgery consists of removal of the cataract and placement of an intraocular lens; improves visual acuity in 95% of cases.

GLAUCOMA

A group of disorders characterized by ↑ intraocular pressure, leading to irreversible damage to the optic nerve.

Open-Angle Glaucoma

↑ intraocular pressure due to abnormal aqueous drainage through the trabecular meshwork of the eye (Figures 15.3 and 15.4). The **most common form of glaucoma,** accounting for >90% of cases. Prevalence is ↑ in first-degree relatives of affected individuals and in persons with diabetes. May also develop after uveitis or trauma. Risk factors include age >65 years, ⊕ family history of glaucoma, black ancestry, and diabetes.

Symptoms

- Insidious onset; patients are often asymptomatic until vision is seriously compromised; **painless.**
- Characterized by **bilateral peripheral vision loss,** leading to ↑ tunnel vision (Figure 15.5).
- Patients may also complain of "halos around lights."

Diagnosis

- On fundal exam, you will see an anatomically normal or "open" anterior chamber angle and "cupping" (hollowed out appearance) of the optic nerve in the setting of ↑ intraocular pressure (see Figure 15.3).
- Periodic ophthalmologic exams are the best way to diagnose the disease, especially in **high-risk** individuals.

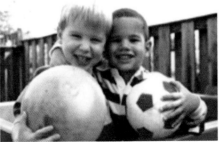

Normal   Cataract

FIGURE 15.2. **Vision with cataract.** (Reproduced from the National Eye Institute.)

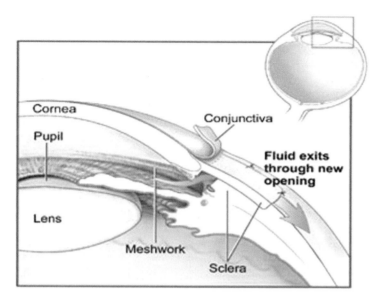

FIGURE 15.3.   **Pathophysiology of open-angle glaucoma.** The fluid leaves the chamber at the open angle where the cornea and iris meet. When the fluid reaches the angle, it flows through a spongy meshwork, like a drain, and leaves the eye. (Reproduced from the National Eye Institute.)

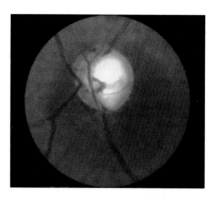

FIGURE 15.4.   **Glaucoma.** Color fundus photograph of a 65-year-old man's left eye shows a left optic nerve with glaucomatous cupping and peripapillary atrophy. The patient had elevated intraocular pressure. (Reproduced with permission from USMLE-Rx.com.)

Management

- **Avoid** anticholinergics medications that can worsen glaucoma.
- **Medications** (Table 15.1). Combining drops from different classes has been shown to have greater reduction in IOP than monotherapy.
- **Surgical treatments:** Surgical intervention improves aqueous outflow; recommended in patients whose intraocular pressure remains ↑ despite medical therapy.

Acute Angle-Closure Glaucoma

An ophthalmologic emergency due to a closed anterior chamber angle. The only type of glaucoma that is curable. Accounts for approximately 10% of glaucoma cases in the United States. More prevalent among persons of Asian descent.

Symptoms

- Rapid onset; usually **unilateral.**
- Presents with **severe pain** and profound vision loss.
- As intraocular pressure ↑, patients may experience nausea, vomiting, and abdominal pain that may be mistaken for an acute abdomen.

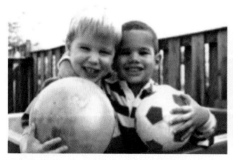
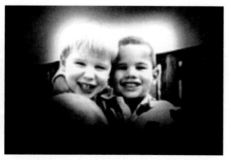

Normal   **Glaucoma**

FIGURE 15.5.   **Vision with glaucoma.** (Reproduced from the National Eye Institute.)

TABLE 15.1. **Antiglaucoma Agents**

MEDICATION CLASS	EXAMPLE	NOTES
β-blockers	Timolol (topical drops)	↓ aqueous production and intraocular pressure May have side effects similar to those of systemic β-blockers
Carbonic anhydrase inhibitors	Acetazolamide (oral) and dorzolamide (topical drops)	↓ aqueous production Topical preparations have largely replaced oral systemic ones Systemic therapy may induce kidney stones or acidosis
Prostaglandin analogs	Bimatoprost (topical drops)	↑ aqueous outflow (generally considered first-line therapy)
Cholinergic agonists	Pilocarpine (topical drops)	↑ aqueous outflow Fewer systemic effects, but ↑ ocular side effects (myopia, fixed pupil) therefore less commonly used
α-adrenergic agonists	Brimonidine (topical drops)	↓ aqueous production and ↑ outflow Use with caution in patients with coronary or cerebrovascular insufficiency

KEY FACT

Don't be tricked by **amaurosis fugax:** painless transient monocular or binocular visual loss; an umbrella term for transient vision loss, includes wide differential.

A **ANSWER 1**

Acute angle-closure glaucoma.

A **ANSWER 2**

Age-related macular degeneration.

Exam

- Exam reveals a red, tender globe that may be firm to touch.
- A steamy or hazy cornea and a nonreactive, dilated pupil may be seen (Figure 15.6).
- Tonometry or palpation of the globe reveals ↑ intraocular pressure.

Differential

Angle-closure glaucoma must be differentiated from acute conjunctivitis, uveitis, and corneal disorders.

Management

- This is a **medical emergency!** You should immediately refer to an ophthalmologist. Delay of treatment can cause irreversible vision loss.
- Immediate reduction of intraocular pressure via IV acetazolamide in conjunction with a topical agent, followed by laser peripheral iridotomy. Usually leads to permanent cure.

AGE-RELATED MACULAR DEGENERATION

Deterioration of the macula, leading to **bilateral central vision loss.** The leading cause of permanent legal blindness in the elderly. May be **atrophic** (dry) or **exudative** (wet); atrophic age-related macular degeneration (AMD) is the **more common** type. Its exact cause is unknown, but risk factors include age >50 years, white race, female gender, ⊕ family history of AMD, and smoking.

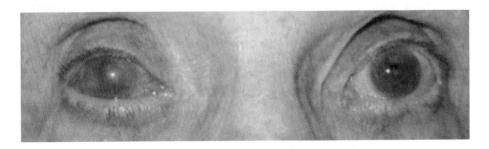

FIGURE 15.6. **Acute angle glaucoma.** The patient awoke with severe right eye pain, headache, ↓ vision, and nausea. Right eye was firm with a pressure of 70 mm Hg. Refractive error was +1.50 to +2.00 sphere in each eye. (Reproduced with permission from USMLE-Rx.com.)

Symptoms/Exam

- Blurred vision is the earliest symptom of atrophic AMD, whereas the perception of straight lines as bent or crooked is the earliest symptom of exudative AMD.
- Reading vision is lost, but peripheral vision is often maintained (eg, patients have difficulty reading but less difficulty driving).
- Small, yellow-white deposits called **drusen** appear underneath the retina (Figure 15.7).

Management

- Limited treatment exists for **atrophic** AMD.
- Antioxidant multivitamins may slow progression in **exudative** AMD.
- Intravitreal injection of VEGF (vascular endothelial growth factor) inhibitors may reduce loss of visual acuity.

KEY FACT

Classic signs and symptoms in retinal detachment are eye flashes, floaters, and a visual field defect.

RETINAL DETACHMENT

Results from separation of the sensory portion of the retina from its pigment epithelium. Most often occurs in people >50 years of age. Risk factors include aging, myopia, cataract surgery, trauma, and a $\oplus$ family history of retinal detachment.

Symptoms/Exam

- Presents with unilateral blurred vision described by patients as a **"curtain coming down"** over the eye.
- Marked by flashes of light and a shower of floaters.
- Exam reveals the retina hanging in the vitreous like a gray cloud.

Diagnosis

Based on an ophthalmoscopic exam in addition to the **clinical triad** of **eye flashes, floaters,** and a **visual field defect.**

Management

You should immediately referral to an ophthalmologist. Treatment is surgical and is directed at closing retinal tears via cryotherapy or laser photocoagulation. Approximately 80% of uncomplicated cases can be cured with a single surgery.

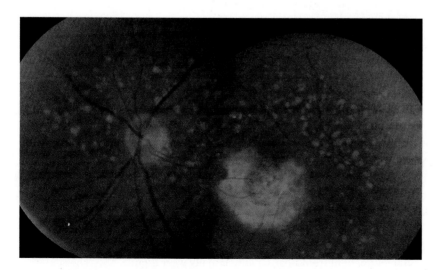

FIGURE 15.7. Macular degeneration. Composite fundoscopic photogram showing drusen (arrow, white spots) associated with atrophy and fibrosis of the macula. (Reproduced with permission from USMLE-Rx.com.)

QUESTION

A new 76-year-old patient arrives in tears. Her companion states that except for minor arthritis pain, she is in excellent health and usually very lively. However, over the last year she has stopped participating in social activities because of her embarrassment at being unable to understand her peers. She often perceives that others are mumbling. What is the most likely diagnosis?

PRESBYOPIA

Natural aging process by which the lens loses its elasticity and therefore ability to accommodate to objects close to eye. Typically begins around age 40 years with difficulty reading and progressively worsens until age 65 years. There is no preventative treatment. Bifocal lenses or reading glasses may be recommended.

HEARING LOSS

Sensorineural Hearing Loss

Caused by disease of the cochlea or the eighth cranial nerve (CN VIII). Affects almost 50% of individuals >75 years of age, making it the most common disability among elderly patients. Timely treatment can help prevent social isolation, depression, and functional dependence on caregivers. Risk factors include older age, noise exposure, and ototoxic medications.

Symptoms/Exam

- Presents with bilateral, gradual, and usually symmetric hearing loss.
- Loss of speech discrimination is experienced in noisy environments; hears "mumbling."
- Patients have ↓ ability to hear high-frequency (>4000-Hz) sounds.
- Otoscopic exam may reveal findings that suggest conductive hearing loss (eg, cerumen impaction) or anomalies of the ear canal or tympanic membrane (eg, otitis media, tumors, tympanosclerosis, perforation).

Differential

Metabolic derangements (eg, diabetes, hypothyroidism, dyslipidemia, renal failure), infections (eg, measles, mumps, syphilis), and radiation therapy are less common but potentially reversible causes of sensory hearing loss.

Diagnosis

Although not sufficient for diagnosis, tuning fork tests (Figure 15.8) can be useful in differentiating conductive from sensorineural hearing losses:
- **Weber test:** A vibrating tuning fork is placed on the forehead.
    - Sensorineural losses: Sound radiates to the better-hearing ear.
    - Conductive losses: Sound appears louder in the poorer-hearing ear.
- **Rinne test:** A vibrating tuning fork is placed alternately on the mastoid bone and in front of the ear canal.
    - Sensorineural losses: Air conduction (AC) exceeds bone conduction (BC) (ie, AC > BC); louder in front of ear, which is normal.
    - Conductive losses: The opposite is true (ie, BC > AC); louder on bone.
- Audiometry is a standardized tool for recording hearing thresholds at different frequencies (see Table 15.2 and Figure 15.9). Frequencies **most important** for human speech are in the 250- to 6000-Hz range.
- You may consider an MRA if the patient is experiencing hearing loss accompanied by pulsatile tinnitus to differentiate carotid vaso-occlusive disease, aneurysm, AVM, or paraganglioma.

Management

- **Hearing aids:** The 1° treatment for presbycusis; however, <50% of elderly patients who might benefit from hearing aids actually wear them.
    - **Behind-the-ear aids:** The most powerful ear-level units; easier to see and manipulate.
    - **In-the-canal aids:** Smaller and more expensive; the best choice for patients with mild to moderate hearing loss.

KEY FACT

Sensorineural hearing loss is the most common type of hearing loss in elderly persons.

ANSWER

Sensorineural hearing loss.

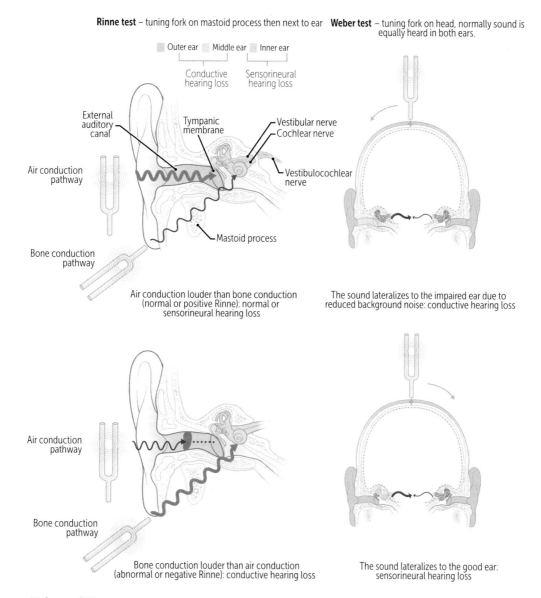

Rinne test – tuning fork on mastoid process then next to ear   Weber test – tuning fork on head, normally sound is equally heard in both ears.

Outer ear   Middle ear   Inner ear

Conductive hearing loss   Sensorineural hearing loss

External auditory canal

Tympanic membrane

Vestibular nerve
Cochlear nerve
Vestibulocochlear nerve

Air conduction pathway

Bone conduction pathway

Mastoid process

Air conduction louder than bone conduction (normal or positive Rinne): normal or sensorineural hearing loss

The sound lateralizes to the impaired ear due to reduced background noise: conductive hearing loss

Air conduction pathway

Bone conduction pathway

Bone conduction louder than air conduction (abnormal or negative Rinne): conductive hearing loss

The sound lateralizes to the good ear: sensorineural hearing loss

FIGURE 15.8.   Weber and Rinne tests. (Reproduced with permission from USMLE-Rx.com.)

- **Aural rehabilitation:** Most patients benefit from this treatment, which includes practical advice on how to optimize communication.

Conductive Hearing Loss

Hearing loss that occurs when sound is not conducted efficiently through the ear canal, tympanic membrane, or ossicles of the middle ear. This type of hearing loss can often be medically or surgically corrected.

Symptoms/Exam

- May present with painless sudden or gradual loss of hearing.
- Exam may reveal **obstruction** (eg, cerumen impaction), middle ear effusion, otosclerosis, and ossicular disruption.

TABLE 15.2. **General Guidelines for the Interpretation of Audiometric Findings**

DECIBEL MEASURE	AUDIOMETRIC FINDING
0-25 dB	Hearing within normal limits
26-50 dB	Mild hearing loss
	Patients will have trouble with soft sounds, with background noise, and when at a distance from the source of the sound
51-70 dB	Moderate hearing loss
	Patients will have significant difficulties with normal conversational-level speech and will rely on visual cues
71-90 dB	Severe hearing loss
	Patients cannot hear conversational speech and miss all speech sounds; however, they can hear environmental sounds, such as dogs barking and loud music
91+ dB	Profound hearing loss
	Patients can hear only loud environmental sounds, such as jackhammers, airplane engines, and firecrackers

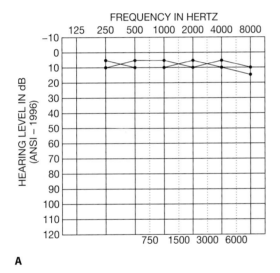

A

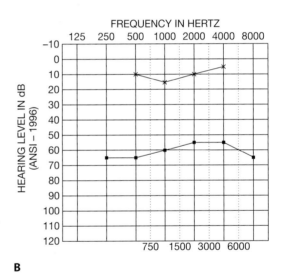

B

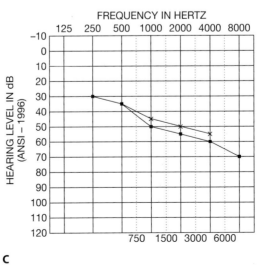

C

FIGURE 15.9. **Common audiograms.** Examples of audiograms: (**A**) Normal audiogram. (**B**) Conductive hearing loss. (**C**) Sensorineural hearing loss. *= bone conduction. ■ = air conduction. (Reproduced with permission from Lalwani A, et al. *Current Otolaryngology—Head and Neck Surgery*, 1st ed. New York: McGraw-Hill, 2004: Figure 44-2.)

Diagnosis

- Weber and Rinne tests may help differentiate conductive from sensorineural hearing loss (see above).
- Audiometry.

Management

Treatment is geared toward correcting the underlying cause.

Dementia

Acquired and significant impairment of memory or another cognitive domain that **interferes with activities of daily living.**

Other cognitive domains:
- Aphasia: Loss of the ability to understand and/or produce language.
- Apraxia: Difficulty with carrying out learned actions or movements in the absence of motor or sensory impairment.
- Agnosia: Failure to recognize or identify objects despite intact sensory function.
- Impaired executive function: Includes the abilities to initiate, monitor, plan, and organize behaviors.

KEY FACT

Dementia is not an inherent aspect of aging.

Types of dementias:
- **Alzheimer disease (AD):**
  - Accounts for 66% of dementia cases; affects 6% to 8% of individuals ≥65 years of age and 30% of those ≥85 years of age.
  - The two greatest risk factors for AD are advanced age and ⊕ **family history** of AD.
- **Vascular dementia:**
  - Accounts for 15% to 25% of dementia cases.
  - Common risk factors for vascular dementia include hypertension, hyperlipidemia, diabetes mellitus, smoking, advanced age, and male sex.
- **Other (less common) dementias:**
  - Lewy body dementia: Cognitive fluctuations, visual hallucinations, **parkinsonism features,** neuroleptic sensitivity, becoming more prevalent.
  - Frontotemporal dementia: **Personality** and social behavior changes, nonfluent speech.
  - Neurodegenerative conditions, such as Huntington disease, and metabolic abnormalities.
  - Chronic traumatic encephalopathy (dementia pugilistica), ↑ evidence for early-onset dementia in setting of contact sports (boxers, football) and motor vehicle accidents: personality changes, depression, suicidality.

KEY FACT

If initial symptom is memory loss of recent events/names, think Alzheimer; if initial symptom is impaired judgment/ability to make decisions, think vascular; if initial symptom is sleep disturbance/visual hallucinations, think Lewy body.

Symptoms/Exam

Presents with **gradual, progressive memory loss** (may be stepwise, with periods of plateaus in vascular dementia). Other common features include:
- Word-finding and concentration problems.
- Emotional lability, personality changes, social withdrawal.
- Difficulties with dressing, cooking, balancing checkbook, maintaining hygiene.
- Visuospatial disturbances.

Diagnosis

- Complete history and physical; assess for mood disorders.
- Brief quantitative screening tests of cognitive function, such as the Montreal Cognitive Assessment (**MOCA**) **or the Mini Mental Status Exam (MSSE) and clock**

QUESTION

A 78-year-old woman is brought by her son who has noticed changes in her behavior over the last several months. He says she has gotten lost while driving in her neighborhood. Some days she seems normal; other days, she is confused, unable to hold a conversation, and easily agitated. Recently, she started seeing small animals that no one else sees. You note a shuffling gate and slowed speech; no resting tremor. She can recall one of three objects on mental status exam and has great difficulty with clock drawing. What is the most likely diagnosis?

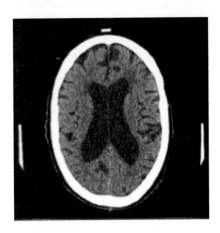

FIGURE 15.10. **Normal pressure hydrocephalus.** Head CT of a 60-year-old woman with slowly developing urinary incontinence, gait instability, and dementia shows dilatation of the lateral ventricles out of proportion to the level of diffuse brain atrophy. (Reproduced with permission from USMLE-Rx.com.)

KEY FACT

Remember: The classic presentation of normal pressure hydrocephalus is *wobbly*, *wet*, and *wacky*—gait apraxia, urinary incontinence, and dementia.

ANSWER

Lewy body dementia.

KEY FACT

Common misdiagnoses of delirium include schizophrenia, depression, dementia, and anxiety.

drawing, may be useful and provide a baseline for future comparison. Accuracy depends on age and educational background.

- **Labs:** CBC, glucose, metabolic panel, albumin, LFTs, TSH, vitamin B_{12}, UA. Consider syphilis screen if patient is at risk for 3° syphilis.
- **Imaging:** Routine brain imaging is controversial. If obtained, noncontrast CT is usually adequate and can help identify subdural hematomas, hydrocephalus (Figure 15.10).

Management

- Discontinue nonessential medications, especially sedatives, hypnotics, and anticholinergics.
- Identify and treat coexisting depression, malnutrition, thyroid dysfunction, occult infections.
- Evaluate for home safety and minimize social isolation; consider screening for caregiver stress.
- **Medications:**
  - Cholinesterase inhibitors may modestly slow decline in function and improve cognition in patients with mild to moderate AD and may also be useful in other types of dementia.
  - NMDA **(N-methyl-D-aspartic acid)** antagonists (eg, memantine, amantadine) may provide modest benefit to patients with moderate to severe AD.
  - Behavioral symptoms of dementia, such as paranoia, agitation, and irritability, are best managed by nonpharmacological strategies such as reducing overstimulation.

Delirium

Acute changes in mental status, marked by inattention, poor concentration, and **fluctuating** levels of consciousness. Commonly occurs in hospitalized elderly patients and very common in ICU setting; one-third of patients >70 years of age admitted to a general medical facility experience delirium.

Symptoms/Exam

- ↓ ability to focus, sustain, or shift attention.
- Rapid onset, fluctuating course.
- Rambling, irrelevant, or incoherent speech.
- Confusion.
- May have ↑ or ↓ level of arousal.
- **Hyperactive delirium:** Agitation prominent, may be mistaken for anxiety.
- **Hypoactive delirium:** Psychomotor activity is slowed. More common! Worse prognosis.

Diagnosis

- **Obtain a thorough history** from individuals close to the patient to determine the frequency and duration of mental status changes. Get a baseline mental status. Ask about alcohol, prescription and illicit drug use, as withdrawal can precipitate delirium.
- **Review medications.** Steroids, benzodiazepines, hypnotics, anticholinergics, quinolones, and TCAs are common causes of delirium.
- Review complete physical exam, with assessment of vital signs and O_2 saturation.
- **Labs:** CBC, serum glucose and electrolytes, UA. Consider blood cultures and arterial blood gas levels.

- **Additional tests:** ECG and CXR may reveal cardiac or pulmonary causes of delirium. LP may also be considered to rule out infections of the central nervous system.
- **Imaging:** Head CT may be indicated for high-risk patients (eg, those with head trauma or focal neurologic findings) or when etiology cannot be established.

Management

- Identify and treat underlying causes.
- Minimize physical and chemical restraints as much as possible.
- Encourage consistent presence of family or caregivers familiar to the patient, as well as clocks, calendars, and encourage exposure to daylight by opening blinds to help with orientation.
- Encourage patients to wear eyeglasses and hearing aids, if indicated.
- Target medications for delirium to specific behaviors (eg, physical aggression, distressing hallucinations) only after nonpharmacologic measures have been attempted.
- Low-dose antipsychotics such as haloperidol are preferred in hyperactive delirium. Use the minimal dose necessary.
- Benzodiazepines are last-line therapy, as they may worsen delirium. Preferred for patients with Parkinsonian features.
- May take weeks or months to fully resolve.

Parkinsonism

A syndrome characterized by **resting tremor, bradykinesia, muscular rigidity,** and **loss of postural reflexes.** A common disorder in patients >60 years of age; affects both sexes and all racial groups. Results from the depletion of dopamine in the **substantia nigra,** leading to unopposed cholinergic activity.

Parkinsonism may be due to Parkinson disease or other neurodegenerative disorders (Table 15.3) or 2° to drugs, small vessel disease of the brain, trauma, or metabolic disturbances.

TABLE 15.3.   Clinical Features of Parkinson-Plus Syndromes

SYNDROME	KEY FEATURES
Dementia with Lewy bodies	Cognitive decline, **visual hallucinations,** misidentification of family/friends, marked **daily fluctuations** in mental status
Progressive supranuclear palsy	Cognitive decline
	Extraocular abnormalities, especially **vertical gaze**
	Prominent **rigidity** of the entire body, leading to frequent **falls** and a characteristic **facial appearance** ("wide-eyed" scared expression)
Corticobasal degeneration	Cognitive decline, **"alien limb"** phenomenon; **limb apraxia;** inability to perform learned motor tasks (eg, brush teeth, salute)
Multiple system atrophy	Encompasses a group of Parkinson-plus syndromes (Shy-Drager syndrome, olivopontocerebellar atrophy, striatonigral degeneration)
	Autonomic dysfunction, especially orthostatic hypotension
	Ataxia; in coordination with mild parkinsonism
	Isolated parkinsonism; no tremor; **no response to levodopa**
Parkinsonism-dementia-amyotrophic lateral sclerosis complex	High prevalence in Guam
	TRAP symptoms, dementia, progressive paralysis
	Cause unknown, treat symptoms

KEY FACT

Patients with delirium during hospitalization have longer stays, higher mortality rates, and ↑ risk for deconditioning, pressure ulcers, atelectasis, and malnutrition.

MNEMONIC

Parkinsonism symptoms:

TRAP

Tremor
Rigidity
Akinesia/bradykinesia
Postural instability

Symptoms/Exam

- Presents with resting tremor or "pill rolling" that is **less severe during voluntary movement.**
- Bradykinesia commonly manifests as ↓ arm swing while walking.
- Rigidity is evident during passive movement of limbs (eg, "cogwheeling").
- Shuffling gait and impaired postural reflexes are seen.
- Masklike facial expressions are seen, with ↓ frequency of eye blinking.
- Seborrhea of the scalp and face is common.

Diagnosis

Clinical: Based on symptoms and neurologic exam.

Management

- Discontinue drugs that can worsen parkinsonism (eg, antipsychotics, metoclopramide).
- Regular exercise and physical therapy may aid with balance; occupational therapy may help patients use adaptive strategies and equipment to carry out activities of daily living.
- **Medications:**
    - **Levodopa/carbidopa:** First-line treatment that has been shown to improve all major features of parkinsonism. Levodopa, a precursor of dopamine, is administered with carbidopa, a decarboxylase inhibitor that inhibits peripheral conversion of dopamine, thereby reducing the amount of levodopa required for treatment while lowering the risk of side effects.
    - **Monoamine oxidase inhibitors:** Selegiline may be used as an adjunct to levodopa by inhibiting the degradation of levodopa; sometimes used to improve declining response to levodopa.
    - **Dopamine agonists:** Pramipexole and ropinirole may be considered for initial monotherapy in mild disease to delay the use of levodopa and appearance of levodopa-related dyskinesias and motor fluctuations.
    - **Amantadine:** An antiviral medication that may be used to treat dyskinesias in patients with advanced disease.
    - **Anitcholinergics:** Useful for tremor in younger patients; avoid in elderly patients due to potential adverse effects on cognition.
- **Surgical measures:** Patients who become unresponsive to medical treatment or have intolerable side effects may be helped by brain stimulators or thalamotomy or pallidotomy.

MNEMONIC

Causes of reversible urinary incontinence:

DIAPPERS

Delirium

Infection

Atrophic vaginitis/urethritis

Pharmaceuticals (most commonly alcohol, anticholinergics, diuretics, opiates, sedatives)

Psychological

Excess urine output (hypercalcemia, hyperglycemia, diuretics, caffeine, nocturnal mobilization of peripheral edema)

Restricted mobility

Stool impaction

KEY FACT

Urge incontinence is common in both men and women. Think "overactive": urgency, frequency, nocturia.

Urinary Incontinence

A disorder characterized by the unintentional loss of urine. Causes are multifactorial:

- **Transient factors** include inadequate mobility, motivation, or dexterity; confusion; and medications.
- **Chronic factors** include detrusor overactivity/underactivity, insufficient sphincter tone, or outlet obstruction.
- Urinary incontinence ↑ risk of decubitus ulcers and can cause loss of self-esteem and social isolation.

URGE INCONTINENCE

The **most common** type of incontinence in geriatric patients. Due to **detrusor overactivity.**

Symptoms/Exam

- Patients feel an **abrupt urge** to urinate, but cannot get to the toilet in time. May have nocturia.
- Pelvic and rectal exam should be performed.

Differential

Mixed, overflow, or stress incontinence; diuretic effect of caffeine or medications.

Diagnosis

- **Bladder diary** to establish severity of problem, exacerbating factors.
- UA to rule out UTI.
- Consider PSA testing in men if appropriate and after informed discussion with patient.
- Postvoid residual >200 mL indicates urinary retention.
- **Cystoscopy** indicated in patients with **hematuria** (gross or microscopic) or **pelvic pain** to rule out irritative processes such as stones or cancer.

Management

- First line: **Nonpharmacologic**:
  - Frequently scheduled voids.
  - Bladder retraining, such as urge suppression exercises.
  - Behavior modifications, such as reducing or eliminating caffeine and alcohol and late-night fluid intake, and weight loss.
- Pharmacologic:
  - **Anticholinergics** such as **oxybutynin** and **tolterodine (may cause less dry mouth)** antagonize acetylcholine at muscarinic receptors, leading to bladder smooth muscle relaxation.
  - β-adrenergic agonists, mirabegron, activates β-3 receptors, relaxing detrusor muscle; takes weeks to obtain effect.
  - Onabotulinumtoxin A injection, inhibit release of acetylcholine, therefore relaxing detrusor muscle (third-line).
  - Estrogen (intravaginal, systemic) **not** FDA approved. Systemic estrogen can worsen incontinence.
  - **Surgery:** Neuromodulation of the sacral nerve may be helpful in severe, otherwise refractory cases.

STRESS INCONTINENCE

Involuntary loss of urine during a stress maneuver due to weak pelvic floor muscles or insufficient internal urethral sphincter strength. More common in women, although it may develop in men following prostate surgery.

Symptoms/Exam

- Symptoms with sneeze, cough, laugh.
- Nocturnal symptoms are uncommon.
- Pelvic exam may reveal weak pelvic floor muscle strength or cystocele.

Diagnosis

Look for evidence of pelvic prolapse and causes of intrinsic sphincter deficiency such as use of α-adrenergic antagonists (eg, terazosin), radiation, or surgical trauma.

Management

- First line: Nonpharmacologic:
  - Treat chronic cough if it is a precipitant.
  - Kegel exercise to strengthen pelvic floor muscles. Reinforce these exercises, as patients often give up too early.
- Second-line treatment:
  - Pessaries may benefit women with stress incontinence exacerbated by bladder or uterine prolapse.
  - **Surgery offers highest cure rates.** Options include bladder neck suspension, suburethral slings, and tension-free vaginal tape.
  - Although rarely primary treatment, periurethral injection of collagen-like substance is a short-term alternative that focally expands pressure to the proximal and mid-urethra.
  - Some recent evidence indicating use of **duloxetine** has shown benefit, but is not FDA approved and many patients stop use due to side effects or lack of effect.

PELVIC ORGAN PROLAPSE

Occurs with the descent of the bladder, uterus, or vagina from the anatomic location toward or through the vaginal opening (also known as genital prolapse). Prolapse is the most common indication for hysterectomy in the United States for women over the age of 55. Risk factors include multiparity, genetic predisposition, advancing age, prior pelvic surgery, menopause, obesity, chronic constipation with straining, repeated heavy lifting, pregnancy, and connective tissue disorders.

Symptoms

- Usually asymptomatic. May complain of feeling a bulge of tissue that protrudes to or past the vagina. May also experience pelvic pressure with straining, urinary incontinence, and/or difficulty with bowel movements.
- Speculum exam, bimanual exam, and rectovaginal exam identify pelvic abnormalities.

Diagnosis

May stage the pelvic organ prolapsed by the Baden-Walker System and Pelvic Organ Prolapse-Quantification System (Table 15.4).

Management

- Asymptomatic or mildly symptomatic women: Recommend weight management, avoidance of heavy lifting and straining with bowel movements, and pelvic floor muscle training (Kegel exercises).

TABLE 15.4.   Pelvic Organ Prolapse Staging Systems

BADEN-WALKER SYSTEM		PELVIC ORGAN PROLAPSE-QUANTIFICATION SYSTEM	
GRADE	DESCRIPTION	STAGE	DESCRIPTION
0	No prolapse	0	No prolapse
1	Descent halfway to hymen	I	>1 cm above hymen
2	Descent to hymen	II	<1 cm proximal or distal to hymen plane
3	Descent halfway past hymen	III	>1 cm below hymen plane, protrudes <2 cm from total vaginal length
4	Maximal descent	IV	Eversion of lower genital tract

- Symptomatic: Obliterative or reconstructive surgery. Pessaries can improve symptoms for women awaiting surgery, poor surgical candidates, or women who decline surgery.

INCOMPLETE EMPTYING OR OVERFLOW INCONTINENCE

Unpredictable dribbling of urine or weak urine stream due to **impaired detrusor activity and/or outlet obstruction.** The second most common cause of incontinence in older men. Underactive bladder may be due to medications (eg, calcium channel blockers, anticholinergics) or detrusor denervation or injury. Outlet obstruction may be due to enlarged prostate gland, tumors, urethral stricture, or chronic constipation.

Symptoms/Exam

Nocturnal enuresis due to pelvic floor relaxation at night.

Diagnosis

- UA and cytology.
- Digital rectal examination: Assess for fecal impaction and abnormalities of the prostate.
- Postvoid residual: If >200 mL, consider renal ultrasound to rule out hydronephrosis.
- Consider PSA testing in men; indications for PSA testing same, despite urinary symptoms.
- Cystoscopy may help identify masses.
- Urodynamic testing may reveal detrusor underactivity.

Management

- First-line treatment:
  - Lifestyle modifications, pelvic floor exercises as above.
  - If possible, discontinue anticholinergics and narcotics that promote urinary retention.
  - Address constipation, if present.
- Pharmacologic options:
  - α-blockers prazosin and terazosin induce internal sphincter relaxation and may relieve retention associated with benign prostatic hyperplasia.
  - 5α-reductase inhibitors such as finasteride may partially relieve symptoms associated with BPH, but require months for onset of effect.
- Third-line treatment:
  - Acute urinary retention and acontractile bladders may require indwelling or intermittent catheterization.
  - Surgical decompression may be required for obstruction, such as cystocele or uterine prolapse.
  - Sacral neuromodulation, percutaneous tibial nerve stimulation.

Constipation

Attributable partly to normal physiologic changes such as ↑ rectal compliance and weakening of pelvic floor and abdominal muscles. Often exacerbated by underlying medical and surgical conditions.

- **1° constipation** is functional constipation:
  - Normal transit: Hard stool, normal frequency.
  - Slow transit: Abnormal innervation, infrequent defecation, bloating, abdominal pain.

KEY FACT

About one-third of adults ≥60 years report at least occasional constipation, and in nursing home residents, the prevalence is 50% or more.

- Disorders of defecation: ↓ smooth muscle contraction in rectum or inability to relax muscles (older adults may have rectal receptors that have ↓ response to stretch).
- 2° **constipation,** due to another cause such as medications, chronic disease, and psychosocial reasons.

Symptoms/Exam

- Characterized by ↓ stool frequency, difficult passage of feces, and/or a feeling of incomplete evacuation.
- Severe fecal impaction can cause symptoms of intestinal obstruction, colonic ulceration, overflow fecal incontinence, and paradoxical diarrhea.
- Exam may reveal hemorrhoids, anal fissures, and rectal prolapse (from excessive straining).

Diagnosis

- Identify misperceptions about normal bowel movement frequency.
- Thorough physical exam, including rectal exam.
- Basic metabolic panel and TSH tests to exclude metabolic factors.
- Abdominal x-ray to identify the distribution of stool and findings that warrant surgical consultation.
- If persistent, colonoscopy to evaluate for structural lesions.

Management

Nonpharmacologic (behavioral):

- ↑ hydration and foods high in fiber; fiber supplementation if needed.
- ↑ physical activity, however evidence shows it may not improve symptoms of constipation in nursing home patients.
- Stop constipating medications, if possible; such as opiates, iron supplementation, clonidine, antihistamines.

Pharmacologic:

- Daily osmotic laxatives such as **polyethylene glycol** (more effective, fewer side effects), lactulose, and sorbitol are useful for chronic slow-transit constipation.
- Stool softeners (eg, docusate) are helpful for patients who are on opiates or who are bedridden.
- Stimulant laxatives (eg, senna, bisacodyl) are best reserved for short-term use.
- Enemas when fecal impaction is present.
- Newer agents such as linaclotide (increases intestinal fluid secretion and motility), lubiprostone (a chloride channel activator that moves water into the intestinal lumen), and peripherally acting μ-opioid antagonists (ie, methylnaltrexone or alvimopan) have shown benefit.

Falls

The number one cause of injuries and deaths from injury in older Americans. Major cause of morbidity and mortality among elderly patients, especially women. Falls impact quality of life. Fear of falling in older adults can lead to limitation of activities and social engagements, which can result in further physical decline, depression, social isolation, and feelings of helplessness. Prevention of falls should focus on modifiable risk factors (Tables 15.5 and 15.6).

Complications: Falls commonly lead to fractures of the wrist, vertebrae, and hip. Older persons have a 20% ↑ in mortality rate in the first year following a hip fracture.

TABLE 15.5.   Risk Factors and Preventive Interventions for Falls

RISK FACTOR	PREVENTIVE INTERVENTION
Poor vision	Eye exam (corrective lenses; cataract extraction)
Use of psychoactive medications	Review medications for effects on vestibular system, dementia; ↓ polypharmacy (select the least centrally acting drugs; prescribe the lowest effective dose); avoid sedative drugs
Proprioceptive dysfunction	Screen for cervical spondylosis and vitamin B_{12} deficiency
Difficulties with gait and balance	Refer for physical therapy
Postural hypotension and syncope	Assess medications and consider carotid and cardiac ultrasounds to assess for carotid artery and aortic valve stenosis; rehydration
Problems with feet and/or shoes	Foot evaluation; timed up and go test
Home hazards	Home safety assessment

Data from the CDC. https://www.cdc.gov/steadi/pdf/risk_factors_for_falls-a.pdf. Accessed February 2017.

HIP FRACTURE

Hip fractures cause significant morbidity and are associated with ↑ mortality. Much more common in women. Typically occur after fall, however other risk factors include ↓ bone mineral density, reduced level of activity, and chronic medication use.

Symptoms/Exam

- Pain in groin. Unable to bear weight on the affected extremity.
- Affected limb is typically external rotated and abducted, may appear shorter.

Diagnosis

- Plain radiograph confirms diagnosis (Figure 15.11).
- If high suspicion for fracture and x-ray is normal, obtain MRI.

Management

- Surgery unless patient has significant comorbidities or reduced life expectancy.
- Bisphosphonates to reduce risk of recurrent fracture.
- Extensive rehabilitation.

Pressure Ulcers

Skin breakdown often attributable to ↓ subcutaneous fat, poor nutrition, and poor circulation in the setting of prolonged pressure and friction over bony prominences such as the ischial tuberosities and sacrum (Figure 15.12). Immobilization and incontinence are major risk factors for the development of pressure ulcers.

Symptoms/Exam

Staging is as follows:
- **Stage 1:** Nonblanchable erythema of intact skin.
- **Stage 2:** Partial-thickness superficial skin loss up to subcutaneous tissue.

TABLE 15.6.   Intrinsic Versus Extrinsic Risk Factors for Falls

INTRINSIC
Advanced age
Previous falls
Muscle weakness
Gait and balance problems
Poor vision
Postural hypotension
Chronic conditions (arthritis, diabetes, stroke, Parkinson disease, incontinence, dementia)
Fear of falling

EXTRINSIC
Lack of stair handrails
Poor stair design
Lack of bathroom grab bars
Dim lighting or glare
Obstacles and tripping hazards
Slippery or uneven surfaces
Psychoactive medications
Improper use of assistive device

Data from the CDC. https://www.cdc.gov/steadi/pdf/risk_factors_for_falls-a.pdf. Accessed February 2017.

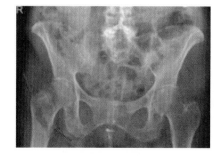

FIGURE 15.11.   Hip fracture. Frontal radiograph of the pelvis shows an intertrochanteric fracture of the right femur (arrows). (Reproduced with permission from USMLE-Rx.com.)

 KEY FACT

About 12% to 17% of patients with a hip fracture die within the first year.

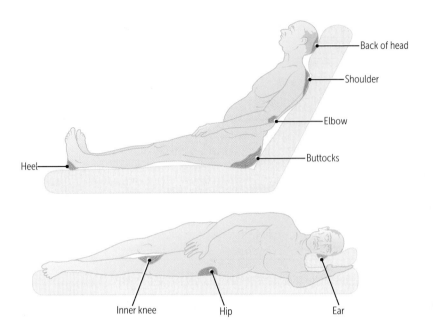

FIGURE 15.12. **Common sites of pressure ulcers.** Bony areas, such as back of the head, ears, shoulders, elbows, buttocks, hips, inner knees, and heels are most commonly affected. (Reproduced with permission from USMLE-Rx.com.)

- **Stage 3:** Full-thickness skin loss through subcutaneous tissue.
- **Stage 4:** Tissue loss down to the level of muscle, tendon, or bone.

Differential

Infectious ulcers, thermal burns, malignant ulcers (cutaneous lymphoma, basal cell carcinoma, or squamous cell carcinoma), rectocutaneous fistula, ulcers due to vascular disease.

Management

- ↓ pressure, friction, and shearing forces via frequent repositioning and use of protective devices such as pillows, foam or sheepskin, and special mattresses.
- ↓ moisture by treating bladder and bowel incontinence.
- Ensure adequate nursing care to keep affected areas clean.
- Optimize nutrition.
- Mobilize the patient as soon as possible.
- When ulcers are not healing or have persistent exudates after 2 weeks of optimal cleansing and dressing changes, consider antimicrobials (topical for superficial infection, systemic for deep tissue infections).

Insomnia

Impaired ability to fall and stay asleep. Up to 50% of elderly people report sleep problems. Factors that contribute to sleep disorders include the following:

- **Psychiatric:** Bereavement, social isolation, anxiety, depression.
- **Neurologic:** Dementia, leading to nocturnal agitation.
- **Medication:** Including sedative-hypnotics, bronchodilators, diuretics, decongestants.
- **Pain syndromes:** Neuropathic pain, arthritic pain, malignancy syndromes.
- **Respiratory:** Dyspnea from cardiac and pulmonary conditions.
- Alcohol.
- Caffeine.

Sleep consists of alternating types: non–rapid eye movement (NREM) and rapid eye movement (REM) sleep.

- Majority of time is spent in NREM sleep.
- NREM sleep has three stages: stages 1 and 2, defined as light sleep, and stage 3 consisting of deep restorative sleep.
- Age-related changes in normal sleep: ↓ REM sleep, ↑ in lighter stages of sleep.

Symptoms/Exam

Presents with difficulty falling asleep, intermittent wakefulness during the night, early-morning awakening, and daytime sleepiness.

Diagnosis

- Evaluate for stress, depressed mood, level of physical activity, and dietary habits.
- Consider sleep apnea and/or restless leg syndrome in the patient and/or **patient's partner.**
- Overnight polysomnography.

Management

- Identify sleep hygiene patterns that may worsen insomnia and recommend the following (CBT):
  - Adherence to regular sleep time and morning rise time.
  - Limitation of daytime napping and go to bed when sleepy.
  - Avoidance of caffeine, alcohol, and nicotine in the evening.
  - Limitation of nighttime fluid intake.
  - Limitation of noise, uncomfortable beds, pets in bed, and inappropriate temperature settings.
  - Go to another room if unable to fall asleep within 15 to 20 minutes.
- Pharmacological Agents:
  - Melatonin; limited effects on initial sleep latency and total sleep time.
  - Sedating antidepressants, such as trazodone, have been shown to ↓ sleep-onset latency and ↑ total sleep time.
  - Benzodiazepines, nonbenzodiazepines (ie, zolpidem), and antihistamines can contribute to confusion and ↑ the likelihood of falls! **Avoid!**

KEY FACT

Older adults need 7 to 9 hours of sleep per night. It is a misconception that as we get older, our sleep needs decline. However, it can be harder for men and women ages >65 years to stay asleep throughout the night.

KEY FACT

CBT (via you or other trained professional) is superior to medication.

Postherpetic Neuralgia

Exquisite pain that persists after the initial rash of herpes zoster has healed. Can occur at any age, but has a peak incidence in patients 50 to 70 years of age. The duration and severity of postherpetic neuralgia (PHN) ↑ sharply with age.

- **Symptoms/Exam:** Vary but can include constant pain; deep, aching, burning pain; spontaneous intermittent lancing pain; or hyperesthesia. **Pain is unilateral.** There are no specific exam findings.
- **Diagnosis:** History of a vesicular rash that resolves and is followed by the pain syndrome.
- **Management:** PHN is difficult to treat. The most effective treatment is prevention with early and aggressive antiviral therapy. Capsaicin ointment, lidocaine patches, gabapentin, pregabalin, and TCAs are helpful. Narcotics and regional anesthetic blocks ± steroids can also be considered for resistant cases.
- **Prevention:** One dose of live attenuated varicella virus vaccine is recommended for patients ≥60 years of age to ↓ risk of herpes zoster and subsequent PHN.

Polypharmacy

Defined as problems that occur when patients are taking more medications than needed, rendering them prone to dosage errors, adverse drug reactions, and interactions. Changes in physiologic function and pharmacokinetics ↑ sensitivity to medications, thereby ↑ the possibility of iatrogenic illness. Such factors include the following:

- **Distribution:**
    - ↓ in total body water, leading to ↑ concentration of water-soluble drugs.
    - ↑ in body fat, leading to longer half-lives of fat-soluble drugs.
    - ↓ albumin levels limits protein binding of some drugs (eg, warfarin, phenytoin), leaving more free drug available.
- **Metabolism:**
    - **Phase I:** Hepatic enzyme activity (eg, cytochrome P-450) is ↓ and thus affects the metabolism of drugs with high 1st-pass metabolism (eg, propranolol).
    - **Phase II:** Conjugation by acetylation, glucuronidation, or sulfation is not affected by aging.
    - **Excretion:** ↓ GFR leads to ↓ excretion of drugs.

Symptoms/Exam

May present with delirium, nausea, anorexia, weight loss, hypotension, fatigue, and acute renal failure.

Diagnosis

- Adverse drug reactions must be considered as a potential cause of ill presentations in elderly patients.
- Obtain a thorough history of both prescribed and OTC medications, including antihistamines that can have anticholinergic effects.

Management

- Ensure that the symptom requiring treatment is not due to another drug.
- Use drug therapy only after nonpharmacologic methods have been tried.
- Simplify dosage schedule (ideally once daily), reduce number of pills, and avoid frequent medication changes.

KEY FACT

When starting medications, start low and go slow! Except mirtazapine (start higher).

Palliative and End-of-Life Care

Palliative care focuses on improving quality of life for the patient and family during serious illness, including relief of pain and other distressing symptoms. Palliative care may be used during, but is not limited to, the end of life.

ETHICAL AND LEGAL ISSUES

End-of-life care is guided by the same ethical principles that inform other types of medical care. In addition, there are three unique ethical considerations that are relevant to end-of-life care:

- **Medical futility:** A unilateral decision by the physician to forgo futile interventions. This decision may create conflict between the physician and the patient or family, but such conflict can usually be resolved through timely, frequent, and consistent communication.
- **Withdrawal of care:** The principle that the patient/family has the right to stop unwanted treatments once begun as well as to refuse those treatments before they are started.

- **Doctrine of double effect:** The argument that the potential to hasten imminent death is acceptable if it comes as an unintended consequence of the original intention to provide comfort and relieve suffering.

Decision-Making Capacity

Consider a patient's decision-making capacity intact when he/she can communicate a choice that takes into account the risks, benefits, and consequences of that choice. Must be consistent with the patient's values and goals. It is often the physician or psychiatrist's responsibility to determine mental capacity.

Informed Consent

A process by which a patient is given information about the nature of the intervention, the expected risks and benefits, the likely consequences, and the alternatives to the interventions.

Advance Directives

Documents that allow patients to express their preferences and values to guide care in the event they can no longer make informed decisions. Types of advance directives include the following:

- **Living will:** Allows patients to direct their physicians to withhold or withdraw life-sustaining treatment in the event they develop a terminal condition or enter a persistent vegetative state.
- **Durable power of attorney for health care:** Allows patients to designate a surrogate to make proxy decisions in the event they themselves are unable to communicate their wishes **or** lose decision-making capacity. Applies to all health situations, not just terminal illness.
- **Do not resuscitate/intubate (DNR/DNI) orders:** Allows patients to request to not receive CPR/intubation if their heart stops beating or they stop breathing. DNR/DNI orders are accepted by doctors and hospitals in all states. Only 15% of all patients who undergo CPR in the hospital survive to hospital discharge. Patients should be informed of mortality outcomes as well as the potential consequences of surviving CPR (eg, neurologic disability, damage to internal organs, and the likelihood of requiring other aggressive interventions).
- **POLST (physician orders for life-sustaining treatment):** These forms, also called MOST (medical orders for scope of treatment) forms, are now used in most states. Completed by patients and their physicians, these forms designate a patient's wishes regarding resuscitation, extent of medical treatment, and artificial nutrition.

HOSPICE CARE

- Patient and family centered; emphasizes the provision of comfort and pain relief rather than an attempt to cure illness and prolong life.
- Requires physicians to estimate the patient's probability of **survival as <6 months.**

SYMPTOM MANAGEMENT

Common end-of-life symptoms that should be addressed to maximize quality of life and comfort include the following:

Pain

Assess for pain frequently. Consider use of numeric and visual facial pain scales. Allow the patient to set goals of pain management.

- **First-line treatment:**
  - Opioid medications, usually morphine is utilized.
  - Regularly assess and treat side effects of opioids such as nausea and constipation.

KEY FACT

There is no maximum allowable dosage for opioids; doses should be titrated to achieve adequate pain relief.

Dyspnea

A sensation of dyspnea is common among dying patients. Identify treatable causes (eg, pneumonia, pleural effusion). Management includes:

- **Buccal morphine sulfate** is highly effective; benzodiazepines may help anxiety.
- Consider supplemental O_2, using a fan, or open windows for fresh air.

Nausea and Vomiting

- If opioid related, consider substituting an equianalgesic dose of another opioid or a sustained-release formulation; can also add a dopamine antagonist antiemetic (eg, haloperidol) to block the chemoreceptor trigger zone.
- If due to an intra-abdominal process such as constipation, gastroparesis, or gastric outlet obstruction, consider laxatives, prokinetic agents, NG suction, high-dose corticosteroids, and ondansetron.
- Around-the-clock dosing of antiemetics and as-needed benzodiazepines are also highly effective.

Constipation

Opioids, poor dietary intake, and physical inactivity make constipation common among the dying.

- Anticipate and prevent constipation via **prophylactic bowel regimens** of stool softeners and stimulant laxatives when opioid treatment is begun.
- Consider simple considerations such as privacy, undisturbed toilet time, and a bedside commode in appropriate patients.

Delirium and Agitation

Many terminally ill patients experience delirium before death. Manage as follows:

- Nonpharmacologic strategies to help orient patients may be sufficient to ↓ delirium when no other reversible causes are identified.
- Haloperidol, risperidone, or quetiapine can be highly effective.
- It may be acceptable to do nothing if the delirium does not negatively affect the family or patient.

NUTRITION AND HYDRATION

- Individuals at the end of life may refuse nutrition and hydration. Reassure the family that this is normal and the patient is not in distress.
- Eating without hunger and artificial nutrition can cause potential complications such as nausea, vomiting, choking, and aspiration.
- IV hydration is not recommended. However, you may use moist oral swabs for dry mouth.
- Starvation is associated with **ketonemia,** which can cause a sense of well-being, analgesia, and mild euphoria.

WITHDRAWAL OF SUPPORT

- Requests for withdrawal of care from informed and competent patients or their surrogates must be respected.
- Physicians may determine medical futility and cease further medical intervention.
- Educate the patient and family on the expected course of events following withdrawal of support.

PSYCHOLOGICAL, SOCIAL, AND SPIRITUAL ISSUES

- Family meetings may help family members and patients during end-of-life transitions.
- Remain attentive to patients' spiritual need to understand the underlying meaning of their lives and their experience in the world.
- Attempt to understand how cultural beliefs and ethnic traditions can affect the experience of dying.

Elder Abuse

An intentional or unintentional act that causes harm to an elderly person. It is estimated that between 1 and 2 million elderly Americans are abused each year; however, it is often unreported. Abuse may be verbal, physical, or sexual; it may also be in the form of neglect and financial exploitation. Domestic and institutional **risk factors** for abuse include isolation, poverty, physical or emotional dependence of the victim on the caregiver, lack of community resources, a low staff-to-patient ratio, and caregiver or staff burnout. Table 15.7 lists the types of elder abuse and their clinical presentations.

Symptoms/Exam

- Symptoms are wide ranging and may include unexplained withdrawal from normal activities, depressed mood, or a strained or tense relationship with the caregiver or spouse.
- Exam may reveal poor hygiene, unusual weight loss, bedsores, bruises, pressure marks, broken bones, and abrasions.

Diagnosis

Ask screening questions **while the patient is alone.** Inquire about perceived safety and violence in the family. Ask about the patient's dependency on caregivers, friends, and family.

TABLE 15.7.   **Types and Characteristics of Elder Abuse**

TYPE	DESCRIPTION
Domestic	Maltreatment of an older adult living at home or in a caregiver's home
Institutional	Maltreatment of an older adult living in a residential facility
Self-neglect	Behavior of an older adult who lives alone that threatens his or her own health or safety
Physical abuse	Intentional infliction of physical pain or injury
Financial abuse	Improper or illegal use of the resources of an older person without his/her consent, benefiting a person other than the older adult
Psychological abuse	Infliction of mental anguish (eg, humiliating, intimidating, threatening)
Neglect	Failure to fulfill a caretaking obligation to provide goods or services (eg, abandonment, denial of food or health-related services)
Abandonment	Desertion of an elderly person by someone who has assumed responsibility for providing care to that person
Sexual abuse	Nonconsensual sexual contact of any kind

Management

- Document the type, frequency, and severity of abuse. **Assess the decision-making capacity of the victim.**
- Health care providers are **mandated by law** to report suspected elder mistreatment. Reports should be given to the state or county division of Adult Protective Services. In the absence of such services, the reporter should contact the county or state extension office of Child and Family Services.
- **If the patient has the capacity** to make decisions and refuses intervention:
  - Educate the patient about the incidence of mistreatment of elderly persons and the tendency for mistreatment to ↑ in frequency and severity over time.
  - Provide written information about emergency assistance numbers.
  - Develop and review a safety plan.
  - Refer the patient to agencies that provide respite care, support for personal care, and transportation.
- **If the patient does not have the capacity** to make decisions, the physician should initiate the process of separating the victim from the perpetrator while arranging supportive services for the whole family, including the abuser.

CHAPTER 16

Reproductive Health

Caroline Morgan, MD

Maternity Care

Any medical visit with a female patient of childbearing age is an opportunity to offer basic counseling on preconception health, an essential conversation given that nearly 50% of pregnancies are unplanned.

DIAGNOSIS OF PREGNANCY

Common symptoms of pregnancy include breast tenderness, fatigue, and nausea or vomiting. Signs on physical exam in the early first trimester include Chadwick sign (blue cervix) or Goodell sign (cervical softening), and palpable uterine enlargement.

Diagnose with urine qualitative hCG assay (98% sensitivity 7 days after implantation), serum quantitative β-hCG assay (sensitivity 4-5 days after implantation), or pelvic ultrasound (a gestational sac is usually visible 5-6 weeks after the last menstrual period [LMP]).

The estimated date of delivery can be established by the following in the first trimester:
- LMP + 40 weeks, adjusting for cycle length if different from 28 days.
- Ultrasound measurement of crown-rump length in millimeters, most reliable method.

For ultrasonography dating in the second trimester, also consider the following:
- Biparietal diameter and head circumference.
- Femur length.
- Abdominal circumference.

PRENATAL CARE IN THE FIRST TRIMESTER

The goals of the initial prenatal visit are four-fold:
- Identify patients with undesired pregnancies and refer for adoption counseling/abortion if applicable.
- Identify any medical or psychosocial problems that merit immediate attention.
- Establish the gestational age of the pregnancy.
- Begin patient education.

Prenatal Risk Assessment and Lab Workup

- **Physical exam:** A full exam, including a thyroid, breast, and pelvic exam, along with BP screening, performed within 1 to 2 weeks of diagnosis. After 9 to 12 weeks of gestation, fetal heart tones auscultated at each visit with a Doppler ultrasound.
- **Medical history:** Metabolic and autoimmune diseases, cardiac disease; **reproductive history,** including gynecologic or pregnancy complications and DES exposure; **medication use** (prescription drugs, OTC medications, and herbal supplements, teratogenic medications).
- **Family history:** CF, thalassemia, sickle cell anemia, birth defects, endocrine disorders, thromboembolic disease, and multiple gestation.
- **Psychosocial history:** Domestic violence, financial stability, emotional support, and barriers to care; **substance use** (EtOH, tobacco, illicit drugs).
- **Initial labs:**
  - CBC, ABO/Rh, rubella titer, hepatitis B antigen, RPR, Pap smear, chlamydia screening in women <25 years of age or at risk, gonorrhea in women at risk, and HIV testing.

- Maternal serum antibody test (if Rh ⊖, give RhoGAM at 28 weeks, or with any bleeding during pregnancy, and also postpartum, to prevent Rh isoimmunization).
- Complete UA with culture.
- For diabetic screening in high-risk patients, 1-hour 50-g oral glucose tolerance test (OGTT).
- Pelvic ultrasound for dating if the LMP is unknown.
- Urine dipstick at each visit to screen for proteinuria and glucosuria.

Prenatal Counseling

- **Overview of prenatal care:** Patients should be counseled regarding the frequency of prenatal visits, routine pregnancy monitoring, how to reach after-hours care, and other resources that may be available (eg, childbirth classes).
- **Nutrition:** Patients should follow a healthy, balanced diet, aiming for BMI-adjusted weight gain: 25 to 35 pounds for BMI 20 to 25; 10 to 15 pounds for a BMI >26; 35 to 45 pounds for a BMI <19.8. They should also be counseled to avoid uncooked food, unpasteurized dairy products, mercury-containing fish, and excess vitamin A. A daily prenatal vitamin with at least 400 µg of folic acid can help prevent neural tube defects.
- **Drug/alcohol cessation:** Alcohol use is associated with growth restriction, small-for-gestational-age babies, fetal alcohol syndrome, and other effects of fetal exposure to alcohol. Some illicit drugs are associated with preterm birth, poor growth, and neonatal abstinence syndrome. Substance use treatment can be highly effective and should be initiated promptly. Opioid use disorders should be treated with methadone or buprenorphine.
- **Tobacco cessation:** Smoking during pregnancy is associated with low birth weight, prematurity, and an ↑ risk of miscarriage and thromboembolic events. Nicotine patches or gum may be used to aid in tobacco cessation; the use of bupropion is not well studied in pregnancy.
- **Safety:** Screen all patients for domestic violence. Patients should avoid trauma (no contact sports; use seat belts), environmental toxins (organic solvents, lead, radiation), extremes of temperature (no hot tubs), and prolonged immobility. Toxoplasmosis and *Listeria* precautions should also be discussed (eg, avoid raw meat/fish, unpasteurized dairy products, and cat litter), as should safe sex practices.
- **Genetic counseling:** All women should be offered nuchal translucency testing for Down syndrome and quadruple screening with serum AFP, hCG, estriol, and inhibin A. If these tests suggest a high risk of genetic disorders, additional testing and services should be offered, including genetic counseling, cell free fetal DNA testing, amniocentesis, chorionic villus sampling, and a detailed anatomic survey by ultrasound.

EARLY FETAL DEVELOPMENT

Milestones of first-trimester fetal development are outlined in Table 16.1.

COMMON PROBLEMS IN THE FIRST TRIMESTER

Hyperemesis Gravidarum

Persistent vomiting with weight loss and ketonuria, usually starting at <10 weeks of gestation. Affects 1 in 200 pregnancies and is especially associated with molar pregnancies and multiple gestations. Advanced maternal age and nicotine use may be protective.

KEY FACT

The following tests may be appropriate in pregnant women with certain risk factors:
- **Hepatitis C antibody** (IV drug use, tattoos, or received blood products before 1992)
- **PPD ± CXR** (eg, immigrants and those with known exposure)
- **Toxoplasmosis titer** (exposure to cat feces or undercooked meat)
- **CMV/parvovirus titer** (eg, those who work at day care centers)

KEY FACT

Pregnant women should not receive live attenuated vaccines for MMR and varicella; recommend immunization postpartum. Gamma-globulin for protection from rubella is not recommended, given that herd immunity should protect most patients in the United States from contracting the disease.

KEY FACT

The flu vaccine is recommended during all stages of pregnancy.

KEY FACT

Screen all women at 11 to 16 weeks' gestation for asymptomatic bacteriuria on urine dipstick. If present, treat for a UTI.

TABLE 16.1. **Fetal Development Milestones**

WEEKS	MILESTONES
1-2	Implantation with the beginning of placental development
3-4	Gestational sac with distinct ectoderm, mesoderm, and endoderm layers
4-5	Primitive brain
5-6	Fetal pole with cardiac activity
4-8	Primitive eyes, ears, abdominal organs, and limb buds
7	Fetal movement is visible
8-9	Spine/limb formation and organogenesis are complete
10	The palate is formed
12	Breathing, swallowing, sucking motions; the fetus is able to move the head, arms, hands, legs, and feet; formation of fingernails and toenails
14	Blinking, meconium accumulation, cardiac/digestive systems fully functional

MNEMONIC

Causes of recurrent miscarriage:
RIBCAGE

Radiation
Immune reaction
Bugs (infection)
Cervical incompetence/**C**lotting disorder
  (eg, Factor V Leiden, lupus anticoagulant)
Anatomic anomalies (eg, uterine septum)
Genetic (eg, aneuploidy, balanced
  translocation)
Endocrine

KEY FACT

Elevated β-hCG levels probably account for the ↑ incidence of hyperemesis gravidarum in molar and multiple-gestation pregnancies.

KEY FACT

Patients with >2 spontaneous abortions require workup for thromboembolic disorders and chromosomal anomalies.

Symptoms/Exam

- Presents with persistent vomiting accompanied by weight loss >5% of prepregnancy weight.
- Often orthostatic blood pressures, and with signs of hypovolemia on exam.

Differential

Normal nausea of early pregnancy; GI disorders (gastroenteritis, hepatitis, appendicitis, biliary disease); metabolic disorders (DM, porphyria); pyelonephritis or other infections; neurologic or psychiatric disease; medication side effects; preeclampsia or HELLP syndrome if diagnosed after 20 weeks; fatty liver of pregnancy.

Diagnosis

- **Labs:** Urine ketones, TSH/T_4, and serum electrolytes.
- **Imaging:** Ultrasound to rule out molar pregnancy or multiple gestation.

Management

- Initial treatment consists of avoiding triggers; eating small, salty meals with clear fluids; consuming ginger; and using Sea-Bands and acupressure.
- Antiemetics (eg, vitamin B_6 (pyridoxine), doxylamine, H_2 blockers, promethazine, ondansetron) may be of benefit.
- Patients with severe dehydration and/or >5% weight loss should be hospitalized with IV/enteral fluids and nutrition.
- Corticosteroids are the last resort for treatment.

Complications

Hypokalemia, metabolic alkalosis, Wernicke encephalopathy, Mallory-Weiss esophageal tears. Mild hyperthyroidism and hyperparathyroidism may also be associated with the condition.

First-Trimester Vaginal Bleeding

Vaginal bleeding that occurs prior to 14 weeks of gestation can range from spotting to life-threatening hemorrhage. See Table 16.2 for the causes of first-trimester bleeding.

- Immediate goals of management are to maintain maternal hemodynamic stability and rule out ectopic pregnancy or trophoblastic disease. In the case of spontaneous,

TABLE 16.2.   **Common Causes of First-Trimester Bleeding in an Intrauterine Pregnancy**

CAUSE	DEFINITION/PRESENTATION	DIAGNOSIS/TREATMENT
Physiologic bleeding	Vaginal spotting in the early first trimester without any other cause No cramping or other symptoms; closed cervix on pelvic exam	Pelvic exam; ultrasound for prolonged spotting; expectant management Differential includes threatened SAB, ectopic pregnancy, and gynecologic pathology
Spontaneous abortion (SAB)	The most common complication of early pregnancy (occurs in roughly 20% of recognized pregnancies); defined as expulsion of an embryo/fetus <500 g (usually at <20-22 weeks) Moderate bleeding, cramping, and passage of tissue; an open cervix is seen on pelvic exam	Pelvic exam; ultrasound with serial serum β-hCG if the history of tissue passage is uncertain; D&C for prolonged or heavy bleeding Risk factors include advanced maternal age, prior SAB, multiparity, toxin/teratogen exposure, and invasive intrauterine procedures
Threatened abortion	Vaginal bleeding with a closed cervix but no passage of tissue Cramping is variable; fetal cardiac activity is present, and uterine size is appropriate for gestational age	Pelvic exam; ultrasound and/or β-hCG; expectant management The differential includes SAB, physiologic bleeding, gynecologic pathology, and ectopic pregnancy Most threatened abortions do **not** result in loss of pregnancy
Inevitable abortion	Usually painful uterine cramps, ↑ bleeding, and a dilated cervix with gestational tissue often visible at the cervical os	Pelvic exam; removal of tissue at the os may stop bleeding D&C is indicated for significant cramping or blood loss; otherwise, treat with expectant management or misoprostol
Incomplete abortion	Embryonic demise with partial passage of tissue Cramping/bleeding is variable; uterine size is less than dates; retained placental tissue may be visible; usually occurs at >12 weeks	Expectant or medical management can be offered D&C indicated for significant cramping or blood loss or for retention of gestational products for a prolonged period
Septic abortion	Uterine infection Fever, chills, pelvic pain, bleeding, purulent vaginal discharge, a boggy and tender uterus with a dilated cervix, and signs of sepsis	Usually a complication of nonsterile elective abortion or other invasive procedures Stabilize with IV fluids; broad-spectrum antibiotics; D&C
Missed abortion ("blighted ovum" or anembryonic pregnancy)	Embryo/fetus demise prior to 20 weeks with retention of pregnancy Inadequate growth and absent fetal heart tones or empty gestational sac on routine monitoring; closed cervix on exam	Ultrasound to confirm diagnosis; may choose between expectant management, medical management with misoprostol, or D&C/D&E for prolonged retention/unsuccessful medical management/patient preference

incomplete, or missed abortion, uterine evacuation may be performed if the patient desires or if bleeding does not resolve spontaneously or with the administration of misoprostol.

Ectopic Pregnancy

An ectopic pregnancy occurs when an embryo implants outside of the uterus, usually in a fallopian tube, and sometimes in the peritoneal cavity (Figure 16.1). Tubal pregnancies never survive to term. If left untreated, a tubal pregnancy will lead to rupture of the fallopian tube, an **obstetric emergency.** Risk factors for ectopic pregnancy include:

- Previous ectopic pregnancy.
- Current use of an IUD does not ↑ the risk of ectopic pregnancies, but if a woman becomes pregnant with an IUD inserted, she is more likely to have an ectopic pregnancy than a pregnant woman without an IUD.

MNEMONIC

Risk factors for ectopic pregnancy:

PID

Prior ectopic pregnancy/**P**rior abdominal or gynecologic surgery

IUD/**I**nfection (history of PID): Note that an IUD itself is not a risk factor for an ectopic; rather, if a woman with an IUD has a ⊕ pregnancy test, it is more likely to be an ectopic than if she did not have the IUD

DES exposure in utero/**D**amaged tubes (eg, from prior PID)

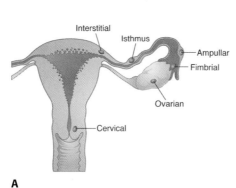 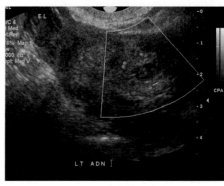

A   **B**

FIGURE 16.1. **Ectopic pregnancy.** (**A**) Locations of embryo implantation outside of the uterus. (**B**) Pelvic ultrasound shows a left adnexal structure with peripheral vascularity in a woman with abdominal pain and $\oplus$ hCG. (Reproduced with permission from USMLE-Rx.com.)

- Prior abdominal/gynecologic surgery or invasive procedures.
- Prior history of PID.
- *In utero* DES exposure.
- Tubal/uterine pathology or unusual anatomy.

Symptoms/Exam

Presents with pelvic pain, vaginal bleeding (variable), and nausea/vomiting.

Diagnosis

- **Imaging:** Ultrasound shows an empty uterus and may reveal an enlarged adnexal mass (see Figure 16.1B).
- **Labs:** $\oplus$ qualitative or quantitative β-hCG ± abnormal doubling time for β-hCG in early pregnancy).

Management

- Give IM methotrexate if the ectopic pregnancy is small (<3 cm), unruptured, and without fetal cardiac activity, and if the patient is stable and likely to be adherent. Follow with serial β-hCG measurements to ensure resolution. Methotrexate may be repeated in 1 week if β-hCG remains elevated.
- Laparoscopic injection of methotrexate is appropriate if the patient is hemodynamically unstable and/or unable or unlikely to follow-up with serial labs.
- Surgery may be necessary if medical treatment is unsuccessful.

Hydatidiform Molar Pregnancy

A nonmalignant subtype of gestational trophoblastic disease in which an abnormal fertilization event leads to a tumor of fetal origin. Rule out gestational trophoblastic disease in any patient with a $\oplus$ pregnancy test and significant vaginal bleeding. Molar pregnancies can be complete (no normal fetal tissue is present) or partial (some fetal tissue is present). Risk factors include nulliparity, a history of prior gestational trophoblastic disease, and extremes of maternal age (<20 or >35 years).

Symptoms/Exam

Presents with vaginal bleeding ± anemia; pelvic pressure or pain; hyperemesis gravidarum; hyperthyroidism; and/or early-onset preeclampsia.

Diagnosis

- **Imaging:** Ultrasound reveals enlarged ovaries with theca-lutein cysts, and an enlarged uterus containing a heterogeneous mass with anechoic areas (Figure 16.2).

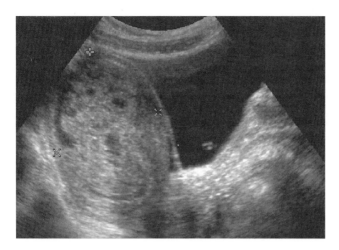

FIGURE 16.2. **Molar pregnancy.** Sagittal ultrasound shows the uterus to be distended by a heterogeneously echogenic mass with multiple hypoechoic foci. (Reproduced with permission from USMLE-Rx.com.)

- **Labs:** CBC reveals anemia; β-hCG is elevated. Tissue pathology confirms the diagnosis.

Management

Hemodynamic stabilization; expeditious uterine evacuation; serial β-hCG measurements to ensure resolution; CXR. Consider a repeat pelvic ultrasound.

PRENATAL CARE IN THE SECOND AND THIRD TRIMESTER

The second trimester is the time of most rapid fetal growth. Continued self-care and good nutrition are key to ensuring a healthy pregnancy.

Physical Examination

- **Fundal height measurement:** By 20 weeks, the uterine fundus should be palpable at the umbilicus. After 20 weeks, fundal height (in centimeters) should correspond to gestational age (in weeks) ± 2 cm until the fetus descends into the pelvis at 34 to 36 weeks.
- BP screening; fetal heart rate auscultation (normal is 120-160 bpm); examination for the presence of edema.
- Leopold maneuvers to determine fetal position after 36 weeks.
- If planning induction, a digital cervical exam to assess cervical ripening.

Laboratory Studies

- At each visit: Urine dipstick for glucosuria and proteinuria.
- At 15 to 18 weeks: Offer a "quadruple screen" to measure maternal serum α-fetoprotein, hCG, unconjugated estriol, and inhibin A levels; findings help predict the risk of Down syndrome, neural tube defects, and trisomy 18.
- At 24 to 28 weeks: 1-hour 50-g OGTT.
- Check hematocrit; treat with iron if anemic.
- Where applicable, obtain a test of cure for UTIs or genital tract infections; repeat gonorrhea/chlamydia screen in high-risk patients.
- Periodic urine toxicology screens are necessary for high-risk patients.
- Ultrasound for routine anatomic survey is recommended by many providers, although there is no evidence that this measure has any effect on morbidity or mortality.
- At 36 weeks: Vaginal/rectal swab for group B streptococcus (GBS).

MNEMONIC

The ABCs of second- and third-trimester prenatal visits:

Amniotic fluid leakage?
Bleeding vaginally?
Contractions?
Dysuria?
Edema?
Fetal movement?

QUESTION

A 20-year-old woman presents after several days of ↑ right lower abdominal pain. Her LMP was >6 weeks; a urine pregnancy test is ⊕. Pelvic ultrasound reveals an empty uterus and ectopic tubal pregnancy with visible fetal pole, a tubal mass size of 2.0 cm, and no cardiac activity. How should she be treated?

Counseling

- **Second trimester:**
    - Nutrition, weight gain, and exercise recommendations.
    - Ongoing screening for domestic violence.
    - Education on maternal physiologic changes.
    - Influenza vaccine when seasonally available.
- **Third trimester:** As above, plus the following.
    - **Fetal kick counts:** To monitor fetal well-being.
    - **Travel:** Caution patients to avoid airline travel after 35 to 36 weeks.
    - **Sex:** Sexual activity may stimulate uterine contractions, but is safe in uncomplicated pregnancies with intact membranes.
    - **Work:** Most women are eligible for disability or family leave for the last 3 to 4 weeks of pregnancy. Patients should also avoid excessive exertion.
    - **Labor plans:** Discuss emotional support (including plans for a doula if available), anesthesia options, fetal monitoring during labor, the labor process, and orientation to the hospital or birth center.
    - **Postpartum birth control:** Discuss options; obtain signed consent for tubal ligation if desired.
    - **Breastfeeding:** Encourage all patients to try breastfeeding. Inform patients about the advantages of breastfeeding for the infant and for the mother.
    - **Other postpartum measures:** Discuss routine postpartum and newborn care as well as postpartum follow-up.

Fetal Development

Table 16.3 lists significant milestones associated with second- and third-trimester fetal development.

Antenatal Testing

Methods and indications for antenatal testing are as follows.
- **Biophysical profile (BPP):** Series of biophysical variables measured by ultrasound that, taken together, can help predict fetal well-being. The scoring includes the following criteria:
    - **Fetal tone:** Two points for movement extension and flexion of a joint, including opening and closing a hand, in 30 minutes.

ANSWER

Administer methotrexate with serial serum β-hCG levels (to ensure resolution of the tubal pregnancy). If methotrexate is unsuccessful or there are signs of hemodynamic instability, immediate surgical intervention is indicated.

TABLE 16.3.   Second- and Third-Trimester Milestones

WEEK	MILESTONES
18	Sleep/wake cycles, hair growth, egg development in females, fully formed placenta
20	Rapid brain and bone growth; testicular descent in males; thumb sucking
22	Continuing growth; ability to hear maternal sounds
24	Tooth buds; beginning of lung maturation
26	Brain growth; eyes open
28	Rhythmic breathing motions; disappearance of lanugo; fat accumulation
30	Head hair develops; lack of space "fetal position"; brain development
32	Continued brain growth; immune system development
34	Vertex position; lungs fully mature
36	Descent into the maternal pelvis begins
38	Vernix (sebaceous secretion protecting the skin from the amniotic fluid) is gone

- **Fetal movements:** Two points for two episodes of gross limb or body movements in 30 minutes.
- **Fetal breathing motions:** Two points for one or more episodes of >20 seconds in 30 minutes.
- **Nonstress test (NST) assessment of fetal heart rate:** Two points in a term pregnancy for a "reactive" NST (two accelerations of 15 bpm lasting 15 seconds during a 20-minute period).
- **Measurement of amniotic fluid index (AFI):** Two points for one or more fluid pockets >2 cm vertically.
- **Modified BPP:** Consists of NST and AFI; currently indicated on a biweekly basis after 36 to 37 weeks of gestation for pregnancies complicated by gestational diabetes, a hypertensive disorder, multiple gestation, cholestasis of pregnancy, poly- or oligohydramnios, preeclampsia, or other serious medical or obstetrical conditions.
  - An abnormal NST/AFI should be followed by a full BPP.
  - If the BPP is normal (10/10), the NST/AFI should be repeated in 2 to 3 days. If the BPP is 8/10 due to inadequate fluid, rule out ruptured membranes, hydrate, and repeat the NST/AFI in 2 to 3 days.
  - A BPP <8/10 with adequate amniotic fluid indicates a pregnancy at risk for fetal asphyxia. The patient should be admitted for observation, a BPP should be repeated, and a contraction stress test (CST) should be conducted (see below).
  - **CST:** A CST is performed to evaluate fetal ability to tolerate labor. External fetal heart monitors are placed, and either nipple stimulation or IV Pitocin is used to stimulate uterine contractions until either three strong uterine contractions occur in 10 minutes with no decelerations in fetal heart rate **or** >2 fetal heart rate decelerations occur.
  - One fetal heart rate deceleration associated with uterine contraction is considered an equivocal test and should be repeated.
  - A ⊕ CST is a contraindication to labor, and operative delivery should be considered.

SECOND- AND THIRD-TRIMESTER ISSUES

Third-Trimester Bleeding

Third-trimester bleeding most commonly results from placenta previa, placental abruption, and vasa previa. Table 16.4 outlines the etiologies, presentation, risk factors, and treatment of these conditions. Low-lying placentas (ie, a placenta in the lower uterine segment, but not covering or immediately adjacent to the os) are also at ↑ risk for bleeding (Figure 16.3).

Intrauterine Growth Restriction

Fetal weight below the 10th percentile for gestational age. Etiologies for true growth restriction are classified as fetal, maternal, or placental. Fetal factors include congenital anomalies, genetic syndromes, and multiple gestations; maternal factors include substance use disorder, tobacco and alcohol use, poor nutrition, hypoxemia, thrombotic and hypertensive disorders, and infections. Placental causes include abruption, hematoma, structural anomalies, and a two-vessel cord.

Symptoms/Exam

Uterine fundal measurements >2 cm less than expected for gestational age; confirm with ultrasound. If dates are unknown, serial ultrasounds may be needed every 2 weeks for evaluation.

TABLE 16.4. Presentation and Management of Third-Trimester Bleeding

CAUSE	DEFINITION	PRESENTATION	RISK FACTORS	MANAGEMENT
Placenta previa	Placental tissue completely or partially covering the internal cervical os Diagnosed by ultrasound	Asymptomatic, or presents with generally painless vaginal bleeding late in the second or third trimester Incidence is 1 in 4000 pregnancies	Advanced maternal age, multiparity, multiple gestation, uterine anomalies, prior uterine surgery May be complicated by placenta accreta (placenta ingrown into the uterine wall)	**If no bleeding:** Complete pelvic rest (no intercourse, tampons, or douching) until resolution of the previa is confirmed on serial ultrasounds or until cesarean delivery **If actively bleeding:** Admit and stabilize the mother; immediate C-section delivery if fetal/maternal status is nonreassuring **If bleeding resolves:** Conservative inpatient management with bed rest, corticosteroids, and serial ultrasounds; C-section once fetal lung maturity is confirmed at approximately 34 weeks
Placental abruption	Separation of the placenta prior to delivery of the infant An **obstetric emergency;** second-trimester abruption is associated with an extremely poor fetal prognosis	Constant severe uterine contractions ± vaginal bleeding (80%); CBC and coags may suggest occult bleeding or consumptive coagulopathy; nonreassuring fetal heart tracing Partial abruption may be difficult to distinguish from early labor Diagnosis is clinical; ultrasound is insufficiently sensitive to rule out abruption	Abdominal trauma, maternal hypertension, smoking, advanced maternal age, thrombophilic disease, ↑ parity, cocaine or methamphetamine use, polyhydramnios with sudden rupture of membranes, preterm **premature rupture of membranes** (PROM), multiple gestation, previous abruption	Stabilize the mother (IVs, type and cross, transfuse PRN); continuous fetal monitoring **If nonreassuring maternal/ fetal status:** Immediate C-section **If term and stable:** May deliver vaginally in the OR **If preterm and stable:** Inpatient conservative management
Vasa previa	Amniotic blood vessels presenting in front of the fetal head	Painless vaginal bleeding with ROM, often with fetal heart rate anomalies (a sinusoidal pattern is classic)	Low-lying or multilobed placentas; multiple gestations; in vitro fertilization	**If term and/or unstable:** Immediate C-section **If preterm and stable:** Inpatient conservative management; C-section when fetal lungs are mature Transvaginal ultrasound with color Doppler and/or Apt/ Kleihauer-Betke tests to determine the origin of bleeding if the diagnosis is unclear Rule out DIC

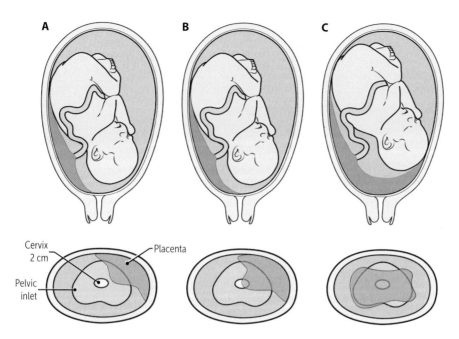

FIGURE 16.3. **Placenta previa.** (A) Marginal placenta previa. (B) Partial placenta previa. (C) Complete placenta previa. (Reproduced with permission from USMLE-Rx.com.)

Diagnosis

- Detailed fetal anatomic surveys by ultrasound can confirm the diagnosis, distinguish symmetric from asymmetric growth restriction, and evaluate for placental causes of intrauterine growth restriction (IUGR).
- Determine fetal karyotype, especially in severe cases and/or those associated with polyhydramnios.
- Obtain maternal serum infection titers if rubella, CMV, or syphilis is suspected.
- Doppler flow velocimetry of the umbilical artery can determine the systolic-to-diastolic ratio to rule out placental insufficiency.

Management

- Give corticosteroids for lung maturity if the fetus is preterm; follow with antenatal testing.
- Deliver by 40 weeks or sooner if there is evidence of placental insufficiency or non-reassuring antenatal testing.

Gestational Diabetes Mellitus (GDM)

Glucose intolerance beginning or first recognized during pregnancy. Women with a family history of diabetes and a personal history of glucose intolerance, polycystic ovarian syndrome (PCOS), obesity, glucocorticoid use, or prior macrosomic infants are at high risk. Hispanic, Native American, and African American women are also at ↑ risk.

Symptoms/Exam

Often asymptomatic. May present with polydipsia/polyuria or frequent infections, especially UTIs or yeast infections, obesity and acanthosis nigricans (see the Endocrinology chapter).

Diagnosis

- Screen everyone at 24 to 28 weeks with a 1-hour 50-g OGTT. Screen earlier in high-risk patients. If ⊕ (>140 mg/dL), follow up with a 3-hour tolerance test within 1 week.

KEY FACT

Any one of the diagnostic criteria for GDM is sufficient to make the diagnosis.

QUESTION

A 35-year-old G8P6 with no history of prenatal care presents to labor and delivery complaining of heavy vaginal bleeding. Her BP is 90/60 mm Hg, pulse 115 bpm, and temperature 37°C (98.6°F); a fetal strip shows ↓ variability and tachycardia. The patient has a scar from a prior C-section and has a steady flow of bright red blood from her vagina. How should she be treated?

Diagnostic criteria:

- Random blood glucose >200 mg/dL on two separate occasions **or**
- Fasting blood glucose >126 mg/dL on two separate occasions **or**
- A 100-g OGTT with abnormal values: >95 mg/dL fasting, >180 mg/dL at 1 hour, >155 mg/dL at 2 hours, or >140 mg/dL at 3 hours.

Management

- Offer nutritional counseling. Aim for 30 kcal/kg/day in women of normal weight, with carbohydrates no more than 40% of total caloric intake.
- Encourage regular blood sugar monitoring and exercise regimens; offer diabetic education.
- If fasting blood glucose is >95 mg/dL **or** postprandial glucose is >130 mg/dL on >2 occasions, start insulin (bedtime NPH for high fasting glucose at a starting dose of 0.2 U/kg; meal time regular/lispro for high postprandial glucose at a starting dose of 1.0-1.5 U/10 g of carbohydrates).
- **Peripartum management:** IV saline, NPO, and hourly blood glucose monitoring with a goal of 70 to 110 mg/dL. Most laboring diabetic patients do not need insulin.
- **Postpartum management:** Continue diet and exercise counseling, weight control, and diabetic education, as women with GDM have a significantly ↑ risk of type 2 DM. Check a 2-hour 75-g glucose tolerance test 6 weeks postpartum, and check HbA$_{1c}$ yearly thereafter.

Complications

Preeclampsia, polyhydramnios, fetal macrosomia with ↑ risk of birth trauma/operative delivery, neonatal metabolic complications and ↑ perinatal morbidity, subsequent maternal development of type 2 DM.

Macrosomia

Fetal weight at term exceeding 4.5 kg. Incidence is roughly 9% in the United States. May be associated with maternal DM and congenital anomalies, although many cases of macrosomia are simply constitutionally large infants.

Symptoms/Exam

Maternal impression of ↑ fetal weight; uterine fundal height >2 cm greater than the number of weeks of gestation.

Diagnosis

Clinical assessment by Leopold maneuvers; ultrasound (fetal abdominal circumference is the most accurate parameter).

Management

- Maintain tight control of maternal diabetes if applicable.
- Induction or elective C-section at term should be considered only in severe cases.
- In the case of vaginal births, prepare for shoulder dystocia.

Complications

Shoulder dystocia, maternal traumatic injury; ↑ morbidity is associated with a fetal weight >4 kg.

Polyhydramnios

An accumulation of excess amniotic fluid. Affects 0.2% to 1.6% of pregnancies, with potential causes including fetal malformations (especially those that cause problems with fetal breathing or swallowing), fetal anemia, maternal DM, and multiple gestations.

Symptoms/Exam: Presents with a uterine size measuring large for dates; may be accompanied by ↓ fetal movement.

MNEMONIC

Cornerstones of GDM management:
DIABETIC

Diet
Information
Antenatal testing
Baby growth monitoring
Exercise
Test home blood glucose
Insulin
Check postpartum blood glucose

KEY FACT

Treatment of GDM helps prevent macrosomia, dystocia, assisted deliveries, and maternal preeclampsia.

KEY FACT

Maternal assessment is a more accurate measure of fetal weight than Leopold maneuvers or ultrasound.

ANSWER

Initial management of this patient, who has a presumed diagnosis of placenta previa, includes placement of two large-bore IVs, typing and crossing of 2 to 4 units of blood, a call to anesthesia for a stat C-section, and expeditious ultrasound determination of placental position where possible.

Diagnosis

- Ultrasound to evaluate AFI, as well as fetal surveillance for fetal GI obstruction (eg, esophageal or duodenal atresia or gastroschisis) or neurologic abnormalities.
- Glucose challenge test if not already done.
- Kleihauer-Betke test to look for fetomaternal hemorrhage.
- Maternal serology for infectious agents and hereditary metabolic abnormalities; amniocentesis for karyotype analysis if severe.

Management

- Monitor AFI every 1 to 3 weeks.
- Amnioreduction is appropriate for cases that are symptomatic and severe.
- Give indomethacin in preparation for delivery if severe and/or preterm and give steroids to accelerate fetal lung maturity.

Complications

Maternal respiratory compromise, preterm labor, preterm PROM, fetal malposition, umbilical cord accidents, postpartum hemorrhage.

Oligohydramnios

Inadequate amniotic fluid. Incidence of approximately 1 in 200 pregnancies. Oligo-hydramnios is usually idiopathic, but can be asszociated with the following:
- Uteroplacental insufficiency (maternal hypertension, medications, placental abruption or infarction).
- Fetal factors, such as intrauterine fetal demise, chromosomal/congenital anomalies, and twin-twin transfusion.
- Postdate pregnancy and unrecognized rupture of amniotic membranes should also be considered.

Symptoms/Exam

Presents with a uterine size measuring small for dates and ↓ fetal movement.

Diagnosis

Inadequate AFI measured on ultrasound; consider amniocentesis for karyotype analysis.

Management

- Maternal hydration; amnioinfusion if necessary for adequate ultrasound assessment of the fetus. Antepartum surveillance with biweekly AFI measurements.
- Labor induction is indicated at term or earlier if there is evidence of nonreassuring fetal status.

Complications

Meconium aspiration, cord accidents, fetal growth restriction.

Preterm Labor

Uterine contractions leading to cervical change prior to 37 weeks of gestation. Approximately 10% of births in the United States are preterm. Preterm labor is the second leading cause of perinatal mortality (after congenital anomalies) and is the leading cause of perinatal morbidity. See the Mnemonic for risk factors.

Diagnosis

- UA and culture to rule out pyelonephritis; sterile speculum exam to rule out preterm PROM (pooling/ferning/nitrazine).
- Obtain cervical swabs for gonorrhea, chlamydia, and bacterial vaginosis.
- Obtain a fetal fibronectin (fFN) specimen between 24 and 34 weeks.
- Ultrasound to measure cervical length.
- Serial sterile vaginal exams if membranes are unruptured to evaluate cervical change.

KEY FACT

Most idiopathic cases of polyhydramnios resolve spontaneously.

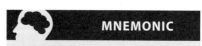

MNEMONIC

Risk factors for preterm labor:
PIMS

Placental abruption, **P**olyhydramnios, **P**lacenta **P**revia
Infection (bacteriuria/pyelonephritis, STIs, bacterial vaginosis, periodontal disease), **I**nadequate cervix
Multiple gestation, **M**ultiple years (advanced maternal age)
Socioeconomic: **S**ingle, **S**ad (anxiety/depression), **S**tress, or **S**ubstance use, tobacco, poor nutrition, African American, extreme physical exertion

MNEMONIC

Contraindications to tocolysis:

OH SH**

Pregnancy **O**ver (intrauterine fetal demise or lethal anomaly)

Hypertension (severe preeclampsia or eclampsia)

Small baby (IUGR)

Hemorrhage (especially with maternal hemodynamic instability)

Infection (chorioamnionitis)

Troubled baby (nonreassuring fetal heart tracing)

Management

- **Initial management of preterm contractions:** See Figure 16.4.
- **Active management of preterm labor:**
  - Give antibiotics to treat any UTI or genital infections as indicated; GBS prophylaxis.
  - Administer corticosteroids (betamethasone 12 mg once per day × 2; maximum benefit is derived 48 hours after the first dose) if prior to 34 weeks' gestation.
  - Bed rest (unproven benefit); tocolytics prolong labor 48 hours to 7 days, but have not been shown to improve outcomes (Table 16.5). They are standard of care and should be used to give time for the administration of steroids, transfer to an appropriate facility, or resolution of a known cause of preterm labor (ie, trauma, abdominal surgery).

Premature Rupture of Membranes

Rupture of amniotic membranes before the onset of uterine contractions occurs in 1 in 10 pregnancies. Most patients will enter labor spontaneously within 24 hours of PROM. Risk factors are similar to those for preterm labor and include genital tract infection, a prior history of PROM, smoking, cervical insufficiency, polyhydramnios, multiple gestation, and antepartum hemorrhage.

- **Symptoms/Exam:** Presents with leaking or gushing of clear fluid from the vagina and pooling of amniotic fluid in the vaginal vault. Avoid a digital cervical exam until the patient is in labor!
- **Diagnosis:** ⊕ **nitrazine testing** (blood or semen may also turn nitrazine paper ⊕); **ferning** of amniotic fluid; pooling of fluid in the vaginal vault.
- **Management:** Expectant management for 24 hours, after which labor should be induced if it has not started spontaneously. An algorithm for the treatment of PROM is outlined in Figure 16.5.
- **Complications:** Chorioamnionitis, endometritis, preterm delivery.

Hypertensive Disorders of Pregnancy

A spectrum of complex multisystem diseases of uncertain etiology that complicate up to one in five pregnancies and are associated with greatly ↑ fetal and maternal morbidity and mortality. Milder forms (eg, transient gestational hypertension) are often a precursor to more severe forms (eg, preeclampsia).

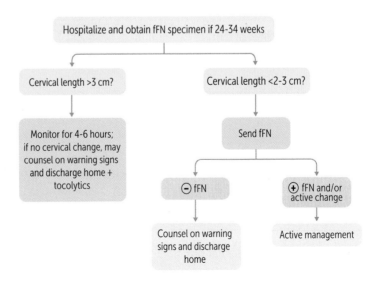

FIGURE 16.4. Treatment of preterm contractions. (Reproduced with permission from USMLE-Rx.com.)

TABLE 16.5.   **Guidelines for Treatment With Tocolytics**

MEDICATION	CLASS	LOADING DOSE	MAINTENANCE DOSE	SIDE EFFECTS/COMPLICATIONS
Terbutaline	B_2-adrenergic agonist	2.5-5.0 µg IV	Up to 25 µ/min or until contractions abate	Contraindicated in women with cardiac disease
Magnesium sulfate		4-6 g IV	IV infusion 2-4 g/hr; monitor serum magnesium levels and DTRs	Magnesium toxicity (loss of DTRs, respiratory paralysis, cardiac arrest)
Nifedipine	Calcium channel blocker	30 mg PO	20 mg q 4-8 hr	Fewest side effects
Atosiban	Oxytocin receptor antagonist	Not available in the United States	Not available in the United States	Considered first-line treatment outside the United States owing to favorable side effects; efficacy is similar to that of terbutaline

Transient Gestational Hypertension

BP >140/90 mm Hg on two occasions 6 hours apart, with onset after 20 weeks of pregnancy, in the absence of other causative factors. Risk factors include a prior or family history of hypertension.

Diagnosis

- Elevated BP, defined above.
- Obtain CMP, CBC, and urine dipsticks to test for proteinuria. Consider 24-hour urine collection for baseline protein level in case preeclampsia is suspected later in pregnancy.

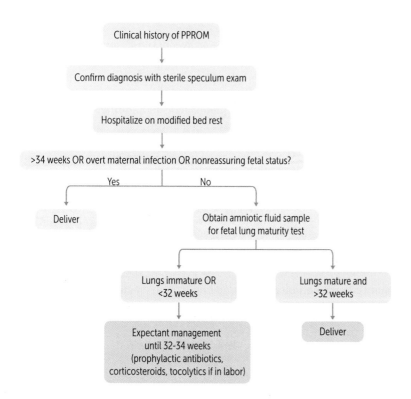

FIGURE 16.5.   **Treatment of premature rupture of membranes.** (Reproduced with permission from USMLE-Rx.com.)

Management

- Diet and exercise counseling.
- Labetalol or methyldopa if systolic BP persistently elevated above 160 mm Hg.
- Antepartum NST/AFIs.
- In severe cases, consider delivery by 38 to 39 weeks.

Preeclampsia

Persistent high BP that develops **after 20 weeks of pregnancy** or during the postpartum period that is associated with proteinuria or the new development of ↓ blood platelets, kidney or liver problems, fluid in the lungs, or signs of brain dysfunction such as seizures and/or visual disturbances. Risk factors include primigravidity, a history of preeclampsia, obesity, preexisting hypertension or renal disease, multiple gestations, diabetes, advanced maternal age, antiphospholipid antibody syndrome, chronic autoimmune disease, and a partner with a prior history of fathering a preeclamptic pregnancy.

Symptoms/Exam

May present with edema, blurry vision, epigastric pain, nausea, headache, and hyperactive deep tendon reflexes (DTRs).

Diagnosis

BP >140/90 mm Hg. Can be diagnosed without proteinuria (>300 mg/24 hours with onset). Preeclampsia with severe features is diagnosed in the presence of any of the following: BP >160/110 mm Hg, CNS or pulmonary symptoms, thrombocytopenia, IUGR, hepatic involvement, renal insufficiency, cerebral or visual disturbances, oliguria, or proteinuria >5 g/24 hours.

Screen with a urine dipstick for proteinuria on each visit; obtain 24-hour urine protein if dipstick is elevated. LFTs, CBC with smear, creatinine, uric acid.

Management

- Give labetalol, hydralazine, or nifedipine to control BP; supplement with antepartum surveillance and frequent weight checks. Deliver at term; consider magnesium sulfate ($MgSO_4$) for seizure prophylaxis.
- **Preeclampsia with severe features:**
  - Immediate delivery with continuous fetal monitoring; consider a 48-hour delay only to give steroids for fetal lung maturity.
  - Restrict fluids and monitor urine output; control BP with hydralazine or labetalol; give $MgSO_4$ for seizure prophylaxis; monitor magnesium q 4 to 6 h; repeat LFTs and creatinine. Aggressive furosemide treatment is appropriate in the presence of pulmonary edema.
- Daily low-dose aspirin to help prevent preeclampsia in very high-risk women, and the use of magnesium sulfate for severe preeclampsia, eclampsia, or HELLP syndrome.

Complications

Pulmonary edema, neurologic deterioration, coma, seizure, stroke.

Eclampsia

- **Onset of tonic-clonic seizures in a preeclamptic patient in the absence of any other cause.** Approximately 1 in 50 patients with preeclampsia with severe features patients will progress to seizures.
- **Management:** Check ABCs; stabilize the mother; administer $MgSO_4$ (6 g IV) for seizure control accompanied by fetal monitoring. If $MgSO_4$ is not effective, consider benzodiazepines.

KEY FACT

Management of preeclamptic patients should include frequent assessment of DTRs and pulmonary status, as neurologic complications and pulmonary edema can progress rapidly.

KEY FACT

Treat magnesium toxicity with calcium gluconate if patient has a PIV, and with calcium chloride if the patient has central line access.

KEY FACT

In patients with prior history of preeclampsia or other risk factors, 60 to 80 mg daily aspirin starting at 12-weeks' gestation may help prevent preeclampsia.

HELLP Syndrome

Hypertensive disorder characterized by **H**emolysis, **E**levated **L**iver enzymes, and **L**ow **P**latelets. Incidence is approximately 1 in 1000 pregnancies. Develops in up to 10% to 20% of women with preeclampsia. Usually diagnosed in the third trimester but may present earlier or even postpartum.

Symptoms/Exam

May present with nausea/vomiting, edema, headache and blurry vision, and ↓ urine output.

Differential

Acute fatty liver of pregnancy; gastroenteritis or appendicitis; cholecystic or hepatic disease; HUS/TTP.

Diagnosis

- Look for the presence of preeclampsia.
- **Labs:** Hemolytic anemia, platelet count <100,000, and either LDH >600 and total bilirubin >1.2 or AST >70. Creatinine monitoring for kidney function.
- **Imaging:** Obtain CT/MRI if hepatic infarction, rupture, or hematoma is suspected.

Management

- Hospitalize and stabilize the mother; assess the fetus.
- Consider corticosteroids for fetal lung maturity if <34 weeks.
- Hypertensive medications to control maternal BP; platelet transfusion if platelet count is <20,000 or there is maternal bleeding.
- Expeditious delivery is indicated at >34 weeks of gestation and in the setting of nonreassuring fetal status or severe maternal disease to prevent complications (see the Mnemonic).

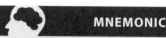

MNEMONIC

Complications of HELLP syndrome:

The 4 H's

Hepatic failure
Hepatic infarction
Hematoma
Hepatic rupture

Cholestasis of Pregnancy

A syndrome of pruritus and ↑ serum bile acids that typically develops after 30 weeks of gestation. Cholestasis of pregnancy is associated with fetal prematurity and sudden intrauterine demise; its pathogenesis is unknown.

- **Symptoms/Exam:** Presents with intolerable itching, especially on the palms and soles, that usually worsens at night. May present with jaundice.
- **Diagnosis:** Bile acids. Total bilirubin, alkaline phosphatase, and AST/ALT may also be high.
- **Management:** Synthetic bile acids; cholestyramine; hydroxyzine for symptomatic relief. Deliver by 38 weeks or sooner if severe, and fetal lung maturity is established.

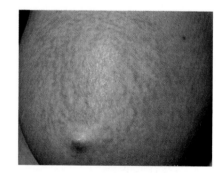

FIGURE 16.6. **Pruritic urticarial papules and plaques of pregnancy.** (Reproduced with permission from Wolff K, et al. *Fitzpatrick's Dermatology in General Medicine,* 7th ed. New York: McGraw-Hill, 2008.)

Pruritic Urticarial Papules and Plaques of Pregnancy

The most common dermatosis of pregnancy, with an incidence of 1 in 160. The cause is unknown. Usual onset is in the late third trimester. There is no associated risk of ↑ fetal/maternal morbidity.

- **Symptoms/Exam:** Presents with extreme pruritus, with erythematous papules coalescing to plaques within striae (Figure 16.6). Usually starts on the abdomen and spreads to the extremities.
- **Differential:** Pemphigoid gestationis, viral syndromes, allergic reactions, cholestasis.
- **Management:** Topical steroids; antihistamines for symptomatic relief.

 QUESTION

A 36-year-old G3P1 with a history of gestational hypertension presents to labor and delivery at 36 weeks' gestation with a complaint of intense frontal headaches, progressive pedal edema, and nausea over the last week. Her BP is 176/92 mm Hg, her cervix is favorable, and her urine dip reveals 2+ proteinuria. External fetal monitoring shows a reactive strip. How should she be managed?

Melasma

Hyperpigmentation related to normal hormonal changes in pregnancy. Also caused by OCPs. See the Dermatology chapter for management.

Breech Presentation

Nonvertex presentation of the fetus occurs in 3% to 4% pregnancies at term, with the frequency ↓ as the pregnancy approaches term. Risk factors include placental or uterine anomalies, fetal anatomic anomalies, multiple gestation, poly- or oligohydramnios, and a short umbilical cord. Frank, complete, and footling breech presentations are illustrated in Figure 16.7.

Symptoms/Exam

- The fetal head is not palpable on cervical exam.
- Breech position is found by Leopold maneuvers.

Diagnosis

Confirm the position with ultrasound.

Management

- **If diagnosed prior to onset of labor,** external cephalic version at 36 to 39 weeks.
- **If cephalic version is unsuccessful,** schedule a C-section at 39 to 40 weeks if the hospital is unable to perform a vaginal breech delivery.
- **If presentation is in active labor,** proceed to C-section.
- Women with a strong preference for vaginal delivery may, in consultation with a physician who is well trained in breech vaginal deliveries, pursue that option.

Complications

Labor dystocia; maternal and/or fetal birth trauma. External cephalic version is associated with a risk of placental abruption, cord accident, or fetal distress.

Multiple-Gestation Pregnancies

Although the incidence of monozygotic (identical) twins has remained constant at roughly 1 in 250, dizygotic (fraternal) twinning varies from 1 in 30 to 1 in 100, depending on the population. Risk factors include high parity, family history of twins, assisted reproductive technology, advanced maternal age.

Symptoms/Exam

- Presents with ↑ uterine size for dates and >1 fetal heart tone heard on Doppler.
- Associated with prolonged or more severe nausea than is typical with a singleton pregnancy.

Diagnosis

- Early ultrasound to establish amnionicity/chorionicity; level 2 ultrasound to detect congenital anomalies.
- Serial ultrasound should be obtained through the second and third trimesters every 4 to 6 weeks (for uncomplicated twin pregnancies) to look for discordant growth or twin-twin transfusion problems.

Management

- Recommend an extra 300 kcal daily over singleton pregnancies and a 35- to 45-pound weight gain by term for uncomplicated twin pregnancies.
- Antepartum testing with biweekly **NST/AFI** after 36 weeks has not been shown to be effective, but is nevertheless recommended by the American College of Obstetricians and Gynecologists (ACOG).

MNEMONIC

Complications of multiple-gestation pregnancies:

PAPA PIG

Preterm labor
Antepartum hemorrhage
Preeclampsia
Abortion (intrauterine fetal demise)
Polyhydramnios
IUGR
Gestational diabetes

KEY FACT

If division of the embryo occurs . . .
- Up to 3 days after fertilization: Diamniotic/dichorionic
- Between 4 and 8 days: Diamniotic/monochorionic
- Between 8 and 12 days: Monoamniotic/monochorionic (high risk for morbidity/mortality)
- After 13 days: Conjoined twins (extremely high risk; refer to a perinatologist)

ANSWER

Severe preeclampsia at term requires hospital admission, obstetrical consultation, initiation of 24-hour urine collection and GBS swab if this has not previously been done, induction of labor, and IV magnesium for seizure prophylaxis. If <34 weeks, treat with betamethasone as well.

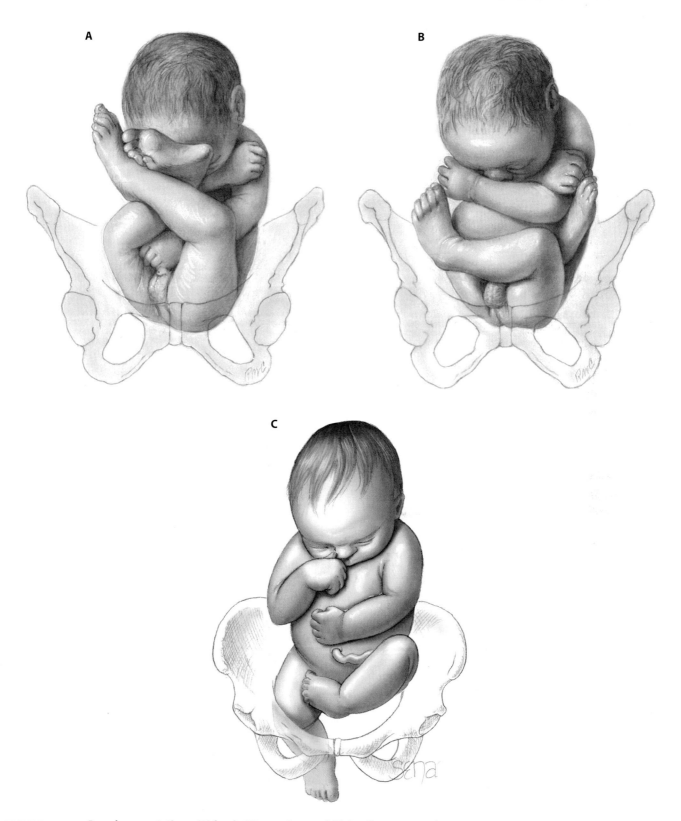

FIGURE 16.7.   **Breech presentations: (A) frank, (B) complete, and (C) footling presentations.** (Reproduced with permission from Cunningham FG, et al. *Williams Obstetrics*, 23rd ed. New York: McGraw-Hill.)

- Perform elective induction/C-section at 37 to 38 weeks if fetal lungs are mature; epidural anesthesia and continuous monitoring are recommended.
- Route of delivery depends on presentation, risk factors, and maternal preference. If twin A delivers vaginally, the position of twin B should be evaluated by ultrasound prior to delivery.

Complications

↑ risk of all pregnancy complications except macrosomia and postterm pregnancy. Preterm delivery is most common.

MANAGEMENT OF LABOR AND DELIVERY

Labor is separated into three stages: cervical dilation and effacement, descent and delivery of the fetus, and delivery of the placenta. Initial assessment of a patient presenting in labor should include the following:

- Brief physical exam, including a sterile vaginal exam for cervical dilation and effacement (unless ROM is suspected).
- Assessment of fetal presentation, position, and station.
- Determination of amniotic membrane status (intact vs ruptured); sterile speculum exam if ROM/PROM is suspected (defer the digital vaginal exam).
- Assessment of the quality and quantity of uterine contractions (an adequate number of uterine contractions in active labor is defined as 3-5 regular intense contractions every 10 minutes, each >60 Montevideo units of pressure above baseline).
- Assessment of vaginal bleeding.
- Initial assessment of fetal heart rate tracing with NST.

Stage I: Cervical Dilation and Effacement

Routine expectant management of normal stage I labor includes vaginal exams every 4 hours to monitor progress, intermittent fetal heart rate monitoring (every 15 minutes during active and transitional phases), and analgesia as needed. Labor can be plotted on a Friedman curve to monitor progress and facilitate prompt recognition of a protraction or arrest disorder (Figure 16.8). Phases within stage I are:

- **Latent phase (cervical dilation 0-3 cm):** Characterized by loss of the cervical mucous plug ("bloody show") and by slow, irregular uterine contractions. May last for days in nulliparous women and up to 14 hours in multiparous women.
- **Active phase (cervical dilation 3-9 cm):** Characterized by increasingly intense, regular uterine contractions, usually with spontaneous ROM. Cervical dilation should progress at a rate of ~ 1 cm/hr in nulliparas and at ~ 1.2 cm/hr in multiparas.
- **Transition (cervical dilation 9-10 cm):** Characterized by continued intense uterine contractions; cervical dilation may slow during this phase.

Stage II: Descent and Delivery of the Fetus

Routine expectant management of a normal second stage of labor includes serial vaginal exams to monitor progress, more frequent fetal heart rate monitoring (every 5 minutes), analgesia as needed, and preparation for delivery of the fetus. The second stage is characterized by an ↑ in bloody show, continuing intense uterine contractions, intrapelvic pressure, and a maternal urge to push. Accurate assessment of fetal position and station is important for anticipation of potential problems during stage II. Additional considerations are as follows:

- **Duration:** Stage II should last no longer than 1 hour in multiparas and 2 hours in nulliparas, although the presence of epidural/spinal anesthesia may prolong the second stage.

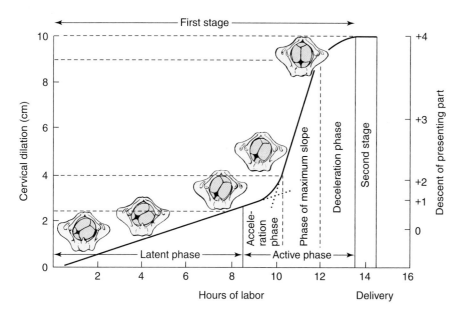

FIGURE 16.8. **Friedman curve showing normal progression of stage I labor in nulliparous women.** (Reproduced with permission from Morgan Jr GE, Mikhail MS, Murray MJ. *Clinical Anesthesiology,* 4th ed. New York: McGraw-Hill, 2006.)

■ **Assessment of fetal position:** The fetus undergoes a series of position changes during the end of stage I and stage II as it progresses through the birth canal (Figure 16.9). Most babies are born either right or left occiput anterior (ROA or LOA). Occiput posterior (OP) babies are associated with protracted labors and with an ↑ likelihood of maternal birth trauma. The key to determining position lies in palpation of the sutures of the fetal head.

■ **Assessment of fetal station** (3+, 3, 2, 1, 0, −1, −2, −3): Refers to the relative position of the fetal head and maternal ischial spines in centimeters (0 = fetal head level with ischial spines).

Stage III: Delivery of the Placenta

The third stage of labor should last no longer than 30 minutes. Active management with oxytocin and controlled traction is associated with ↓ rates of postpartum hemorrhage. Signs of imminent placental delivery include cord lengthening, a gush of blood indicating placental separation, and a ↓ in uterine fundal height.

Fetal Monitoring

Assessment of fetal heart rate during labor is a controversial practice, but has become accepted as the standard of care. Initially developed in an attempt to ↓ the rate of cerebral palsy and hypoxic birth injury, continuous electronic fetal monitoring has not been shown to be of benefit, and in uncomplicated labor it is associated with ↑ risk of operative delivery. Intermittent fetal auscultation can replace continuous FHR assessment in institutions that have sufficient nursing staffing and training.

■ **Monitoring techniques:** Performed with an external ultrasound monitor or internal placement of fetal scalp electrodes (more accurate, but more invasive and requires ROM).

■ **Monitoring recommendations:**

■ **Intermittent auscultation or external fetal monitoring:** Appropriate for uncomplicated labors. Performed every 15 minutes in the active phase of stage I and every 5 minutes in stage II.

KEY FACT

OP babies are less likely to be born via normal spontaneous vaginal delivery and have an ↑ rate of C-section and assisted/operative deliveries.

KEY FACT

The cardinal movements of labor.

How to get engaged:
Descend to the floor.
Flex your knee.
Look down (internal rotation) at the ring you are about to give your beloved.
Extend your hand to give your beloved the ring.
Look up (external rotation) to see what the answer will be.
Straighten up (restitute) when the answer is yes!

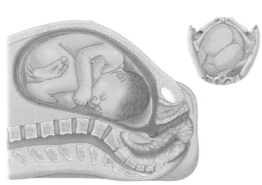

1. Head floating, before engagement

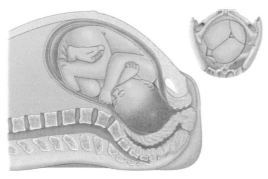

2. Engagement, descent, flexion

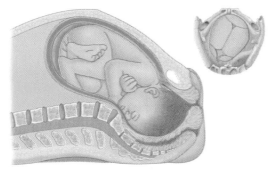

3. Further descent, internal rotation

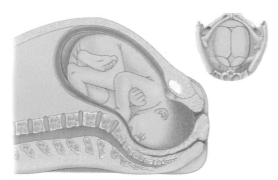

4. Complete rotation, beginning extension

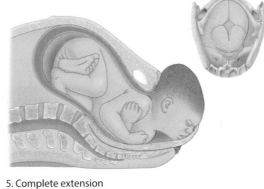

5. Complete extension

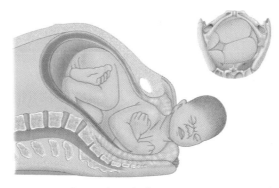

6. Restitution (external rotation)

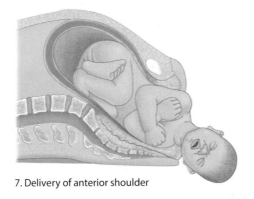

7. Delivery of anterior shoulder

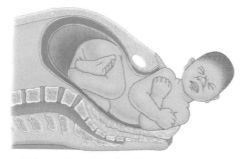

8. Delivery of posterior shoulder

FIGURE 16.9. Cardinal movements of labor. Cardinal movements consist of engagement, descent, flexion, internal rotation, extension, external rotation, restitution, and expulsion. (Reproduced with permission from Cunningham FG, et al. *Williams Obstetrics,* 22nd ed. New York: McGraw-Hill, 2005:418.)

- **Continuous external fetal monitoring:** Indicated if the mother is receiving IV Pitocin for labor induction or augmentation or with conditions known to be associated with ↑ fetal morbidity/mortality.
- **Continuous internal fetal monitoring:** Use if fetal heart rate tracing cannot be consistently followed with external monitoring or if fetal heart rate tracing is not reassuring.

- Categories of fetal heart tracing:
  - **Category 1, normal.** Baseline pulse of 110 to 160 bpm, with moderate variability. Early decelerations may be present, but no other decelerations. FHR accelerations may or may not be present.
  - **Category 2, indeterminate.** Any of the following may be present: Absent or minimal variability, marked variability, tachycardia, bradycardia without absent variability, absence of accelerations with stimulation, recurrent variable decelerations with minimal or moderate variability, recurrent late decelerations (Figure 16.10) with moderate variability, prolonged deceleration >2 minutes but <10 minutes, recurrent variable decelerations (Figure 16.11) with slow return to baseline or overshoot.
  - **Category 3, abnormal.** Either of the following: Sinusoidal pattern **or** absent variability with recurrent late decelerations or bradycardia.

Management of category 2 fetal heart rate tracing consists of IV fluid, moving the mother onto her left side, oxygen administration, discontinuation of exogenous Pitocin, and treatment of underlying conditions. An internal fetal scalp electrode should be placed for continuous accurate monitoring. Consider terbutaline administration to stop contractions. Consider warm saline amnioinfusion for concerning or recurrent decelerations on fetal heart tracing.

Category 3 fetal heart tracing is an indication for immediate delivery.

Fetal Heart Rate

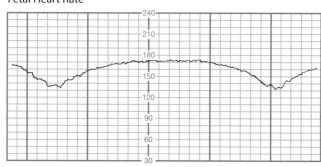

Tocometer

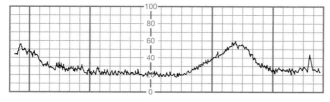

FIGURE 16.10.   Late decelerations on fetal heart rate tracing indicate uteroplacental insufficiency and fetal acidemia. Upper image shows a fetal heart rate with minimal variability and late decelerations reaching their nadir after maximal uterine contraction and slowly resolving. The bottom image displays a tocometer measuring the timing of uterine contractions. In this case, abruption was the cause and immediate C-section was performed. The umbilical artery pH was 7.05. (Reproduced with permission from Cunningham FG, Leveno KJ, Bloom SL, et al. *Williams Obstetrics,* 23rd ed. New York: McGraw-Hill, 2008.)

Fetal Heart Rate

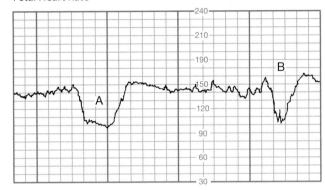

Tocometer

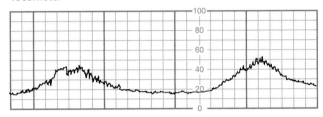

FIGURE 16.11. **Variable decelerations on fetal heart tracing suggest cord compression and are not an indication of fetal distress.** Top image shows FHR with steep decelerations that resolve rapidly. Bottom image shows tocometer indicating timing of uterine contractions. (Reproduced with permission from Cunningham FG, Leveno KJ, Bloom SL, et al. *Williams Obstetrics*, 23rd ed. New York: McGraw-Hill, 2008.)

Labor Arrest and Protraction Disorders

A protraction disorder is defined as slower-than-normal labor. Complete cessation of progress is termed arrest of labor.

Management of Stage I Protraction/Arrest

- Assess maternal/fetal well-being.
- Perform digital cervical exam every 1 to 2 hours.
- Perform amniotomy if membranes are still intact.
- Oxytocin administration: Indicated if uterine contractions are inadequate. Titrate the dose to effect.
- Intrauterine pressure catheter (IUPC): Recommended for greater accuracy of oxytocin titration.
- Adequate uterine contractions are defined as at least three contractions every 10 minutes, each more than 60 Montevideo units above baseline and lasting approximately 10 seconds (200 Montevideo units in a 10-minute period).
- Consider C-section in the setting of complete arrest despite 4 hours of adequate uterine contractions, especially in the setting of fetal intolerance of labor.

Management of Stage II Protraction/Arrest

- Observation is adequate as long as maternal/fetal status is reassuring and some progress has been made.
- Oxytocin administration with IUPC, as above, is appropriate in the presence of inadequate uterine forces.
- Attempt operative vaginal delivery (see below).
- Perform C-section if in complete arrest, operative vaginal delivery is unsuccessful, or in fetal intolerance of labor.

MNEMONIC

Causes of protraction and arrest disorders:

The 3 P's

Power (eg, hypocontractile uterine activity, epidural anesthesia, chorioamnionitis)

Passenger (eg, fetal macrosomia, malposition [especially occiput posterior fetus], postdate pregnancy)

Pelvis (eg, pelvic contraction, cephalopelvic disproportion, short maternal stature, obesity)

Pain Control During Labor and Delivery

Labor pain is caused primarily by distention of mechanoreceptors in the uterus and cervix during stage I and by stretching and/or tearing of the birth canal and pelvic ligaments during stage II. Fetal malpresentation and nulliparity are physiologic risk factors for ↑ pain, but fear or emotional distress can exacerbate pain as well. A feeling of control over the labor process can greatly improve patients' experience of labor; thus, early education about the labor process and pain control options, along with encouragement of maternal involvement in the decision-making process, is key. Treatment options are as follows.

- **Nonpharmacologic options:** Presence of a doula/labor support person, acupuncture, hypnosis, visualization, breathing exercises, family support, movement, bathing in warm water.
- **Pharmacologic options:** Vary according to stage.
    - **Stage I:**
        - Nalbuphine IV 10 to 20 mg q 3 to 4 hr.
        - Fentanyl 25 to 100 µg IV/IM q 1 to 2 hr.
        - Epidural anesthesia (continuous drip of local anesthetic and opiate, eg, bupivacaine and fentanyl). Requires bed rest, urinary catheter placement, and continuous fetal monitoring.
        - Spinal anesthesia (opioid injection alone during early labor, or combination opioid/local anesthetic later in labor and/or for C-section). Requires bed rest, urinary catheter placement, and continuous fetal monitoring.
    - **Stage II:**
        - Pudendal block (10 mL 1% lidocaine injected posterior to both ischial spines).
        - Local anesthetic into the perineum, especially if an episiotomy is to be performed.
        - Epidural/spinal anesthesia may be initiated during the second stage (see above), but is less desirable given the prolonged latency of medications and the potential for fetal respiratory depression.

Induction of Labor

Indicated when prolonging the pregnancy puts the mother, the fetus, or both at risk. The most common indication is for postterm pregnancy (40-42 weeks), but induction may be necessary at any gestational age. If possible, fetal lung maturity should be established either by accurate pregnancy dating or by amniocentesis, and, if necessary, corticosteroids should be administered for fetal lung maturity.

To choose a method for induction, check the Bishop score (Table 16.6).

- **Bishop score >6:** Associated with a higher chance of success. Start IV Pitocin; cervical ripening agents are not needed.

TABLE 16.6.   **The Bishop Scoring System**

CERVIX	SCORE			
	0	1	2	3
Position	Posterior	Midposition	Anterior	—
Consistency	Firm	Medium	Soft	—
Effacement	0-30	40-50	60-70	≥80
Dilation	Closed	1-2	3-4	≥5
Station	−3	−2	−1, 0	+1, +2

MNEMONIC

Contraindications to spinal/epidural:

BK PAIN

Blood pressure too low (uncorrected hypovolemia)
"**K**oagulopathy" (bleeding disorder)
Pressure (↑ ICP)
Anatomic back problems
Infection of the soft tissue overlying the epidural injection site
No (the patient refuses)

KEY FACT

Regional anesthesia:
- Does not lead to ↑ C-section rate, but does ↑ risk of vacuum or forceps delivery.
- Not statistically significantly different from childbirth without an epidural in terms of maternal satisfaction, ie, pain relief, long-term backache, or different APGAR scores.

- **Bishop score <6:** Consider a cervical ripening agent such as misoprostol and placement of a Foley bulb into the cervical os. Failure rate is 10% to 50%. Continuous fetal monitoring necessary throughout induction.

PERIPARTUM COMPLICATIONS

Group B Streptococcus (GBS) Infection

GBS is normal vaginal flora, but used to be the most common cause of neonatal sepsis. It is transmitted during passage through the birth canal. Risk factors for neonatal sepsis with GBS are preterm delivery, prolonged ROM, and maternal colonization with GBS.

Diagnosis

- Universal screening should be performed at 35 to 37 weeks.
- If GBS bacteriuria found on urine culture during this pregnancy, no need for vaginal swab, as the mother is considered ⊕.
- In threatened preterm labor, collect cultures and start treatment during tocolysis. If ⊖, discontinue treatment and rescreen at 35 to 37 weeks.

Management

See Figure 16.12 and Table 16.7.

Shoulder Dystocia

Failure of the fetal shoulders to deliver spontaneously 1 minute after the delivery of the baby's head, usually because the baby's anterior shoulder is stuck behind the maternal pubic bone. **Considered an obstetric emergency,** shoulder dystocia occurs in 0.5% to 2.9% of deliveries, with most cases affecting babies weighing >4 kg. Other risk factors include maternal obesity, maternal diabetes, and vacuum or forceps delivery.

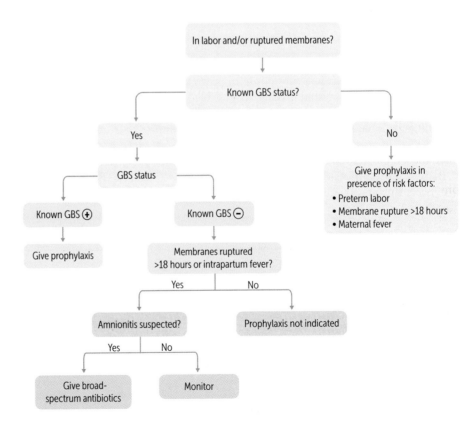

FIGURE 16.12. **Antibiotic prophylaxis for GBS infection.** (Reproduced with permission from USMLE-Rx.com.)

TABLE 16.7. **GBS Prophylaxis Regimens**

	MEDICATION	INITIAL DOSE	MAINTENANCE DOSE
Preferred regimen	Penicillin G	5 MU IV	2.5 MU IV q 4 hr until delivery
Alternative regimen	Ampicillin	2 g IV	1 g IV q 4 hr until delivery
Penicillin-allergic patients with low risk of anaphylaxis	Cefazolin	2 g IV	1 g q 8 hr until delivery
Penicillin-allergic patients with high risk of anaphylaxis	Clindamycin	900 mg IV	900 mg IV q 8 hr until delivery

- **Symptoms/Exam:** Anticipate shoulder dystocia if there is prolonged fetal descent and/or "turtling" of the fetal head.
- **Management:** See HELPER mnemonic.
- **Complications:** Fetal hypoxia, fetal clavicular fracture, Erb palsy, and maternal perineal laceration.

Genital Tract Lacerations

Injury to the birth canal during vaginal delivery is the one of the most common obstetric complications. Perineal midline tears are most common, but periurethral, labial, and cervical lacerations also occur frequently. Risk factors include primiparity, precipitous delivery, fetal macrosomia or malpresentation, operative vaginal delivery, and maternal connective tissue disorders.

Symptoms/Exam

Categorized by the extent of injury as follows:
- **First degree:** Laceration of the vaginal mucosa only.
- **Second degree:** Extension of the laceration into the vaginal deep tissue.
- **Third degree:** Extension of the laceration into the external rectal sphincter muscle.
- **Fourth degree:** Extension of the laceration through the rectal mucosa.

Management

Surgical repair. If minor, healing by 2° intention.

Complications

Postpartum hemorrhage, urinary or fecal incontinence, fistula formation.

Chorioamnionitis

Infection of the amniotic membranes. Also known as amnionitis or intrapartum fever. The most common pathogens are gram-negative rods and anaerobes (*Bacteroides, Mycoplasma, Ureaplasma, Gardnerella,* GBS). Risk factors include nulliparity, preterm or prolonged ROM, genital tract infections, internal monitoring, digital cervical exams in women with ruptured membranes, and meconium-stained amniotic fluid.
- **Symptoms/Exam:** Presents with maternal fever >38°C (100.4°F), uterine tenderness, and foul-smelling amniotic fluid. Exam reveals maternal and/or fetal tachycardia.
- **Diagnosis:** CBC; culture of amniotic fluid.
- **Management:** Treat with broad-spectrum antibiotics (ampicillin and gentamicin) along with continuous fetal monitoring.

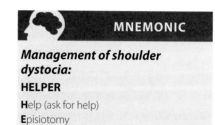

MNEMONIC

Management of shoulder dystocia:
HELPER
Help (ask for help)
Episiotomy
Legs up (perform McRoberts maneuver)
Pressure (suprapubic)
Enter the vagina to rotate with Wood's screw maneuver or to deliver the fetal arm
Return the fetal head to the pelvis for C-section (Zavanelli maneuver)

MNEMONIC

Procedure for vacuum delivery:
ABCDEFGH

Address the patient/ensure adequate **A**nalgesia
Bladder must be emptied
Cervix completely dilated, 0 station or more
Determine position of fetal head
Equipment check
Find **F**lexion point, apply vacuum, and engage
Gentle traction downward
Halt if three pulls without movement, three pop-offs, or 20 minutes

KEY FACT

Operative vaginal delivery should **not** be undertaken unless the provider is willing to abandon the attempt should it prove unsuccessful.

- **Complications:** Fetal sepsis, fetal neurologic damage, ↑ C-section rate, wound infection, endomyometritis, postpartum hemorrhage.

Operative Vaginal Delivery

Vacuum or forceps application to assist in vaginal delivery. Criteria for operative delivery include a completely dilated cervix and a term fetus in vertex position and **at least 0 station,** with no shoulder dystocia anticipated. Complications include maternal birth trauma, fetal cephalohematoma, subgaleal hematoma, fetal retinal hemorrhage, and fetal intracranial hemorrhage.

Cesarean Section

Approximately 20% to 25% of babies in the United States are delivered via C-section. Table 16.8 lists indications for C-section. Preoperative preparation includes informed consent (with consent for tubal ligation if desired by patient); placement of a Foley catheter; spinal/epidural anesthesia (general anesthesia if emergent); removal of fetal monitors; sterile prep/drape.

- **Complications:** Bleeding; infection; damage to the abdominal organs, especially the uterus, ureters, and bladder; prolonged maternal recovery time; anesthesia risks; and neonatal injury or respiratory depression.

Vaginal Birth After C-Section

Due to the risk of uterine rupture, vaginal birth after C-section is performed only in hospitals with 24-hour on-site anesthesia and obstetric services, and with patients with a history of no more than one low transverse or low vertical uterine incision. Requires continuous monitoring, avoidance of prostaglandin cervical ripening agents, and very close monitoring if oxytocin augmentation is used.

- **Complications:** Signs of uterine rupture include fetal bradycardia, constant severe abdominal pain, vaginal bleeding, loss of uterine tone, a change in uterine shape, and hypovolemia.

Meconium-Stained Amniotic Fluid

Meconium-stained amniotic fluid occurs in roughly 14% of deliveries, and is associated with neonatal meconium aspiration syndrome. Risk factors include postdate gestation and nonreassuring fetal status.

- **Diagnosis:** Clinical, by the characteristic thick "pea soup" appearance of amniotic fluid.
- **Management:** If there is no spontaneous cry at delivery, attempt intubation with a meconium suction device × 2 before initiating the Neonatal Advanced Life Support (NALS) protocol (Figure 16.13).

Placental Pathology

The placenta is the site of maternal and fetal nutrient exchange and contains many clues to intrauterine pathology. Examine the weight/appearance of placental parenchyma and membranes, cord length, and number of vessels. Order a full pathology

TABLE 16.8. Indications for Cesarean Section

FETAL	MATERNAL
Malpresentation	Failure to progress
Intolerance of labor	Placenta or vasa previa
Fetal congenital anomalies	1° HSV infection
Estimated fetal weight >4.5 kg	Medical contraindications to labor
	Uterine/cervical abnormalities

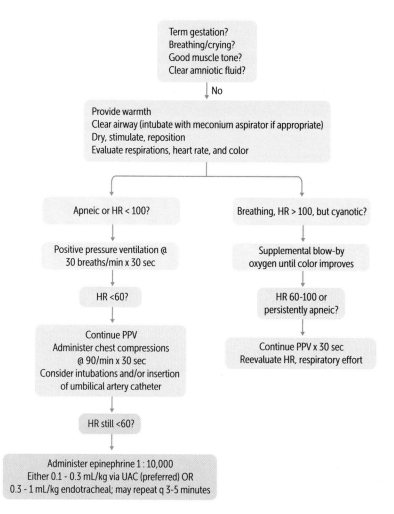

FIGURE 16.13. **Neonatal Advanced Life Support protocol.** (Reproduced with permission from USMLE-Rx.com.)

exam if: abnormal placental appearance; preterm or postterm birth; stillbirth; fetal infection, hydrops, or congenital anomalies; oligo- or polyhydramnios; antepartum hemorrhage; or severe hypertensive disorders. Abnormalities include the following.

- Cord abnormalities:
  - **Hypo- or hypercoiled cord/short cord:** Associated with poor fetal growth.
  - **Long cord:** Presents with a knotted or compressed cord.
  - **Abnormal cord insertion** (eg, marginal or velamentous): Associated with cord trauma or thrombi.
  - **Abnormal number of vessels:** Associated with congenital anomalies and IUGR.
- Membrane abnormalities:
  - **Abnormal color:** Associated with infection, meconium, or hemorrhage.
  - **Abnormal membrane insertion:** May be circummarginate (in which membranes originate from the inside margin of the placental disk) or circumvallate (in which membranes are grooved from abnormally deep implantation in the disk).
- Parenchymal abnormalities:
  - **Small placenta:** Associated with inadequate placental perfusion.
  - **Missing lobe:** Presents with retained placental tissue in the uterus.
  - **Calcified placenta:** Associated with postterm pregnancy.
  - **Placenta succenturiata:** An additional lobe; associated with a retained placental lobe or with placenta or vasa previa.

- **Duplex placenta:** Complete separation into two lobes; associated with velamentous cord insertion.
- **Circumvallate placenta:** A small chorionic plate with growth of extrachorial placental tissue; associated with premature separation and second-trimester bleeding.

ROUTINE POSTPARTUM CARE

Routine care during the 6 weeks after delivery focuses on mother-baby bonding, breastfeeding, and parent education. While most obstetrical problems resolve after delivery, keep in mind the possibility of persistent gestational diabetes, postpartum depression, eclampsia, venous thromboembolism, infection, or hemorrhage.

Postpartum Physical Exam

- Immediate assessment after birth: Evaluation of the extent of bleeding, palpation of the uterine fundus for size and firmness, and assessment of the cervix and perineum for the presence of trauma (see the discussion on repair of vaginal lacerations).
- Pelvic exam at approximately 6 weeks postpartum.

Postpartum Labs

- Recheck hematocrit if there was postpartum hemorrhage.
- For women with GDM, a fasting blood glucose should be obtained the day after delivery, and a 2-hour 75-g glucose challenge obtained 6 weeks after delivery to ensure resolution of GDM.

Postpartum Counseling

- Ask about common discomforts (eg, urinary retention, constipation, perineal care).
- Determine the frequency of breastfeeding and commonly encountered problems.
- Counsel patients about routine newborn care, including stooling and urination patterns, how to take the baby's temperature, anticipate URIs, and car safety seats.
- Offer information about postpartum depression, family support, and emotional self-care.
- Discuss birth control methods. Estrogen-containing combined hormonal contraceptives are Category 3 on the CDC medical eligibility criteria for contraception during the first 21 days after pregnancy because of the risk of blood clots and ↓ breast milk supply. Progesterone-only contraceptives do not have these same risks and are Category 2.
- Discuss the duration of normal bleeding and recommend pelvic rest for 6 weeks.

POSTPARTUM COMPLICATIONS

Endometritis

Uterine infection after delivery, usually caused by *Bacteroides*, *Enterobacter*, group A or B streptococcus, or *Chlamydia trachomatis* (late endometritis). Incidence after a vaginal birth is <3%, but is higher after a C-section; risk factors include operative delivery, prolonged ROM, and amnionitis.

- **Symptoms/Exam:** Presents with fever, abdominal pain, and uterine tenderness without any other identifiable cause.
- **Differential:** UTI, retained placental products, wound/episiotomy infection, pelvic abscess, septic pelvic thrombophlebitis, drug fever, pulmonary embolism.

MNEMONIC

Postpartum physical exam assessment:
BUBBBLES

Breast
Uterus
Bowel
Blues
Bladder
Lochia
Episiotomy
Surgical site (for cesarean section)

MNEMONIC

Causes of postpartum hemorrhage:
The 4 T's

Tissue (retained placenta)
Tone (uterine atony)
Trauma (traumatic delivery, episiotomy)
Thrombin (coagulation disorders, DIC)

- **Diagnosis:** CBC; UA and urine culture. Consider CXR and ultrasound.
- **Management:** Ampicillin, gentamicin, and clindamycin **or** ticarcillin/clavulanate. Continue antibiotics until the patient is afebrile for 24 to 48 hours.

Hemorrhage

Blood loss of 500 mL 0 to 24 hours after delivery or blood loss sufficient to make the patient symptomatic (eg, lightheadedness, dizziness, tachycardia). Risk factors include prolonged or very rapid labor, large baby, multiple gestations, nulliparity or grand multiparity, use of endogenous oxytocin, uterine infection, retained placenta, or lacerations of the cervix and vagina. The most common causes are uterine atony and retained tissue or blood clot.

Symptoms/Exam

- Cervical and perineal exam for continued vaginal bleeding due to lacerations; do a bimanual exam to assess uterine tone.
- Placental exam, uterine sweep, and ultrasound can assess for clots and retained tissue.

Diagnosis

Through accurate assessment of blood loss postpartum (providers consistently **underestimate** blood loss for vaginal and cesarean deliveries).

Management

- **Retained placental tissue:** Evacuation or curettage.
- **Genital tract laceration:** Expeditious repair!
- **Uterine inversion** (Figure 16.14): Give terbutaline to relax the uterus; then replace the uterus in the pelvis. Do **not** remove the placenta while the uterus is inverted!
- **Uterine atony:** See the mnemonic "**Arm Pits Help Me Pack Blood In.**"

MNEMONIC

Treatment of uterine atony:
Arm Pits Help Me Pack Blood In

Arm (bimanual pressure)

Pits (Pitocin; may be given IV or IM)

Help (call for help) and **He**mabate (250 µg IM q 1.5-3.5 hr unless asthmatic)

Methergine (200 µg IM unless hypertensive) and misoprostol 800 to 1000 µg

Pack (the uterus)

Blood (type and cross; transfusion PRN)

Into the OR for emergent uterine ligation/hysterectomy; **in**terventional radiology for embolization

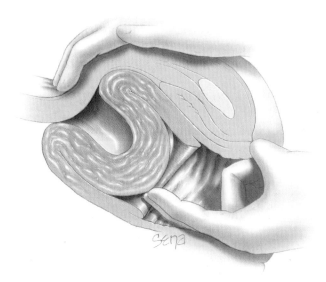

FIGURE 16.14. Partial uterine inversion. Partial uterine inversion is diagnosed by a crater-like depression on abdominal palpation and vaginal palpation of the fundal wall in the lower segment and the cervix. (Reproduced with permission from Cunningham FG, Leveno KJ, Bloom SL, et al. *Williams Obstetrics,* 23rd ed. New York: McGraw-Hill, 2008.)

Retained Placenta

Diagnosed when the third stage of labor lasts >30 minutes or when the placental exam confirms retention of placental tissue. Occurs in 1% to 2% of deliveries and is associated with uterine abnormalities and placenta accreta.

Diagnosis

Ultrasound to determine whether the placenta is detached from the uterine wall.

Management

- **If the placenta is completely detached from the uterine wall:** Manual traction on the umbilical cord.
- **If the placenta is partially or completely adherent to the uterine wall:** Attempt manual removal.
- May require general anesthesia in the OR.

Complications

Postpartum hemorrhage, intrauterine infection.

Breastfeeding Issues

Exclusive breastfeeding is recommended for the first 6 months of life and partial breastfeeding thereafter for the first year, although can be continued. Common problems encountered include the following:

- **Engorgement:** Treat with frequent and complete feeds along with cool compresses.
- **Plugged ducts:** Presents with a palpable tender lump. Treat with frequent feeds. Aspiration may be required.
- **Mastitis:** Presents with a hard, red, tender area associated with fevers, chills, and malaise. Treat with frequent feeds along with dicloxacillin for 10 to 14 days.
- **Poor latch:** Improper seal of the infant's lips around the nipple. Address with a lactation consult.
- **Nipple soreness/trauma:** Keep nipples clean with water and saline; air dry; use lanolin cream and/or mupirocin (Bactroban) ointment for refractory cracking or soreness. Consider treating for a yeast infection with topical antifungals if the patient has pink skin surrounding the nipple or complains of stabbing pain during breastfeeding.

INFECTIONS IN PREGNANCY

Urinary Tract Infections and Asymptomatic Bacteriuria

UTIs complicate roughly 5% of pregnancies, and are caused by the same pathogens as those that affect nonpregnant patients. Risk factors include bladder/kidney anomalies, gestational diabetes, and multiparity. Rapid progression to pyelonephritis is the main risk of UTIs in pregnancy.

Diagnosis

Obtain a clean-catch urine culture; perform routine screening at the first prenatal visit.

Management

- Treat with 7 days of antibiotics (nitrofurantoin, amoxicillin, cephalosporins, or sulfisoxazole); adjust treatment in accordance with culture and sensitivity.
- Obtain follow-up urine cultures.
- Hospitalize for IV antibiotics if pyelonephritis is suspected.
- GBS bacteriuria requires intrapartum antibiotic prophylaxis.

KEY FACT

Avoid TMP (a folic acid antagonist) in the first trimester, sulfonamides in the third trimester (may cause jaundice), and fluoroquinolones and tetracyclines throughout the pregnancy (potential teratogens).

Complications

Pyelonephritis, which is associated with ↑ risk of preterm delivery and hypoxic fetal events, in addition to severe sepsis and perinephric abscesses in the mother Bacteriuria is also associated with an ↑ risk of preterm birth and perinatal mortality.

Bacterial Vaginosis

Overgrowth of normal vaginal bacterial flora; occurs in 10% to 25% of pregnant women.

- **Symptoms/Exam:** Generally asymptomatic; exam reveals a vaginal discharge with a fishy odor.
- **Diagnosis:** ⊕ KOH "whiff test"; clue cells on wet mount; vaginal discharge with pH >4.5.
- **Management:** Oral or topical metronidazole. Generally, treatment is indicated only in symptomatic women. If bacterial vaginosis is found incidentally on Pap, you should only treat women who are at high risk for preterm labor.
- **Complications:** Higher incidence of preterm PROM; spontaneous abortion; preterm birth.

HIV Infection in Pregnancy

Ideally detected during routine screening of all pregnant women at the first prenatal visit. If the patient has had no prenatal care, obtain a rapid HIV test at the time the patient presents to the hospital in labor. Management of HIV-infected pregnant women includes:

- Consultation with an HIV specialist.
- Referral to mental health and substance use disorder treatment resources as well as behavioral interventions, as applicable.
- Assessment of current disease status with a CD4 cell count and viral load.
- Antiretroviral treatment, as this dramatically reduces the risk of vertical transmission from 25% to 30% to <5%.
- Antibiotic prophylaxis as indicated for opportunistic infections (as with nonpregnant patients).

Prevention of Perinatal HIV Transmission

- Give maternal intrapartum IV zidovudine and proceed to elective C-section in the presence of a viral load >1000 copies/mL.
- Administer immediate antiretroviral prophylaxis/treatment to the infant in consultation with an HIV specialist.
- Avoid fetal scalp electrodes, episiotomy, or artificial ROM.
- Wash the baby **immediately** after birth.
- Breastfeeding is not recommended for HIV-positive mothers in the United States because of the risk of viral transmission. In developing countries, breastfeeding is still recommended because it is protective against gastroenteritis and other infections that are more common and morbid in these countries.

Varicella-Zoster Infection

Infection with varicella-zoster virus (VZV), or "chickenpox," affects 1 to 5 in 10,000 pregnancies and is transmitted via respiratory droplets.

- **Symptoms/Exam:** Typical symptoms of fever, malaise, myalgias, and vesicular rash may be more severe in pregnant women.
- **Diagnosis:** By viral titer.
- **Management:** Administer VZIG to neonates at risk and to nonimmune pregnant women who have been exposed to VZV. Avoid varicella vaccination during pregnancy.

KEY FACT

All pregnant women and postpartum women within 2 weeks of childbirth who test ⊕ for influenza are given antiviral treatment; oral oseltamivir is preferred.

KEY FACT

HIV-positive mothers who are stable on antiretroviral therapy and have a depressed viral load may deliver vaginally and do not require intrapartum IV AZT administration.

QUESTION

A 27-year-old G3P2 with poorly controlled GDM presents to the ED at 30 weeks' gestation with 12 hours of lower abdominal pain radiating to the back, accompanied by fever, chills, nausea, and vomiting. Her urine is cloudy, with 25 to 50 WBCs/hpf. How should she be treated?

- **Complications:** Maternal varicella pneumonia (40% mortality), congenital varicella syndrome, neonatal varicella infection.

STIs in Pregnancy

See the STI section in this chapter for diagnosis and treatment of the following conditions (exception noted for genital herpes). STIs in pregnancy are ideally detected during routine screening of all pregnant women at the first prenatal visit. Consider retesting later in pregnancy for patients at high risk.

Genital Herpes Simplex Infection

Requires treatment to prevent systemic neonatal herpetic infection from passage through the birth canal. Neonatal herpes has a 50% mortality rate.

- During pregnancy, treat genital HSV outbreaks with acyclovir (400 mg PO BID or TID) or valacyclovir (500 mg PO once per day) × 7 to 14 days for the first outbreak.
- Begin suppressive therapy at 36 weeks.
- A C-section should be performed if a 1° genital HSV outbreak occurs during labor.
- Consider C-section for any patient with active genital lesions.

Syphilis

Perinatal transmission in mothers with 1° or 2° syphilis is 50%. Complications include perinatal death, preterm birth (especially in the setting of a Jarisch-Herxheimer reaction), congenital anomalies, IUGR.

Gonorrhea and Chlamydia

Cervical infections associated with an ↑ risk of PROM and preterm labor, chorioamnionitis, endometritis, and neonatal ophthalmologic infection. Public health reporting is mandatory in most states for confirmed diagnosis of either pathogen.

OTHER MEDICAL ISSUES IN PREGNANCY

Depression in Pregnancy/Postpartum Depression

Three percent to 5% of pregnant women and 1% to 5% of postpartum women experience major depression. Risk factors include a prior or family history of depression, social and psychological stressors, and intrapartum or neonatal complications.

Differential

Bipolar disorder, hypothyroidism, generalized anxiety disorder, recreational substance use.

Diagnosis

CBC, TSH, CMP; urine toxicology screen.

Management

- Counseling; family support; physical activity; SSRIs (fluoxetine and sertraline are the best studied).
- Hospitalization may be necessary if the depression is severe and/or associated with psychosis.

Complications

- Use of SSRIs is associated with persistent pulmonary hypertension of the newborn and may be associated with "neonatal behavioral syndrome," which consists of self-limited tremors, mild tachypnea, and, rarely, seizures.

ANSWER

Appropriate management of pyelonephritis includes hospital admission, IV fluid administration, fetal monitoring, and IV antibiotics until the patient has been afebrile for 24 hours. Urine should be sent for culture, and antibiotic treatment should be adjusted per culture and sensitivity results.

- On the other hand, untreated depression is associated with: preterm birth; low birth weight; impaired maternal-infant bonding; poor nutrition; suicidal/homicidal ideation and attempts; postpartum psychosis.
- Paroxetine is contraindicated because of its association with fetal cardiac abnormalities.

Thromboembolic Disease

Pregnancy is a hypercoagulable state, and DVT or pulmonary embolism occurs in 0.2% of pregnancies. Risk factors include inherited thrombophilia, C-section, preterm delivery, and multiple births.

Symptoms/Exam

- **DVT:** Presents with lower extremity swelling or pain.
- **Pulmonary embolism:** Presents with dyspnea or cough.

Diagnosis

- D-dimer has excellent ⊖ predictive value.
- Lower extremity Doppler ultrasound for suspected DVT; V/Q scan for pulmonary embolism.

Management

- Anticoagulation with low-molecular-weight or unfractionated heparin up to 4 to 6 weeks postpartum.
- May switch to warfarin postpartum; titrate to an INR of 1.5 to 2.5.
- IVC filter for patients in whom anticoagulation is contraindicated.

Medications in Pregnancy

Categorized by their safety in pregnancy as well as in lactation. See Table 16.9.

KEY FACT

SSRIs, with the exception of paroxetine (associated with congenital abnormalities), are first line for intrapartum and postpartum depression. Most research is around safety/efficacy of fluoxetine, sertraline, and escitalopram. TCAs are contraindicated in breastfeeding.

KEY FACT

If a patient already carries a diagnosis of hypothyroidism, she will likely require ↑ supplementation in pregnancy. To start, continue prepregnancy dose + two extra doses per week. Use TSH to monitor and to guide medication adjustments.

TABLE 16.9.   **Medications Not Contraindicated in Pregnancy**

CATEGORY	EXAMPLES
Analgesics	Acetaminophen, narcotics (except if used on a long-term basis or in high doses at term)
Antimicrobials	Penicillin, cephalosporin, erythromycin, azithromycin, nystatin, clotrimazole, metronidazole, nitrofurantoin
Cardiovascular	Labetalol, methyldopa, hydralazine, heparin
Dermatologic	Erythromycin, clindamycin, benzoyl peroxide
Endocrinologic	Insulin, levothyroxine, glyburide
ENT	Chlorpheniramine, diphenhydramine, dextromethorphan, guaifenesin, intranasal steroids
GI	Antacids, simethicone, H_2 blockers, metoclopramide, docusate, doxylamine
Psychiatric	Fluoxetine, desipramine, doxepin
Pulmonary	Albuterol, cromolyn, inhaled steroids, short-term prednisone

Women's Health

CONTRACEPTION

Planning when and if to have children is an important part of overall health maintenance for men, women, and adolescents.

Emergency Contraception

Postcoital contraception that ↓ the chance of pregnancy if used after unprotected sex or method failure (eg, a condom slips off or doses of oral contraceptives are missed).

- The sooner after intercourse emergency contraception (EC) is used, the more effective it is.
- **Only** works before implantation and does not interrupt or terminate an established pregnancy. Like other hormonal birth control methods, its 1° mechanism of action is preventing ovulation. It may also prevent fertilization or implantation.
- May be most needed at night or on weekends, when clinics are closed. To prevent medication delays, consider providing advance prescriptions (and refills) at routine office visits. Advance provision has been found to be safe and effective and does not ↑ high-risk sexual behavior.
- Clinical exam and pregnancy testing are not needed before giving EC. No scheduled follow-up is required. Clinical evaluation is indicated if menses is delayed by a week or more or if lower abdominal pain or persistent irregular bleeding develops; rule out pregnancy, spontaneous abortion, or ectopic pregnancy.
- Levonorgestrel (Plan B) and ulipristal (Ella) are two products approved specifically as EC and can be obtained over-the-counter by patients ≥18 years. Younger patients need prescriptions. Levonorgestrel is FDA approved for up to 3 days after intercourse, and effective up to 5 days; ulipristal is FDA approved for up to 5 days after unprotected intercourse and is more effective in women with obesity.
- If these products are not available, high doses of combined or progestin-only OCPs can be prescribed.
- There are no evidence-based contraindications to EC.
- Common side effects: nausea, vomiting, and irregular bleeding.
- Table 16.10 outlines EC options along with their indications and effectiveness.

Combined Hormonal Methods

- OCPs, the weekly patch (Ortho Evra), and the monthly ring (NuvaRing) all work by releasing estrogen and progestin into the bloodstream, suppressing ovulation, thickening cervical mucous, and inhibiting endometrial proliferation.
- Greater than 99% effective with perfect use, 92% for typical use.

KEY FACT

The effectiveness of a pregnancy prevention method is defined as the percentage of women who do not experience unintended pregnancy within the first year of use.

KEY FACT

Certain antiepileptics (including carbamezapine, phenobarbitol, phenytoin, topiramate) induce hepatic metabolism of estrogen and progestin, leading to potential failure of OCPs. They do not affect IUDs.

TABLE 16.10.   **Emergency Contraception Options**

	PROGESTIN ONLY (EMERGENCY CONTRACEPTION)	COMBINED HORMONAL ("YUZPE METHOD")	COPPER IUD (PARAGARD)
How supplied	Two pills of Plan B (0.75 mg of levonorgestrel) or 40 pills of Ovrette (norgestrel); one pill of Ella (30 mg of ulipristal)	Multiple pills from OCP pack (each dose is equivalent to 100-120 µg of ethinyl estradiol and 0.50-0.75 mg of levonorgestrel)	Inserted by provider
Effective if used	Within 5 days	Within 5 days	Within 5-8 days
Pregnancy rate following use	1%-4%	1%-4%	<1%

- Combined hormonal methods are contraindicated in:
    - DVT, pulmonary embolism, thrombophlebitis, or a thromboembolic disorder.
    - Uncontrolled hypertension, especially if >160/100 mm Hg, or with vascular disease.
    - A history of MI, CVA, CAD, or valvular heart disease with thrombogenic complications.
    - Diabetes of >20 years' duration or with vascular involvement (nephropathy, neuropathy, or retinopathy).
    - Heavy tobacco use (>15 cigarettes per day) in patients >35 years of age. Use caution in all smokers >35 years of age.
    - History of estrogen-dependent cancer, including breast cancer.
    - Migraines with aura, or any migraines in patients >35 years of age.
    - Hepatic adenoma, hepatic carcinoma, or acute or chronic hepatocellular disease with abnormal liver function.
    - Planned surgery with prolonged immobilization.
    - Pregnancy.
    - Undiagnosed abnormal vaginal bleeding.
- Use caution with breastfeeding mothers in the first 6 weeks postpartum and in all women in the first 3 weeks postpartum (in view of ↑ DVT risk).
- Noncontraceptive benefits include reduction in ovarian and endometrial cancer risk, regulation and reduction of menstrual bleeding, treatment of dysmenorrhea, reduced PMS/premenstrual dysphoric disorder (PMDD), treatment of pelvic pain due to endometriosis, prevention of menstrual migraines, reduced ovarian cysts (not used to treat existing functional ovarian cysts), and treatment of acne or hirsutism.
- Patients with menses-related conditions can use combined hormonal contraceptives continuously (skipping the withdrawal bleed). This may ↑ the rate of breakthrough bleeding.
- Combined hormonal contraceptives can be started on any day of the menstrual cycle. For convenience, some people start on the first day of menses or the first Sunday after the beginning of menses. The Quick Start method, in which the patient takes her first dose during the visit with the provider, has been proven to ↑ adherence.
- If starting on the first day of a regular menstrual cycle, no backup method is needed. All others should use a barrier method or abstain for 7 to 14 days.
- Counseling to patient if she misses pill(s):
    - Missed single pill: Take the missed dose immediately and the next dose at the usual time.
    - Missed two pills: Take two pills immediately and two pills the next day.
    - Missed three or more pills: Discard pack of pills, allow withdrawal bleed then start new pack.
- Serious complications—including MI, CVA, and DVT—are exceedingly rare.

Progestin-Only Methods

- Available as medroxyprogesterone injected every 3 months (Depo-Provera IM or Depo-SubQ Provera 104) or as progestin-only pills ("minipills") taken daily.
- Associated with an effectiveness of >99% with perfect use versus 92% (for pills) and 97% (for injections) with typical use.
- Safe for breastfeeding mothers and their babies.
- Irregular spotting and amenorrhea are common.
- Depo-Provera users may have more weight gain than with other methods.
- When Depo-Provera is stopped, it usually takes 7 to 12 months for fertility to return.
- Currently breast cancer is the only absolute contraindication. Use **caution** if patients have a history of the following conditions:
    - Multiple risk factors for cardiovascular disease.
    - Uncontrolled severe hypertension (160/110 mm Hg).
    - Current DVT or pulmonary embolism.

KEY FACT

OCPs are not recommended in patients who have migraines with aura (category 4 contraindication, because of the ↑ risk of stroke) or in patients with acute hepatitis C.

KEY FACT

Eighty-five percent of women will become pregnant within 1 year of having regular sexual intercourse with no method of family planning, making "chance" 15% effective at preventing pregnancy!

MNEMONIC

Pill/patch/ring warning signs for serious complications:
ACHES

Abdominal pain
Chest pain
Headache
Eye problems
Severe leg pain

QUESTION 1

A 31-year-old woman presents 5 weeks after the birth of her first baby with concerns of becoming pregnant after she and her partner had sex without a condom or any birth control. Breastfeeding is going well, and she occasionally supplements with formula. She feels strongly that they are not yet ready to have another baby. How would you counsel her?

QUESTION 2

A teenage girl would like to start OCPs. What do you need to examine?

- Ischemic heart disease or CVA.
- Migraine with focal neurologic symptoms.
- Unexplained vaginal bleeding prior to evaluation.
- Past breast cancer.
- Hepatic adenoma, hepatic carcinoma, active hepatitis, or severe cirrhosis.
- Postpartum <6 weeks and breastfeeding.
- Long-term use of Depo-Provera (>2 years), especially in teens, may lead to ↓ bone mineral density (BMD). Although BMD appears to return to baseline after cessation of Depo-Provera, it should only be used long term if other methods are unacceptable. All users should take adequate calcium and vitamin D and to engage in weight-bearing exercise.
- Progestin-only pills must be taken at the same time every day to be effective.

Intrauterine Contraception

- Copper-T (ParaGard) and levonorgestrel-releasing (Mirena and Skyla) intrauterine devices have >99% effectiveness with perfect and typical use.
- Mirena approved for use up to 5 years, but probably effective for 7 years; Skyla is approved for use up to 3 years. ParaGard approved for use up to 10 years, but appears effective for 12 years. Fertility returns to baseline after the device is removed.
- Counsel patients to use condoms if they are at risk for STIs. Intrauterine contraceptives (IUCs) do not ↑ the risk of acquiring STIs or PID. With monofilament strings, modern IUCs do not cause the ascending infection that older devices are known for. Mirena ↓ risk of PID through its effect on cervical mucus. PID complicating IUC insertion is uncommon, and the risk of PID ↑ only for the first 20 days after insertion.
- *Actinomyces israelii*, a gram-positive anaerobe found in the GI tract, is more common in the genital tract of IUC users than in nonusers. It is considered a colonizing type of bacteria and does not need to be treated unless the patient has symptoms of infection.
- Candidates for IUC use:
  - Multiparous and nulliparous women.
  - Women who desire long-term contraception.
  - Women who are not candidates for combined hormonal contraception for medical reasons.
  - High-risk sexual activity and young age are **not** contraindications to IUC placement.
- Contraindications include the following:
  - Pregnancy.
  - Active infection (endometritis, PID, cervicitis).
  - Anatomic abnormalities or fibroids that distort the uterine cavity enough to make insertion difficult (most fibroids **are** compatible with IUC insertion).
  - Current gynecologic cancer.
  - Breast cancer (Mirena only).
  - Unexplained vaginal bleeding prior to evaluation.
  - Allergy to any component of IUC or Wilson disease (for copper-containing IUC device).
  - For Mirena, all cautions of progestin-only methods apply.
- IUCs ↓ the risk of ectopic pregnancy and are not contraindicated in women with a history of ectopic pregnancy or PID. If a pregnancy occurs, there is an ↑ likelihood that it will be ectopic if an IUC is in place.
- Light or absent menses are common with Mirena, making it a good treatment for menorrhagia and dysmenorrhea. Irregular spotting, especially in the first 6 months, is common.
- Heavier menses and cramps are expected with ParaGard.
- Routine prophylactic antibiotics during insertion are not indicated.
- Risks associated with IUC use include uterine perforation, lack of visible strings, creating difficult removal of IUC, and expulsion of IUC.

KEY FACT

If a patient using an IUC presents with PID, you do *not* need to remove the IUC device. Treat the infection with appropriate antibiotics, and leave the IUC device in place.

KEY FACT

Contraindications to Mirena are severe cirrhosis, liver cancer, and breast cancer.

KEY FACT

If a Mirena is inserted <7 days after menses, no backup method is needed; if inserted >7 days after menses, use backup contraception for 1 week.

ANSWER 1

Since she is not breastfeeding exclusively, she should not rely on lactational amenorrhea to prevent pregnancy. You can offer several options for emergency contraception that are safe during breastfeeding and are available in the office. After that, she may choose from many maintenance birth control methods that will be safe for both her and the baby. She should take a urine pregnancy test in 2 to 3 weeks.

ANSWER 2

Blood pressure. OCPs are contraindicated in severe HTN. You do not need to perform a Pap or other physical exam before providing OCPs unless they are otherwise indicated.

Male Condoms

- Latex condoms are 98% effective with perfect use and 85% with typical use. All condom types have similar contraceptive effectiveness, but animal skin condoms do not protect against STIs (Table 16.11).
- Educate patients about proper condom use and emergency (postcoital) contraception as a backup method. Avoid use with oil-based lubricants, which may weaken condom.
- Advantages include instant reversibility and protection against STIs.
- Disadvantages include lack of control by the female partner, possible diminishing of sexual pleasure for one or both partners, and relatively low effectiveness with typical use.

Vaginal Barriers

- Women have a variety of choices if they wish to use a barrier method that is inserted prior to sexual contact (Table 16.12).
- All vaginal barrier methods confer some degree of protection against STIs, but only the female condom provides protection equivalent to or better than the male condom.
- Educate patients about proper use, cleaning, and storage, as well as the use of postcoital EC as a backup method.

Vaginal Spermicides

- Sold as foams, creams, jellies, films, or suppositories.
- When used alone, they are 82% effective with perfect use and 71% effective with typical use.

Implants

- Implanon is a matchstick-sized single-rod implant that releases progestin slowly, providing up to 3 years of contraception.
- Greater than 99% effective with perfect and typical use.
- Indications and contraindications are the same as other progesterone-only products.
- Norplant, a progestin-releasing method that involved six implanted rods, is no longer distributed.

Sterilization

- Female sterilization can be accomplished by bilateral tubal surgery. Effectiveness is >99%.
- Male sterilization is by vasectomy and is also >99% effective. Vasectomy is considered safer than tubal sterilization, as it is a less invasive procedure performed using local anesthesia.
- Sterilization is considered permanent. Patients should be sure they do not want to have children in the future, as reversal procedures are not reliable.

TABLE 16.11.   Condom Choices

	LATEX	SYNTHETIC	ANIMAL SKIN
Acceptable for latex-allergic users	No	Yes	Yes
Effective pregnancy prevention	Yes	Yes	Yes
Effective STI prevention	Yes	Yes	No
Acceptable lubricant	Water-based	Any	Any

TABLE 16.12. **Vaginal Barrier Choices**

	DIAPHRAGM	FEMALE CONDOM	SPONGE	CERVICAL BARRIERS
Acceptable for latex-allergic users	No	Yes	Yes	Yes
Acceptable lubricant	Water-based	Any	Any	Any
Effectiveness (perfect use)	94%[a]	95%	91% nulliparous; 80% parous	Estimated 91%-98%
Effectiveness (typical use)	80%[a]	79%	84% nulliparous; 68% parous	Data not available
STI prevention	±	+	±	±
How to obtain	Fitted and prescribed by provider	OTC	OTC	Fitted and prescribed by provider

[a]When used as recommended with spermicidal jelly.

Abstinence

- The only way to absolutely guarantee against pregnancy is the complete avoidance of penile-vaginal contact.
- Most currently abstinent patients will become sexually active in the future and may still wish information about other family planning methods.
- Those choosing abstinence can still be at risk for nonconsensual intercourse and should be aware of the availability of emergency (postcoital) contraception.

Fertility Awareness

- Methods that chart fertility based on menstrual cycle timing or physical signs (cervical mucus, basal body temperature, breast and other body changes). Can be used to plan or prevent pregnancy.
- Ninety-one percent to 99% effective with perfect use. Seventy-five percent effective with typical use.

Lactation

- Exclusive breastfeeding with associated amenorrhea is >98% effective at preventing pregnancy for the first 6 months of breastfeeding or until menses return.
- Pumping and supplementing both ↓ the contraceptive effectiveness of breastfeeding.
- Nonhormonal and progestin-only methods are safe for breastfeeding mothers and their infants.
- Estrogen in combined hormonal contraceptives (pills, ring, patch) may ↓ milk production. For nursing mothers who choose an estrogen-containing method, it may be best to delay initiation until 6 weeks postpartum after optimal breastfeeding is established.

Withdrawal

- Coitus interruptus, in which the male partner withdraws his penis from his partner's vagina prior to ejaculating, ↓ the risk of pregnancy but does not prevent STIs.
- Provides approximately 96% effectiveness with perfect use and 73% with typical use.
- Disadvantages include lack of control by the female partner, possible diminishing of sexual pleasure for one or both partners, and possible transmission of sperm to female prior to ejaculation.
- Educate patients about emergency (postcoital) contraception as a backup method.

KEY FACT

Cervical mucus monitoring is the most effective method of natural family planning, up to 92% to 95% in real practice.

ABORTION

Pregnant women should be offered all options: continuing the pregnancy and parenting, continuing the pregnancy and placing the baby for adoption, or terminating the pregnancy. Half of all pregnancies in the United States are unintended, and half of these are electively terminated. It is estimated that up to 40% of women have an abortion in their lifetimes. Nearly all (approximately 91%) abortions in the United States are obtained in the first trimester. Up to the point of viability, abortion is legally protected. When performed by a trained provider, it is extremely safe, with overall complication rates <1%.

First-Trimester Abortion With Aspiration

- Dilation followed by aspiration, with or without sharp curettage, is the most common abortion procedure up to approximately 12 weeks' gestation and can be performed by electric suction or with a handheld manual vacuum aspirator.
- Analgesia includes local paracervical block plus the option of systemic agents such as NSAIDs, benzodiazepines, and/or opioids.
- Perioperative antibiotics ↓ the risk of infection.
- The most common complications are incomplete abortion (continued pregnancy or retained tissue) and infection (combined <1%). Perforation and the need for hospitalization are extremely rare (<0.1%). Mortality is <1 in 100,000.

First-Trimester Abortion With Medication

- A regimen of mifepristone (formerly RU-486) followed by misoprostol is FDA approved for pregnancy termination up to 7 weeks' (post-LMP) gestation. It is commonly used up to 9 weeks' gestation, based on abundant evidence of effectiveness and safety.
- In commonly used and evidence-based regimens, the patient takes mifepristone either vaginally or bucally in the provider's office and is then given misoprostol to take at home. Heavy cramping and bleeding follow the misoprostol, and the patient typically passes the pregnancy within several hours.
- Oral NSAIDs and acetaminophen-opioid combinations are offered as analgesia.
- Prophylactic antibiotics are often used, but their benefit is uncertain.
- Potential side effects: Pain, nausea, vomiting, diarrhea, dizziness, fatigue, headache, and warmth or chills. Complications include continuing pregnancy (1%-4%), infection, and heavy bleeding.
- If gestational cardiac activity is detected on vaginal ultrasound 2 weeks after treatment initiation, medical abortion is considered failed and surgical abortion is needed.
- Good patient follow-through is important for medical abortions, so selecting patients who can understand instructions and will be able to follow them is important. Patients must have access to emergency medical treatment if necessary, and surgical curettage should be available.

Second-Trimester Abortion

- Dilation and evacuation (D&E), which combines vacuum aspiration with forceps extraction, is the most commonly used procedure in the United States.
- Analgesia is usually with IV sedation or general anesthesia, but oral analgesics (plus local cervical block) may be adequate for early second-trimester procedures.
- After the first trimester, maternal morbidity and mortality associated with abortion ↑ with gestational age. Second-trimester abortion nonetheless remains very safe, with mortality (approximately 3 per 100,000) lower than that associated with childbirth.

KEY FACT

Contrary to popular myth, abortion does not ↑ a woman's risk of breast cancer or future pregnancy complications.

KEY FACT

With an early abortion, keep in mind the possibility of an ectopic or heterotopic pregnancy. Neither uterine aspiration nor mifepristone treats an ectopic pregnancy!

KEY FACT

All abortion patients with Rh-positive blood type should receive Rh(D) immune globulin (RhoGAM). Use 50 μg for women who are <12 weeks' pregnant and 300 μg for those >12 weeks.

KEY FACT

Hormonal contraceptive methods can be started at the time of or immediately following an abortion procedure. IUDs can be placed at the conclusion of an aspiration procedure.

QUESTION

A 40-year-old mother is concerned because her period, which she reports comes every 28 days "like clockwork," is 5 days late. Since the birth of their third child 6 years ago, she and her husband have been practicing natural family planning. A sensitive urine pregnancy test is ⊕; a pelvic exam reveals a small uterus consistent with a 5-week pregnancy. You provide supportive counseling and discuss her options. After several days, she and her husband decide to terminate the pregnancy medically. What medical regimen do you offer?

Postabortion Care

- Pelvic rest is recommended for 2 weeks following an abortion.
- Postabortion bleeding may continue for up to 2 to 4 weeks. Patients with excessive bleeding should be assessed for retained products of conception. Monitor for anemia.
- Menses usually return to normal within 4 to 6 weeks of the abortion.
- Follow-up 2 weeks after an uncomplicated abortion. At this visit, address contraceptive needs, offer testing and treatment for STIs, and discuss general social support issues, including patients' remaining questions or feelings about the abortion.

SEXUALLY TRANSMITTED INFECTIONS

The most common STIs are usually asymptomatic in women, so it is important to offer testing to high-risk patients. Routine screening for STIs is recommended for pregnant women and for women or men who are at high risk on the basis of the following risk factors:

- A history of a prior STI or a current diagnosis of another STI.
- New or multiple sex partners, or patient's partner has multiple partners.
- Age <24 years. (See the Community and Preventive Medicine chapter for STI screening in women.)

Symptoms/Exam

- Evaluation of all patients of reproductive age should include a sexual history.
- The specific symptoms, signs, and diagnostic tests for each STI are listed in Table 16.13.

Management

Patients with any STI should make sure their sexual partners are also treated to prevent reinfection.

Prevention

- Complete sexual abstinence is the only way to ensure prevention of STIs.
- Consistent use of latex condoms is the next best protection against STIs.
- All children, as well as adults with risk factors, should be vaccinated against HBV.
- Check HPV vaccination status, ensure that all female and male patients complete the vaccination series. (See the Community and Preventive Medicine chapter for HPV vaccination recommendations.)

Complications

- Gonorrhea and chlamydia infections, even without frank PID, ↑ the risk of tubal scarring, which can lead to infertility and ectopic pregnancy.
- PID can lead to multiorgan systemic illness and even death.
- Untreated syphilis and HIV are fatal.
- Untreated STIs in pregnant women can be transmitted to newborns.

VULVOVAGINITIS

Caused by normal flora that have overgrown rather than STIs, unless trichomoniasis. Patients' partners generally do not require treatment.

TABLE 16.13. **Presentation, Diagnosis, and Treatment of Common STIs**

STI	SYMPTOMS	EXAM	DIAGNOSIS	TREATMENT
Gonorrhea (GC) (*Neisseria gonorrhoeae*); gram–negative intracellular diplococci	Usually asymptomatic in women, or may present with purulent discharge	Exam reveals **mucopurulent discharge** and a friable cervix	Test sample from urine or cervical swab using nucleic acid amplification tests, genetic probe, or culture	Ceftriaxone, cefixime Consider treating presumptively for chlamydia
Chlamydia (*Chlamydia trachomatis*); obligate intracellular bacterium	Usually asymptomatic in women, or may present with purulent discharge	Exam reveals **mucopurulent discharge** and a friable cervix	Test sample from urine or cervical swab using nucleic acid amplification tests, genetic probe, or culture	Azithromycin 1 g PO × 1 Doxycycline 100 mg PO BID × 7 days (avoid in pregnancy)
Trichomoniasis (*Trichomonas vaginalis*); flagellated protozoan	Presents with a copious greenish-yellow vaginal discharge	Exam reveals a frothy greenish-yellow fluid in the vagina, "strawberry cervix"	Wet mount reveals motile trichomonads and white blood cells	Metronidazole 2 g PO × 1 Alternatively, metronidazole 500 mg PO BID × 7 days
Pelvic inflammatory disease (PID); polymicrobial, including *C trachomatis* and *N gonorrhoeae*	Presents with lower abdominal pain ± fever ± nausea and anorexia	Exam reveals diffuse abdominal tenderness ± rebound with cervical motion tenderness ± adnexal tenderness	Clinical diagnosis GC and chlamydia cultures may or may not be ⊕	Ceftriaxone, doxycycline, ± flagyl; can be treated as outpatient in stable cases Consider inpatient IV treatment Broad-spectrum antibiotics, including coverage for GC, chlamydia, and anaerobes
Genital herpes (HSV-1 or 2)	Presents with painful vesicles (pain may precede eruption) ± systemic symptoms (fever, myalgia) ± vaginal discharge May also be asymptomatic or present with nonspecific symptoms	Exam reveals tender grouped vesicles on an erythematous base; ruptured vesicles appear as shallow ulcers or abrasions Inguinal lymphadenopathy is also seen	Mainly clinical Consider viral culture or Tzanck smear from vesicular fluid	Oral acyclovir, valacyclovir, or famciclovir Treatment resolves lesions but does not cure HSV; recurrence is common Suppressive therapy for frequent outbreaks or during pregnancy Topical therapy not effective
Genital warts (HPV)	Presents with painless growths on the genitals, anus, or perineum (see Figure 16.15)	Exam reveals fleshy, skin-colored "cauliflower" papules or plaques on the vulva, vagina, or cervix	Clinical diagnosis Rarely may need biopsy	Options include topical imiquimod or podofilox applied by the patient; podophyllin; cryotherapy; trichloroacetic acid; electrocautery; or excision Treatment resolves lesions; recurrence is common

(continues)

TABLE 16.13. **Presentation, Diagnosis, and Treatment of Common STIs** *(continued)*

STI	SYMPTOMS	EXAM	DIAGNOSIS	TREATMENT
Syphilis (*Treponema pallidum*)	1°: **Painless** genital ulcer 2°: Fever, malaise, diffuse rash **Latent:** Asymptomatic 3°: Aortic aneurysm rupture, CNS symptoms	1°: Nontender **chancre** 2°: Nonspecific maculopapular rash involving palms and soles of feet; **condylomata lata** **Early latent (<1 y:** 4-fold in titer **Late latent (>1 y or unknown):** Serology remains ⊕ 3°: Aortitis, gummas, meningitis, encephalitis, tabes dorsalis, Argyll Robertson pupil	Start with nonspecific RPR or VRDL (may be false ⊕) FTA-ABS or darkfield microscopy to confirm; LP if neurosyphilis is suspected	Penicillin 2.4 MU IM × 1 for new infections; × 3 for infections of >1 y duration In penicillin-allergic patients, consider desensitization For neurosyphilis, IV penicillin G (3-4 MU IV q 4 hr × 10-14 days)
Chancroid (*Haemophilus ducreyi*)	Presents as a **painful** genital ulcer	Exam reveals a tender papule, pustule, or ulcer with an erythematous edge Tender inguinal lymphadenopathy is also seen	Mainly clinical Gram stain may help (streptobacillary chains) Rule out HSV and syphilis	Azithromycin, ceftriaxone, ciprofloxacin (avoid in pregnancy)
Granuloma inguinale (*Calymmatobacterium granulomatis*); gram-negative intracellular bacterium	Presents as painless; progressive to ulcerative lesions	Exam reveals painless nodule that progresses to beefy red ulcer	Diagnosis requires visualization of dark-staining Donovan bodies on tissue biopsy	Bactrim, doxycycline, tetracycline
HIV/AIDS	Acute retroviral syndrome 3-6 weeks after infection; opportunistic infections	Exam findings vary, depending on the cause of presentation	Serology: ELISA and Western blot; rapid test is available	HAART; appropriate prophylaxis (see the Infectious Disease chapter)
Hepatitis B (HBV)	Presents as acute hepatitis with flulike symptoms and jaundice	Exam reveals acute hepatitis with jaundice and hepatomegaly	HBsAg (may be used alone for screening)	See the Infectious Disease chapter
Pubic lice or "crabs" (*Phthirus pubis*)	Presents with an itch in the pubic hair May also affect the axillae and other hair-covered areas	Tiny white nits are attached to hair; adult lice may be seen	Clinical diagnosis Lice may be viewed under the microscope	Topical permethrin, malathion, or lindane; decontaminate bedding and clothing
Molluscum contagiosum (caused by *Poxvirus*)	Presents with multiple small bumps that are painless and nonpruritic	Dome-shaped pearly papules with **central umbilication** are seen	Clinical diagnosis Giemsa stain of material expressed from the lesion contains inclusion bodies	Most resolve spontaneously and do not require treatment Options include imiquimod, cryotherapy, curettage, and electrodesiccation

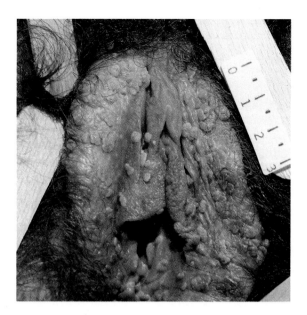

FIGURE 16.15. **Multiple genital warts on the vulva.** (Reproduced with permission from Wolff K, et al. *Fitzpatrick's Color Atlas & Synopsis of Clinical Dermatology,* 5th ed. New York: McGraw Hill, 2005:888.)

Symptoms/Exam

The specific presentation of each cause of vulvovaginitis is given in Table 16.14. The diagnosis should be considered for any of the following:

- Unusual vaginal discharge.
- Unusual vaginal/vulvar odor.
- Vaginal/vulvar itch or irritation.

Prevention

- Douching ↑ the risk of bacterial vaginosis and should be discouraged.
- Patients with bacterial vaginosis and candidiasis should ↓ vulvar warmth and minimize moisture (eg, losing weight, wearing cotton underpants, and loose-fitting clothing).

Complications

Bacterial vaginosis and trichomoniasis have been associated with an ↑ risk of preterm labor.

Gynecologic Cancers

OVARIAN CANCER

Develops from three types of tissue: epithelial, stromal, and germ cell. Usually diagnosed in late stages, it is the leading cause of gynecologic cancer death. Risk factors include advancing age (greatest risk in postmenopausal women), family history of breast or ovarian cancer, early menarche, late menopause, and nulliparity. Use of hormonal contraception provides significant and long-lasting protection. A history of tubal ligation and, to a lesser degree, hysterectomy appears to be protective.

KEY FACT

All patients treated for gonorrhea and chlamydia infections need rescreening 3 months after treatment due to the high rates of repeat infection.

KEY FACT

If you have a high suspicion for syphilis and the test is ⊖, repeat RPR in 2 weeks.

KEY FACT

Clinical judgment is the only information required for empiric treatment of PID. CT is a poor quality diagnostic tool; lab results often take days to return; laparoscopy with biopsy is invasive and lengthens time from presentation to treatment.

QUESTION 1

A 23-year-old woman presents for a routine checkup and Pap smear. She is sexually active only with her boyfriend of 1 year and uses OCPs. She expresses concern about several small, painless growths on her labia. Her external genital exam reveals multiple nontender, cauliflower-like, skin-colored papules. Speculum and bimanual exams are unremarkable. What is the most likely diagnosis?

QUESTION 2

A patient presents with throat pain, cervical lymphadenopathy, erythema, and exudates. Test results for *Streptococcus pyogenes* and mononucleosis are ⊖. What STI do you need to consider?

TABLE 16.14.   **Presentation and Treatment of Vulvovaginitides**

CAUSE	SYMPTOMS	EXAM	BEDSIDE TESTS	TREATMENT
Bacterial vaginosis (*Gardnerella* and other spp)	Presents with a malodorous discharge	Discharge is thin and yellowish-gray A fishy odor may be noticeable without KOH	pH >4.5 Wet mount shows **clue cells** (see Figure 16.16) KOH whiff test is ⊕ for a fishy amine odor	Metronidazole 500 mg PO BID × 7 days is most effective Metronidazole gel 5 g PV once per day × 5 days Clindamycin 5 g PV QHS × 7 days
Yeast infection (*Candida albicans*)	Presents with vaginal itching and burning accompanied by a cheesy white discharge	Exam reveals a white discharge adherent to the introitus; the discharge is thick and cottage cheese–like The perineum and vulva may be red and tender	pH 3.5-4.5 KOH prep shows "budding" hyphae	Intravaginal azole antifungals; oral fluconazole (avoid in pregnancy) Antifungal cream may be applied externally for symptom relief
Trichomoniasis (*Trichomonas vaginalis*)	Presents with a copious green discharge	Exam reveals a discharge that is frothy green	See Table 16.13	See Table 16.13
Atrophic vaginitis	Vaginal irritation and pain with intercourse in postmenopausal women	Exam reveals a clear, thin discharge and a pale vaginal epithelium with patches of erythema	pH >7	Water-based moisturizing preparations or estrogen vaginal cream If vaginal bleeding is present, rule out malignant causes

ANSWER 1

HPV-associated genital warts (Figure 16.15). You offer the patient treatment options of topical medications or cryotherapy, as well as testing for other STIs.

ANSWER 2

Gonorrhea pharyngitis. Because concomitant chlamydia cervicitis is possible, presumptively treat both.

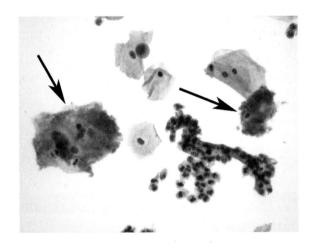

FIGURE 16.16.   **Clue cells of bacterial vaginosis.** Clue cells (arrows) can be seen on Pap smears of patients with bacterial vaginosis. The image shows the organisms coating squamous cells forming a purple, velvety coat. (Reproduced with permission from USMLE-Rx.com.)

Symptoms/Exam

- Initially asymptomatic, or may present with pelvic fullness, ↑ abdominal size, bloating, urinary urgency, frequency, incontinence, early satiety, weight loss, fatigue, constipation, or dyspareunia.
- Acute abdominal pain from a torsed or ruptured mass (rare presentation).
- Irregular menses or postmenopausal bleeding.
- Abdominal pain and swelling may be from invasive tumor or from 2° ascites.
- Bimanual and rectovaginal exams may reveal a solid, irregular, fixed pelvic mass.

Differential

Consider the broad differential diagnosis of abdominal pain and bloating.

Diagnosis

- Pelvic ultrasound reveals a solid or cystic mass with extramural fluid, wall thickening, septa, and papillary projections, Doppler flow to the solid component of the mass with ↑ number and tortuosity of vessels ± ascites.
- CA-125: Useful for tracking disease course, but is nonspecific, therefore not useful for screening asymptomatic women.

Management

- Surgical excision and "debulking" of tumor burden.
- Chemotherapy if indicated.
- Women with a known hereditary syndrome (eg, Lynch syndrome or BRCA mutations) may choose prophylactic oophorectomy.

UTERINE CANCER

Endometrial cancer is the most common gynecologic malignancy in the United States. Often causes early symptoms, thus tends to be diagnosed at a curable stage. Uterine sarcomas (rare) are more likely to be diagnosed late. Universal screening is not recommended. Women with hereditary nonpolyposis colorectal cancer should have annual screening with endometrial biopsy beginning at age 35.

- Type I (endometrioid) accounts for >75% of cases and has a good prognosis. Usually results from unopposed estrogen stimulation of the endometrium, leading to hyperplasia.
- Type II lesions are not related to estrogen exposure or endometrial hyperplasia. Usually diagnosed at a more advanced age and with a poorer prognosis. Includes serous, clear cell, mucinous, squamous, and adenosquamous carcinomas.

Symptoms/Exam

- Commonly presents with postmenopausal bleeding, or in premenopausal women with heavy or irregular menses.
- Rule out cancer in women >35 years of age with suspected anovulatory uterine bleeding and postmenopausal women with benign endometrial cells on Pap smear.
- Uterus may be enlarged or normal. On general physical exam, look for signs associated with ↑ risk.

Differential

- Benign causes of irregular or postmenopausal bleeding, such as atrophic vaginitis, endometrial hyperplasia, polyps, fibroids, trauma, infection, and hormonal medications.
- Other gynecologic cancers.

 KEY FACT

There is no effective way to screen for ovarian cancer, but suspicious symptoms should be evaluated by pelvic exam ± transvaginal ultrasonography and CA-125. In fact, USPSTF recommends **against** screening.

 KEY FACT

The use of OCPs significantly reduces the risk of endometrial and ovarian cancer.

 MNEMONIC

Risk factors for endometrial cancer:

ENDOMET

Elderly
Nulliparity
Diabetes
Obesity
Menstrual irregularity
Estrogen monotherapy
Hyper**T**ension

 QUESTION 1

Five hours after receiving penicillin treatment for syphilis, your patient returns to the clinic with fever, myalgias, and malaise. What do these symptoms represent?

 QUESTION 2

A 19-year-old woman complains of 1 week of yellow-gray vaginal discharge with a fishy odor that is not remediated with douching. She has no urinary symptoms or vaginal itching or burning. She is not sexually active and denies a history of STIs. Speculum exam reveals copious discharge but an otherwise normal vulva, vagina, and cervix. Bimanual exam is unremarkable. Litmus paper applied to the discharge shows a pH of 5. Saline wet mount reveals epithelial cells with peripheral stippling. KOH applied to the slide releases a strong amine "fishy" odor but is ⊖ for hyphae. What is the mostly likely diagnosis?

Diagnosis

- Suspicious symptoms should be evaluated with endometrial biopsy. Transvaginal ultrasound can be helpful in postmenopausal women. However, if the stripe is >3-4 mm, do a saline infusion hysteroscopy. If the saline hysteroscopy shows an area of focal hypertrophy, biopsy the focal area. If the saline hysteroscopy shows global hypertrophy, do an EMB.
- D&C ± hysteroscopy is more sensitive but also more invasive, and can be used if EMB is ⊖ but symptoms persist.
- Pelvic masses suspicious on imaging but ⊖ on endometrial sampling should be excised to evaluate for sarcoma. Most are found incidentally at the time of surgery for fibroids or other benign indications.

Management

- Staging: Surgically based.
- Total abdominal hysterectomy with bilateral salpingo oophorectomy almost always indicated.
- Radiation, chemotherapy, and/or hormonal agents as indicated by the stage and type of cancer.

CERVICAL CANCER

Infection with a high-risk subtype of HPV is necessary for the development of cervical cancer. Risk factors include early sexual activity, multiple sexual partners, partner with high number of sexual partners, STIs, previous history of squamous dysplasias of cervix/vagina/vulva, immunosuppression, and smoking. Two major histologic types of invasive cervical cancer are squamous cell carcinoma (80% of cases) and adenocarcinoma or adenosquamous carcinoma.

Symptoms/Exam

- Preinvasive lesions (dysplasia and carcinoma in situ) are asymptomatic.
- Invasive carcinoma generally leads to abnormal vaginal bleeding ± a foul-smelling discharge.
- Advanced disease may lead to pelvic pain, lower extremity edema, or urinary symptoms.
- Invasive lesions may be invisible to the naked eye on speculum exam.
- Tumors may appear ulcerated, necrotic, or exophytic.
- Bimanual ± rectovaginal exam may reveal cervical distortion or a frank mass.
- Look for signs of disease extension such as inguinal lymphadenopathy, leg edema, ascites, or hepatomegaly.

Differential

- Benign causes of abnormal bleeding and discharge, such as atrophic vaginitis, endometrial hyperplasia, polyps, fibroids, trauma, infection, and hormonal medications.
- Other gynecologic cancers.

Diagnosis

Colposcopy with directed biopsy and endocervical curettage.

Management

- Low-grade lesions can be followed without therapy, as >90% will spontaneously regress.
- High-grade preinvasive lesions can be ablated or excised with cryotherapy, loop electrosurgical excision procedure (LEEP), or conization.
- Invasive disease requires radical hysterectomy and/or radiation therapy.

KEY FACT

All women aged ≥21 years should be routinely screened for cervical cancer. Cervical cytology (Pap smear) is the standard-of-care screening test.

ANSWER 1

The patient is having a Jarisch-Herxheimer reaction, a transient, acute, febrile reaction within a few hours of treatment of syphilis. Treat with salicylates/antipyretics; this reaction has no clinical significance and is self-limited.

ANSWER 2

Bacterial vaginosis, based on the presentation, the presence of "clue cells" on microscopy (Figure 16.16), and a ⊕ "whiff test." You offer the patient treatment with metronidazole and advise against douching.

Complications

- Most superficial therapies are safe and have little or no effect on future pregnancies.
- LEEP may modestly ↑ the risk of PROM and preterm delivery in future pregnancies.
- Conization ↑ the risk for cervical stenosis or incompetence.
- Pelvic radiation and radical surgery may have serious adverse effects.

VULVAR AND VAGINAL CANCER

Rare cancer (2° vaginal cancers are more common than 1°), but care should be taken not to miss the diagnosis, as the presenting symptoms can be nonspecific. In utero exposure to diethylstilbestrol (DES) is an important risk factor for clear cell adenocarcinoma of the vagina. Other risk factors include HPV exposure, smoking, and advanced age.

Symptoms/Exam

- Many patients are asymptomatic.
- Presenting symptoms: Vulvar itching most common in vulvar cancer; vaginal discharge most common in vaginal cancer.
- Less commonly, patients will see or feel a lesion.
- External genital and speculum exams may reveal a lesion that can vary in color, texture, and appearance.
- Paget disease of the vulva, often associated with an underlying adenocarcinoma, appears as a well-demarcated, scaly lesion that may look like eczema.
- Skin cancers, including melanoma, may present on the vulva.

Differential

Genital warts; vaginitis; benign skin lesions, including lichen sclerosus and lichen planus.

Diagnosis

- Vaginal malignancies may be detected on Pap smear.
- Biopsy, often guided by colposcopy, required for definitive diagnosis.

Management

Surgical excision ± radiation.

GESTATIONAL TROPHOBLASTIC NEOPLASIA

Malignancy arising from fetal tissue. This diagnosis includes a persistent or invasive mole and malignant choriocarcinoma. Most cases are curable, but metastases may be fatal.

Symptoms/Exam

- Presents with persistent pregnancy symptoms and irregular vaginal bleeding for >6 weeks following cessation of a term, preterm, ectopic, or molar pregnancy.
- Metastatic disease may present with pulmonary, GI, or neurologic symptoms.
- Exam reveals an enlarged uterus, adnexal fullness due to ovarian cysts, and RUQ pain from hepatic involvement.

Differential

Normal pregnancy; other pelvic masses.

KEY FACT

Malignant melanoma is the second most common vulvar cancer. In patients at ↑ risk for melanoma, the full-body skin check should truly include the entire body!

QUESTION

A 60-year-old woman with a long-standing history of genital lichen sclerosus presents with ↑ vulvar itching, pain, and dysuria. What is the likely diagnosis?

Diagnosis

- Look for a rapidly rising β-hCG.
- Ultrasound reveals a "snowstorm" appearance (Figure 16.18).
- Pathologic diagnosis is made after surgical treatment. The characteristic "bunches of grapes" appearance is caused by hydropic villi.
- Staging based on age, β-hCG level, type of previous pregnancy, duration of disease, site of metastasis, and number of metastases.

Management

- D&C curative in many cases. Rarely, hysterectomy is necessary.
- Nonmetastatic disease: Methotrexate may be used.
- Metastatic disease: Requires combination chemotherapy.
- Follow β-hCG levels to resolution; plateau or rise in β-hCG levels is a marker of persistent disease.

Complications

Molar pregnancy carries 1% risk of recurrence with future pregnancies. Since choriocarcinoma may metastasize to the lungs, vagina, brain, liver, kidney, or GI tract, recommend CXR, CT of chest/abdomen/pelvis, and brain CT.

Menstrual Disorders

DYSMENORRHEA

Pain during menses resulting from uterine contractions caused by the release of prostaglandins. 1° dysmenorrhea affects women with normal pelvic anatomy; risk factors include age <20, nulliparity, heavy menses, depression, and smoking. 2° dysmenorrhea can be caused by endometriosis, adenomyosis, pelvic infection, IUC use, cervical stenosis, congenital vaginal or uterine abnormalities, or fibroids.

ANSWER

Squamous cell carcinoma in situ arising in an area of lichen sclerosus (Figure 16.17) can be confirmed with biopsy of the lesion. Although itself a benign condition, lichen sclerosus leads to vulvar cancer in 4% to 6% of affected women.

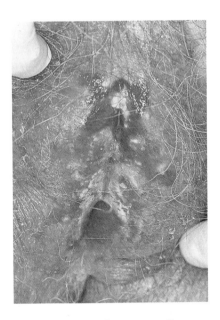

FIGURE 16.17.   **Squamous cell carcinoma of the vulva arising in an area of lichen sclerosus.** (Reproduced with permission from Wolff K, et al. *Fitzpatrick's Color Atlas & Synopsis of Clinical Dermatology,* 5th ed. New York: McGraw Hill, 2005:1047.)

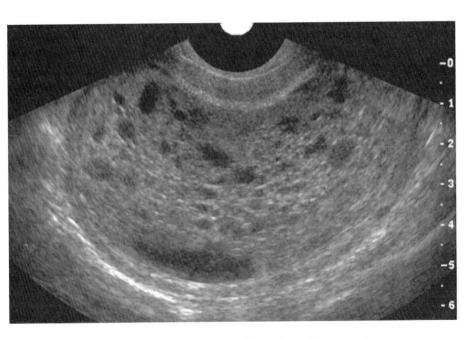

FIGURE 16.18.   **Complete hydatidiform mole.** Image shows "snowstorm" appearance on ultrasound. (Reproduced with permission from USMLE-Rx.com.)

Symptoms/Exam

- Presents with crampy pelvic pain beginning at the onset of menses and lasting 1 to 3 days.
- A pelvic mass, abnormal vaginal discharge, and pelvic tenderness not limited to the time of menses suggest 2° dysmenorrhea.

Diagnosis

- Can be treated empirically if the history and physical are consistent with 1° dysmenorrhea.
- A **speculum and bimanual exam** should be done on sexually active patients to evaluate for STIs or anatomic abnormality.
- Ultrasound is useful in evaluating 2° dysmenorrhea; laparoscopy with histologic confirmation is best for the diagnosis of endometriosis.

Management

- NSAIDs: Best first-line treatment, as they have an analgesic effect while also ↓ the volume of menstrual flow.
- Levonorgestrel IUCs ↓ dysmenorrhea.
- **Combined hormonal contraceptives** ↓ prostaglandin release during menses. Extended-cycle use (ie, 12 continuous weeks of active hormones followed by 1 week off) ↓ the number of menstrual periods.
- Depot medroxyprogesterone acetate leads to amenorrhea in most women.
- Danazol or leuprolide acetate can suppress the menstrual cycle, but both drugs are expensive and have side effects. Reserved for refractory cases of 2° dysmenorrhea.
- Alternative therapies that may be effective include topical heat, magnesium and calcium supplementation, vitamin E, thiamine, omega-3 fatty acids, and acupuncture.
- Hysterectomy is indicated only for severe, refractory cases.

KEY FACT

Risk factors for endometriosis include early menarche, ↑ frequency of cycles, heavy prolonged cycles, and low parity.

KEY FACT

NSAIDs are first-line treatment for dysmenorrhea, as they ↓ both pain and volume of menstrual flow. However, if endometriosis, treat with levonorgestrel IUCs, OCPs, or depot medroxyprogesterone acetate.

KEY FACT

If starting iron supplementation for patients with menorrhagia, counsel to take iron with vitamin C to improve absorption, and not with coffee, tea, or calcium.

ABNORMAL UTERINE BLEEDING

Bleeding that deviates from the patient's normal pattern. Prior to the onset of menses, any vaginal bleeding is considered abnormal, except self-limited, physiologic withdrawal bleeding in some newborns. In women of childbearing age, abnormal uterine bleeding encompasses bleeding between cycles as well as any change in menstrual frequency, duration, or amount of flow. Bleeding may be classified as **ovulatory** or **anovulatory,** based on the timing, duration, and amount of flow.

Symptoms/Exam

Clinical presentation varies by the pattern of abnormal bleeding and associated symptoms and exam findings (Table 16.15).

- **Ovulatory bleeding—menorrhagia** (excessive or prolonged bleeding during menses)—etiologies include:
  - **Anatomic lesions:** Cervical disease (polyps, inflammation, cancer), PID, IUC use, uterine disease (fibroids, cancer).
  - **Concurrent disease:** Foreign body, coagulopathy, or thyroid, hepatic, or renal disease.
  - **Medications:** Anticoagulants, antipsychotics, corticosteroids, herbal supplements (ginseng, gingko, soy), SSRIs, tamoxifen.
- **Anovulatory bleeding—metrorrhagia** (irregular bleeding between ovulatory cycles), **menometrorrhagia** (irregular, noncyclic bleeding characterized by heavy flow or duration), or **oligomenorrhea** (cycles lasting >35 days)—etiologies include:
  - **Endocrine dysfunction:** PCOS, hypothyroidism, or excess androgen, cortisol, or prolactin.
  - **Hypothalamic cause:** Situational stress, excess exercise, or weight loss.
  - **Functional cause:** Puberty, perimenopause.

TABLE 16.15. **Exam Findings Associated With Abnormal Uterine Bleeding**

SYMPTOMS/FINDINGS	CONDITION
Weight loss, stress	Hypothalamic suppression
Galactorrhea, headache, visual disturbance	Pituitary adenoma
Pelvic pain	Ectopic pregnancy, PID, trauma, miscarriage
Nausea, weight gain, fatigue, urinary frequency	Pregnancy
Weight gain, fatigue, constipation, cold intolerance	Hypothyroidism
Weight loss, palpitations, heat intolerance	Hyperthyroidism
Bleeding tendency, easy bruising	Coagulopathy
Jaundice, abdominal pain	Liver disease
Hirsutism, acne, acanthosis nigricans, ± obesity	PCOS
Postcoital bleeding	Cervical dysplasia, endocervical polyp

- Other causes of abnormal uterine bleeding:
    - Polymenorrhea: Cycles <21 days; usually due to luteal phase dysfunction.
    - Mid-cycle spotting: Physiologic spotting just before ovulation.
    - Pregnancy: Ectopic pregnancy, threatened abortion, incomplete abortion.
    - Postmenopausal bleeding: Unpredictable bleeding that occurs >1 year after cessation of menses or in a menopausal woman who has been receiving hormone therapy for ≥12 months. Pathology may be **vaginal** (atrophic vaginitis), **cervical** (polyps, erosion, cancer), or **uterine** (polyps, fibroids, cancer).

Diagnosis

- One of exclusion: abnormal uterine bleeding may be due to hormonal imbalances either at the pituitary level (anovulatory bleeding) or at the level of the endometrial lining (ovulatory bleeding).
- **Always rule out pregnancy,** iatrogenic causes, genital tract pathology, and systemic conditions.
- **Labs:** urine hCG, CBC, LFTs, PT, PTT, TSH, prolactin, blood glucose, DHEA, free testosterone, Pap smear, gonorrhea and chlamydia tests.
- **Imaging:** Transvaginal ultrasound; hysteroscopy for cases unresponsive to empiric treatment.
- Endometrial assessment to rule out cancer (see Uterine Cancer section above).

Management

- **Acute anovulatory bleeding:** To stop bleeding, give high-dose oral or IV estrogen to build up the endometrial lining. Oral medroxyprogesterone or IM progesterone can also be used to convert proliferative endometrium to secretory endometrium. D&C or hysteroscopy is appropriate in refractory cases.
- **Chronic anovulatory bleeding:** Treat the underlying cause, and add monthly progesterone therapy or combination hormonal contraceptives both to promote regular endometrial shedding and to prevent endometrial hyperplasia.
- **Ovulatory bleeding:** Treat the underlying cause and associated anemia. NSAIDs, combined hormonal contraceptives, or a levonorgestrel-releasing IUC can ↓ the duration and quantity of bleeding. Consider myomectomy in refractory cases associated with fibroids.
- Surgical options such as endometrial ablation or hysterectomy may be indicated in severe cases.

AMENORRHEA

Absence of menses. **1° amenorrhea** is defined as failure of menses to appear by age 16 in a patient with normal 2° sexual characteristics or by age 14 in a patient with no 2° sexual characteristics. **2° amenorrhea** is defined as the absence of menses for 3 consecutive months in women with previous normal menstruation or for 9 months in women with prior oligomenorrhea.

Etiologies of **1° amenorrhea** include the following.
- **Hypothalamic/pituitary:**
  - **Hypothalamic dysfunction:** May be due to organic illness, vigorous exercise, stressful life events, or anorexia nervosa.
  - **Genetic gonadotropin deficiency:** Kallmann syndrome.
  - **Hypothalamic lesions:** Craniopharyngioma.
  - **Pituitary tumors:** Prolactinoma.
  - **Endocrinopathies:** Cushing syndrome; hypothyroidism.
  - **Hyperandrogenism:** From adrenal, ovarian, or exogenous sources.
- **Ovarian:** Turner syndrome; ovarian failure due to autoimmunity; ovarian steroidogenic enzyme deficiencies.
- **Uterine:** Congenital absence or malformation of the uterus; imperforate hymen.
- **Pseudohermaphroditism:** Absent uterus and intra-abdominal or cryptorchid testes due either to an enzymatic defect in testosterone synthesis or to complete androgen resistance (testicular feminization).

Etiologies of **2° amenorrhea** are as follows.
- Pregnancy.
- **Hypothalamic/pituitary:**
  - Emotional stress, illness, dieting, exercise, medications (phenothiazine, OCPs), anorexia nervosa, intensive exercise leading to extreme weight loss.
  - Cushing syndrome; hypothyroidism.
  - Pituitary tumor (eg, prolactinoma); pituitary infarction (eg, Sheehan syndrome).
  - Granulomatous disease (sarcoidosis).
- **Ovarian:**
  - PCOS.
  - Premature ovarian failure (autoimmune, radiation therapy, chemotherapy, endometriosis, oophoritis, idiopathic).
  - Hyperandrogenism (from adrenal, ovarian, or exogenous sources).
- **Uterine:** Asherman syndrome (involves extensive intrauterine scarring and synechia formation); cervical scarring leads to closure of the os.

Symptoms/Exam
- **Obtain a detailed history.** Ask about the following:
  - Menstruation: Age at menarche, the character of normal cycles, and the timing of missed cycles, as well as a pregnancy history.
  - Psychosocial history: Situational stresses, emotional problems, dieting and nutritional issues, bulimia, weight loss, and exercise.
  - Medications, especially antipsychotics and OCPs.
  - Hormonal symptoms: Hot flashes, skin changes, hirsutism, headaches, breast changes, galactorrhea, and changes in libido.
  - Previous CNS or pelvic chemoradiation.
  - Family history: Genetic defects or infertility; menstrual and pubertal history of the patient's mother and sisters.
- Table 16.16 outlines exam findings that commonly occur in association with amenorrhea.

KEY FACT

If concerned about 2° amenorrhea, test TSH, LH, and FSH. Try medroyprogesterone provocation first. If this is does not induce menstruation, do a functional anatomy evaluation and test estrogen levels.

MNEMONIC

Causes of 2° amenorrhea:
SOAPH

Stress
OCPs
Anorexia
Pregnancy, **P**COS, **P**rimary ovarian failure
Hypothalamic amenorrhea,
    Hyperprolactinemia

TABLE 16.16.   **Exam Findings Associated With Amenorrhea**

FINDINGS	RELATED DIAGNOSIS
Obesity, hirsutism, acne	PCOS
Webbed neck, widely spaced nipples, short stature	Turner syndrome
Hypertension, buffalo hump, central obesity, easy bruising, striae	Cushing syndrome
Pubic hair with absent uterus	Müllerian agenesis
Virilization, clitoral hypertrophy	Androgen-secreting tumor
Galactorrhea, visual field defects	Pituitary tumor
Enlarged thyroid	Hypothyroidism
Imperforate hymen, transverse vaginal septum	Outflow tract obstruction
Anosmia	Kallmann syndrome

Diagnosis

- 1° amenorrhea:
  - **Labs:** FSH, LH, prolactin, testosterone, TSH, free T4, hCG. Virilized or hypertensive patients should have serum electrolytes and further hormonal evaluation.
  - **Imaging:** MRI of the hypothalamus and pituitary is indicated in girls with low to normal FSH and LH as well as high prolactin levels.
  - Karyotyping can diagnose X chromosome mosaicism in patients with a normal uterus and high FSH without classic features of Turner syndrome.
- 2° amenorrhea:
  - Measure urine or serum hCG. If ↑, the most likely cause is pregnancy (although false ⊕ results are possible with ectopic hCG secretion, as occurs in choriocarcinoma or bronchogenic carcinoma).
  - Progestin challenge can be attempted. If withdrawal bleed occurs, the patient is likely anovulatory. If no withdrawal bleed occurs, an estrogen/progestin challenge can be used to distinguish a hypothalamic/pituitary disorder from outflow tract obstruction.
  - Labs that can be helpful include prolactin, FSH, LH, TSH, potassium, and renal and liver function tests.
  - MRI is indicated for ↑ prolactin or hypopituitarism.
  - In hirsute or virilized women, check serum testosterone.
  - In patients with signs of hypercortisolism, a 1-mg overnight dexamethasone suppression test is needed.

Management

- Treatment directed by underlying cause.
- **2° amenorrhea:** For reversible causes, withholding therapy periodically is recommended to determine if periods return.
  - **Hypothalamic dysfunction:** Periods usually return when precipitants (exercise, dieting, situational stress) are withdrawn. Patients with anorexia nervosa often need to reach 90% of their normal weight prior to the return of menses. Chronic amenorrhea can be treated with medroxyprogesterone or combined hormones to bring on withdrawal bleeding every 1 to 3 months and ↓ the risk of endometrial cancer.

KEY FACT

1° amenorrhea is most commonly a chromosomal abnormality that leads to anatomic or hormonal abnormalities, so perform a karyotype + pelvic ultrasound.

KEY FACT

If the patient has nipple discharge, test prolactin levels (prolactin inhibits gonadotropins). In patients with ↑ prolactin levels, order an MRI of the pituitary to rule out adenoma.

- **Pituitary disease:** Bromocriptine, a dopamine agonist, is used for hyperprolactinemia; larger pituitary tumors may require surgical intervention. Patients with destructive pituitary lesions may need replacement of estrogen, progesterone, thyroid hormone, or adrenal steroids.
- **Ovarian causes:** Estrogen/progesterone replacement is indicated for ovarian failure.
- **Uterine disease:** Asherman syndrome can be treated with dilation and recurettage to sever bridging synechiae and with glucocorticoids to inhibit the formation of new scar tissue.

Complications

Infertility, endometrial cancer, osteoporosis, heart disease.

POLYCYSTIC OVARIAN SYNDROME

Characterized by androgen excess, insulin resistance, and gonadotropin abnormalities, PCOS is the most frequent cause of anovulatory infertility.

Symptoms/Exam

May present with menstrual irregularities, infertility, hirsutism, acne, obesity, possible ovarian enlargement, and acanthosis nigricans.

Differential

- Pregnancy, premature ovarian failure, medications (progestational agents), pituitary adenoma, thyroid disorders, adrenal tumors, Cushing syndrome, congenital adrenal hyperplasia.
- In patients with rapidly progressive hirsutism, ↑ DHEA levels suggest a virilizing adrenal tumor.
- If congenital adrenal hyperplasia is suspected in patients with hypertension and potassium abnormalities, check serum 17-hydroxyprogesterone levels at 8 AM.
- Patients with physical findings of cortisol excess (eg, hypertension, easy bruising, central obesity, proximal muscle weakness) should have an overnight dexamethasone suppression test to rule out Cushing syndrome.

Diagnosis

- Primarily clinical, consisting of a combination of oligomenorrhea and hyperandrogenism. Lab tests are not necessary if diagnosis is clear, although pregnancy must be ruled out.
- Lab findings can include ↑ testosterone, androstenedione, LH, estradiol, estrone, and fasting insulin; an ↑ ratio of LH to FSH (>3:1); and ↑ sex hormone-binding globulin.
- Other useful tests include hCG to rule out pregnancy, TSH, prolactin, fasting glucose, and a lipid panel.
- Diagnosis by ultrasound consists of one or both ovaries with 12 or more follicles <10 mm in diameter, but imaging is not necessary or sufficient for the diagnosis.

KEY FACT

PCOS is largely a clinical diagnosis, combining oligomenorrhea and clinical or laboratory hyperandrogenism.

Management

- **Oligomenorrhea:**
  - Combination OCPs (choose the least androgenic progestins; avoid norgestrel and levonorgestrel) prevent pregnancy and endometrial hyperplasia, normalize menstrual cycles, and treat hirsutism and acne.
  - Monthly DMPA is an option for contraception and endometrial protection, but does not suppress ovarian androgen production.

- **Hirsutism:** Treat with antiandrogens such as spironolactone in combination with OCPs, or use OCPs with a progestin with antimineralocorticoid activity. Topical eflornithine cream is FDA approved for management of hirsutism. Management with shaving, waxing, plucking, bleaching, thermolysis, electrolysis, depilatory creams, and laser removal may be helpful.
- **Anovulation/infertility:** Weight loss; clomiphene citrate ± metformin. Surgical options (which are rarely used) include ovarian cautery and laser vaporization.
- **Weight loss:** ↑ serum androgen, insulin, and LH. Diet and exercise are recommended for all patients; metformin can help with weight loss.

Complications

Chronic anovulation and amenorrhea, with associated long-term exposure to unopposed estrogen, can lead to endometrial hyperplasia and endometrial cancer. Women with PCOS have ↑ risk of diabetes (check fasting glucose or glucose tolerance test), metabolic syndrome, insulin resistance, and nonalcoholic fatty liver disease.

Other Gynecologic Conditions

OVARIAN MASSES

Types of benign ovarian masses include ovarian cysts, germ cell tumors (mature teratomas = dermoid cysts), stromal cell tumors (thecomas, fibromas), and epithelial cell tumors (serous or mucinous adenomas and Brenner tumors). Most ovarian masses are found on physical exam in both symptomatic and asymptomatic women or are discovered incidentally on imaging. The risk of malignancy ↑ significantly with age, from 13% in premenopausal women to 45% following the onset of menopause. Malignant adnexal lesions include 1° ovarian carcinoma and metastatic disease from the uterus, breast, or GI tract. Additional considerations are as follows:

- Newborns can have small functional cysts due to maternal hormones for a few months.
- In girls <9 years of age, 80% of adnexal masses are malignant (usually germ cell tumors).
- In reproductive-age women, most adnexal masses are follicular and corpus luteum cysts of the ovary and benign tumors such as mature teratomas, endometriomas, and serous or mucinous cystadenomas.
- Nonmalignant masses in postmenopausal women include ovarian fibromas.

Symptoms/Exam

- May see urinary frequency, pelvic pressure or pain, dyspepsia, abdominal bloating, early satiety, constipation, and changes in stool caliber. Patients with ovarian cancer often complain of vague GI symptoms. However, most patients are asymptomatic.
- Evaluate for cervical, supraclavicular, and groin lymphadenopathy. Breast exam, as the ovary is a common site of metastasis for breast carcinoma. Bimanual and rectovaginal exams.

Diagnosis

- **Imaging:** Ultrasound is the most important diagnostic study to determine size, whether cystic or solid, and other signs suggestive of malignancy such as internal septae/papillae or the presence of ascites. Signs suggestive of benign mass include unilocular, thin-walled sonolucent cysts with smooth, regular borders.
- **β-hCG level** to rule out ectopic pregnancy, nongestational choriocarcinomas. Serum tumor markers are useful in certain instances:
  - **α-fetoprotein:** For endodermal sinus tumors.
  - **LDH:** For dysgerminomas.

KEY FACT

First-line treatment of PCOS is OCPs. When selecting an OCP, consider the patient's symptoms and medications. Of note, drospirenone-containing OCPs combined with spironolactone can lead to hyperkalemia. Metformin for metabolic/glycemic abnormalities and menstrual irregularities and to ↑ insulin sensitivity (particularly in patients trying to get pregnant). Spironolactone for hirsutism and acne.

KEY FACT

Several disorders associated with PCOS can lead to ↑ risk of endometrial cancer: Obesity, hyperinsulinemia, type 2 DM, anovulatory cycles, and high androgen levels.

- **Serum CA-125:** ↑ in malignant conditions such as serous epithelial ovarian, breast, colon, lung, and pancreatic cancers. In the setting of a postmenopausal woman with an ultrasonographically suspicious pelvic mass, the PPV for malignancy is 97%. Because it can be elevated in benign conditions, CA-125 is not recommended as a routine screening test (the PPV in healthy patients is only 2.3%).

Management

- **Prepubertal patients:** All adnexal masses in prepubertal girls must be evaluated with ultrasound and referral.
- **Premenopausal patients:** Premenopausal women with cysts <10 cm can be followed. If cyst persists >12 weeks, referral is recommended. Monophasic OCPs can suppress symptomatic functional cysts. All solid adnexal masses call for immediate surgical exploration, as does the presence of ascites.
- **Postmenopausal patients:**
  - Asymptomatic ovarian cysts <5 to 10 cm in diameter and a normal serum CA-125 can be followed with serial ultrasounds, because of the very low risk of malignancy. Larger cysts should be evaluated laparoscopically.
  - Symptomatic patients with an ultrasonographically suspicious mass and ↑ serum CA-125 should be referred for surgical evaluation.

OVARIAN TORSION

Rotation of an ovary on its ligamentous supports, often resulting in impairment of the ovary's blood supply. Can be complete or partially torsed. Usually occurs in a pathologically enlarged ovary. Most common in the early reproductive years, with more than half of all cases affecting patients with ovarian masses. (The masses are usually benign; malignant tumors often have adhesions that fix the ovary.) Pregnant women with enlarged corpus luteum cysts, women undergoing ovulation induction, and patients with a history of pelvic surgery, especially tubal ligation, are at ↑ risk for ovarian torsion. Prepubertal patients with congenitally elongated fallopian tubes and normal ovaries are also at ↑ risk.

Symptoms/Exam

- Sudden-onset, severe, unilateral pelvic pain that radiates to the back or thigh. Pain can also be mild or bilateral. Most patients complain of nausea and vomiting. Onset often occurs during exercise.
- Most patients have a unilateral, tender adnexal mass, but up to 30% can have no tenderness on exam. In advanced cases, fever and peritoneal signs can be present.

Differential

Appendicitis, diverticulitis, endometriosis, mesenteric ischemia, bowel obstruction, ovarian cyst, PID, tubal ovarian abscess, ectopic pregnancy, renal calculi, UTI.

Diagnosis

- **Labs:** Rule out other diagnoses with a pregnancy test, UA, and gonorrhea and chlamydia cultures.
- **Imaging:** Ultrasound usually shows ovarian enlargement or an ovarian mass. Doppler flow imaging can be useful, but flow can be normal during transient periods of detorsing. CT can be used to rule out other causes of pain.

QUESTION 1

A healthy 25-year-old woman asks you for a CA-125 test to screen for ovarian cancer. Should you order one?

QUESTION 2

A 36-year-old woman with mild pelvic pain and moderately heavy periods but no anemia is found on pelvic ultrasound to have multiple small uterine fibroids. How would you manage this patient?

Management

- Laparoscopy can be used for confirmation of diagnosis as well as for treatment; conservative treatment consists of uncoiling the torsed ovary.
- Salpingo-oophorectomy is necessary in cases with severe vascular compromise, peritonitis, or tissue necrosis.

Complications

Delayed diagnosis and treatment can lead to infarction and necrosis of the ovary.

VULVODYNIA

A syndrome of unexplained vulvar pain, often accompanied by physical disabilities, limitations in daily activities such as sitting or walking, sexual dysfunction, and psychological distress.

Symptoms/Exam

- Usually acute in onset, vary by subtype. May become chronic and last months or years.
- Discomfort is often described as stinging or burning, or, alternatively, a feeling of rawness or irritation. Itching may be prominent, and pain may be associated with menses, intercourse, or tampon use.
- History of vaginal infections, cryotherapy or laser therapy, and use of medications must be obtained.
- Look for thickened or scaly lesions (papulosquamous vulvar dermatoses), blisters or ulcers (vesiculobullous vulvar dermatoses), or plaques (possible neoplasms), and assess for skin lesions elsewhere on the body.
- Of note, some people have minimal findings.

Differential

Allergic vulvitis, chronic candidal vulvitis, lichen planus, lichen sclerosus, vulvar atrophy, vulvar intraepithelial neoplasia.

Diagnosis

- Pelvic exam to assess for **erythema, edema,** and **vaginal discharge.**
- Fungal and bacterial cultures; KOH microscopic exam; biopsy of suspicious areas with acetowhitening and colposcopy to rule out dermatoses or neoplasm.
- Swab test: Palpation of the vestibulum with a moist, cotton-tipped swab to assess for point tenderness. The vestibule is tested between the hymen and Hart's line.

Management

- **Oral medications:** Fluconazole for cyclic vulvovaginitis; TCAs, SSRIs, or gabapentin for essential vulvodynia; calcium citrate for cyclic vulvovaginitis or vulvar vestibulitis.
- **Topical medications:** Lidocaine or cromolyn cream; estradiol cream for vulvar vestibulitis; corticosteroids for papulosquamous dermatoses.
- Intralesional interferon injection for **vulvar vestibulitis.**
- Low-oxalate diet; physical therapy with biofeedback to ↓ vaginal spasms and strengthen weakened pelvic floor muscles; support groups.
- **Surgery:** Vulvar vestibulectomy and excited dye laser surgery are reserved for severe cases in which all medical therapies have failed.

ANSWER 1

No. The positive predictive value (PPV) in this patient is only 2.3%.

ANSWER 2

As her symptoms are mild, the patient can be reassured and treated conservatively with NSAIDs and OCPs to ↓ menstrual flow. If she develops more severe symptoms, the ultrasound should be repeated and surgery considered.

VULVAR CUTANEOUS CONDITIONS

Lichen Sclerosus

Chronic, progressive, inflammatory disorder of skin commonly seen on the vulva with extragenital lesions. Onset commonly seen in postmenopausal women, but may occur at all ages. Etiology is unclear. ↑ risk of developing squamous cell carcinoma.

Symptoms/Exam

- Commonly presents with intense vulvar pruritus. May be associated with dyspareunia, burning sensation, and irritation. May also be asymptomatic.
- May initially appear as white, thickened, and excoriated skin with edema of labia minora; progresses to thinned and crinkling "cigarette paper" appearance on skin. Vaginal epithelium usually spared. Perianal involvement usually observed (figure-of-eight appearance). May observe clitoral hood phimosis and labia minora fusion.

Differential

Atopic and contact dermatitis, lichen planus, lichen simplex chronicus, genital atrophy, vulvodynia, psoriasis, vulvar intraepithelial neoplasia, vulvar cancer, contact dermatitis, scabies, pediculosis, vulvovaginal candidiasis, tinea cruris.

Diagnosis

Shave vulvar biopsy.

Management

- High-potency topical steroid (eg, clobetasol propionate) to reduce symptoms, prevent architectural damage, and reverse histologic changes.
- Immunosuppressants (tacrolimus) are considered second-line therapy.
- Surgery is not curative; reserved for treatment of malignancy or release of labial adhesions.
- Lifelong monitoring for possible malignancy.

Vulvar Lichen Planus

Inflammatory condition of keratinized and mucosal surfaces. May be the result of an autoimmune disorder. Chronic and recurrent. Of the three types, erosive, papulosquamous, and hypertrophic, the erosive type is the most common form and may lead to destruction of vulvar architecture. Peaks between ages 30 and 60 years.

Symptoms/Exam

- Itching, dyspareunia, burning, vaginal discharge, postcoital bleeding, pain.
- White, lacy, or fernlike striae (Wickham striae) on mucosal membranes. May observe typical pruritic, purple, shiny papules. Genital skin may appear dusky pink without scales.
- The erosive form may have painful, erythematous erosions and denuded epithelium.

Differential

Lichen sclerosus, mucous membrane pemphigoid, pemphigus vulgaris, Behçet syndrome, desquamative inflammatory vaginitis.

Diagnosis

Punch biopsy.

Management

High-potency topical steroids, oral steroids, topical and oral cyclosporine, topical immunosuppressant (tacrolimus). Surgery reserved for release of labial adhesion.

QUESTION

A 35-year-old woman presents with chronic vulvar pain and itching. On exam, she is found to have a ⊕ swab test for vestibular point tenderness, and there are no signs of fungal or bacterial infection. How should you manage this patient?

Vulvar Lichen Simplex Chronicus

Eczematous disease caused by chronic scratching that may occur consciously or unconsciously while sleeping. Usually a response from heat, excessive sweating, irritation from clothing or lotions, soaps, or perfumes. May also occur as a 2° reaction from candidiasis, tinea, HPV, psoriasis, scabies, or neoplasia.

Symptoms/Exam

Intense pruritus in vulvar area. Itchy, scaling, lichenified plaques. In chronic conditions, skin may appear thickened and leathery, associated with hypo/hyperpigmentation.

Differential

Lichen sclerosus, psoriasis, neoplasia, contact dermatitis.

Diagnosis

Vulvar biopsy.

Management

- Treat the underlying disorder.
- Moderate-potency topical steroids; oral steroids. Must break the itch-scratch cycle.
- Amitriptyline and SSRIs may be effective in controlling subconscious scratching.

MENOPAUSE

Cessation of menses for 12 months without another cause. Occurs from gradual depletion of functioning ovarian follicles. After menopause, ovaries lose the ability to produce estrogen. The average age of menopause is 51 years. Most women experience vasomotor symptoms for about 2 years after their LMP, but 25% of women are asymptomatic.

Symptoms/Exam

- **Hot flashes:** Worsened by eating, exertion, emotional stress, and alcohol.
- **GU symptoms:** Vaginal atrophy leading to dryness, pruritus, and dyspareunia; urethral atrophy leading to stress incontinence, frequency, urgency, and dysuria.
- **Mood changes:** Irritability, anxiety, depression, sleep disturbance.
- **Perimenopause:** Syndrome before menopause. Characterized by variable cycle length, and often accompanied by the symptoms of menopause.
- Exam reveals ↓ breast size, vaginal dryness, and urogenital atrophy.

Differential

Premature ovarian failure (cessation of menses in women <40); infections such as TB; malignancy.

Diagnosis

↑ serum FSH can indicate menopause, although is insensitive and rarely needed for diagnosis.

Management

- Hormone replacement therapy (HRT):
  - Associated with a significant ↓ in hot flash severity and frequency; improves GU symptoms and can prevent osteoporosis.
  - Slight ↑ risk of coronary disease, stroke, DVT, and breast cancer, and most appropriately used as a short-term treatment aimed at symptom relief. To prevent endometrial cancer, women with a uterus must be treated with a combination of estrogen and progestin.

KEY FACT

HRT is best used as short-term treatment at the lowest effective dosage for menopausal symptom relief, as it ↑ the risk of coronary disease, breast cancer, and blood clots.

ANSWER

Treatment for vulvar vestibulitis includes oral calcium citrate, topical estradiol cream, and in severe cases, intralesional interferon injection.

- Contraindicated in patients with a history of breast cancer, premalignant breast lesions, endometrial cancer, unexplained vaginal bleeding, DVT or pulmonary embolism, liver disease, or CAD.
- Symptoms of **vaginal atrophy** can be controlled with topical estrogen cream, vaginal estradiol rings, and vaginal lubricants.
- **Other oral medications** that may ↓ hot flashes are gabapentin, clonidine, SSRIs, including paroxetine and fluoxetine, and SNRIs like venlafaxine.
- Phytoestrogens, including soy and red clover, have not consistently been shown to help relieve menopausal symptoms, and studies of black cohosh have also yielded conflicting results.
- **Lifestyle interventions:** Lowering room temperatures, consuming cold food and drinks, weight control, regular physical activity, tobacco avoidance, and relaxation techniques.

Complications

Long-term complications related to menopause and ↓ estrogen include cardiovascular disease and osteoporosis.

KEY FACT

Alternatives to HRT in the treatment of hot flashes include lifestyle changes, SNRIs (eg, venlafaxine), gabapentin, and clonidine.

Sexual Dysfunction

FEMALE SEXUAL DYSFUNCTION

Distress and impairment resulting from a disturbance in sexual desire and/or from emotional and physiologic changes in the sexual response cycle. Affects approximately 25% to 40% of women. Factors that predict sexual functioning include a general state of well-being and a quality relationship with a partner. Dysfunction is generally **not** related to hormone levels. Subtypes include the following:

- **Hypoactive sexual desire disorder/low libido:** Absence of sexual fantasies and lack of desire to engage in sexual activity.
- **Sexual arousal disorder/excitement phase dysfunction:** Inability to respond to sexual stimulation despite genital vasocongestion and lubrication.
- **Orgasmic dysfunction:** Inability to have an orgasm despite normal sexual desire and ability to enjoy intercourse.
- **Pain associated with sex:** Dyspareunia, vaginitis, incompletely ruptured hymen, Bartholin gland cyst, postepisiotomy pain, vulvovaginal atrophy, vulvar vestibulitis, vaginismus (involuntary spasm of musculature of the outer third of the vagina, making penetration impossible or painful), PID, ovarian cyst, endometriosis, fibroids, relaxation of pelvic support.

KEY FACT

Hypoactive sexual desire disorder is present in 5% to 15% of women. Diagnosed by recurrent deficiency or absence of desire or by distress associated with the thought of sexual activity. Treatment includes topical testosterone (patch or gel).

Symptoms/Exam

Pelvic exam may reveal vulvovaginitis, cervicitis, uterine masses or tenderness, cervical motion tenderness, or rectocele or cystocele.

Diagnosis

Primarily based on complete history that explores the following:

- **Interpersonal relationships** (quality and conflict) and sexual history—concerns, degree of satisfaction, sexual orientation, relationship issues, partner performance and satisfaction, contraception, and safe sex practices.
- **Psychology:** Depression, anxiety, past sexual or physical abuse, substance abuse.
- **Sociocultural influences:** Stress, fatigue, lack of privacy, religion, lack of education about sex and sexuality.
- **Physiology:** Medication use, medical/neurologic problems, gynecologic/urologic problems, estrogen or androgen deficiency to rule out 2° causes of sexual dysfunction (eg, Cushing disease, Addison disease, DM, hyperprolactinemia, hypothyroidism, hypopituitarism, degenerative joint disease, MS, temporal lobe lesions, CAD).

KEY FACT

Female sexual function is more commonly related more to a state of well-being and relationship quality than to hormone levels.

MNEMONIC

Sexual response cycle:
EXPLORE
EXcitement
PLateau
Orgasm
REsolution

- **Labs:** CBC, ESR, FSH, estradiol, testosterone, TSH, prolactin, cervical cultures.
- **Imaging:** Pelvic ultrasound if exam is suspicious for a pelvic mass.

Management

- Treat the underlying cause. Counseling, sex therapy, and adjustment of life situation may be of benefit.
- **Estrogen** may be helpful for women with vaginal dryness or atrophy.

ERECTILE DYSFUNCTION

KEY FACT

For low libido, low testosterone, repletion may be indicated. But first, check hemoglobin and hematocrit, because testosterone replacement can induce polycythemia.

Repeated inability to achieve or sustain a penile erection sufficient for sexual intercourse. Affects up to 10% of men; more common in older men and smokers. Screen for cardiovascular risk factors in men with ED; symptoms of ED present 3 years earlier than symptoms of CAD on average (↑ risk of coronary, cerebrovascular, and peripheral vascular diseases). Up to 50% of ED is due to organic causes (Table 16.17).

Symptoms/Exam

- Preservation of morning erections suggests psychogenic disease.
- Assess for atherosclerotic risk factors.
- **Vital signs:** Look for orthostatic changes in BP; BMI (obesity is a risk factor).
- **Skin:** Signs of endocrinopathies include palmar erythema, dryness, hyperpigmentation, and spider angiomata.
- **GU exam:** Inspect the penis for tumors, inflammation, discharge, phimosis, testicular masses, atrophy, or asymmetry. Perform a prostate exam.
- **Vascular exam:** Assess peripheral pulses and evaluate for femoral and aortic bruits.
- **Neurologic exam:** Assess for pain sensation in the genital and perianal areas.
- **Other:** Perform a thyroid exam; palpate the spine for tenderness and evidence of cord compression; examine for gynecomastia.

TABLE 16.17. Etiologies of Erectile Dysfunction

PHYSIOLOGY	EXAMPLES/COMMENTS
Psychogenic disorders	Performance anxiety, depression, mental stress
Diabetes mellitus	ED is seen in up to 50% of DM cases
Peripheral vascular disease	High cholesterol, high BP
Endocrine disorders	Hypogonadism, hyperprolactinemia, thyroid abnormalities, Addison disease, Cushing disease, acromegaly
Surgery or injury	Pelvic surgery, spinal cord injury
Drugs of abuse	Amphetamines, cocaine, marijuana, chronic alcoholism, tobacco, opiates, barbiturates
Medications	Antihypertensives (thiazides, β-blockers, clonidine, methyldopa), antiandrogens (spironolactone, H_2 blockers, finasteride), antidepressants (TCAs, SSRIs, MAOIs, lithium), antipsychotics, benzodiazepines, opiates, antihistamines
Cancer	Prostate cancer
Penile and urethral lesions	Pelvic fracture, hypospadias, priapism, Peyronie disease, phimosis

Diagnosis

- Based on thorough history: Sexual, medications, substance use, psychiatric, medical, surgical.
- **Labs:** Depending on clinical presentation, consider fasting glucose of HbA_{1c} and lipids, TSH, and morning total testosterone.
- Nocturnal penile tumescence testing; Doppler ultrasonography.

Management

- Offer psychological support.
- Adjust contributory medications.
- Address the underlying cause, especially nicotine dependence.
- First-line medications include oral phosphodiesterase type 5 inhibitors (sildenafil, vardenafil, and tadalafil, which has the longest duration of action). Side effects include flushing, headache, dyspepsia, and visual disturbance (sildenafil only); contraindicated if patients are on nitrates because of the risk of hypotension.
- Testosterone replacement.
- Phosphodiesterase type 5 inhibitors are effective in the treatment of ED associated with diabetes and spinal cord injury, and in treatment of ED from sexual dysfunction related to antidepressants.
- Men with hypogonadism may benefit from testosterone to improve ED and libido. Because of ↑ risk of adenocarcinoma of the prostate, monitor hemoglobin, serum transaminase, and PSA levels and perform digital rectal exam.
- Other treatments include intracavernosal injection with alprostadil and/or papaverine, transurethral alprostadil, penile prostheses, and vacuum constriction devices.
- Inform patients about potential risk of prolonged erections and seek immediate medication evaluation for erections lasting >4 hours.

Infertility

Defined as the inability to conceive after 1 year of regular, unprotected vaginal intercourse. In 20% of cases, no cause is found; 40% are due to male factors, 40% to female factors, of which 20% is combined (Table 16.18).

Symptoms/Exam

- Patients may present with a wide array of concerns that they associate with impaired fertility. Inquire about the frequency and timing of intercourse and how long the couple has been trying to conceive.
- Take a complete menstrual and reproductive history. Irregular menses may indicate anovulatory cycles. Prior conception rules out 1° infertility. A history of STIs or endometriosis predisposes women to 2° infertility.
- Perform a complete GU exam to look for anatomic abnormalities, such as undescended testis or varicocele in men or large fibroids in women.
- Examine patients for 2° sexual characteristics as well as for signs of endocrine/metabolic disorders, such as gynecomastia in men or hirsutism or extreme body weight in women.

Diagnosis

- Semen analysis to evaluate ejaculatory function, sperm count, morphology, and motility.
- TSH, FSH, free testosterone, DHEA, and an oral glucose tolerance test if suspected hormonal/metabolic causes in female partner.
- Midcycle progesterone or home luteinizing hormone urine test kit to determine whether the woman is ovulating. Daily basal body temperature readings can also be of benefit—sustained rise of >0.4°F suggests that ovulation has occurred.

KEY FACT

Patients on nitrates should not take sildenafil, vardenafil, or tadalafil owing to the risk of hypotension.

KEY FACT

Infertility is often the presenting complaint of endometriosis (presence of endometrial tissue on the ovaries, fallopian tubes, or other abnormal sites). Women with endometriosis may also have dysmenorrhea, menorrhagia, dyspareunia, low back pain that worsens during menses, rectal pain, and painful defecation.

QUESTION 1

A 68-year-old male smoker with hypertension and diabetes asks you to prescribe sildenafil for erectile dysfunction. The patient takes an ACEI, a diuretic, aspirin, a statin, metformin, and insulin. What do you tell him?

QUESTION 2

A 38-year-old husband and 33-year-old wife present to your clinic because of the inability to conceive after 2 years of trying. The woman has been pregnant once and had an abortion. She reports regular menses every 30 days. The man has two children from a previous marriage. Both travel frequently for work and have gone 2 to 3 weeks at a time without having intercourse. How would you proceed?

TABLE 16.18. **Causes of Infertility**

	MALE FACTORS	FEMALE FACTORS
Anatomic (congenital or acquired)	Varicocele Cryptorchidism History of orchitis	Gonadal dysgenesis Uterine anomalies Endometriosis Prior surgery affecting the reproductive organs Prior tubal inflammation such as that associated with PID Asherman syndrome (uterine synechiae)
Endocrine/ metabolic	Hypothalamic or pituitary dysfunction Hyperprolactinemia Thyroid disease Adrenal disease	Hypothalamic or pituitary dysfunction Hyperprolactinemia Thyroid disease Premature ovarian failure Androgen excess Extremes of body weight
Functional	Erectile dysfunction Ejaculatory dysfunction ↓ libido	Sexual dysfunction ↓ libido
Exposures	Chemical, radiation, or heat effects on testes Exogenous androgens	DES in utero Exogenous androgens Chemical or radiation effects on ovaries

- If concern for ↓ ovarian reserve, **obtain a day-3 FSH.**
- May consider imaging with ultrasound, hysterosalpingography, or hysteroscopy to rule out anatomic causes in female partner.

Management

- Treatment should be targeted to the couple-specific cause of infertility.
- Lifestyle changes to maximize fertility: Avoidance of alcohol and tobacco, ↓ caffeine, and optimizing weight, as well as timing intercourse to ovulation.
- Anovulation can be treated with clomiphene citrate.
- PCOS-related infertility should be addressed with weight loss. If this is unsuccessful, clomiphene citrate ± metformin may be useful.
- Couples with irreversible or unidentified causes of infertility may still be able to conceive using intrauterine insemination, in vitro fertilization, or other assisted reproductive therapies.
- Couples may consider adoption as an alternative.
- Psychosocial support throughout the workup and treatment: Infertility and assisted reproductive therapy can be stressful and emotionally trying.

Men's Health

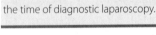

EPIDIDYMITIS

Infectious or noninfectious (eg, trauma or autoimmune disease) inflammation of the epididymis. Most common cause of scrotal inflammation in men. The usual route of

KEY FACT

Medical treatment for endometriosis does not restore fertility. For infertile women with advanced endometriosis, surgical ablation of lesions is often performed at the time of diagnostic laparoscopy.

KEY FACT

Women with PCOS or metabolic syndrome ↑ their chance of conceiving by improving their insulin sensitivity, eg, with metformin.

ANSWER 1

Although sildenafil is absolutely contra-indicated only in patients taking nitrates, before writing the prescription, you should make sure that the patient understands the risks of sexual activity with his multiple cardiac risk factors.

ANSWER 2

Provide education about fertile times of the month and encourage them to keep a journal of fertile periods and sexual activity. It would also be appropriate to provide preconception counseling. Given the couple's history of prior pregnancies and the wife's regular menstrual cycle, they have a high likelihood of being able to conceive together.

infection is retrograde ascent of bacteria. In men <35 years, usually sexually transmitted (chlamydia but sometimes gonorrhea); in older men, usually due to UTI or prostatitis (*Escherichia coli*, sometimes other coliforms).

Symptoms/Exam

- Painful, swollen scrotum usually acute in onset (<6 weeks). Pain localized to the posterior testis but may radiate to the groin, abdomen, or flank.
- Dysuria, urinary frequency, fever, chills, and malaise are common.
- Urethral discharge is possible.
- Exam reveals a swollen, tender mass attached to the testicle and tender spermatic cord. Inflammation may extend locally. May see swollen, tender lymph nodes.
- Normal cremasteric muscle reflex.
- ⊕ Prehn sign (relief of pain with elevation of testis).
- Reactive hydrocele may be seen.

Diagnosis

- UA and culture may be normal or reveal bacteriuria, pyuria, and hematuria.
- CBC and blood culture if patient is febrile or toxic.
- Urine nucleic acid amplification tests or urethral culture for gonorrhea and chlamydia. Offer testing for other STIs.
- Ultrasound with Doppler is not necessary, but reveals enlarged, thickened epididymis with ↑ blood flow.

Management

- Start empiric treatment based on likely pathogens before test results return. If patient is 14 to 35 years old with suspicion of sexual transmission, prescribe antibiotics to cover N *gonorrhoeae* (ceftriaxone) and C *trachomatis* (doxycycline or azithromycin). TMP-SMX or a fluoroquinolone if you suspect enteric gram-negative organisms or *Staphylococcus*.
- Hospitalization for IV therapy in patient with intractable pain, vomiting, failed outpatient therapy, or toxic-appearance.
- NSAIDs, scrotal elevation, limitation of activity, and cold packs.

Complications

Sepsis, abscess, infertility, and extension of infection. Follow with periodic exams to exclude an underlying testicular mass. Prepubescent boys need urology referral to rule out urogenital abnormalities. Evaluate for urethral obstruction due to enlargement of prostate in men >50 years.

PROSTATITIS

An inflammatory disorder of the prostate that may be irritative or infectious. It may present as an acute febrile illness with risk of sepsis or may have a chronic, lingering course. Bacterial prostatitis stems from enteric gram-negative organisms (*E coli*, *Klebsiella*, *Proteus*, *Pseudomonas*), gram-positive organisms (*Staphylococcus*, *Enterococcus*), and/or gonorrhea or chlamydia.

Symptoms

- Perineal, rectal, and/or low back pain. Pain may radiate to head of penis.
- May be acute in onset, with fever, chills, malaise, and myalgias, or chronic, with fewer systemic symptoms.
- Urinary urgency, frequency, retention, nocturia, hesitancy, straining to void, incomplete voiding, and dysuria are seen.
- Painful ejaculation is common.

KEY FACT

Hematospermia is usually self-resolving and benign. But still, test for STIs.

MNEMONIC

Differential diagnosis of scrotal swelling:

THE THEATRES

Torsion
Hernia
Epididymitis/orchitis
Trauma
Hydrocele, varicocele, hematoma
Edema
Appendix testes (torsion, hemorrhage)
Tumor
Recurrent leukemia
Epididymal cyst
Syphilis, TB

KEY FACT

If you suspect acute prostatitis, avoid prostate massage and urethral catheterization if possible, as they may ↑ the risk of bacteremia.

QUESTION 1

A 30-year-old woman and her partner are trying to conceive. They have been having intercourse timed around ovulation for 1 year, and she has regular menses. Semen analysis is normal. What do you do next?

QUESTION 2

A 65-year-old man presents with dysuria and deep rectal pain for the last 2 months. He is generally healthy and has no new sexual partners and no other urinary symptoms. On DRE, his prostate is found to be normal in size, shape, and consistency, and is nontender. Urine culture is ⊖. Exam of expressed prostatic secretions reveals multiple WBCs, but culture is ⊖. What is the likely diagnosis, and how would you treat this patient?

Exam

- Acute prostatitis: the prostate feels boggy, swollen, warm, and tender, and the patient is febrile and appears toxic.
- Chronic prostatitis: may present with a normal exam.

Differential

- Voiding symptoms may indicate UTI or BPH.
- Pain may be isolated prostatodynia, with no exam or lab findings.
- Prostatic abscess, which is rare in nondiabetics, presents with high fever and non-response to treatment and requires surgical drainage.
- If the patient is not responding to antibacterial therapy, consider prostatic abscess, as above, and TB and *Cryptococcus*, especially in immunocompromised patients.
- Consider fistula, foreign body within urinary tract, kidney stones, and bladder cancer.

Diagnosis

- Bacterial prostatitis: UA reveals bacteriuria, hematuria, and pyuria.
- Urine culture and sensitivity identifies the causal organism. If ⊖ in chronic prostatitis, prostatic secretions may be expressed by massage.
- In acute prostatitis, CBC reveals leukocytosis, and blood cultures may be ⊕.

Management

- Acutely ill patients may require hospitalization and IV antibiotics. Ampicillin and an aminoglycoside are recommended until cultures can guide therapy.
- If infectious but IV therapy is not required, treat for at least 4 to 6 weeks with TMP-SMX, amoxicillin, or a fluoroquinolone.
- Adjuvant therapy includes analgesics (usually NSAIDs) and stool softeners for comfort.
- If chronic symptoms persist and cultures are ⊖, treatment is symptomatic with analgesics, anti-inflammatory agents, β-blockers, and sitz baths.

Complications

- Acute prostatitis can lead to bacteremia and sepsis.
- Acute episodes may recur or become low-grade chronic prostatitis. A full month of therapy may ↓ risk of recurrence. Occasionally, patients may require chronic suppressive antibiotic therapy.
- Chronic prostatitis is the most common cause of recurrent UTI in men.

ANSWER 1

Test luteal phase progesterone. If >5 on day 21 of cycle, refer for hysterosalpingography and possibly laparoscopy. If <5, check TSH, LH, FSH, and estradiol.

ANSWER 2

The patient has chronic nonbacterial prostatitis. Treatment is symptomatic, consisting of NSAIDs and sitz baths; β-blockers or antispasmodics may provide additional relief.

URETHRITIS

Classified as gonoccocal or nongonoccocal inflammation of the urethra. 1° pathogens are *C trachomatis* and *N gonorrhoeae*. Common nongonoccocal organisms include *Mycoplasma genitalium* and *Ureaplasma*; less common organisms include *Trichomonas*, HSV, and adenovirus.

Symptoms/Exam

Urethral discharge, penile itching or tingling, dysuria, urgency, hematuria. May also see ulcers and inguinal lymphadenopathy.

Differential

UTI, pyelonephritis, HSV, prostatitis, epididymitis, orchitis.

Diagnosis

- Presence of urethral discharge.
- UA with positive leukocyte esterase or >10 WBCs.
- Urine nucleic acid amplification tests or urethral culture for gonorrhea and chlamydia. Offer testing for other STIs.
- Consider *Mycoplasma*, *Trichomonas*, or *Ureaplasma* cultures from urethra or urine for recurrent infection.

Management

- Treat gonorrhea with ceftriaxone. Treat chlamydia, *Mycoplasma*, and *Ureaplasma* with azithromycin. Chlamydia may also be treated with doxycycline. *Trichomoniasis* may be treated with metronidazole.
- If infections are not present, suggest fragrance-free soaps and lotions; ↑ water intake and ↓ carbonated beverages; ↓ frequency of masturbation or intercourse; no spermicide use.
- Treat partner for STIs. Abstain from sex for at least 1 week following therapy initiation.
- CDC recommends annual screening for men who have sex with men, including urethral/urine DNA testing for chlamydia and gonorrhea, rectal testing for chlamydia and gonorrhea, and DNA swab or culture for pharyngeal gonorrhea. Pharyngeal chlamydia testing is not recommended.
- CDC recommends annual screening in both men and women <25 years with urine, urethral, or vaginal GC/CT DNA testing.

BALANITIS

Inflammation of the glans penis, usually related to fungal organisms but sometimes due to bacteria from skin or sexually transmitted organisms. The condition is more common in uncircumcised men and diabetics.

Symptoms/Exam

- Presents with burning, irritation, and redness of the head of the penis; dysuria.
- A white, cheesy discharge may be seen if the cause is fungal.
- Exam reveals a tender, erythematous, and swollen glans, prepuce, and urethral opening.
- Papules, pustules, or ulcerations may be seen (Figure 16.19).
- If the patient is uncircumcised, retract the foreskin to reveal an adherent, cheesy discharge.

Differential

In prepubertal boys, rule out sexual abuse.

Diagnosis

- The history and exam are usually diagnostic.
- Consider skin culture for fungus and bacteria; consider testing for STIs.

Management

- Topical antifungals if a fungal source is suspected or proven.
- Recommend hygiene measures (keep the area clean and dry; avoid unnecessary foreskin manipulation) to prevent recurrence.
- Aggressive glycemic control in diabetics.
- Antibacterials against skin or STI organisms.
- If fungal infection recurs, consider treating the sexual partner to prevent reinfection.
- If balanitis recurs frequently in an uncircumcised patient, consider circumcision.

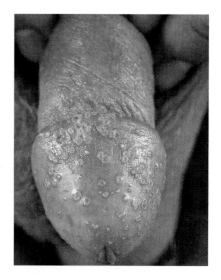

FIGURE 16.19.   Candidal balanitis.
(Reproduced with permission from Wolff K, et al. *Fitzpatrick's Color Atlas & Synopsis of Clinical Dermatology*, 5th ed. New York: McGraw-Hill, 2005:727.)

 KEY FACT

Diabetes is the most common condition underlying balanitis. Don't miss an opportunity to diagnose diabetes or motivate good glycemic control!

ORCHITIS

Infection of the testes, primarily caused by the mumps virus. Other causes include nonmumps viruses, or, rarely, TB, fungi, or local bacterial spread from epididymitis.

Symptoms/Exam

- Presents with abrupt onset of painful, tensely swollen testicle.
- If caused by mumps, associated symptoms include parotitis, fever, and malaise.
- May see reactive hydrocele.
- Normal cremasteric muscle reflex.

Diagnosis

- History and exam are usually diagnostic.
- Testicular masses of unknown etiology should be evaluated with ultrasound.
- In mumps, generalized symptoms and parotitis precede orchitis by 4 to 6 days.

Management

- Supportive care with analgesics, limitation of activity, scrotal support, and cold packs.
- If symptoms do not improve, consider abscess or other causes of testicular mass.

Complications

Mumps orchitis leading to impaired fertility in 10% of men affected and testicular atrophy in 30% to 50%.

BENIGN SCROTAL MASSES

Hydrocele, varicocele, and spermatocele are relatively common scrotal swellings.

Symptoms/Exam

- Present with scrotal swelling or lump, scrotal discomfort or heaviness, occasionally with inguinal or low back pain.
- Hydrocele surrounds or sits below the testis and can be separated from it on exam; is painless, unilateral, fluctuant.
- Spermatocele consists of one or several cysts of the epididymis and sits just above and attached to the testis.
- Varicocele consists of dilated veins of the spermatic cord, more commonly on the left side; feels like a "bag of worms" on palpation. Enlarges when standing or with Valsalva maneuver, and may disappear when the scrotum is elevated or when the patient is lying down.
- Hydrocele and spermatocele transilluminate; varicocele does not.

Differential

Inguinal hernia and malignancy must be considered as sources of a scrotal mass.

Diagnosis

If exam is not definitive, imaging (usually ultrasound) is required to rule out testicular cancer.

Management

- **Hydrocele and spermatocele** usually do not require treatment. If they become large or uncomfortable, surgical repair is offered.
- **Varicocele repair** may be advised to prevent infertility if the mass was detected incidentally; watchful waiting may be appropriate if semen parameters are normal.

KEY FACT

The key to preventing mumps is vaccination. All children should receive two doses of MMR vaccine by kindergarten. Offer MMR to adults without proven immunity.

Complications

By reducing spermatogenesis, varicocele may contribute to male fertility problems.

TESTICULAR TORSION

Inadequate fixation of the testis to the tunica vaginalis leads to the testis twisting around the spermatic cord, compromising blood flow to the testis. A surgical emergency, as cessation of blood supply for 4 to 6 hours will lead to ischemia and permanent loss of the testicle. Most common in infants, teens, and men <30 years of age.

Symptoms/Exam

- May present with testicular pain, abdominal pain, nausea, and vomiting. Scrotal pain is not always present.
- Affected testicle is tender (with testicular elevation) and swollen, which may progress to reactive hydrocele and scrotal wall erythema. High-riding testicle; may be transversely oriented.
- Absent cremasteric muscle reflex.

Differential

Torsion of the appendix testis, appendicitis, epididymitis.

Diagnosis

- If torsion is considered, **do not delay consulting urology.**
- Ultrasound may help distinguish among the causes of scrotal pain but can be falsely ⊖ for torsion (approximately 10% of the time). Ultrasound with Doppler may reveal normal-appearing testicle with ↓ blood flow.
- UA is ⊖.

Management

- Immediate surgical repair is the definitive treatment. Bilateral surgical fixation may be done to prevent recurrence. If surgical treatment is not available, manual detorsion may be attempted.
- Torsion of the appendix testis does not require treatment, but surgical exploration may be needed to rule out testicular torsion.

Complications

- May lead to testicular infarction and impaired fertility if not corrected in time.
- If not surgically fixed, the testes have ↑ risk of recurrent torsion on the ipsilateral or contralateral side.

BENIGN PROSTATIC HYPERTROPHY

Enlargement of the prostate gland, common as men age and can cause partial urethral obstruction, leading to urinary symptoms and occasionally impaired renal function. The severity of symptoms may not correlate with the size of the gland felt on exam.

Symptoms/Exam

- Presents with urinary frequency (≤ every 2 hours) due to incomplete emptying; urinary hesitancy (difficulty initiating stream) or weak stream; and urinary dribbling or incontinence. Nocturia is common.
- Intermittence of voiding (starting and stopping urine flow during voiding) is also seen.
- The gland feels smooth and symmetrically enlarged on DRE, and the bladder may be distended.

KEY FACT

Since testicular torsion can lead to complete loss of blood supply to the testicle if not surgically corrected, the "acute scrotum" should be treated as an emergency. If the ultrasound is inconclusive, suspicion for torsion is still an emergent surgical consult.

MNEMONIC

Differential diagnosis of scrotal swelling:

THE THEATRES

Torsion
Hernia
Epididymitis/orchitis
Trauma
Hydrocele, varicocele, hematoma
Edema
Appendix testes (torsion, hemorrhage)
Tumor
Recurrent leukemia
Epididymal cyst
Syphilis, TB

KEY FACT

The symptom severity of BPH may not correlate with gland size on exam. Once other causes of symptoms have been ruled out, treatment should be guided by the history.

Differential

Prostate cancer, UTI, prostatitis, neurogenic bladder, medications (antihistamines, diuretics, opiates, TCAs).

Diagnosis

- The history and exam are usually diagnostic.
- Postvoid residual urine volume and urodynamic studies can be used to indicate the degree of obstruction.
- PSA may be ↑, but is nonspecific.
- Serum creatinine and other signs of renal impairment may be ↑ due to obstruction and resultant hydronephrosis.

Management

- Treatment is primarily symptomatic, and is aimed at preventing or treating clinically significant urinary obstruction.
- α-blockers (doxazosin, terazosin, prazosin, tamsulosin) relieve symptoms by relaxing the smooth muscles of the bladder neck.
- 5-reductase inhibitors (finasteride, dutasteride) shrink the prostate gland. Six to 12 months of treatment is generally needed before the size reduction corresponds with a change in symptoms; thus, they do not acutely relieve symptoms.
- These two classes of medications can safely be used in combination.
- Transurethral resection of the prostate (TURP) and other minimally invasive surgical techniques have proven effective. Side effects of TURP include sexual dysfunction, hemorrhage, strictures, and hyponatremia associated with hypotonic saline during the procedure.
- Open prostatectomy is the treatment of last resort.

Complications

- Obstruction, leading to hydronephrosis and chronic renal insufficiency; recurrent UTI may result from incomplete bladder emptying.
- Complete inability to urinate that requires urgent bladder catheterization may occur.

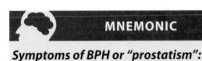

MNEMONIC

Symptoms of BPH or "prostatism":
HI FUN

Hesitancy
Intermittence, **I**ncontinence
Frequency, **F**ullness
Urgency
Nocturia

BENIGN PENILE CONDITIONS

Peyronie disease, leading to "crooked" erections that may be painful due to thickening of the corpora tunica. **Priapism** is a prolonged, painful erection. It is most commonly related to medications such as chlorpromazine and sildenafil or to hematologic conditions such as sickle cell disease and leukemia. **Penile trauma** during erection can lead to rupture of the tunica albuginea, sometimes called penile fracture.

Symptoms

- Peyronie disease presents as a bent angle of the shaft that is often accompanied by pain during erection. The patient may also note subcutaneous nodules.
- The painful, prolonged erection of priapism may be accompanied by fever and inability to urinate.
- Penile fracture is an acutely painful sensation that usually occurs during sexual activity and may be accompanied by a popping sound.

Exam

- Peyronie disease includes palpable, nontender plaques just beneath the skin of the penile shaft, usually on the dorsum.
- Priapism presents with an erect or semierect penis that may last for hours to days.

- Penile fracture is usually accompanied by a subcutaneous hematoma and by swollen "eggplant deformity" of the penis.

Diagnosis

- The history and exam are diagnostic.
- With penile injury, surgical exploration may be required to determine the extent of trauma.

Management

- Peyronie disease can be managed with verapamil injection, shock wave therapy, radiotherapy, or surgery. Many cases resolve without treatment.
- Priapism should be relieved as quickly as possibly to prevent cellular damage that can lead to functional impairment. Treatment is intracavernosal injection of a sympathomimetic drug and/or aspiration and irrigation. Surgical shunting is an option if these therapies are not successful.
- Penile trauma may require surgical repair. Rupture of the tunica albuginea is a surgical emergency.

Complications

- Peyronie disease may progress and lead to worsening pain and sexual dysfunction.
- Prolonged priapism can lead to erectile dysfunction.
- Untreated trauma to the corpora cavernosa or urethra can lead to permanent sexual and urinary dysfunction.

PENILE CUTANEOUS CONDITIONS

Noninfectious lesions are categorized as inflammatory and papulosquamous lesions. See Table 16.19.

PROSTATE CANCER

Most common malignancy among US men, and second most common cause of cancer death. Most cases remain latent, with only 10% progressing to clinically significant disease.

Symptoms/Exam

- Often asymptomatic, or may lead to urinary obstruction with symptoms of prostatism.
- Bony metastases can lead to vertebral or hip pain.
- DRE reveals areas of induration or nodules if the tumor is on the posterior aspect of the prostate.
- Anterior tumors will produce a normal exam.
- Palpate vertebrae for bony tenderness from metastases.

Differential

BPH.

Diagnosis

- There is insufficient evidence to support routine screening, but experts recommend discussing the risks and benefits of screening with all men starting at age 55 years, or at a younger age if risk factors such as African American race or family history are present. Screening should not be offered to men >70 years.
- If PSA or DRE raises concern, ultrasound-guided biopsy is indicated.

KEY FACT

Discuss the risks and benefits of prostate cancer screening with men starting at age 55 and ending at age 70. It is not clear that benefits of screening outweigh harms in most people.

TABLE 16.19. **Penile Cutaneous Lesions**

	INCIDENCE	SYMPTOMS/EXAM	DIFFERENTIAL DIAGNOSIS[a]	TREATMENT
Psoriasis	Occurs in up to 40% of men; 16-22 years and 57-60 years	Penile pruritus; triggered by stress, alcohol/tobacco use, acute infections, α-blockers, lithium. May note extragenital psoriasis	Carcinoma in situ	Topical corticosteroids, tacrolimus, pimecrolimus, vitamin D_3 analogs
Lichen sclerosus	May occur at all ages; average age 42 years	May be asymptomatic; urinary retention, painful erections, phimosis, pain, itching, bleeding. Hypopigmented lesion with skin similar to crinkled paper. May note erosions, atrophy, or bullae	Carcinoma in situ, scleroderma, leukoplakia	Topical corticosteroids, circumcision if limited to glans penis and prepuce, surgery if patient has persistent disease. Retinoids if local therapy fails. Lifelong monitoring for possible malignancy
Lichen nitidus	Occurs in boys and young men	Usually asymptomatic, or, rarely, pruritus. Discrete hypopigmented papules	Pearly papules, HSV	Observation; may resolve spontaneously. Treatment for cosmesis (corticosteroids, vitamin A analogues, cyclosporine, itraconazole, phototherapy)
Lichen planus	Occurs in 25% of men. Relatively uncommon	Pruritus, soreness, and occasionally ulceration. Raised, violaceous, flat-topped, polygonal papules. May observe fine white streaks (Wickham straie)	2° syphilis	Topical corticosteroids or circumcision if isolated only on prepuce
Angiokeratomas	Common in white men >40 years	Asymptomatic, or, rarely, pruritus, pain, intermittent bleeding. Well-circumscribed red or blue papules on glans penis, scrotum, thighs, and abdominal wall	Pearly papules, penile cancer	Observation. For symptomatic or bleeding lesions, treat with surgery, cryoablation, electrocautery, and laser ablation

[a]Diagnosis is based on physical exam. Biopsy and/or further evaluation performed if lesions are atypical.

Management

- Depends on stage at diagnosis and patient's comorbidities. May include surgery, radiation, hormonal therapy, or watchful waiting.
- Close attention to pain control is essential, including management of bone pain from metastases with analgesics and bisphosphonates.

Complications

Treatment (surgery or radiation) may lead to impaired sexual function and/or incontinence.

TESTICULAR CANCER

Can occur at any age, but most commonly seen at ages 20 to 35 years. Risk factors include cryptorchidism (undescended testicle), family history, infertility, tobacco use, white race, and exposure to DES in utero. USPSTF and American Cancer Society recommend against routine screening and self-examination in low- and high-risk asymptomatic men. All scrotal masses should be evaluated to rule out cancer.

Symptoms/Exam

- May be asymptomatic, or may present with a painless mass in the scrotum.
- Patients may have a dull ache/pain, swelling, or hardness in the lower abdomen or scrotum.
- Symptoms of metastasis include neck mass, abdominal mass, lumbar back pain, hemoptysis, dyspnea, cough, or GI symptoms.
- Exam reveals a firm, hard, or fixed nodular mass on the testis that does **not** transilluminate. May be accompanied by epididymitis. Palpate for inguinal lymphandenopathy.

Differential

Isolated epididymitis; benign scrotal mass; hydrocele; swelling of testicular appendix; varicocele.

Diagnosis

- Evaluate any suspicious history or exam findings with ultrasound and possible referral to urology.
- Serum tumor markers: β-hCG, LDH, and α-fetoprotein.
  - Nonseminoma: ↑ α-fetoprotein and β-hCG.
  - Seminoma: Normal α-fetoprotein and usually ↑ β-hCG.
  - Metastasis: ↑ LDH.

Management

- Staging determined by TNMS (tumor, regional nodes, metastasis, serum tumor markers) system.
- Depends on the tumor type. Orchiectomy ± lymph node dissection in most cases. May include chemotherapy.
- Cure rates are high, with roughly 95% 5-year survival.
- After diagnosis, CT of chest/abdomen/pelvis to detect metastasis.

Complications

Impaired fertility after germ cell tumor; ↑ risk of cardiovascular disease and 2° malignancies (leukemia and gastric cancer due to chemotherapy and radiation). Due to ↑ risk of infertility from therapy, recommend sperm banking. ↑ risk of cancer in contralateral testicle.

PENILE CANCER

A rare squamous cell cancer occurring largely in uncircumcised men. Incidence peaks in men >70 years old. Appears to be associated with high-risk HPV infection. Risk factors include smoking, advanced age, presence of foreskin, phimosis, smegma, poor hygiene, and lichen sclerosus.

KEY FACT

There is no effective screening test for testicular cancer, but all suspicious masses should be considered cancerous until proven otherwise.

Symptoms/Exam

Presents with an ulcer, erosion, or nodule on the glans or prepuce or, rarely, on the shaft. Often accompanied by phimosis, which masks the lesion. Retract the foreskin to thoroughly examine the glans, prepuce, and shaft.

Differential

Genital warts, HSV, Peyronie disease.

Diagnosis

Any suspicious lesion should be referred for biopsy.

Management

Depends on the stage at diagnosis.
- Local excision ± lymph node dissection ± radiation.
- Adjuvant chemotherapy may be advised.
- Amputation of the penis is standard treatment for higher-staged tumors.

Complications

Urinary and sexual function after treatment depends on the extent of surgery and radiation required.

Sports Medicine and Musculoskeletal Disorders

Emilia De Marchis, MD

The Preparticipation Physical Evaluation

Goal: Screen athletes for injuries, illnesses, and other factors that might place them or others at risk during sports. Should occur 6 weeks prior to starting activity.

- **History:** Most important and highest-yield part of the preparticipation physical evaluation (PPE). Screen for:
    - General:
        - Recent or current illnesses, infections, or fever.
        - Prior surgeries.
        - Prior injuries.
        - Current medications, supplements.
        - Rapid weight changes (up or down).
    - Family history:
        - Heart disease, including hypertrophic or dilated cardiomyopathy, long QT syndrome, Marfan syndrome, arrhythmias.
        - Sudden death in a family member <50 years of age (hypertrophic cardiomyopathy [HCM] is autosomal dominant).
    - Cardiovascular:
        - History of heart murmur, elevated blood pressure, seizure.
        - Episodes of dizziness, palpitations, chest pain, or syncope/presyncope with exertion, in addition to unexplained syncope/presyncope.
    - Pulmonary:
        - Asthma or coughing/shortness of breath during or after exercise (may point to exercise-induced bronchospasm).
    - Neurologic:
        - Prior concussion, including any head trauma, loss of consciousness, confusion, memory loss, or headache with exertion.
    - Gynecologic:
        - Menstrual history in females (screen for female athlete triad: disordered eating, amenorrhea, osteoporosis).
- **Exam:** Evaluate for medical conditions that would prevent or restrict participation, or potentially worsen with participation. Table 17.1 describes the standard components of a PPE.
- **Studies:**
    - No routine diagnostic testing is recommended (including blood/urine testing).
    - If history and/or exam is concerning for structural heart disease, arrhythmia, genetic/congenital heart disease, then standard evaluation generally includes a 12-lead ECG, ± stress echocardiography and graded exercise testing. Consider event monitor if history is concerning for arrhythmia. Concerning cardiac findings include:
        - Systolic murmurs of grade 3/6 or more (concern for atrial stenosis, mitral regurgitation).
        - Any diastolic murmur (concern for aortic regurgitation, mitral stenosis).
        - Any murmur that grows louder with ↓ venous return, eg, Valsalva maneuver, standing from squatting to standing (concern for HCM).
        - An S4 gallop (concern for HCM).
- An S3 gallop can be normal in younger patients and in high-output states, such as pregnancy.

Concussion Management

A concussion, also known as mild traumatic brain injury (MTBI), is an alteration in cerebral function due to force on the brain. Features include the following:

- Caused by direct or indirect (rotational) force to head.
- Short-term impairment with spontaneous improvement.

TABLE 17.1.   **Components of the Preparticipation Physical Evaluation**

SYSTEM	COMPONENT
Vitals	Routine vital signs (height, weight, pulse, BP, oxygen saturation)
	Screen for eating disorders, Marfan features
Cardiovascular	Palpate pulses (including femoral to screen for aortic coarctation), auscultate for murmurs in both sitting and standing positions
Musculoskeletal	Assess range of motion, strength, flexibility (general, neck, shoulder/upper extremity, and back), gait/lower extremity, and asymmetry of muscle bulk/scarring/posture
	Use the duck walk as a quick way to assess multiple joint range of motion and flexibility
	Have patient lean forward to touch his/her toes to assess for scoliosis
Skin	Assess for contagious lesions and rashes; especially relevant for close contact sports, eg, wrestling
Vision and hearing	General screening; automatically refer if vision <20/40
Abdomen	Check for masses and evidence of hepatosplenomegaly
Genitourinary—males only	Check for testicular abnormalities and hernias; note Tanner stage
Neurologic	Rule out problems with coordination, gait, and mental processing

Based on data from Wilson PE, Matthews DJ. Rehabilitation and Sports Medicine. In Hay WW, et al. *Current Pediatric Diagnosis and Treatment,* 18th ed. New York: McGraw-Hill, 2007.

- No imaging abnormality (if obtained; not required for diagnosis).
- ± loss of consciousness.

Symptoms/Exam

- Early: Headache, dizziness, nausea, confusion, amnesia, double or blurry vision, vertigo, nausea/vomiting, ± loss of consciousness.
- Late (hours to days): Irritability, photo-/phonophobia, changes in sleep pattern, difficulty concentrating, memory problems, ↑ emotionality, and easy fatigability.
- Exam may reveal delayed verbal and motor responses, a vacant stare, disorientation, slurred or incoherent speech, incoordination, and memory deficits.

Differential

Skull fracture, intracranial injury (subdural/epidural hematoma). Also consider migraine, heat stroke, hypoglycemia, dehydration, infection.

Diagnosis

- Clinical; **any abnormalities found on neurologic exam are not normal** and should be emergently evaluated in the emergency department.
- Consider head CT or MRI if patient has persistently altered mental status (GCS <15), concern for skull fracture, 2+ episodes of vomiting, age ≥65, hypocoagulability (eg, anticoagulant use), seizures, worsening of symptoms, amnesia ≥30 minutes before injury, or any focal neurologic findings (eg, unequal pupil size).
- Consider 24-hour inpatient observation if GCS <15, hypocoagulability, seizure, or lack of responsible caregiver.

Management

- Complete mental and physical rest until asymptomatic (including no homework or screen time).

 KEY FACT

Amnesia is thought to be a better indicator of concussion severity than loss of consciousness.

 QUESTION

You are team physician for a high school football team. During a game, one of the players sustains a forceful tackle and falls to the ground unresponsive. You run onto the field and find him dazed but coherent. He reports a headache and dizziness. His teammates report that the player appeared unconscious for a few seconds. After clearing his C-spine, you help the player off the field and conduct a neurologic exam, which is normal. After 10 minutes, the player states that he feels fine and that his headache and dizziness are gone. He asks to return to the game. What do you do?

MNEMONIC

Inspection "SEADS":
Swelling
Erythema
Atrophy
Deformity
Scars

MNEMONIC

In v**AR**us stress, there is more **A**i**R** between the knees.

■ Return to play: Allow slow progression of activities through the following stages: light aerobic activity, sport-specific exercise, noncontact drills, full-contact drills, and then normal game play. Each stage should last at least 1 day. Athletes must remain asymptomatic to progress to the next stage and should begin this process only after successful return to academics.

General Approach to the Joint Exam

■ **Inspection:** Surface anatomy (muscle wasting, symmetry), alignment (eg, genu valgum).
■ **Palpation:** Identify landmarks, localize tenderness, compare temperature with the contralateral side (to detect the warmth of infection or posttraumatic inflammation or to gauge the coolness of vasoconstriction or vascular compromise), and check pulses.
■ **Manipulation:** Test range of motion (ROM), tone, muscle strength, sensation, reflexes, stability, and special tests.
■ **Special terms:** In the forearm and hand, different terms are used to specify location:
  ■ **Volar** = anterior (palmar surface; also sole of foot); **dorsal** = posterior.
  ■ **Ulnar** = medial; **radial** = lateral (remember the anatomic position of the hand).

Axial alignment is described in terms of the angle made by the proximal and distal segments.
■ **Valgus alignment:** Two limb segments create an angle that points toward midline.
■ **Varus alignment:** Two limb segments create an angle that points away from midline.

General Approach to Overuse Injuries

Repetitive stress across a bone, tendon, or muscle without adequate healing time can lead to tissue injury and degradation. The process can be largely inflammatory, as in carpal tunnel syndrome and de Quervain tenosynovitis; largely degenerative, as in lateral epicondylitis; or due to incomplete remodeling, as seen in stress fractures.

If you encounter multiple stress fractures, especially in a female athlete, you should workup for osteoporosis along with questioning regarding the female athlete triad (disordered eating, amenorrhea, osteoporosis).

TENDINOPATHIES

Repetitive stress along a tendon (eg, Achilles, patellar, medial and lateral elbow, rotator cuff) can lead to collagen degeneration or tendinosis. Many studies have cast doubt on the role of inflammation (tendinitis). Overloading of the tendon due to poor biomechanics (eg, muscle imbalances, foot overpronation) and repetitive stress can cause collagen breakdown and/or inflammation.

Management
■ Early treatment = rest, cryotherapy/ice, unloading devices (eg, counterforce straps for the elbow and patellar tendon; heel lifts for the Achilles tendon), and physical therapy (PT).

- Role of NSAIDs and corticosteroid injections is controversial, but can often provide short-term relief.
- Healing is slow and can take 6+ months.
- Surgical debridement is a last resort and not always effective.
- Eccentric exercises are activities that lengthen the muscle while the patient is contracting the muscle (example: downward motion of squatting or downward motion of calf raises).
- Use splints with caution: Splinting for only 2 weeks can cause significant loss of ROM. Encourage early mobilization when possible.
- In children, bones grow first, pulling on muscles and tendons, risking injury to muscles, tendons or growth plates. Growth plates are weaker than tendons/ligaments, which ↑ the chance of an avulsion fracture.

Principles of Imaging

STANDARD VIEWS

Radiographs must include a minimum of two views, AP and lateral, to fully evaluate patients for fractures. Table 17.2 describes additional views by anatomic location. Table 17.3 describes the Ottawa rules for ruling out the need for imaging of the knee, ankle, and foot in specific scenarios.

KEY FACT

Most effective treatment for tendinopathies is physical therapy, focusing on eccentric exercises.

KEY FACT

Plain films are not recommended in the first 6 weeks of evaluation/treatment of low back pain, unless there are red flags such as concerns for infection, malignancy, or cauda equina.

KEY FACT

A fracture with any overlying laceration or abrasion should be considered an open fracture and requires further evaluation with orthopedic consult (the old term for this was a compound fracture).

TABLE 17.2. Radiologic Views and Key Points

REGION	VIEWS
Wrist	For acute wrist injuries, always include oblique view
	To improve sensitivity of detecting sdcaphoid fractures, include PA films in ulnar deviation, and pronated and supinated oblique view
	To evaluate for scapholunate joint widening, obtain AP with patient's fist clenched
Elbow	Consider axial view to evaluate olecranon fossa, oblique view to evaluate radial head, and stress views for joint instability
	Look for an anterior **sail sign** (fat pad displaced by effusion), which suggests fracture (Figure 17.1)
Cervical spine	AP and lateral view must include C1-C7 to fully clear C-spine
	The swimmer's view (arm overhead) may help visualize C7
	Use odontoid view to rule out traumatic fractures or congenital abnormalities
	Oblique views give additional information on neural foramina narrowing
Shoulder	For acromioclavicular (AC) joint: AP, axillary and Zanca view (AC joint, 10-15° cephalic)
	For glenohumeral joint or proximarl humeral fractures: AP, scapular Y and axillary
	For clavicle, include serendipity view (40° cephalic)
Hip/pelvis	AP and frog-leg lateral views (to evaluate anterosuperior aspect of femoral head)
	In osteoarthritis, get weight-bearing films
Knee	Weight-bearing AP in full extension, 45° flexion (Rosenberg), and 40° flexion (notch/tunnel view) if osteoarthritis is suspected
	Include notch/tunnel view to evaluate osteochondritis dissecans: include axial (merchant) or sunrise view to evaluate the patellofemoral joint, use sunrise view also to evaluate patellar fracture
Ankle and foot	Oblique (mortise) ankle view evaluates ankle joint integrity (symmetry of the mortise space)
	Olique view of foot shows articulation of calcaneus, talus, navicular, and cuboid bones

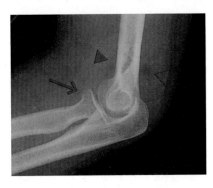

FIGURE 17.1. Elbow effusion and fracture. Displacement of the anterior and posterior fat pads (arrowheads) at the elbow joint on a lateral radiograph indicates the presence of a joint effusion, raising concern for fracture. The arrow denotes a subtle associated fracture of the head. (Reproduced with permission from USMLE-Rx.com.)

KEY FACT

Open fractures are an orthopedic emergency. Patients should be taken to the OR within 24 hours to reduce infection risk: treatment includes surgical irrigation and debridement, in addition to repair of fracture. Patients should receive antibiotics and tetanus prophylaxis.

KEY FACT

Image the contralateral, unaffected joint in children with suspected fracture involving growth plate, to allow for comparison of the normal growth plate, given normal variability with age.

KEY FACT

Always refer supracondylar humerus fractures given the high risk of neurovascular injury.

MNEMONIC

Salter-Harris categories:

SALTER

Type I **S**lipped: separation of physis
Type II **A**bove: fracture lies above the physis
Type III **L**ower: fracture below the physis in the epiphysis
Type IV **T**hrough: fracture through the metaphysis, physis, and epiphysis
Type V **ER**ased/crushed: the physis has been crushed

TABLE 17.3. Ottawa Rules for Knee, Ankle, and Foot Imaging

LOCATION	CRITERIA
Knee	Age ≥55 years
	Tenderness at fibular head
	Isolated tenderness of patella
	Inability to flex knee to 90°
	Inability to bear weight for 4 steps immediately after injury and in examination room
Ankle	Bone tenderness over posterior edge/tip of lateral malleolus
	Bone tenderness at posterior edge/tip of medial malleolus
	Inability to bear weight immediately and in examination room
Foot	Bone tenderness at base of 5th metatarsal
	Bone tenderness at navicular
	Inability to bear weight immediately and in examination room

If no criteria are met, then imaging is not indicated.

IMAGING OF FRACTURES

Fracture Categories

Fractures are categorized by location (eg, distal radius, tibial plateau), type (Table 17.4 and Figure 17.2), and degree of displacement (Table 17.5).

Pediatric Fractures

Until late adolescence, tendons and ligaments are stronger than bones, so fractures are more common and true sprains are infrequent. Children's bones are more malleable, creating a few fracture terms specific to pediatrics (Figure 17.3). See Table 17.6 for a list of common pediatric fractures.

TABLE 17.4. Fracture Types

TYPE	DESCRIPTION
Transverse	Perpendicular to the shaft of the bone
Oblique	Slanting or inclined fracture line
Spiral	Multiplanar fracture line, caused by a torsional force
Comminuted	Multiple fragments
Segmental	Large, well-defined fragments (a type of comminuted fracture)
Intra-articular	Extends into the joint space; the general rule is that if the fracture includes more than one third of the joint space, it requires surgical evaluation for possible fixation
Avulsion	Bony fragment pulled away from its native bone
Compression	Impaction of bone, such as in the vertebrae or proximal tibia
Pathologic	Fracture through bone weakened by tumor or disease (eg, osteoporosis)

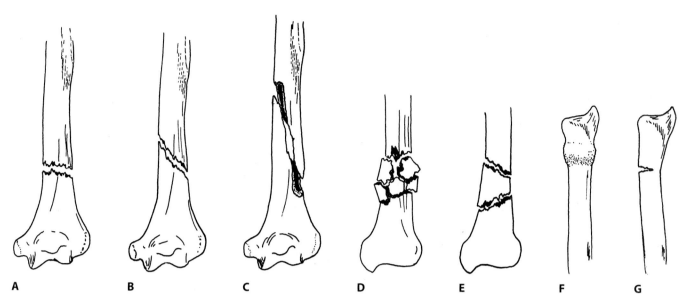

FIGURE 17.2. **Fracture classification.** (**A**) Transverse. (**B**) Oblique. (**C**) Spiral. (**D**) Comminuted. (**E**) Segmental. (**F**) Buckle (torus). (**G**) Greenstick. (Reproduced with permission from Tintinalli JE, et al. *Tintinalli's Emergency Medicine: A Comprehensive Study Guide*, 6th ed. New York: McGraw-Hill, 2004, Fig. 267-2.)

Shoulder Injuries

- **Inspection:** Note supraspinatus and infraspinatus atrophy seen on the posterior shoulder with **suprascapular nerve entrapment** or chronic rotator cuff tears.
- **Palpation:** Check for acromioclavicular (AC) joint tenderness (separation, arthritis).
- **ROM:** Watch for scapular dyskinesis or winging on abduction and forward flexion (rotator cuff dysfunction).

Table 17.8 outlines special tests that can aid in the evaluation of injuries to the shoulder.

KEY FACT

Cervical disc disease, apical lung tumor, pleural disease, myocardial ischemia, and subdiaphragmatic processes should be considered as causes of referred shoulder pain.

TABLE 17.5. **Degrees of Fracture Displacement**

TERM	DEFINITION
Displaced	When one fragment shifts in relation to the other through translation, angulation, shortening, or rotation
Nondisplaced	A fracture in which the fragments are in anatomic alignment
Translation	Movement in the AP (volar/dorsal in the forearm) or medial-lateral plane (ulnar/radial in the forearm)
Angulated	Malalignment described using the direction the apex is pointing, eg, apex dorsal angulation
Bayonetted	The distal fragment longitudinally overlaps the proximal fragment
Distracted	The distal fragment is separated from the proximal fragment by a gap

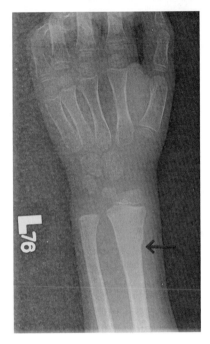

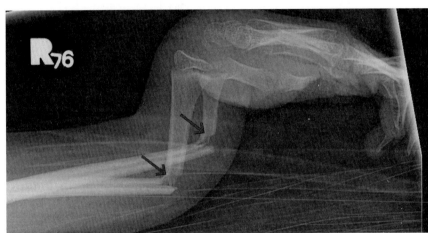

A   **B**

FIGURE 17.3.   **Pediatric fractures. (A)** Buckle (torus) fracture (arrow) of the distal radius after trauma. **(B)** Greenstick fractures of the distal radius and ulna after a motor vehicle accident. Note the intact periosteum and cortex (arrows) opposite the side of fracture through the cortex and periosteum. (Reproduced with permission from USMLE-Rx.com.)

TABLE 17.6.   **Common Pediatric Fractures**

PEDIATRIC FRACTURE	MECHANISM	TREATMENT
Buckle (torus) fracture	Impaction fracture, identified by a focal widening (or outward buckling) of the cortex of a long bone Periosteum bends but does not break Most common in distal radius or ulna	Immobilize in cast 3-5 weeks
Greenstick fracture	Periosteum buckles on one side and breaks on the other, which can cause angulation that may need to be reduced	Reduce with casting Reimage in 10-14 days
Salter-Harris fracture	Physeal (growth plate) fracture, unique to children Classify using the Salter-Harris system (see Table 17.7)	Alignment with closed versus open reduction, then immobilize
Clavicular fracture	Most common long bone fracture in children Can be due to birth trauma and can result in brachial nerve palsies Most frequently occurs at middle 1/3 of clavicle, with superior displacement of proximal end due to pull of sternocleidomastoid	Figure-of-eight versus arm sling
Nursemaid's elbow	Radial head subluxation; due to pulling/lifting by hand Child is in pain and refuses the bend the elbow	Manually reduce with supination of elbow at 90° flexion Do not immobilize
Supracondylar humerus fracture	Most common pediatric elbow fracture, with peak at ages 5-8 years ↑ risk of Volkmann's contracture due to proximity to brachial artery, which, if injured, can cause compartment syndrome of forearm	Always test radial artery to check for brachial artery entrapment Immobilize in cast If significantly displaced, may require closed reduction with percutaneous pinning

Modified from Le T, Bhushan V, Chen V, King M. *First Aid for the USMLE Step 2 CK,* 9th ed. New York: McGraw-Hill, 2016, Table 2.13-25.

TABLE 17.7. **Salter-Harris Fracture Classification**

TYPE	LOCATION	OUTCOME	IMAGE
I	Through the physis	Associated with the best prognosis (difficult to distinguish from normal growth plate)	
II	Through the physis and metaphysis	Growth arrest may occur	
III	Through the physis and epiphysis	Growth arrest is rare, but joint surface involvement requires close maintenance of anatomic reduction (referral)	
IV	Through the metaphysis, across the physis, and through the epiphysis	Associated with a risk for both growth arrest and articular cartilage damage (referral)	
V	Crush injury to the physis	Usually diagnosed retrospectively if growth arrest or angular deformity has occurred	

TABLE 17.8.   Special Tests for the Diagnosis of Shoulder Injury

EXAM	TECHNIQUE	INDICATIONS
Hawkins test	With the patient's elbow and shoulder flexed to 90°, the examiner passively internally rotates the shoulder by stabilizing the elbow and pushing down on the wrist	Pain points to rotator cuff tendinosis/impingement
Neer impingement sign	The examiner performs maximal passive forward flexion with internal rotation while stabilizing the patient's scapula with the other hand	Pain points to rotator cuff tendinosis/impingement
Jobe test (empty can)	The arms are abducted 90° and brought forward 30°, thumbs down; the patient resists downward pressure	Pain points to supraspinatus tendinosis; weakness suggests tear
O'Brien test	Forward flex the shoulder to 90° with the elbow extended and the arm 15° toward the midline; the patient resists downward force with the thumb down and the thumb up	Deep pain with the thumb down that improves with the thumb up suggests superior glenoid labrum (SLAP) lesions
Apprehension test (crank test)	The shoulder is in 90° abduction and slight extension with the elbow flexed; the examiner externally rotates the arm	Simulates the most common position of subluxation/dislocation; pain or anxiety suggests anterior instability
Cross-body adduction test	Bring shoulder across body	Assess stability of AC joint, squeezing acromion and clavicle; painful in cases of separation or arthritis
Speeds test	The shoulder is in 60° front flexion with forearm supinated and elbow fully extended; the examiner forcefully presses down on patient's arm at the forearm	Assess for biceps tendonitis
Yergason test	The examiner palpates the bicipital groove, the patient's arm is relaxed at the patient's side and the elbow is flexed to 90°; the examiner's other hand applies downward pressure on the forearm while patient resists	Assess for biceps tendonitis

MNEMONIC

Rotator Cuff Muscles:

SITS:

Supraspinatus (abduction)
Infraspinatus (external rotation)
Teres minor (external rotation)
Subscapularis (internal rotation)

KEY FACT

Pain on abduction suggests subacromial impingement syndrome; weakness suggest rotator cuff tear.

KEY FACT

Refer complete rotator cuff tears for surgery.

ROTATOR CUFF TEARS AND IMPINGEMENT SYNDROME

Symptoms/Exam

Rotator cuff impingement and tearing usually begin in the supraspinatus tendon as it passes under the acromion. Patients are usually >50 years of age and will often have significant pain with abduction above the head and internal rotation (reaching up the back). Can occur in young athletes. Will often hear a "pop" (eg, baseball pitchers). **Hawkins** and **Neer** tests are ⊕.

Diagnosis/Management

If weakness on exam and lack of full improvement with rehabilitative exercises (eg, initial treatment with 6 weeks PT) ± subacromial corticosteroid injection, suspect a tear rather than isolated impingement. Tears are diagnosed with MRI and often require surgical repair.

ADHESIVE CAPSULITIS (FROZEN SHOULDER)

- Idiopathic loss of both active and passive motion of the shoulder; usually resolves over **6 months to 2 years.**
- Usually results from prolonged immobility from another shoulder injury. Significant association with **diabetes, especially type 1;** 40% to 50% of people with diabetes will develop bilateral disease. People without diabetes are also at ↑ risk for occurrence in the other shoulder.

- Characterized by progressive/painful initial "freezing" phase, presenting with complaints similar to those of rotator cuff pathology (differentiated by loss of **passive** ROM), followed by a "thawing" phase with improvement in pain and ROM.
- Treat initially with NSAIDs and stretching (such as arm pendulum and wall push-ups). Can use glenohumeral corticosteroid injections; surgery rarely required.

ACROMIOCLAVICULAR JOINT PATHOLOGY

- Degenerative **arthritis** of the AC joint is often a component of rotator cuff pathology and shoulder pain seen in patients >50 years of age. For this reason, a distal clavicle resection often accompanies surgical repair of the rotator cuff.
- AC injuries (**shoulder separations**) usually occur from a fall onto the lateral aspect of the shoulder with an adducted arm, causing stress and tearing of the AC ligaments ± the coracoclavicular (CC) ligaments. Remember, this is not the same thing as a shoulder dislocation, which involves the glenohumeral joint (see Glenohumeral Dislocations below). AC injuries are classified as types I–VI (Rockwood classification; see Table 17.9).

GLENOHUMERAL DISLOCATIONS

- The shoulder is most vulnerable when abducted and externally rotated. A fall or tackle with the arm in this position can cause an **anterior dislocation.** Posterior dislocations are less common, but can occur with a grand mal seizure or an electrical shock.
- With anterior dislocation, patients hold the arm abducted/externally rotation; with posterior dislocations, patients hold arm adducted/internally rotated.

QUESTION

A mother brings in her 2-year-old son and states that he is refusing to use his left arm. He is holding his hand in a slightly flexed and pronated position. He was having a tantrum in a store when she picked him up by his hands to get him off the floor. The child does not appear to be in severe pain, but he does not move his left arm despite attempts to have him reach for a toy with that arm. Given the history and exam, you suspect a subluxation of the radial head (nursemaid's elbow). What do you do?

KEY FACT

In patients who have difficulty brushing their hair or pain at night when rolling onto their shoulder, suspect impingement syndrome.

KEY FACT

Anterior dislocations of the shoulder can injure the axillary nerve, causing difficulty with abduction.

TABLE 17.9.   Rockwood Classification of Acromioclavicular Injury

TYPE	INJURY	EXAM/IMAGING	TREATMENT
Type I	Sprained AC ligaments, intact CC ligaments	Tenderness/swelling but no step-off on palpation; normal imaging	Nonoperatively with sling for comfort, analgesics, and ice for weeks, followed by rehabilitative exercises; 4-6 weeks to heal
Type II	Torn AC ligaments, sprained CC ligaments	Partial separation/instability of clavicle from acromion with horizontal stress; widening of AC joint on stress radiographs and palpation	Nonoperative as above; 8 weeks to heal
Type III	Disruption of AC and CC ligaments	Complete separation of the clavicle from the acromion superiorly, with instability on horizontal and vertical stress	Conservatively or surgically; 12 weeks to heal
Type IV	Posterior displacement into trapezius muscle	Not reducible on exam; posterior dislocation on axillary imaging	Operative reduction
Type V	Rupture of muscle/fascia surrounding distal clavicle	Distal clavicle elevated 1-3 times width of clavicle	Operative reduction
Type VI, rare	Inferior displacement of distal clavicle under conjoined tendon into subacromial/ subcoracoid position	Associated with rib fractures/neurovascular injury	Operative reduction

ANSWER

The child's arm must be reduced. Hold the child's hand, stabilizing his elbow while supinating and flexing the forearm. Immediately, the child begins using his arm again. You tell the mother that he is at risk of recurrence and advise her to avoid pulling him by his arms.

KEY FACT

Glenohumeral dislocations are the most common type of major joint dislocation.

KEY FACT

Anterior dislocations of SC joint are generally easy to reduce, but at risk of redislocation.
Posterior dislocations of SC joint should be reduced with a vascular surgeon available, given risk to underlying great vessels.

KEY FACT

Humerus fractures can damage the radial nerve, causing radial nerve palsy and resulting in wrist drop and inability to extend thumb.

Management

- Reduction, followed by sling (4 weeks) and then PT for strengthening.
- Surgical repair of the capsule integrity is required for recurrent dislocations; consider especially in young athletes given high recurrence rate.
- Recurrence rates after 1° traumatic dislocation are 65% to 95% in patients <20 years of age; 60% in patients 20 to 40 years of age; and 10% in patients >40 years of age.

SLAP LESIONS

- SLAP = injury or tear of the Superior Labrum from Anterior to Posterior. The superior labrum is the upper portion of the cartilaginous ring that surrounds the glenoid fossa, ↑ its depth and adding to shoulder stability.
- Most common in throwing athletes, such as baseball pitchers. Patients experience a sense of catching or popping in the shoulder, with loss of force ± pain.
- Requires MRI or MR arthrography to diagnose. First-line therapy is NSAIDs and PT.
- Surgical repair required for severe symptoms that fail conservative management.

STERNOCLAVICULAR INJURIES

- Often associated with trauma (landing on lateral shoulder) or overuse; patients often note popping/pain over medial aspect of the clavicle.
- Acute dislocation of SC joint present with localized tenderness of medial clavicle. Exam may demonstrate asymmetry.
- Treatment is reduction.

FRACTURES OF THE SHOULDER

- **Clavicle fractures:** Caused by fall onto lateral aspect of the shoulder or a direct blow. Eighty percent affect the middle third of the clavicle. Treat nonoperatively with either an arm sling or a figure-of-eight harness for 2 to 6 weeks (3-4 weeks for children <12 years of age). Surgical referral if displacements are greater than the width of the clavicle or for shortening >20 mm.
- **Scapula fractures:** Caused by high-energy trauma, such as significant falls and motorcycle accidents. Ninety percent associated with other injuries, such as rib fractures, pneumothorax, pulmonary contusion, and injuries of the head, spinal cord, or brachial plexus. Treat with a sling for comfort and early ROM.
- **Proximal humerus fractures:** Common in elderly patients with osteoporosis, especially women; often due to direct trauma in younger patients. Most are minimally displaced and can be treated with a sling (for 6-8 weeks) and early mobilization.

Elbow and Forearm Injuries

EPICONDYLITIS/ELBOW TENDINOSIS

Repetitive stress across the common tendon of the wrist flexors (medial) or extensors (lateral) leading to collagen breakdown and failure of tendon healing, resulting in a tendinosis. A degenerative problem, not inflammatory.

Medial epicondylitis = **golfer's elbow;** lateral epicondylitis = **tennis elbow.**

Symptoms/Exam

- Activity-related pain (over medial vs lateral elbow) progressing to pain at rest and functional strength loss.

- Tenderness over the medial versus lateral tendon origins, and pain with resisted wrist flexion/pronation (for medial epicondylitis) or resisted wrist and middle finger extension/supination (for lateral epicondylitis).

Diagnosis

Clinical diagnosis based on the history and exam. Consider MRI for persistent cases.

Management

- PT with focus on stretching and strengthening is superior to rest, NSAID, steroid injection, or bracing alone.
- NSAIDs can control pain and allow for rehabilitative exercises. Corticosteroid injections can provide short-term relief for lateral epicondylitis, however there is a risk for tendon rupture if steroid is injected into the tendon itself. This risk ↑ with multiple injections.
- Ice/heat, high-voltage electrical stimulation, and ultrasound can aid in pain relief.
- Control force loads across the tendon, with use of counterforce strap bracing and improvements in technique.
- Consider surgical debridement of the tendon if conservative measures fail, although its effectiveness is inconsistent. Counsel patients that conservative measures may take weeks to months to succeed.

> **KEY FACT**
>
> Unlike lateral epicondylitis, corticosteroid injections for medial epicondylitis are not recommended for short-term pain relief due to risk of injury to ulnar nerve.

ULNAR NERVE COMPRESSION

Chronic or posttraumatic compression of the ulnar nerve near or at the elbow, can lead to an ulnar neuritis. May occur in multiple sites, the most common of which is the cubital tunnel ("funny bone"), where the nerve passes through the groove on the posterior aspect of the medial epicondyle.

> **KEY FACT**
>
> Elbow dislocation can injure the ulnar nerve, causing difficulty with finger abduction, resulting in claw hand.

Symptoms/Exam

- Aching pain in the medial aspect of the elbow, along with numbness and tingling into the fourth and fifth fingers.
- Weakness of the intrinsic muscles of the hand occurs late, which can interfere with activities such as opening jars or turning a key.
- Pain and paresthesias in ulnar distribution with tapping on the nerve in the cubital tunnel (**Tinel test, do not** confuse with a Tinel test for carpal tunnel syndrome).

> **KEY FACT**
>
> Most common elbow dislocation = posterior.

Diagnosis

Nerve conduction velocity studies can confirm the clinical diagnosis and may provide an objective measure of nerve impairment.

Management

- Activity modification to limit elbow flexion and direct pressure on the ulnar nerve.
- Nighttime splint can be used to prevent full flexion (stretches ulnar nerve).
- Surgical decompression or transposition of the nerve can be considered if 3 to 4 months of conservative measures fail.

> **KEY FACT**
>
> Ulnar neuropathy most commonly occurs at the elbow, but can also occur at the wrist (due to chronic wrist extension).

Complications

Loss of grip and pinch strength, with numbness in the ring and little fingers, which can become permanent in long-standing cases.

OLECRANON BURSITIS

- Caused by repeat friction of olecranon against hard surface, or trauma; most common type of bursitis and common cause of painless elbow swelling.
- Exam notable for soft, fluctuant area of swelling over olecranon.

- Aspirate bursitis if concern for infection; never inject corticosteroids if any concern for infection.
- Obtain radiographs only if concern for fracture or dislocation (eg, bursitis 2/2 trauma).
- Treat with compression and ice; avoid impact over olecranon.

Hand and Wrist Injuries

Table 17.10 outlines special tests that may facilitate the diagnosis of wrist and hand injuries.

CARPAL TUNNEL SYNDROME

Compression of the **median nerve** in the carpal tunnel at the wrist due to direct trauma, repetitive use, or anatomic anomalies. Most commonly affects middle-aged or pregnant women. May lead to thenar atrophy (Figure 17.4).

Symptoms/Exam

- Vague ache into the thenar eminence and sometimes the forearm.
- Numbness, tingling and pain in a median nerve distribution (thumb, index, long, and radial half of the ring fingers).
- Late symptoms: weakness, dropping objects, persistent numbness, and thenar atrophy.
- Reproduction of these symptoms with the Tinel and/or Phalen test is suggestive.
- ↓ 2-point discrimination can be seen on sensation testing.

Differential

- **Diabetic neuropathy.**
- **Flexor carpi radialis tenosynovitis:** Tenderness near the base of the thumb.
- **Cervical radiculopathy affecting the C6 nerve:** Neck pain and numbness in the thumb and index finger only.
- **Hypothyroidism:** Rule out with TSH.
- **Arthritis of the wrist or CMC joint of the thumb:** Painful, limited ROM; evident on radiographs.

TABLE 17.10.   **Special Tests for the Diagnosis of Wrist and Hand Injuries**

EXAM	TECHNIQUE	INDICATIONS
Finkelstein test	With the hand in a neutral position, the patient flexes the thumb across the palm and then ulnar-deviates the wrist	Pain along the first dorsal compartment indicates de Quervain tenosynovitis
Tinel test	Examiner taps over the median nerve in the wrist	Pain and tingling into the hand suggests carpal tunnel syndrome
Phalen test	Patient compresses the backs of the hands against each other so that the wrists are flexed 90° for 1 min (more sensitive than Tinel)	Reproduction of the patient's symptoms and aching or tingling in a median nerve distribution suggest carpal tunnel syndrome
Thumb grind test	Axial compression and rotation of first MCP joint	⊕ in first CMC osteoarthritis, but ⊖ in de Quervain tenosynovitis

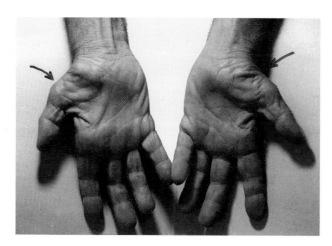

FIGURE 17.4. **Carpal tunnel syndrome.** Thenar muscle atrophy (arrows) secondary to median nerve compression. (Reproduced from Wikimedia Commons; courtesy of Dr. Harry Gouvas.)

Diagnosis

EMG (median nerve conduction velocity study) confirms the diagnosis and indicates severity (important if surgery is being considered, not required for diagnosis). Up to 25% of patients with carpal tunnel syndrome have normal EMG results.

Management

- Wrist splints at night and for provocative activities, and ergonomic modifications as needed.
- Corticosteroid injection into the carpal canal (avoid the median nerve) for short-term relief.
- Consider surgical decompression for failure of conservative treatment or if weakness or atrophy present.

DE QUERVAIN TENOSYNOVITIS

Swelling and stenosis of the sheath that surrounds the thumb extensor tendons. More common in middle-aged women. Often precipitated by repetitive use of the thumb and activities requiring a forceful grip (eg, cleaning tasks, racket sports).

- Presents with pain, tenderness ± swelling over the radial styloid, especially with use of the thumb and ulnar deviation of the wrist (pulls tendons through the inflamed sheath).
- ⊕ **Finkelstein** test is pathognomonic; ⊖ grind test.
- Avoid activities that provoke pain. Consider a thumb spica splint to immobilize the wrist and thumb.
- Consider corticosteroid injection into the tendon sheath for acute relief.
- Surgical decompression is appropriate if no improvement with conservative measures.

SCAPHOLUNATE SPRAINS

Usually caused by falls onto an outstretched hand (FOOSH).

Symptoms/Exam

- Pain in the wrist with movement, grip, lifting.
- Obtain radiographs: Must rule out carpal dislocation, carpal instability, scaphoid fracture, displaced intra-articular distal radius fracture. ↑ gap between scaphoid and lunate bones 2 to 3 mm in AP film = David Letterman sign = scapholunate dissociation (Figure 17.5).

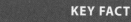

KEY FACT

De Quervain's tenosynovitis is common postpartum from repetitively picking up an infant.

KEY FACT

The lunate is the most commonly dislocated carpal bone.

KEY FACT

Scapholunate advanced collapse (SLAC) of the wrist is the most common degenerative arthritis of wrist. Result of untreated, advanced scapholunate sprain.

KEY FACT

Metacarpal fractures are more common in adults; phalangeal fractures are more common in children.

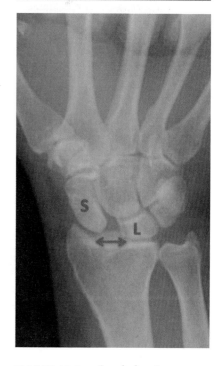

FIGURE 17.5. **Scapholunate dissociation.** Radiograph shows widening of the gap between the scaphoid (S) and lunate (L) bones after a fall on outstretched hand. (Reproduced with permission from USMLE-Rx.com.)

Differential

Triangular fibrocartilage complex (TFCC) tear/sprain: Pain along ulnar aspect of wrist, worse with ulnar deviation.

Management

- Splinting, with active ROM and hand therapy as tolerated.
- Consider early referral to hand surgeon for possible joint fixation, given future risk of scapholunate advanced collapse (SLAC) of the wrist.

THUMB AND FINGER INJURIES

Table 17.11 describes common injuries of the thumb and fingers.

HAND AND WRIST FRACTURES

In a fall onto an outstretched hand (FOOSH), approximately 80% of the force goes through the radial side of the wrist. Subtypes of wrist fractures include:

- **Distal radius fractures:** Most frequently occurring fracture in adults.
  - **Colles fracture:** Fall onto an extended wrist; distal fragment of the radius is tilted dorsally. Treat with closed reduction and long arm cast; open reduction if intra-articular fracture.
  - **Smith fracture:** Fall onto a flexed wrist; distal fragment of the radius is tilted volarly. Less angulation is tolerable in this direction.
  - **Galeazzi fracture:** Diaphyseal fracture of radius with dislocation of distal radial-ulnar joint. Caused by direct blow to radius. Treat with open reduction and internal fixation (ORIF), and casting.
- **Ulnar fractures:**
  - **"Nightstick fracture":** Fracture of ulnar shaft, often from self-defense with arm against blunt force. ORIF if significant displacement.

TABLE 17.11. **Common Thumb/Finger Injuries**

INJURY	MECHANISM	SYMPTOMS/EXAM	TREATMENT
Ulnar collateral ligament (UCL) tear (also known as **skier's** or **game-keeper's thumb**	Fall onto an abducted thumb, causing an acute rupture of the UCL of the thumb MCP joint	Instability of the MCP joint of the thumb accompanied by pain and weakness with pinch grasp Up to 70% of full ruptures are associated with a **Stener lesion,** in which the torn end of the UCL is displaced, preventing healing and requiring surgical repair; suggested by a palpable lump or gross instability	In absence of a Stener lesion, many injuries heal well in a thumb spica cast for 4 weeks, followed by protective splinting during competitive activities for 2-4 months
Mallet finger	Forced flexion of an actively extended DIP joint (eg, "jammed finger"), causing disruption of the extensor mechanism at its insertion into the distal phalanx (see Figure 17.6)	Full passive ROM but an inability to actively extend at the DIP joint Clinical diagnosis, but obtain x-rays to evaluate for bony avulsion versus tendon rupture	**Continuous** extension splinting for at least 6 weeks, followed by 4 weeks of nighttime splinting If the finger is bent at all during the initial 4 weeks, healing can be greatly affected Surgical referral for large bony avulsion or failure to heal with splinting

(continues)

TABLE 17.11.   **Common Thumb/Finger Injuries** *(continued)*

INJURY	MECHANISM	SYMPTOMS/EXAM	TREATMENT
Jersey finger	Forced extension of actively flexed DIP joint (eg, grabbing someone's jersey), causing an avulsion of the flexor digitorum profundus tendon from its insertion on the distal phalanx ~ 75% of cases involve the ring finger	Inability to bend the finger down to the palm of the hand	All cases require surgical repair, but the urgency depends on the degree of tendon retraction (the more retracted, the more urgent)
Boutonnière deformity	Deformed position of a finger caused by acute injury or progressive arthritis Disruption of the central slip of the extensor tendon where it inserts into the middle phalanx If not properly treated, the head of the middle phalanx may buttonhole through the defect between the lateral bands of the extensor tendon mechanism, causing fixed flexion at the PIP joint (see Figure 17.7)	Obtain radiographs to rule out fracture	Treat the finger with extension splinting of the PIP while allowing DIP motion for 6 weeks Surgical repair is required for large bony fragments or with lack of improvement with splinting
Trigger finger (also known as digital flexor tenosynovitis)	Inflammation of the flexor tendon, with thickening and stenosis of the first annular (A1) pulley, causing pain and catching with flexion/extension of the finger Most cases are degenerative, although there is an association with rheumatoid arthritis	Catching as the patient extends a fully flexed finger A nodule (the thickened A1 pulley) is often palpable by the distal palmar crease	Corticosteroid injection into the tendon sheath at the level of the A1 pulley Surgical release is appropriate for stubborn lesions
Boxer fracture	Fracture of the neck of the fifth metacarpal due to punching an object with a closed fist	Radiographs: Up to 40° of angulation tolerated, as long as there is no extensor lag (the patient can fully extend the finger)	Closed reducation and an ulnar gutter splint for 2-3 weeks If >40° angulation, percutaneous pinning Less angulation is tolerated in fractures of the other metacarpals due to less mobility of the bones in the hand structure

- **Monteggia fracture:** Diaphyseal fracture of proximal ulna with subluxation of radial head. Treat with ORIF of shaft fracture and closed reduction of radial head.
- **Scaphoid fractures:**
  - Most commonly fractured carpal bone; most common in young men. Less common in children and older adults because the distal radius is the weak point in these two populations.
  - Clinically presents with snuff box tenderness. If initial x-ray films are ⊖ for fracture, still immobilize the area with thumb spica cast and repeat imaging in 10 to 14 days (many fractures are not initially apparent). Ten percent to 20% of films will be initially ⊖.

QUESTION

A 20-year-old bike messenger fell off his bike and tried breaking his fall with his left hand. Exam reveals tenderness at the proximal base of the thumb, between the extensor policies longus and extensor pollicis brevis/abductor pollicis longus tendons. X-rays of the wrist, including PA, lateral, oblique, and scaphoid views (full wrist pronation with ulnar deviation) are ⊖. What do you tell him?

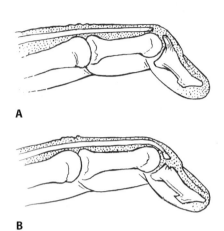

A

B

FIGURE 17.6.   Mallet finger.
Disruption of the extensor mechanism can be due to extensor tendon injury (**A**) or avulsion of bone fragment (**B**) at the dorsal insertion of the extensor tendon. (Reproduced with permission from Knoop KJ, et al. *The Atlas of Emergency Medicine*, 3rd ed. New York: McGraw-Hill, 2010, Fig. 11.50.)

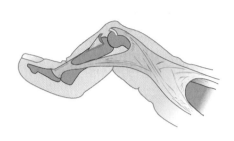
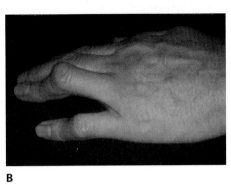

A   **B**

FIGURE 17.7.   Boutonnière deformity. (**A**) Avulsion or laceration of the central extensor mechanism results in a flexion deformity at the PIP joint and hyperextension of the DIP joint—the boutonnière, or buttonhole, deformity. (**B**) Boutonnière deformity in two fingers of a 50-year-old woman with rheumatoid arthritis. (Image A reproduced with permission from Doherty GM. *Current Diagnosis & Treatment: Surgery,* 13th ed. New York: McGraw-Hill, 2010, Fig. 42-15; image B reproduced from Wikimedia Commons; courtesy of Alborz Fallah.)

- If pain persists and radiographs are nondiagnostic, obtain an MRI or CT. Can also consider a bone scan 1 to 2 days after injury.
- Many patients require surgical fixation.

Neck, Back, and Spine Injuries

Low back pain affects 60% to 80% of adults at some point in their lives. Most episodes of back and neck pain resolve within 4 weeks, but you should still fully evaluate each case.

- Exam includes inspection (eg, loss of normal lordosis), palpation (eg, midline tenderness vs paraspinal tenderness), ROM, muscle testing, reflexes, and sensation (Table 17.12).
- **Red flags:** Night pain, weight loss, history of cancer (think tumor); fevers, chills, sweats, injection drug use, immunocompromise (think bone/disc infection); acute bony tenderness (think fracture); morning stiffness lasting >30 minutes in young adults (think seronegative spondyloarthropathy); ↓ dexterity, urinary urgency (think myelopathy); and any neurologic deficit or bowel/bladder involvement (think nerve root compromise).
- **Spurling test:** Patient extends the neck and tilts the head to the side while examiner presses down on the head, narrowing the neural foramen, which worsens or reproduces radicular pain due to disc herniation or cervical spondylosis. Very specific, but not very sensitive.
- **Straight-leg raise:** With patient supine, raise straight leg, placing tension on the L5 and S1 nerve roots and the sciatic nerve. ⊕ with reproduction or worsening of radicular symptoms. Dorsiflexion of the foot should worsen symptoms.

 ANSWER

You tell him that his history and exam (snuff box tenderness) is concerning for a scaphoid fracture. Although imaging was ⊖, he should be placed in a thumb spica cast. X-ray of the wrist should be repeated in 10 to 14 days.

CERVICAL RADICULOPATHY

Pain, tingling, numbness, caused by nerve root compression, eg neural foramen narrowing due to cervical arthritis or cervical disc lesions due to disc degeneration or herniation.

TABLE 17.12.   Nerve Root Testing

NERVE ROOT	MOTOR TESTING	REFLEX	SENSATION
C5	Deltoid, biceps	Biceps	Lateral shoulder
C6	Biceps, wrist extensors	Brachioradialis	Radial side of the forearm, thumb, and index finger
C7	Triceps, wrist flexors, finger extensors	Triceps	Middle finger
C8	Finger abduction and adduction finger flexors	—	Ulnar side of the forearm and ring and pinky fingers
L4	Foot dorsiflexion	Patellar	Medial side of the big toe and lower leg
L5	Big toe dorsiflexion	—	Dorsum of the foot from the lateral side of the big toe to the medial side of the little toe
S1	Foot eversion, plantar flexion	Achilles tendon	Lateral side of the little toe and lower leg

Symptoms/Exam

- Pain radiating to shoulder or down arm; paresthesias in fingers.
- Tenderness of neck, ROM limitations, focal dermatomal sensory loss or pain; diminished reflexes; ± ⊕ Spurling test.

Diagnosis/Management

- Clinical; radiographs needed only if history of trauma, persistent symptoms, or red flags.
- X-ray may show narrowing of disc space, bone spurs.
- Start with conservative treatment: rest, pain relief, stress reduction; consider short course of muscle relaxants.
- Obtain MRI/refer to specialist if any red flags, weakness, progression of neurologic symptoms, or failure of conservative measures after 4 to 6 weeks (including PT).

CERVICAL STRAIN/SPRAIN

- Pain in neck due to irritation/spam of muscles of posterior neck. Often related to poor posture, overuse of one shoulder more than the other, emotional/physical stress, or trauma.
- Pain and stiffness in low neck/upper back/shoulders. ± ROM limitations.
- Diagnosis is clinical; consider x-ray image if history of trauma, abnormal neurologic exam, or failure of conservative measures.
- Conservative management (heat, ROM, NSAIDs, ± PT) and treat underlying cause (eg, ergonomics, stress reduction).

KEY FACT

Cervical radiculopathy is most often due to degenerative disease of the cervical spine; most common in patients 50 to 54 years old

KEY FACT

Most common neurologic deficits in cervical radiculopathy is ↓ deep tendon reflex of triceps.

QUESTION

A 54-year-old painter presents to clinic noting sudden onset pain in his low back. The pain is worse when he bends forward, and is associate with shooting pain down the side of his right leg to his right foot. On exam, when he is lying down and you passively raise his right leg, he is asymptomatic; raising his left leg reproduces the pain in his right leg. What do you tell him?

WHIPLASH

- Hyperextension injury causing excess stretching of muscles/soft tissue of cervical spine.
- Pain in lower neck and shoulders; can radiate to occiput and cause headaches.
- If associated with disc herniation or tracheal/esophageal injury, may be associated with hoarseness or dysphagia.
- Tenderness to palpation of neck, ± mild limitation ROM neck; normal neurologic exam.
- Diagnosis is clinical; plain films, if obtained, will be ⊖.
- Conservative treatment with rest (consider cervical collar), ice, NSAIDs, early ROM, ± PT (early mobilization and early return to normal activity, plus anti-inflammatory medications has best evidence); neck pain can last weeks to months.

TORTICOLLIS

- Horizontal turning of neck; can be congenital or acquired (think abscess vs tumor).
- Contraction of sternomastoid muscle on one side of neck; head tilts to ipsilateral side.
- Refer for emergent evaluation/treatment of possible traumatic injury versus retropharyngeal abscess versus tumor.

Management

- First step is imaging: Plain radiographs (5 view: AP, lateral, open-mouth [odontoid], and left/right oblique views).
- If all plain films are ⊖ and patient has ⊕ neurologic signs/symptoms, or there is concern for infection or tumor: obtain MRI (CT if MRI contraindicated).
- CT scan: Preferable to MRI if concern for facet osteoarthritis (OA) or osseous injuries.

HERNIATED DISC

Bulging or herniation of the **nucleus pulposus** (a gel-like substance that cushions axial compression) through the surrounding **annulus fibrosus** (the outer, ligamentous portion of the intervertebral disc) into the spinal canal → nerve root irritation and compression; also known as herniated nucleus pulposus. Lumbar disc herniations affect 2% of the population, but only 10% to 25% of these patients have symptoms that persist >6 weeks.

Symptoms/Exam

- Abrupt onset of unilateral radicular leg pain, low back pain that is worse with sitting, walking, standing, coughing, or sneezing.
- Most commonly occurs at the L4-L5 or L5-S1 level.

Differential

- **Lateral femoral cutaneous nerve entrapment:** Involves the lateral thigh; sensory only.
- **Spinal stenosis:** Affects older people; associated with relief with flexion. Classic symptom is **pseudoclaudication,** which presents as leg and buttock pain that is exacerbated by walking (worse going downhill).

ANSWER

You tell him that his symptoms and exam (⊕ contralateral straight leg raise) is most consistent with an L5 radiculopathy due to disc herniation, which is usually a self-limiting condition. The contralateral straight leg raise is more specific, but less sensitive for radiculopathy from disc herniation.

- **Cauda equina syndrome:** Bilateral involvement; presents with perianal numbness, with possible ↓ sphincter tone with urinary incontinence or retention. Surgical emergency!
- **Demyelinating conditions:** Can present with clonus.

Diagnosis

- Clinical, largely based on symptoms and exam. Imaging is not needed acutely, as most cases are self-limiting. Obtain plain radiographs to evaluate vertebral alignment and disc space if no improvement in 4 to 6 weeks. Imaging is likely to show degenerative changes in older patients.
- MRI is necessary only for progressive neurologic changes or preoperative planning.

Management

- Acute use of NSAIDs, muscle relaxants, and, if this is insufficient, a short course of opioids, with 1 to 3 days of bed rest if needed, followed by slow progression of activity.
- Short course of oral steroids or an epidural steroid injection may be necessary.
- Surgical evaluation is appropriate for patients who show no improvement or have progressive neurologic symptoms.

DEGENERATIVE DISC DISEASE

Age-related degenerative changes of the intervertebral discs. Degree of degeneration may be modified by factors such as injury, repeat trauma, infection, heredity, and smoking.

- Characterized by recurrent, episodic low back pain that radiates to one or both buttocks ± intermittent sciatica.
- AP and lateral radiographs may reveal anterior osteophytes, loss of disc height, and a "vacuum sign" showing apparent air (nitrogen) in the disc space.

Management

Treatment includes intermittent NSAIDs, weight reduction, and core strengthening; can attempt spinal injections. If no improvement, consider referral for surgical repair (usually spinal fusion).

LUMBAR SPINAL STENOSIS (NEUROGENIC CLAUDICATION)

Narrowing of 1+ levels of the spinal canal with compression of the nerve roots. Up to 30% of adults >60 years of age have lumbar stenosis anatomically, but most are asymptomatic.

Symptoms/Exam

- Radicular symptoms in the calf, buttock, or thigh ± back pain. Starts gradually or following minor trauma and usually progresses from proximal to distal.
- Pain aggravated by extension, and patients have poor walking tolerance.
- Walking and prolonged standing cause fatigue and leg weakness.
- Leg pain due to vascular claudication resolves when the patient stops walking, whereas neurogenic claudication does not immediately subside.

Differential

Vascular claudication, diabetic neuropathy, folic acid or vitamin B_{12} deficiency, infection, tumor, degenerative disc disease.

KEY FACT

In spinal stenosis, walking **down** a hill causes pain to go **up** (↑).

KEY FACT

Encourage patients with acute low back pain to stay active; most pain resolves spontaneously within 4 weeks.

KEY FACT

NSAIDs, opioids, and topiramate are more effective than placebo for short-term treatment of nonspecific low back pain.

KEY FACT

Spinal manipulation therapy results in mild pain relief and improved function in chronic low back pain for up to 6 months.

KEY FACT

Pain bending forward (flexion) = think disc problem.
Pain bending backward (extension) = think facet joint degenerative changes, spinal stenosis, spondylolisthesis.

KEY FACT

Epidural injections are much more likely to improve radicular symptoms than axial back pain.

KEY FACT

In general, paresthesias and dysesthesias are found in neurogenic claudication but not in vascular claudication.

Diagnosis

- Obtain AP and lateral x-ray films to look for contributing degenerative factors such as spondylolisthesis, narrowing of the intervertebral disc spaces, osteoporosis, osteophytic changes, or an old burst fracture of a vertebral body.
- Usually diagnosed on MRI, however MRI is necessary only if considering surgical intervention or to evaluate new red flag symptoms.

Management

- PT focusing on flexion exercises and core/abdominal strengthening.
- Surgical decompression is often needed and can be quite effective.

Hip and Thigh Injuries

Pain from hip pathology, such as OA, localizes to the anterior groin or thigh and is exacerbated with internal rotation of the hip. Lateral hip pain is much more likely to be due to soft tissue pathology, such as trochanteric bursitis/iliotibial band (ITB) tightness. ROM and resisted muscle testing will often identify the source of pain in soft tissue injuries. Special tests are listed in Table 17.13.

ILIOTIBIAL BAND–RELATED PATHOLOGY

The ITB is a large, flat, fascial band that runs from the iliac crest down the lateral thigh and inserts onto the lateral condyle of the tibia at the knee (Gerdy tubercle).

TABLE 17.13.   Special Tests for the Diagnosis of Hip and Thigh Injuries

EXAM	TECHNIQUE	INDICATIONS
Ober test	Patient lies on his or her side with the affected side up. Knee is flexed 90° and the hip is abducted, extended, and then allowed to drop down toward the table	⊕ if the knee does not drop past the midline, suggesting a tight ITB
Trendelenburg test	Patient is observed from behind while standing on 1 foot and then the other; note pelvic stability	⊕ if unsupported hemipelvis droops, suggesting hip abductor weakness on the other side (weakness on the side of the leg the patient is standing on)
FABER (**F**lexion, **AB**duction, **Ex**ternal **R**otation) test	Patient is supine and places the leg of the affected side into the figure-4 position, with the ankle resting above the contralateral knee. Examiner presses down on the ipsilateral knee, stressing the sacroiliac joint and stretching the psoas	Posterior hip pain suggests sacroiliac pathology; anterior pull suggests psoas involvement

Tightness of ITB can cause pain and bursitis as it rubs over bony prominences both proximally (at the greater trochanter) and distally (at the lateral knee).

Iliotibial Band Syndrome

An overuse tendinopathy of the ITB as it passes over the lateral femoral condyle.
- Lateral knee pain and crepitus at the lateral femoral condyle or insertion on the Gerdy tubercle. A tight ITB is seen on the Ober test.
- Check for contributing mechanics such as genu varus, excessive foot pronation or supination, and weak hip abductors/pelvic stabilizers.
- Treat with ITB stretching, foam roller exercises for soft tissue work to relax the ITB, rest, ice, NSAIDs, iontophoresis.

Snapping Hip

A snapping or popping sensation that occurs as a tendon "snaps" across a bony prominence. Most commonly due to the ITB snapping over the greater trochanter, but can also be due to the iliopsoas tendon sliding over the pectineal eminence of the pelvis or to labral tears of the acetabulum.

Symptoms/Exam

- Snapping sensation at the lateral hip that can often be reproduced in the office with rotation of the hip. If the trochanteric bursa has become inflamed, there will be tenderness with palpation.
- Snapping of the iliopsoas tendon felt in the groin as the hip extends from a flexed position (eg, with rising from a chair).

Diagnosis

- If not evident on exam, obtain AP pelvis and lateral hip radiographs to exclude bony pathology.
- If the diagnosis remains unclear, MR arthrography may be needed to rule out a labral tear or an intra-articular loose body.

Management

PT for stretching of the ITB, hip abductors, adductors, and flexors. If injury is painful, corticosteroid injection into the trochanteric bursa or psoas sheath may be needed.

Trochanteric Bursitis (Greater Trochanteric Pain Syndrome)

Inflammation, swelling, and hypertrophy of the greater trochanteric bursa. Can develop with direct injury, ITB tightness/overuse, or due to problems with hip mechanics (eg, lumbar spine disease, intra-articular hip pathology, or significant limb length asymmetries).
- **Symptoms/Exam:** Pain and tenderness at the lateral hip over the greater trochanter. Can have intense pain with rising from a chair or sleeping on the affected side. Point tenderness is diagnostic, but radiographs may be used to rule out bony and articular pathology.
- **Differential:** OA of the hip, trochanteric fracture, sciatica, tumor.
- **Management:** Treat with stretching of the ITB, NSAIDs, rest, activity modification, ± corticosteroid injection.

FRACTURES OF THE HIP AND THIGH

Hip fractures are common in the elderly, occurring with equal frequency in the femoral neck (from twisting injuries) and in the intertrochanteric region (from a fall onto the side). Age is the most important risk factor: the frequency of hip fractures doubles

KEY FACT

In addition to causing hip pain, ITB syndrome is the leading cause of lateral knee pain in runners.

KEY FACT

Patients with a stress fracture of the hip may present with diffuse aching pain in the thigh or groin that is worse with weight-bearing activities.

QUESTION

A 22-year-old professional ballet dancer complains about an audible popping sensation and pain across her thigh and lateral knee when dancing. She notices the feeling when she extends her legs quickly from a flexed position (eg, standing from a squat). She has ↑ the intensity of her workouts, as she is trying to join a dance troupe. On exam, you note a snapping sensation at the lateral hip with rotation of the hip. There is also tenderness to palpation at the trochanteric bursa. What do you tell her?

with each decade >50 years. Other risk factors: being white, female, sedentary, a smoker, and an alcoholic.

- Patients with a displaced fracture will present with the limb externally rotated, abducted, and shortened.
- Femoral neck stress fractures will have gradual onset of groin pain, antalgic gait, and pain on internal rotation.
- AP pelvis and cross-table lateral radiographs are usually diagnostic for complete fractures. Stress fractures may require MRI for diagnosis (Figure 17.8).
  - Most hip fractures require operative management.
  - Compression-side stress fractures (those on the inferior surface) can be managed with non–weight-bearing status until there is radiographic evidence of healing.

Knee and Tibial Injuries

MENISCAL TEARS

The medial and lateral menisci are fibrocartilaginous discs that provide shock absorption and stability between the femur and tibia. The blood supply to the menisci is very poor, so tears do not usually heal, predisposing the knee to degenerative arthritis.

Symptoms/Exam

- Traumatic tears usually occur with a sudden twisting injury and have **slow development** of swelling and stiffness over a few days. Symptoms then wax and wane.
- Pain localized to the medial (more common) or lateral joint line and often recurs with twisting or squatting motions such as getting out of a car.
- Mechanical symptoms such as locking, catching, and popping can also develop.
- Moderate effusion, joint line tenderness, pain with forced flexion, and meniscal rotation signs on exam (**McMurray sign**) are suggestive.

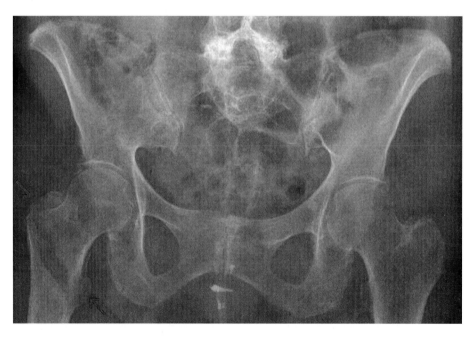

FIGURE 17.8. **Right hip fracture.** AP radiograph of the pelvis clearly demonstrates an intertrochanteric fracture of the right femur (arrows). (Reproduced with permission from USMLE-Rx.com.)

Differential

- **Anterior cruciate ligament (ACL) tear:** Sudden; characterized by larger swelling and instability.
- **Medial collateral ligament (MCL) injury:** Pain with valgus stress.
- **Osteoarthritis:** Loss of joint space, osteophytes, sclerosis, ± subchondral cysts on weight-bearing radiographs.
- **Pes anserine bursitis:** Medial tenderness **below** the medial joint line at the attachment of the sartorius, gracilis, and semitendinosus tendons.
- **Bony pathology:** Tibial plateau fracture; osteonecrosis of the femoral condyle.
- **Patellar subluxation or dislocation:** Tender patellar facets and apprehension sign (while patient is supine and leg is in full extension, apply pressure to the medial patella; test is ⊕ if it causes pain or apprehension).

Diagnosis

- Radiographs to rule out bony conditions.
- MRI is used for diagnosis, as it is highly sensitive and specific for meniscal pathology (Figure 17.9).

Management

- Arthroscopic debridement or repair is the treatment of choice for traumatic tears in the younger, active population.
- For degenerative tears (more likely in the older population) or in the absence of mechanical symptoms, such as catching or locking, conservative measures (eg, rest, ice, NSAIDs, PT, corticosteroid injection) can initially be tried.

LIGAMENTOUS INJURIES

Anterior Cruciate Ligament Tear

The ACL is the 1° stabilizer of the knee, resisting anterior translation of the tibia on the femur. A tear results from forced hyperflexion (eg, in skiing, football, soccer, and basketball). Seventy percent of ACL injuries occur during sports.

Symptoms/Exam

- Forty percent of patients report feeling or hearing a pop (the most reliable factor).
- Rapid development of hemarthrosis, causing significant swelling.
- Instability of the knee or a "wobbly" feeling.
- **Lachman test** is the most sensitive test (87%-98%), showing ↑ anterior tibial displacement and a soft end point.

Diagnosis

The history and exam remain key diagnostic tools, but MRI is increasingly used for confirmation as well as for the evaluation of associated injuries, such as injury of the menisci, posterior cruciate ligament (PCL), and collateral ligaments (Figure 17.10).

Management

- Depends on patient preference, age, activity level, knee instability, and associated injuries.
- Some older, less active patients can have satisfactory outcomes with rehabilitation alone (the ACL does not heal, but patients can develop muscular stability). Younger, more active patients are more likely to need reconstruction to remain active.

Collateral Ligament Injuries

Most often caused by a direct blow to the lateral aspect of the knee, leading to valgus stress and MCL injury. Isolated lateral collateral ligament (LCL) injuries are rare.

KEY FACT

Lateral tibial plateau fractures are more common than medial; check integrity of peroneal nerve.

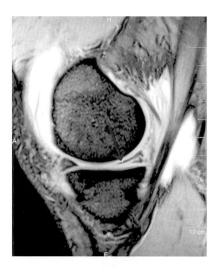

FIGURE 17.9. Meniscal tear. T2-weighted MRI demonstrates high-grade posterior horn of the medial meniscus. (Reproduced from Yaqoob J, et al. Diagnostic accuracy of magnetic resonance imaging in assessment of meniscal and ACL tear: correlation with arthoroscopy. *Pak J Med Sci.* 2015;31(2):263-268.)

KEY FACT

Meniscal repair/debridement ↑ risk of degenerative joint disease later in life, but may be necessary if patient is having locking or catching of the joint, or ongoing severe pain.

KEY FACT

Instability of the knee suggests patellar subluxation or ligament tear.

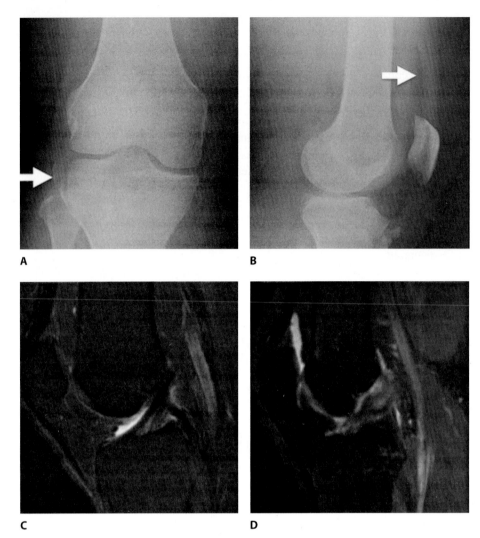

FIGURE 17.10.   **Anterior cruciate ligament tear.** (**A**) Knee radiograph shows large bone fragment off the lateral tibial plateau called a Segond fracture (arrow), which is commonly seen in ACL tears. (**B**) Lateral knee radiograph showing lipohemarthrosis (arrow), a fat/blood level joint effusion. (**C**) Normal MRI of the ACL. (**D**) MRI demonstrating irregularity of the ACL consistent with an ACL tear. (Images A and B reproduced from Wong PKW, et al. What's in a name? Lower extremity fracture eponyms (part 2). *Int J Emerg Med.* 2015;8:25; images C and D reproduced with permission from USMLE-Rx.com.)

- Presents with pain ± laxity on valgus (medial collateral ligament, or MCL) or varus (LCL) stress testing at 30 degrees of flexion (relaxes the cruciate ligaments).
- LCL injuries should be thoroughly evaluated for accompanying injuries (ACL, PCL, posterolateral corner injuries).
- Nonoperative management with a hinged knee brace and ROM exercises usually suffices for isolated MCL or LCL injuries. Rehabilitation can take 6 to 8 weeks.

PATELLOFEMORAL PAIN SYNDROME

Patella-related pain is the single most common cause of knee pain. Patellofemoral pain syndrome is a multifactorial syndrome characterized by diffuse, aching anterior knee pain that worsens with activities that stress the patellofemoral joint (eg, climbing stairs, kneeling, or prolonged sitting [theater sign]).

Symptoms/Exam

- Note any patellar crepitation or tenderness of the patellar retinaculum or facets.
- Evaluate for contributing factors, including ↑ **Q angle** at the knee (angle between the quadriceps and patellar tendon, more common in women because of wider pelvises), patellar tilt or malalignment, excessive lateral patellar mobility, tight hamstrings, weak quadriceps, and excessive femoral anteversion.

Differential

- **Patellar tendinopathy** (also known as **jumper's knee**): Point tenderness over the inferior pole of the patella.
- **Patellofemoral osteoarthritis:** Diagnosed by radiographic changes on sunrise view; affects older patients.
- **Synovial plica:** Redundant fold of synovial lining that can become painfully inflamed and fibrotic, most commonly occurring along the medial border of the patella.
- **Chondromalacia patellae:** Disruption in the articular cartilage of the patella (painful or nonpainful), with possible etiologies including trauma, malalignment, and biomechanical or metabolic factors.
- **Patellar instability/dislocation:** Transient displacement (usually laterally) of the patella, either partially (subluxation) or completely (dislocation), causing acute and/or chronic patellar pain. Associated with a ⊕ **apprehension sign** when displacing the patella laterally.

Diagnosis

Clinical diagnosis; AP, lateral, and sunrise radiographs can reveal articular cartilage loss, tilt, and subluxation.

Management

- Activity modification and an exercise program consisting of quadriceps strengthening (especially the medial quadriceps) and hamstring flexibility. Also attempt to fix contributing mechanical factors such as flat feet or overpronation with orthotic foot inserts. NSAIDs can alleviate discomfort.
- Consider use of a knee sleeve with patellar cutout or a patellar stabilizing brace.

KEY FACT

Knee dislocations can be an orthopedic emergency; 50% are associated with injury to the popliteal artery.

BURSITIS

- Inflammation of a bursae (synovial fluid-filled structure); knee has multiple bursae:
  - Prepatellar bursa
  - Infratpatellar bursa
  - Pes anserine bursa
  - Iliotibial (IT) band bursa
- Characterized by pain over bursa, swelling, ↓ ROM, erythema. ± history of trauma, repeat pressure over bursa, or inflammatory disease.
- Diagnosis is clinical; aspiration required only if concern for infection (septic bursitis).
- Treatment includes decompression, ice, avoiding impact over bursa; if large fluid collection or concern for infection, aspirate bursa. If no concern for infection, can consider corticosteroid injection.
- Treat septic bursitis with 7 to 10 days of antibiotics.

DEGENERATIVE OSTEOARTHRITIS

Loss of hyaline cartilage along knee joint surfaces. Common, affecting one-third of patients >65 years old. Risk factors include: being female, history of inflammatory joint disease obesity, repetitive knee bending, advanced age, prior knee injury.

KEY FACT

Obesity is the strongest modifiable risk factor for osteoarthritis of the knee.

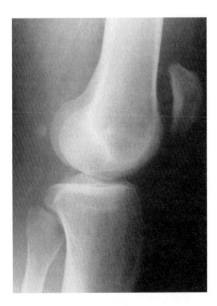

FIGURE 17.11. Patella alta. Note the superiorly dislocated patella. (Reproduced with permission from Tintinalli JE, et al. *Tintinalli's Emergency Medicine: A Comprehensive Study Guide,* 6th ed. New York: McGraw-Hill, 2004, Fig. 274-11.)

Symptoms/Exam

- Knee pain and stiffness with activity/weight bearing, after prolonged sitting, going down stairs, and early in morning; better with rest.
- ± swelling and worse symptoms with weather changes.
- ↓ ROM on exam, varus versus valgus deformity (which can predispose to OA), joint line tenderness.

Differential

- **Soft tissue injury of knee:** Bursitis, ITB syndrome, MCL/LCL instability, meniscal injury.
- **Alternative types of arthritis:** Gout/pseudogout, rheumatoid arthritis, septic arthritis; distinguish by age >50, lab findings (ESR <40 mm/hr) and rheumatoid factor (<1:40 in OA, ⊖ synovial fluid if tapped), and osteophytes on imaging.
- **Referred pain:** Neuropathy, radiculopathy.
- **Avascular necrosis:** Pain with weightbearing, ± rest/night pain; evaluate with imaging.
- **Patellofemoral pain syndrome:** Pain around/under patella, worse with squatting/running/prolong sitting/stairs.
- **Tumor:** Assess for B-symptoms/red flags.

Diagnosis

- Radiographs help evaluate joint space, osteophytes, subchondral sclerosis, and presence of cysts.
- MRIs are required only for preoperative planning or concern for concomitant ligamentous injury.

Management

- Always start with conservative therapy: exercises, weight loss, NSAIDs, PT, knee braces or heel wedges. Can consider topical analgesics, acupuncture (weak evidence), tai chi, ginger. Mixed evidence for hyaluronic acid injections and glucosamine. Early evidence suggests S-adenosylmethionine (SAM-e) may be as effective as NSAIDs (but very expensive), no evidence for chondroitin supplements.
- If no improvement in 4 to 6 weeks, consider corticosteroid injections for short-term relief. Patients should not receive more than four steroid injections to a joint in 1 year. Diabetic patients may have transient hyperglycemia after a corticosteroid injection lasting 2 to 3 days.
- Joint replacement for advanced disease.

QUADRICEPS AND PATELLAR TENDON RUPTURES

Typically occur with a fall onto a partially flexed knee while the quadriceps muscle is forcibly contracting to break the fall. **Patellar tendon ruptures** usually occur in younger patients (<40 years of age) and are frequently associated with sporting activities. **Quadriceps tendon ruptures** typically occur in patients >40 years of age and are three times more common than patellar tendon ruptures.

- Patients often feel a pop at the time of injury and have a palpable defect in one tendon, with an inability to extend the knee against gravity or perform a straight-leg raise.
- Radiographs of the knee can rule out patellar fracture. In a patellar tendon rupture, radiograph will show patella alta (patella has moved up along the thigh; see Figure 17.11), whereas in quadriceps tendon rupture it will show patella baja (patella has moved abnormally low).
- MRI to confirm the diagnosis and for surgical planning.
- **Immediate surgical repair** is indicated for complete ruptures of either tendon.

- Partial tears with little loss of strength and maintenance of the ability to extend the knee can be treated conservatively with a cylinder cast in full extension for 4 to 6 weeks (uncommon).

MEDIAL TIBIAL STRESS SYNDROME (SHIN SPLINTS) AND TIBIAL STRESS FRACTURE

Diffuse stress reaction, leading to fracture if untreated, along the tibia; seen in runners and jumpers (basketball, dancing, racket sports).

Symptoms/Exam

- Onset of symptoms is insidious and associated with ↑ high-impact activity.
  - In tibial stress syndrome, pain often occurs at the beginning of a run, resolves as workout continues, and recurs after the workout.
  - In fracture, the pain is more persistent and may worsen at the end of the run.
- Diffuse pattern of pain and tenderness along the medial border of the middle and distal thirds of the tibia (muscle attachment sites). Pain with resisted plantar flexion and toe walking. Pain may become more focal once fracture develops.

Differential

Chronic exertional compartment syndrome (suggested by localized calf pain that progressively worsens with persistent running and is relieved with cessation of exercise); bony tumor (suggested by unusually severe bone pain and/or night pain).

Diagnosis

Triple-phase bone scan or MRI can distinguish stress syndrome from stress fracture if the exam is unclear.

Management

For tibial stress syndrome, begin with relative rest and cross-training (no immobilization) until pain resolves. Stress fractures require complete rest for 4 to 8 weeks until pain is completely resolved, with slow resumption of activity only if the patient remains pain free. Cryotherapy/ice, NSAIDs and PT (for stretching exercises of calf and plantar flexors of the foot) can also be used for both.

Foot and Ankle Injuries

ANKLE SPRAINS

Partial or complete tearing of 1+ ligaments that support the ankle joint. Most often due to an inversion mechanism, causing injury to the lateral ligaments. The anterior talofibular ligament (ATFL) is the first ligament to be injured, followed by the calcaneofibular ligament (CFL) and finally, in the most severe lateral sprains, the posterior talofibular ligament (PTFL). A syndesmotic ankle sprain (high ankle sprain) involves the ligaments that connect the tibia and fibula; less common but more severe.

Symptoms/Exam

- Lateral ankle swelling and ecchymosis are proportional to the degree of ligament damage and the number of ligaments involved.
- Tenderness of the anterior tibiofibular ligament and pain with the **squeeze test** (compressing the tibia and fibula at midcalf stresses the distal syndesmosis) suggest a high ankle sprain.

QUESTION

A 28-year-old woman presents with pain and tenderness over her tibia when she runs. Previously, she had pain only at the end of her runs, but now is having symptoms with walking. She is training for a marathon and has ↑ her mileage significantly in the last several weeks. She runs only on pavement. On physical exam you find focal tenderness at her midtibia and ↑ pain when you place a tuning fork over the area. X-ray is ⊖, but you still suspect a stress fracture, so you order an MRI, which shows a small hairline fracture in the anterior tibia. How do you counsel this patient?

KEY FACT

For athletes, the tibia is the most commonly involved bone in stress fractures, whereas in military recruits, fractures of the metatarsal and calcaneal bones are more common because of the biomechanics of running versus marching.

KEY FACT

The ATFL is the most commonly sprained ligament in the ankle or foot.

Tell her that rest is the only option for complete healing of the stress fracture. Give her a walking boot and crutches to use for 4 to 8 weeks (healing times vary by location, severity, and the body's healing response). After she is pain free with ambulation, activities may be gradually resumed as long as she remains pain free. Advise her to avoid running on pavement (vs in parks) and tell her not to ↑ her mileage more than 10% a week. Also tell her that if she continues to run with this stress fracture, she is at risk for progression to a complete fracture.

KEY FACT

The most common eversion ankle fracture is a fracture of the lateral malleolus.

KEY FACT

Oral fluoroquinolones can ↑ the risk of tendon rupture and tendinitis.

KEY FACT

Refer all Achilles tendon ruptures to orthopedics immediately.

Differential

- Fracture of the lateral malleolus, calcaneus, talus, or base of the 5th metatarsal.
- Peroneal tendon tear or subluxation (retrofibular tenderness and swelling).

Diagnosis

Need for radiographs to rule out fracture is based on the **Ottawa ankle rules** (Figure 17.12).

Management

- Acutely treat with **RICE** therapy (rest, ice, compression, elevation). Can use NSAIDs for pain. Can use a brace, an air cast, or crutches, depending on severity, with early mobilization and strengthening exercises as swelling ↓.
- Speed of recovery depends on the degree of injury (Table 17.14).
- Residual symptoms can occur in up to 40% of patients.

ACHILLES TENDON RUPTURE

Disruption of the Achilles tendon; most commonly affects middle-aged men who play quick stop-and-go sports such as tennis, squash, and basketball.

- Patient experiences sudden, severe calf pain, with swelling and a palpable defect in the tendon. Patients will say they felt like they were kicked or shot in the back of the ankle. Exam shows lack of plantar flexion with manual squeezing of the calf (⊕ **Thompson test**).
- Differentiate from Achilles tendinosis (gradual onset), medial gastrocnemius tear (more proximal tenderness), DVT (no history of injury, ⊖ Thompson test).
- Nonoperative or surgical repair. Both require a program of graduated casting or bracing to allow for healing.

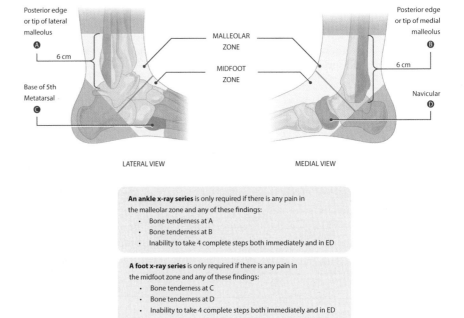

FIGURE 17.12.   Ottawa ankle rules for x-rays in ankle foot trauma. (Reproduced with permission from USMLE-Rx.com.)

TABLE 17.14. West Point Ankle Sprain Grading System

FEATURE	GRADE 1	GRADE 2	GRADE 3
Edema/ecchymosis	Localized/slight	Localized/moderate	Diffuse/significant
Weight-bearing ability	Full or partial without significant pain	Difficult without crutches	Impossible
Ligament pathology	Ligament stretch	Partial tear	Complete tear
Instability testing	None	None or slight	Definite
Time to return to sports	11 days	2-6 weeks	6-12 weeks

ACHILLES TENDINOPATHY

Common overuse injury, especially in running/jumping athletes.
- Pain during/after prolonged walking/running at posterior aspect of distal lower leg versus heel. Worse with hills/stairs, running, jumping.
- Exam may demonstrate swelling/firmness at distal tendon.
- Diagnosis is clinical; radiographs only if chronic to rule out calcific tendinopathy or Haglund deformity (bump on posterior calcaneus, adjacent to Achilles insertion).
- Treat with intense, eccentric strengthening program, in addition to RICE. Consider surgical debridement if chronic.

KEY FACT

Do not offer corticosteroid injections in Achilles tendinopathy due to risk of tendon rupture.

PLANTAR FASCIITIS

Overload injury (inflammation, degeneration, and tearing) of the plantar fascia, most commonly occurring at its calcaneal insertion. Contributing factors include a tight gastrocnemius–soleus complex, tight plantar fascia, a rigid rear foot, and overpronation or supination.
- Symptoms include pain and tenderness at the plantar medial heel that worsens with the **first few steps in the morning,** after rest and with extended walking.
- Diagnosis is clinical. Radiographs are not necessary and will show a plantar heel spur in 50% of patients with plantar fasciitis and 15% of asymptomatic patients. A bone scan can differentiate plantar fasciitis from a calcaneal stress fracture.
- Achilles stretching, activity modification, orthotics, ice massage, NSAIDs, and night splints can help maintain Achilles and plantar stretch. Repetitive corticosteroid injections can cause fat pad insufficiency.
- Symptoms will resolve in 95% of patients within 12 to 18 months. For persistent symptoms, surgical release of plantar fascia is usually effective.

KEY FACT

Plantar fasciitis is the most common cause of foot pain in adults.

MORTON NEUROMA

Perineural fibrosis of the common digital nerve as it passes between the metatarsal heads. Most commonly occurs between the third and fourth toes; five times more common in women (thought to be due to compression from tight shoe wear).
- Forefoot plantar pain ± dysesthesias can be reproduced with pressure to the plantar aspect of the third web space while squeezing the metatarsals together.

- Differentiate form:
  - **Metatarsalgia:** Tenderness over the metatarsal heads.
  - **Hammer toe:** Flexion deformity of the proximal interphalangeal joint.
  - **Metatarsophalangeal (MTP) synovitis:** Tenderness and swelling over the MTP joint.
  - **Stress fracture:** Dorsal metatarsal tenderness.
- Treat by switching to shoes with low heels and a wide toe box; metatarsal pads to spread the metatarsal heads; lidocaine/corticosteroid injection.

FRACTURES OF THE FOOT AND ANKLE

Malleolar Fractures

The ankle joint is considered stable with an isolated malleolar fracture (usually lateral). When combined with an injury to the other side of the ankle (eg, lateral malleolus fracture and deltoid ligament disruption), the ankle joint becomes unstable.

- Patient has history of trauma with swelling, tenderness, and possible deformity at the site of the fracture.
- AP, lateral, and mortise radiographs can evaluate for fracture and widening of the mortise, which suggest an unstable ankle joint.

Management

- **Stable fractures of the distal fibula:** Weight-bearing cast or brace for 4 to 6 weeks.
- **Unstable, nondisplaced fractures:** Non–weight-bearing short- or long-leg cast for a longer period, with close orthopedic follow-up.
- **Unstable, displaced fractures:** Usually require open reduction.

Maisonneuve Fracture

Spiral fracture of the proximal fibula (Figure 17.13), associated with a tear of the tibia-fibula syndesmosis. Associated with fracture of the medial malleolus or rupture

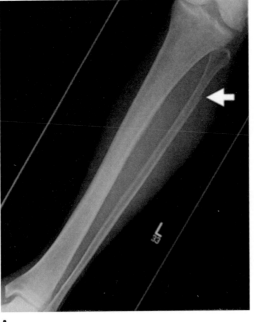
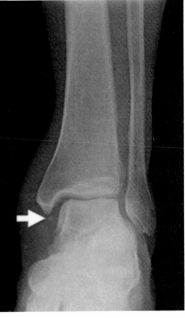

A   B

FIGURE 17.13. **Maisonneuve fracture.** (**A**) Minimally displaced fracture of the proximal fibular shaft (arrow). (**B**) Swelling overlying the medial ankle with small avulsion fracture off the medial malleolus. (Reproduced from Wong PKW, et al. What's in a name? Lower extremity fracture eponyms (part 2). *Int J Emerg Med.* 2015;8:25.)

of the deltoid ligament. Often occurs in athletes who reinjure an inadequately healed ankle sprain.

- Occurs with significant torsional force to the ankle, which is transmitted up the syndesmosis to the proximal fibula.
- Pain at the medial malleolus and proximal fibula.

Fracture of the Base of the Fifth Metatarsal

Three types of proximal fifth metatarsal fractures:

- **Avulsion fracture of the tuberosity:** Most common; usually occurs with high lateral ankle sprains. Generally treated with weight bearing in a walking cast or hard-soled shoes until pain subsides.
- **Jones fracture:** Fracture distal to the tuberosity at the neck. Higher rates of non-union; treat with intramedullary fixation or non–weight-bearing short-leg cast for 6 to 8 weeks.
- **Diaphyseal stress fracture:** Treat with non–weight-bearing short-leg cast for 6 to 8 weeks.

Pediatric Musculoskeletal Injuries

See the Pediatrics chapter for fuller discussions of developmental dysplasia of hip, metatarsus adductus, tapipes equinovarus, genu varum/valgum, tibial torsion, Legg-Calve-Perthes disease, Osgood-Schlatter syndrome, slipped capital femoral epiphysis, septic arthritis, osteomyelitis, scoliosis, and juvenile idiopathic arthritis.

PEDIATRIC INJURIES OF THE BACK AND SPINE

Back pain is uncommon in children and always warrants evaluation if it does not rapidly resolve.

Spondylolisthesis

Slippage of a vertebral body forward in relation to the vertebral body below it. In children, most often a movement of L5 forward on S1, due to a congenital defect or stress fracture through the pars interarticularis of the vertebra (**spondylolysis**) (Figure 17.14).

- Presents with localized back pain at the site of spondylolysis. May have radicular symptoms if slippage is present. Pars injuries are more common in youth sports involving significant hyperextension, such as gymnastics and football.
- "Stork test" can localize a pars defect: patient stands on one leg and extends the back. Test is ⊕ if it causes localized pain on side of spondylolysis. ↑ lordosis, ↓ ROM and tight hamstrings may also be seen.
- Oblique radiographs can show a break in the neck of the **"Scottie dog,"** which represents the pars defect (spondylolysis). If radiographs are ⊖, bone scan and MRI are more sensitive. If spondylolisthesis (slippage) is present, it will be evident on lateral radiographs.
- Treat conservatively (rest, core strengthening and monitoring) unless patient has a documented progression of a slip >50%, in which case bracing or spinal fusion may be considered.

PEDIATRIC OVERUSE INJURIES

Table 17.15 lists the overuse injuries commonly seen in children.

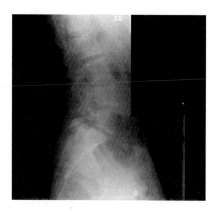

FIGURE 17.14. **Spondylolysis at L5-S1.** Incomplete pars interarticularis on lateral view x-ray in a patient with low back pain. (Reproduced with permission from USMLE-Rx.com.)

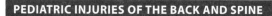

TABLE 17.15. Common Pediatric Overuse Injuries

OVERUSE INJURY	SYMPTOMS/ETIOLOGY	TREATMENT
Sever disease (form of osteochondrosis/ apophysitis)	Heel pain, typically during growth spurts; inflammation of growth plate in heel (calcaneus)	Rest; also consider heel pads, stretches of Achilles tendon, NSAIDs When severe, may consider short-term use of walker boot
Osgood-Schlatter disease	Pain in front of knee, worsens with running/jumping/ kneeling Rupture of the growth plate at the tibial tuberosity → stress on the patellar tendon Occurs in rapidly growing adolescents; 5× more common in athletes, 2-3× more common in boys, typically occurring in ages 10-15 y May be bilateral; usually worse on 1 side	Rest, stretching/strengthening quadriceps/hamstring muscles, NSAIDs, immobilization if severe Will resolve once growth is complete
Sinding-Larsen-Johansson disease	Irritation/injury of growth plate of kneecap; jumper's knee in children	Rest, ice pack, NSAIDs
Medial epicondyle apophysitis ("Little League elbow")	Pain at medial epicondyle where medial apophysis is located Seen in young throwers because of the repetitive valgus stress across the elbow Clinical diagnosis; rule out ulnar nerve involvement and ligamentous instability	Responds well to rest and conservative measures Indications for surgical intervention include ulnar neuropathy with displaced fracture and valgus instability
Osteochondritis dissecans	Presents with gradual onset of vague knee pain; ± swelling after running/jumping Osteonecrosis of subchondral bone (most commonly on the medial femoral condyle) that causes separation from underlying well-vascularized bone → fragmentation of bone and cartilage in the joint Thought to be due to repetitive small stresses to the subchondral bone Usually occurs during childhood, although patients may not become symptomatic until late adolescence or early adulthood Early diagnosis is critical, as the injury has a better potential to heal while the bones are still growing Usually visible on plain radiographs (especially the tunnel view) MRI is used to assess the stability of the fragment as well as the viability of subchondral bone	Younger patients with smaller, stable lesions are most likely to heal well with conservative measures Activity modification (no running or jumping; possible crutch use) minimizes shear forces and allows for new bone formation If the overlying articular cartilage is disrupted, a loose body is present, or the patient is skeletally mature, refer for operative evaluation
Stress fractures	Gradual onset of pain, usually associated with sudden ↑ in activity or intensity of activity → tenderness over affected bone Plain radiographs may be ⊖ for first 2-3 weeks of symptoms	Rest for 6-8 weeks

Supplements and Steroids

Table 17.16 outlines the uses and mechanisms of action of commonly used sports supplements.

TABLE 17.16. **Common Sports Supplements**

SUPPLEMENT	DESCRIPTION	SIDE EFFECTS/LEGALITY
Amino acids	Thought to ↑ growth hormones by ↑ dietary protein, but no evidence of benefit	Minimal adverse effects (GI upset; diarrhea and stomach cramps); legal
Beta-hydroxy-beta-methylbutyrate (HMB)	Thought to ↓ protein breakdown and ↑ synthesis, but no evidence of benefit	Limited long-term evidence of side effects, legal
Carbohydrate-electrolyte drinks	Effective for ↑ energy and ↓ fatigue	Minimal side effects, legal
Chromium	Thought to ↑ lean muscle mass, but no evidence of benefit	Limited long-term evidence of side effects; isolated reports of liver and renal dysfunction and rhabdomyolysis; legal
Creatine	Promotes protein synthesis and provides a quick source of energy for muscle contraction Thought to enhance performance in short-duration, high-intensity exercise such as sprinting and weight lifting; limited evidence	Associated with short-term weight gain due to intracellular water retention; can lead to intravascular dehydration and possible renal injury; legal
Glucosamine and chondroitin	Some evidence that it relieves symptoms of OA Glucosamine thought to promote the formation and repair of cartilage; may be effective in moderate to severe knee OA Chondroitin is a component of cartilage that is thought to promote water retention and elasticity and inhibit the enzymes that break down cartilage; no evidence of benefit in knee OA	Considered safe, without significant side effects; legal
Iron	Not effective in ↑ energy/performance, unless person is deficient	Toxicity if taken above dietary allowance; hemochromatosis if susceptible; constipation; legal
Sodium bicarbonate	Thought to ↑ buffering capacity, but evidence is mixed	Minimal side effects (bloating, diarrhea), legal
Androgens (androstenedione and DHEA)	"Nutritional supplements" (eg, DHEA, a precursor to androgenic steroids) and synthetic agents thought to stimulate muscle growth and strength via ↑ testosterone, but no evidence of benefit	Significant/dangerous side effects: suppression of endogenous testicular function, ↓ spermatogenesis and fertility Chronic use (over years) can cause ↓ testicular size Also associated with gynecomastia, erythrocytosis, hepatotoxicity, ↓ HDL cholesterol, hypertension, virilization of female athletes, premature epiphyseal fusion and stunting of growth, and psychological disorders, including major mood disorders and aggressive behavior ("roid rage"); legal but banned by IOC and NCAA
Caffeine	Effective for ↑ energy and ↓ fatigue	Minimal side effects (anxiety, dependency, withdrawal); legal but banned by IOC and NCAA at urinary concentrations >12 μg/mL

(continues)

TABLE 17.16.   Common Sports Supplements *(continued)*

SUPPLEMENT	DESCRIPTION	SIDE EFFECTS/LEGALITY
Ephedrine/ pseudoephedrine	Thought to ↑ energy and ↓ fatigue, but evidence is mixed	Significant/dangerous side effects (heart palpitations, anxiety/agitation/irritability, tremor, insomnia; case reports of morbidity/mortality related to MI, CVA, seizure, psychosis); legal but banned by IOC and NCAA
Anabolic steroids (oral and injectable)	Evidence for ↑ lean muscle mass	Significant/dangerous side effects, similar to DHEA: associated with gynecomastia, ↓ HDL, hypertension, virilization of female athletes, aggression, azospermia; **illegal**
Blood transfusions/ erythropoietin	Evidence that it ↑ oxygen delivery →↑ endurance	Significant/dangerous side effects: transfusion reactions and infections; ↑ blood viscosity can lead to DVT, PE, coronary and cerebral thrombosis; **illegal** and banned by IOC and NCAA
Human growth hormone (injectable)	Thought to ↑ muscle protein synthesis and strength; limited evidence. Some OTC supplements claiming to ↑ human growth hormone	Significant/dangerous side effects (soft tissue edema, arthralgias, carpal tunnel syndrome), ↑ risk of Creutzfeldt-Jakob disease in human growth hormone from cadaver; **illegal**
International Olympic Committee doping classes	Stimulants, narcotics, anabolic agents, β₂-agonists, β-blockers (used to calm, stop trembling, and ↓ BP and heart rate), diuretics (used to meet weight goals), peptide hormones and analogs (eg, growth hormone and erythropoietin), street drugs	Banned by the IOC for use in athletic competition (except β₂-agonists in the setting of documented asthma)

IOC, International Olympic Committee; NCAA, National Collegiate Athletic Association.

Based on: Jenkinson DM and Harbert AJ. Supplements and Sports. *Am Fam Physician* 2008;78(9):1039-1046.

KEY FACT

SLE can have multiple clinical presentations and is known as one of "the great imitators."

MNEMONIC

Diagnostic Criteria for SLE:
DOPAMINE RASH:

Discoid rash (thick, scaly patches)
Oral ulcers
Photosensitivity rash
Arthritis
Malar rash (butterfly rash)
Immunologic criteria (⊕ anti-dsDNA or ⊕ anti-Sm)
NEurologic or psychiatric symptoms
Renal disease
ANA ⊕
Serositis (pleural, peritoneal, or pericardial)
Hematologic disorders (thrombocytopenia, anemia, or leukopenia)

Rheumatology

Table 17.17 lists common antibodies and their associated pathology.

SYSTEMIC LUPUS ERYTHEMATOSUS

Chronic inflammatory disease that can affect multiple organ systems, including the skin, joints, kidneys, lungs, nervous system, and serous membranes. The disease course can include episodes of remission as well as flare-ups. The female-to-male ratio is 9:1, with onset often in the 20s and 30s. Three times more common among African Americans.

Symptoms/Exam

Nearly 90% of patients have joint symptoms.

Diagnosis

- Diagnostic criteria can be summarized with the mnemonic **DOPAMINE RASH.** At least 4 of the 11 criteria listed must be present for diagnosis.
- ANA testing is highly sensitive but not specific, whereas antibodies to dsDNA and Smith are specific but not sensitive. Titers of dsDNA antibodies generally correlate with disease activity. ANA titers 1:320 are more likely to be clinically relevant. Five percent of the normal healthy population will have a ⊕ ANA titer.

TABLE 17.17.   **Common Antibodies and Their Associated Pathology**

ANTIBODIES	ASSOCIATED CONDITION
ANA, anti-dsDNA, anti-Sm	SLE
Anti-CCP, rheumatoid factor	RA
Anticentromere	CREST syndrome
Antihistone	Drug-induced SLE
Anti-Jo-1	Polymyositis/dermatomyositis
Antimitochondrial	1° biliary cirrhosis
Anti-Scl-70, antitopoisomerase I	Scleroderma
Anti-smooth muscle	Autoimmune hepatitis
Anti-TSHR	Graves disease
MPO-ANCA/p-ANCA	Vasculitis, microscopic polyangiitis
PR3-ANCA/c-ANCA	Vasculitis, especially granulomatosis with polyangiitis (Wegener)
U1RNP antibody	Mixed connective tissue disease

Modified from Le T, Bhushan V, Chen V, King M. *First Aid for the USMLE Step 2 CK*: 9th ed. New York: McGraw-Hill, 201, Table 2.9-8.

Management

- Topical corticosteroids are first line for cutaneous lupus, in addition to sun and stress avoidance and skin protection.
- Pharmacologic treatment depends on the severity of the disease and the degree of organ involvement. Consider NSAIDs for SLE-associated myositis, serositis, and arthritis; topical and systemic steroids; antimalarials for persistent cutaneous lesions; methotrexate and IVIG.

Complications

Organ-specific damage plus accelerated atherosclerosis and opportunistic infections.

Drug-Induced Lupus

- Similar presentation to SLE, but with equal prevalence among men and women. Symptoms resolve with withdrawal of the offending medication.
- Most commonly associated drugs: hydralazine, procainamide, isoniazid, quinidine, methyldopa, and chlorpromazine.

RHEUMATOID ARTHRITIS

Rheumatoid arthritis (RA) is a chronic systemic inflammatory disease that primarily affects the joints. Affects 1% to 2% of the US population, with a female-to-male ratio of 3:1 and a typical age of onset of 20 to 40 years.

Symptoms/Exam

- **Symmetric,** inflammatory joint pain, most commonly of the PIP and MTP joints, wrists, ankles, and knees (Figure 17.15). Inflammatory characteristics include morning stiffness and pain; improvement of symptoms with use of the joint; possible erythema, warmth, and/or swelling of the joint.

KEY FACT

Both SLE and RA affect the MCP and PIP joints; SLE does not deform.

KEY FACT

⊖ ANA titer essentially rules out SLE.

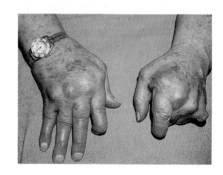

FIGURE 17.15.   **Rheumatoid arthritis.** Typical ulnar deviation of the MCP joints and swelling of the PIP joints in a patient with rheumatoid arthritis. Multiple subcutaneous rheumatoid nodules are also seen, as well as swan neck deformity with DIP flexion and PIP hyperextension (Reproduced with permission from Wolff K, et al. *Fitzpatrick's Dermatology in General Medicine,* 7th ed. New York: McGraw-Hill, 2008, Fig. 161-1A.)

- Patients with long-standing, erosive, RF-positive disease can also develop extra-articular disease, including vasculitis, interstitial lung disease, serositis, ocular disease, Sjogren syndrome, and amyloidosis.

Differential

- Viral infection: **Parvovirus B19, HCV** (usually more pronounced joint pain, less synovitis).
- Other inflammatory syndromes: **SLE, systemic sclerosis, mixed connective tissue disease, Sjogren syndrome** (RA will not have rash, Raynaud phenomenon, or other ⊕ auto-antibodies).
- Other inflammatory arthropathies: **Psoriatic arthritis** and **spondyloarthropathies** (more commonly affect DIP, less symmetry, can involve sacroiliac joint); **gout/pseudogout** (usually oligoarticular); rarely inflammatory **OA** (affects the DIP joints).

Table 17.18 outlines features that distinguish RA from OA, and Figure 17.16 compares the joints most commonly affected in OA and RA.

Diagnosis

- Diagnostic criteria:
  - Presence of synovitis in at least one joint.
  - Absence of an alternative diagnosis that better explains the synovitis.
  - Score of at least six in four domains of the criteria proposed by the 2010 American College of Rheumatology/European League Against Rheumatism Collaborative Initiative (Table 17.19).
- Classic radiographic findings include periarticular osteopenia, joint space narrowing, and juxta-articular erosions (Figure 17.17). X-rays may be normal in early stages.
- RF is ⊕ in 70% to 80% of patients but is not specific. RF can also be ⊕ in viral infections causing joint pain, eg, parvovirus B19, HCV, and mixed connective tissue disease or Sjogren syndrome.

Management

The American College of Rheumatology recommends starting **disease-modifying anti-rheumatic drugs (DMARDs) within 3 months of diagnosis.** DMARDs include systemic and injected steroids, methotrexate, plaquenil, cyclophosphamide, and many other immunomodulators. NSAIDs are appropriate for symptom flares.

TABLE 17.18. Rheumatoid Arthritis Versus Osteoarthritis

	RHEUMATOID ARTHRITIS	OSTEOARTHRITIS
Age of onset	Generally 20s to 40s	Usually old age
Speed of onset	Rapid: weeks to months	Over years
Joints affected	Small and large joints on both sides (symmetrical); wrists, MCP, ankles, knees, shoulders, hips, elbows	Often begins on 1 side of body and usually limited to 1 set of joints (fingers or knees); DIP, PIP, hips, knees
Morning stiffness	Lasts longer than 1 hr, improves with use	Usually worsens as day progresses
Systemic symptoms	Fatigue and general malaise	No systemic symptoms
Synovial fluid/ Imaging	Anti-cyclic citrullinated peptide antibodies	WBC < 2000 cells/mm³ Osteophytes, joint space narrowing on imaging

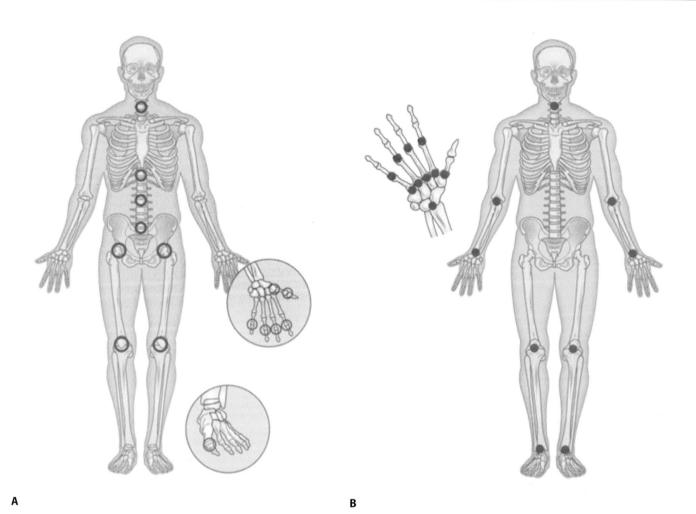

A   B

FIGURE 17.16.   **Joints most commonly affected by osteoarthritis (A) and rheumatoid arthritis (B).** (Reproduced with permission from USMLE-Rx.com.)

TABLE 17.19.   **Classification Criteria for Rheumatoid Arthritis**

Joint involvement	
1 large joint (shoulder, elbow, hip, knee, ankle)	0
2-10 large joints	1
1-3 small joints (MCP, PIP, second to fifth MTP, thumb IP, wrist (does not include DIP, first CMC, first MTP)	2
4-10 small joints, ± large-joint	3
>10 joints, including at least 1 small joint	5
Serology	
Weakly ⊕ RF or weakly ⊕ anti-CCP	2
Strongly ⊕ RF or strongly ⊕ anti-CCP (>3 times upper limit of normal)	3
Acute-phase response: ESR or CRP elevated	1
Duration of symptoms at least 6 weeks	1

Data from 2010 American College of Rheumatology/European League Against Rheumatism Collaborative Initiative.

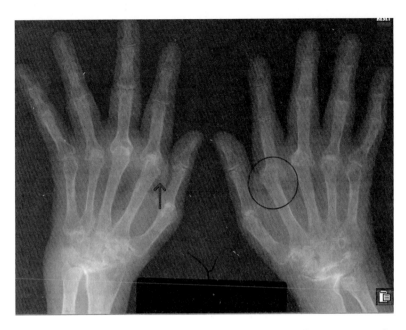

FIGURE 17.17. **Rheumatoid arthritis.** AP bilateral hand radiograph in a patient with advanced RA hows joint space narrowing involving carpal, MCP, and PIP joints as well as subluxation at multiple MCP joints (circle) and periarticular erosions (arrow). (Reproduced with permission from USMLE-Rx.com.)

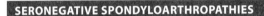

SERONEGATIVE SPONDYLOARTHROPATHIES

Group of disorders characterized by ⊖ serologies for ANA and RF, strong association with the HLA-B27 antigen, and spinal arthritis.

Ankylosing Spondylitis

Chronic inflammation of sacroiliac joints and spine, strong association with HLA-B27.

- Affects 1 in 2000 people, with men having more severe disease than women.
- Progressive pain and stiffening of the spine, with low back pain that is worse in the morning and inactivity but improves with exercise.
- Tenderness of sacroiliac joints with ↓ lumbar lordosis and cervical motion.
- Diagnosed by classic "bamboo-like" appearance of the spine on radiographs (from fusion of vertebral bodies and posterior spine) and/or sacroiliitis on radiographs or MRI. ⊖ RF and ANA, with ↑ ESR and CRP (Figure 17.18).
- NSAIDs are first line initial therapy; also encourage exercise, PT. Consider anti-tumor necrosis factor (anti-TNF) inhibitors in refractory cases. Spinal fusion in severe cases.

Psoriatic Arthritis

Affects 5% to 20% of patients with psoriasis.

- Multiple patterns of presentation, including mono- and polyarticular types. Typically affects DIP joints. Associated with nail disorders (pitting, ridging, onycholysis), psoriatic skin changes, and dactylitis ("sausage-shaped digits").
- X-ray reveals characteristic changes such as marginal erosions and "pencil-in-cup" deformities of the distal digits.

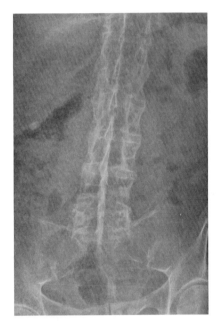

FIGURE 17.18. **Ankylosing spondylitis.** Bamboo spine in a patient with ankylosing spondylitis. (Reproduced from Wikimedia Commons; courtesy of Steven Fruitsmaak.)

KEY FACT

Psoriatic arthritis can occur before or after psoriatic lesions.

- NSAIDs are first line; second line are methotrexate and sulfasalazine. If axial involvement or peripheral disease without improvement on DMARDs, consider anti-TNF medication.

Reactive Arthritis

Develops as autoimmune response within 1 month of an infection with *Salmonella, Shigella, Campylobacter, Yersinia, Chlamydia,* or other pathogens (think GU, GI infections).

- Classic triad of **conjunctivitis, urethritis, and arthritis** (more commonly of the larger peripheral joints than of the spine: knees, ankles, feet); occurs in only one-third of patients. Patients often have heel pain due to reactive arthritis at enthesis of Achilles tendon. May also have systemic symptoms such as fever and weight loss.
- Diagnose via arthrocentesis showing an inflammatory pattern and ⊖ culture.
- Use NSAIDs for symptoms, does not shorten course (symptoms usually resolve in 1 year). Can consider intra-articular corticosteroid injections.
- Always treat underlying disease, as indicated.
- If persistent symptoms, consider sulfasalazine; second line etanercept.
- Rare complications include aortitis, aortic regurgitation.

KEY FACT

To remember the symptoms of reactive arthritis, think "can't see, can't pee, can't climb a tree."

IBD-Associated Arthritis

Twenty percent of patients with IBD (Crohn's disease > ulcerative colitis) develop associated arthritis.

- Peripheral arthritic flares associated with GI disease. Peripheral, asymmetric, oligoarticular, large-joint involvement. Spinal involvement mimics ankylosing spondylitis and is independent of intestinal disease.
- **NSAIDs.** Treatment of GI disease can control peripheral arthritis.

KEY FACT

Most common joint involved in gout is the great toe.
Most common joint involved in pseudogout is the knee.

CRYSTALLINE-INDUCED ARTHROPATHIES

Deposition of crystals in the synovium and other tissues, triggering an inflammatory response. Episodes of abrupt-onset, severe, and usually monoarticular joint pain.

Hyperuricemia

- ↑ the risk of gout, but the majority of patients do not develop gout.
- Due to **overproduction** of uric acid (glycogen storage diseases, psoriasis, myeloproliferative disorders, large tumor burden) or **underexcretion** of uric acid (renal disease, thiazide or loop diuretics, lactic acidosis, alcoholism, ketoacidosis).
- More common in men, patients with diabetes, hypertension, hyperlipidemia, or obesity, and patients of Pacific Islander ancestry.

KEY FACT

Aspirin can cause ↓ excretion of uric acid by the kidney; temporarily discontinue during an acute gout attack.

Calcium Pyrophosphate Deposition Disease

Crystalline arthropathy can lead to a spectrum of disease, ranging from asymptomatic chondrocalcinosis (calcification of the articular cartilage surface) to **pseudogout** (Table 17.20).

Medications that can precipitate a gout flare include:
- Diuretics (including hydrochlorothiazide and furosemide).
- Salicylate-containing drugs (including aspirin).
- Niacin (including vitamin B_3 and nicotinic acid).
- Cyclosporine (used for immune suppression).
- Levodopa (Parkinson disease treatment).

KEY FACT

Rapid or unusual distribution of degenerative joint disease should raise suspicion of calcium pyrophosphate deposition disease.

TABLE 17.20. Gout Versus Pseudogout

	GOUT	PSEUDOGOUT
Etiology	Deposition of uric acid crystals in the synovium, bursae, tendon sheaths, skin, heart valves, and kidneys, which can cause arthritis, tophi, renal stones, and gouty nephropathy	Deposition of calcium-containing crystals in articular cartilage, menisci, synovium, and surrounding tendons/ligaments, which can cause arthritis, chondrocalcinosis
Demographics	Risk ↑ with age; risk factors: male, obesity, postmenopausal females, binge drinking	Risk ↑ with age; can be precipitated by trauma, surgery, postparathyroidectomy, severe illness; associated with hyperparathyroidism, hemochromatosis, hypomagnesemia, hypophosphatemia, hypothyroidism
Symptoms/exam	Acute, exquisitely tender, monoarticular arthritis: "red-hot" swollen joint First MTP joint is most commonly affected, but the knees, ankles, feet, elbows, and hands may also be involved Nodular deposits of uric acid crystals, or **tophi,** may be seen in subcutaneous tissues, tendons, cartilage, and bone	Osteoarthritis-like (50%): chronic, bilateral arthritis Gout-like (25%): acute monoarticular CPPD (20%): chondrocalcinosis on imaging, asymptomatic Pseudorheumatoid (5%): severe destructive arthritis Most commonly affect knees, but can affect wrists, ankles, elbows, toes, shoulders, hip
Diagnosis	⊖ birefringent, needle-like crystals on synovial fluid aspiration; cultures are sterile "Rat-bite" erosions may be seen on joint radiographs (but typically normal for 1st 10 years) (Figure 17.19) Serum uric acid is ↑ in 95% of cases, but is not diagnostic nor required for diagnosis	Weakly ⊕ birefringent rhomboid-shaped crystals on synovial fluid aspiration Radiographs can show the white lines of chondrocalcinosis in joint spaces (punctate or linear densities) Rule out secondary causes with serum calcium, phosphorus, magnesium, alkaline phosphatase, TSH, ferritin, uric acid
Acute treatment	**NSAIDs** such as indomethacin are first-line therapy If contraindicated (renal insufficiency, heart failure, PUD), consider intra-articular or systemic corticosteroids Colchicine is second line	**NSAIDs are first line for acute pain** Corticosteroid injections if <2 joints involved and infection ruled out
Chronic treatment/prevention	Diet modification, weight loss, alcohol avoidance (↓ purine intake) Consider daily allopurinol or colchicine (for both overproducers and underexcretors), or probenecid for underexcretors; goal serum urate <6 mg/dL	Colchicine for chronic cases, although lacking evidence Treat underlying etiology if secondary

INFECTIOUS ARTHRITIS

Most common causes are *Staphylococcus aureus* and *Neisseria gonorrhoeae*. Surgical emergency.

Gonococcal Arthritis (Disseminated Infection)

Arthritis and arthralgias are the principal manifestations of disseminated gonococcal infection, which occurs in 1% to 3% of patients infected with *N gonorrhoeae*. Most common in patients <40 years of age.

- Migratory polyarthralgias and tenosynovitis with fever and a papulopustular rash that can involve the **palms and soles.**
- Blood, rectal, throat, and urethral cultures are 70% to 80% sensitive, whereas synovial fluid culture is <50% sensitive.
- IV antibiotics (third-generation cephalosporin); continue until clinical improvement, followed by oral antibiotics for a 7- to 10-day total course. Treat empirically for chlamydia.

KEY FACT

The knee is the most common site of infectious arthritis.

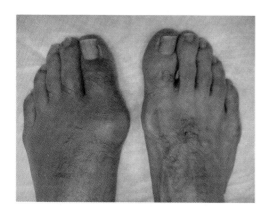

A

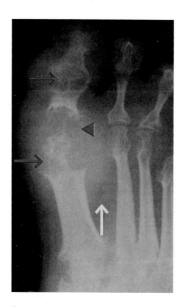

B

FIGURE 17.19. **Gout.** (A) A swollen left 1st MTP joint with overlying erythema and warmth, characteristic of an acute gout attack (podagra). (B) An AP radiograph showing the severe consequences of long-standing gout, including large, nonmarginal erosions with overhanging edges of bone (red arrows), soft tissue swelling, and destruction of the first MTP joint (arrowhead). Note the subtle calcification of a gouty tophus (yellow arrow). (Image A reproduced with permission from LeBlond RF, et al. *DeGowin's Diagnostic Examination*, 9th ed. New York: McGraw-Hill, 2009, Plate 30; image B reproduced with permission from USMLE-Rx.com.)

Nongonococcal Arthritis (Septic Joint)

Inoculation of bacteria into a joint from hematogenous spread, direct penetration of the joint, or spread from an adjacent focus of infection. Most common organisms are gram-positive species (*S aureus* > *Streptococcus*), less commonly gram-negative organisms such as *Escherichia coli* or *Pseudomonas*. ↑ risk with previous joint damage, IV drug use, endocarditis, or prosthetic joints.

Symptoms/Exam

- Presents with acute-onset, monoarticular joint pain with swelling, warmth, and erythema. Patients usually have fevers and chills. Passive ROM of the joint is exquisitely painful.
- Joint aspiration reveals WBC >50,000 cells/mm^3, predominantly neutrophils. Fifty percent of patients have ⊕ blood cultures, and 75% have ⊕ synovial fluid cultures and a ⊕ Gram stain.
- Radiographs can show joint erosions, osteomyelitis, demineralization or periostitis.
- Start IV antibiotics based on Gram stain results; narrow by joint/blood cultures. Often need IV antibiotics for up to 6 weeks. Rapid evacuation of infected synovial fluid, usually through arthroscopic or open surgical debridement.
- Complications include articular destruction, septicemia.

KEY FACT

When considering infections of prosthetic devices, think *Staphylococcus epidermidis*.

Lyme Arthritis

Borrelia burgdorferi is the most common source of Lyme disease. Eighty percent have classic erythema migrans rash, which develops within 1 month of tick bite. Arthritis occurs in ~ 50% of untreated patients, but is rare with treatment.

- Patients experience polyarthralgias, migratory polyarthritis, or oligoarticular arthritis.
- Titers for antibodies to *B burgdorferi* (ELISA first; if ⊕, then Western blot) are diagnostic but have a high false-negative rate; false positives seen in RA, SLE, juvenile rheumatoid arthritis (JRA), and infectious mononucleosis.

- Treat early disease with doxycycline (patients >8 years) or amoxicillin (patients <8 years or pregnant women) for 21 days. Treat late or early disseminated disease with IV antibiotics.
- Complications include meningitis, neuritis, and atrioventricular conduction blocks.

INFLAMMATORY MYOPATHIES

See the Neurology chapter.

SYSTEMIC SCLEROSIS (SCLERODERMA)

Autoimmune disorder characterized by **CREST** syndrome (**C**alcinosis, **R**aynaud phenomenon, **E**sophageal dysmotility, **S**clerodactyly, and **T**elangiectasias). Majority of cases (80%) are limited scleroderma, which has a better prognosis; progressive systemic sclerosis can also have kidney, heart, lung, and GI tract involvement.

- Both types are ANA ⊕, with anticentromere antibodies in limited scleroderma and anti-SCL-70 antibodies in the progressive type.
- Treatment of CREST syndrome is symptomatic (eg, calcium channel blockers for Raynaud phenomenon, ACEI for renal disease, PPI for esophageal dysmotility); progressive disease requires corticosteroids and immunosuppressants.
- Pulmonary hypertension and pulmonary fibrosis are the leading causes of death.

SJOGREN SYNDROME

Autoimmune disorder, T-cell mediated exocrine gland destruction.

- Dry eyes (keratoconjunctivitis sicca), dry mouth (xerostomia) may be associated with fatigue and generalized malaise.
- Symptoms and clinical signs of ocular dryness, dry mouth, and serum findings of autoimmune disease: elevated RF >1:320 or elevated ANA <1:320, or anti-SS-A(Ro) or anti-SS-B(La) antibodies.
- Symptomatic treatment with humidifiers, artificial tears, frequent drinking water, sugarless gums/mints.
- Systemic treatment with NSAIDs and antimalarials.

VASCULITIDES

Group of disorders characterized by inflammatory destruction of blood vessels. Can be primary or secondary.

- Presentation depends on the structures involved.
- 1° vasculitides is can be categorized according to the size of the involved vessels (Table 17.21).
- 2° vasculitides can be due to infection (especially indolent infections such as bacterial endocarditis and HCV), medications, collagen vascular disease, or malignancy.
- Treat with corticosteroids and/or immunosuppressants.

Giant Cell Arteritis (Temporal Arteritis)

Symptoms/Exam

- Gradual onset of constitutional symptoms: fatigue, malaise, fever, weight loss, polymyalgia rheumatica (PMR), followed by development of jaw claudication, new headaches, scalp tenderness, ± diplopia and vision loss due to retinal ischemia, ± changes taste or hearing.
- Tenderness over temporal arteries.

TABLE 17.21.   Classification of Vasculitis

	VESSEL SIZE		
	SMALL	MEDIUM	LARGE
Disorders	Microscopic polyangiitis	Polyarteritis nodosa (PAN)	Takayasu arteritis
	Henoch-Schonlein purpura	EGPA	Giant cell arteritis/temporal arteritis
	Cutaneous leukocytoclastic angiitis	GPA	Behçet syndrome
	Behçet syndrome	Microscopic polyangiitis	
	Hypersensibitiy	Behçet syndrome	
	Cryoglobulinemia		
	Associated with connective tissue disease (SLE, RA)		
	Drug-induced		
	Eosinophilic granulomatosis with polyangiitis (EGPA, Churg-Strauss)		
	Granulomatosis with polyangiitis (GPA)		
Skin	Palpable purpura, digital infarcts	Nodules, ulcers, gangrene, livedo reticularis	Mimics severe atherosclerosis, gangrene
Kidney	Rapidly progressive crescentic glomerulonephritis	HTN, aneurysms	HTN
Cardiovascular	CHF, pericarditis	MI	MI
GI	Pain, nausea/vomiting, GI bleeding	Pain, nausea/vomiting, GI bleeding, infarction, aneurysms	Intestinal angina (pain out of proportion to exam), infarction
Testes	–	Pain (classic for PAN)	–
Peripheral nervous system	Sensory polyneuropathy	Sensory/motor neuropathy; mononeuritis multiplex	–
CNS	Meningitis	TIA	Stroke
Systemic symptoms (fever, weight loss)	++	++++	++

Diagnosis

Must meet three of five criteria:

- Age >50 years.
- New/localized headache.
- Tenderness/↓ pulse of temporal artery.
- ESR >50 mm/hr.
- Temporal artery biopsy with necrotizing arteritis with predominance of mononuclear cells or granulomatous process with multinucleated giant cells.

Management

Prednisone for 2 to 4 weeks; start treatment if high suspicion even before having biopsy results.

KEY FACT

Visual symptoms with giant cell arteritis should be treated emergently with steroids; consider inpatient IV treatment.

Polymyalgia Rheumatica

- Early fever, fatigue, malaise, weight loss, followed by pain, stiffness over shoulder and later over pelvic girdle; difficulty lifting arms over head and/or getting out of chair.
- ESR ↑ >40 mm/hr; frequent association with anemia. Muscle biopsy normal.
- Rapid improvement with low-dose glucocorticoids.
- Low dose prednisone; continue for 6 to 12 months until ESR normal and patient asymptomatic.

FIBROMYALGIA

Poorly understood noninflammatory soft tissue pain disorder. Typically occurs between ages 30 to 60 years. Thought to affect 2% to 8% of the population. Risk factors: female sex, low socioeconomic status, poor functional status, stressful life events.

Symptoms/Exam

- In 50% of patients, symptoms are preceded by a ⊖ event or a flulike illness.
- Chronic: >3 months' duration.
- Widespread musculoskeletal pain.
- Accompanied by severe fatigue, mood and sleep disturbances.

Diagnosis

Based on the presence of: widespread pain and muscle tenderness, severe fatigue, nonrestorative sleep or cognitive symptoms, and duration of symptoms >3 months in the setting of a normal laboratory evaluation (CBC, ESR, or CRP [nonspecific; only test if suspect connective tissue disorder], CK, TSH, renal and liver function) to rule out other causes of chronic fatigue and pain. Sleep study may be indicated to rule out obstructive sleep apnea or narcolepsy as the cause of fatigue.

Differential

- **Chronic fatigue:** Pain is less prominent.
- **Myofascial pain:** Pain is more localized.
- Inflammatory disorders.
- Mood disorders.
- **Common comorbid conditions:** Connective tissue diseases, mood disorders, posttraumatic stress disorder, sleep disorders, Lyme disease, temporomandibular joint disorder, irritable bowel syndrome, interstitial cystitis, and chronic headache.

Management

- Nonpharmacologies therapy:
  - **Aerobic exercise/physical activity:** Gradually ↑ low-impact aerobic exercise, tai chi, and other gentle mindful movement.
  - **Sleep hygiene.**
  - **Self-management support:** Psychoeducation about illness, stress management, psychosocial support; may require job/workplace modifications.
  - **Cognitive behavior therapy.**
  - **Complementary and alternative medicine:** Limited evidence for acupuncture, hypnotherapy, biofeedback, balneotherapy/hydrotherapy, homeopathy, and massage.
- Pharmacologic therapy:
  - **Antidepressants:** Limited evidence for TCAs and SSRI for improving fatigue, pain, sleep, or quality of life. Duloxetine and milnacipran are FDA approved for treatment of fibromyalgia. 2016 Cochrane review demonstrated low-quality evidence for SSRIs (citalopram, fluoxetine, paroxetine studied), but there are

---

KEY FACT

Giant cell arteritis and polymyalgia rheumatica are often seen together.

KEY FACT

Diagnosis of fibromyalgia is by structured symptom history; no longer based on tenderness at trigger points.

KEY FACT

Irritable bowel syndrome may overlap with fibromyalgia.
Up to 70% of patients with fibromyalgia have symptoms of irritable bowel syndrome.

small, statistically significant benefits in pain reduction, global improvement, and depression using SSRI versus placebo.

- Antiepileptics: Limited evidence for pregabalin (FDA approved for treatment of fibromyalgia).
- Muscle relaxants: Limited evidence for cyclobenzaprine in improving pain and sleep, when combined with antidepressants or antiepileptics.
- **Avoid opiates.** 2015 Cochrane review showed no evidence of benefit with controlled-release oxycodone.
- Lack of evidence for benefit with NSAIDs.

NOTES

CHAPTER 18

Emergency/Urgent Care

N. Kenji Taylor, MD, MSc

Trauma Care

Predicated on the concepts of rapid triage, diagnosis, resuscitation, and therapeutic intervention. Evaluation of trauma is categorized by two main surveys:

- **Primary survey (ABCDE):**
    - **Airway:** Establish and ensure a clear airway.
    - **Breathing:** Ventilate with 100% O_2 and check for breathing compromise.
    - **Circulation:** Apply pressure to sites of external bleeding, place two large-bore IV lines, assess blood volume status, and begin fluid resuscitation if signs of hypovolemia.
    - **Disability:** Document functional status and perform a brief neurologic examination.
    - **Exposure:** Completely disrobe the patient and logroll to inspect the back.
- **Secondary survey:**
    - Perform a head-to-toe examination to search for other injuries and set further priorities.
    - May include trauma series imaging, focused assessment with sonography in trauma (FAST), Foley catheter or gastric tube placement, splinting of unstable fractures/dislocations, tetanus prophylaxis, surgical consultation, and medications.

CNS Injury

HEAD TRAUMA

Contributes to about one-third of all injury deaths. Traumatic brain injury can result from **direct injury** caused by the force of an object striking the head or **indirect injury** from acceleration/deceleration forces. Use the Glasgow Coma Scale (GCS) to assess all patients with head trauma (Table 18.1).

Symptoms/Exam

- **Low-risk injuries:** Characterized by minor trauma, scalp wounds, a GCS score of 15, normal neurologic exam, and absence of signs of intracranial injury.
- **Moderate- to high-risk injuries:** Characterized by altered mental status or loss of consciousness, persistent nausea and vomiting, seizures, severe headaches, focal neurologic signs, presence of penetrating skull injuries, evidence of basilar skull fracture (eg, CSF rhinorrhea, Battle sign, hemotympanum, raccoon eyes; Figure 18.1), a GCS score <14.

Diagnosis

Head CT and skull radiographs are generally not indicated in adults unless depressed fracture is suspected or moderate- to high-risk features (as noted above) are present.

Management

- Establish ABCs, including cervical spine immobilization and intubation if the patient is unable to protect the airway.
- Prompt neurosurgical consultation if a high-risk injury is suspected.
- Hyperventilation to maintain a P_{CO_2} of 25 to 30 mm Hg, maintenance of normal cardiac output, mannitol and elevation of the head of the bed to 30 degrees to ↓ ICP.

Complications

Postconcussion syndrome, seizures, neurologic deficits, death.

TABLE 18.1.   Glasgow Coma Scale for All Age Groups

RESPONSE/SCORE	4 YEARS TO ADULT	CHILDREN <4 YEARS	INFANTS
Eye opening			
4	Spontaneous	Spontaneous	Spontaneous
3	To speech	To speech	To speech
2	To pain	To pain	To pain
1	No response	No response	No response
Verbal response			
5	Alert and oriented	Oriented, social, interacts	Coos, babbles
4	Disoriented conversation	Confused speech, disoriented, consolable, aware	Irritable cry
3	Speaking but nonsensical	Inappropriate words, inconsolable, unaware	Cries to pain
2	Moans or unintelligible sound	Incomprehensible, agitated, restless, unaware	Moans to pain
1	No response	No response	No response
Motor response			
6	Follows commands	Normal, spontaneous movements	Normal, spontaneous movements
5	Localizes pain	Localizes pain	Withdraws to touch
4	Withdraws to pain	Withdraws to pain	Withdraws to pain
3	Decorticate flexion	Decorticate flexion	Decorticate flexion
2	Decerebrate extension	Decerebrate extension	Decerebrate extension
1	No response	No response	No response

Space-Occupying Hematomas

Types of space-occupying hematomas include:

- **Epidural:**
    - Arterial blood in the potential space, between the dura and bone, due to disruption of interposed vessels (usually middle meningeal artery).
    - Associated with skull fractures in 85% to 95% of adult cases.
- **Subdural:**
    - Venous blood, usually from bridging veins, below the inner layer of the dura but external to the brain and arachnoid membrane.
    - If untreated, acute subdural hematomas can progress to subacute (3-7 days after injury) and chronic (2-3 weeks after injury) stages.
- **Subarachnoid:**
    - Blood within subarachnoid space resulting from rupture of a berry aneurysm or an AVM.
    - Commonly associated with uncontrolled hypertension, smoking, alcohol use, and cerebral AVMs.

Symptoms/Exam

Headache, nausea, vomiting, seizures, focal neurologic deficits within hours of the injury.

Diagnosis

See Table 18.2 and Figure 18.2. Conventional angiography, MRA, or CT angiography may be used to confirm the presence of an underlying vascular malformation.

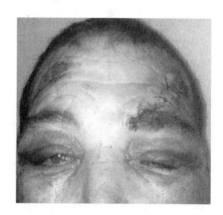

FIGURE 18.1.   Raccoon eyes.
Bilateral periorbital ecchymoses, which is suggestive of basilar skull fracture. (Reproduced from Bouchaouch A, et al. Trauma of the anterior floor of the base of the skull: about a series of 136 cases. *Pan Afr Med J.* 2015;21:155.)

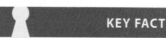

KEY FACT

Think subarachnoid hemorrhage in a patient complaining of **"the worst headache of my life"** or sudden onset like a "thunderclap."

TABLE 18.2.   Evaluation of Space-Occupying Hematomas

	EPIDURAL	SUBDURAL	SUBARACHNOID
Exam	Bradycardia, hypertension due to ↑ICP, anisocoria, skull fractures or lacerations, CSF rhinorrhea or otorrhea, hemotympanum, altered mental status, facial nerve injury, and vertebral column instability	History of blunt trauma; impaired mental status, focal neurologic deficits, Glasgow Coma Scale (GCS) score of <15; photophobia	Prodromal symptoms from minor blood leakage ("sentinel" headache) are reported in 30%-50% of aneurysmal subarachnoid hematomas (SAHs) and are not due to ↑ICP
Differential	Cerebral contusion or laceration, concussion, intracranial epidural abscess, spinal cord disease, spinal epidural abscess, SAH, subdural hematoma	Child or elder abuse, epidural hematoma, meningitis, stroke, subarachnoid hemorrhage, dementia	Encephalitis, hypertensive emergency, meningitis, stroke, TIA, temporal arteritis, tension/migraine/cluster headache
Diagnosis: Noncontrast head CT findings	Hyperdense, lens-shaped mass between the brain and skull (Figure 18.2A)	Hyperdense crescentic mass along the inner table of the skull, most commonly in the parietal region (Figure 18.2B)	Most sensitive within 24 hours of event; shows SAH ± evidence of associated hydrocephalus (Figure 18.2C)
Complications	Posttraumatic seizures, postconcussion syndrome, neurologic deficits, death	↑ICP, brain edema, recurrent hematoma, infection, seizures	Hydrocephalus, rebleeding, intraventricular or intracerebral hemorrhage, cerebral ischemia, hyponatremia from cerebral salt wasting, hypothalamic dysfunction, seizures, ↑ICP, neurologic deficits, death

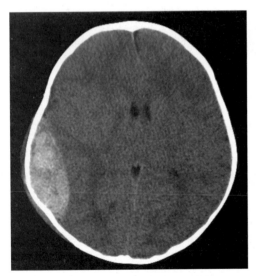

A

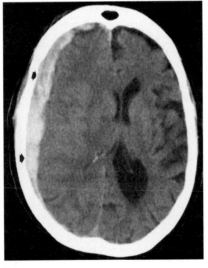

B

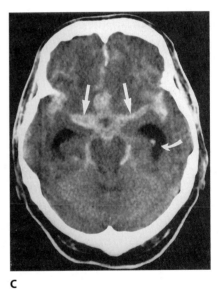

C

FIGURE 18.2.   Space-occupying hematomas. Noncontrast transaxial CT scans show **(A)** a right temporal acute **epidural hematoma,** note the characteristic biconvex shape; **(B)** a right acute holohemispheric **subdural hematoma** (arrows), note the characteristic crescentic shape; and **(C) subarachnoid hemorrhage** filling the basilar cisterns and sylvian fissures (straight arrows). The curved arrow shows the dilated temporal horns of the lateral ventricles/hydrocephalus. (Image A reproduced with permission from Doherty GM. *Current Diagnosis & Treatment: Surgery,* 13th ed. New York: McGraw-Hill, 2010, Fig. 36-8; image B reproduced with permission from Chen MY, et al. *Basic Radiology.* New York: McGraw-Hill, 2004, Fig. 12-32; image C reproduced with permission from Tintinalli JE, et al. *Tintinalli's Emergency Medicine: A Comprehensive Study Guide,* 6th ed. New York: McGraw-Hill, 2004, Fig. 237-4.)

Management

- ABCs, immobilize patient. Consider intubation if GCS <10 to secure airway.
- Neurosurgery emergency consultation.
- Correct coexisting coagulopathy.
- ↓ ICP: Osmotic diuretics (mannitol), hyperventilation to achieve a PCO_2 of 28 to 32 mm Hg; elevation of head of bed to 30 degrees.
- Systemic arterial BP control (mean arterial pressure <130 mm Hg); isotonic fluids; seizure treatment or prophylaxis.
- Although conservative management may be a reasonable option in mild cases, craniotomy, followed by evacuation of the hematoma is the definitive treatment.
- Burr holes are a temporizing option before definitive surgery if clinical concern for herniation.
- Consider ventriculostomy placement if coexisting hydrocephalus.
- SAH: Surgical clipping or endovascular treatment (coiling) of a ruptured berry aneurysm.

KEY FACT

Subdural hematoma is more frequently found in patients >60 years of age. Alcoholics, hemophiliacs, and patients on long-term anticoagulation therapy are at ↑ risk.

NECK TRAUMA

May be classified as penetrating or blunt trauma; one-half of blunt trauma neck injuries are due to motor vehicle accidents. Optimal management of patients with neck trauma is challenging, as seemingly minor injuries can rapidly become life-threatening.

Symptoms/Exam

- Depends on the type of injury, but may include active bleeding, large or expanding hematomas, diminished pulses or bruits, lateralizing signs, tracheal deviation, subcutaneous emphysema, cranial nerve palsies, stridor, hoarseness, vocal cord paralysis, hemoptysis, or hematemesis.
- To clear cervical spine fractures clinically, without imaging, patients must meet all of the National Emergency X-Radiography Utilization Study (NEXUS) criteria (see Mnemonic).

MNEMONIC

NEXUS criteria for C-spine imaging:

NSAID

Neurological deficit
Spinal tenderness (midline)
Altered mental status
Intoxication
Distracting injury (another injury that prevents complete evaluation of the main injury)

Diagnosis

- Three-view radiographs showing all seven cervical vertebrae, the C7-T1 interspace, and a lateral view. If visualization of C-spine on x-ray is incomplete or equivocal findings are noted, CT imaging is indicated (Figure 18.3).
- A full spine series is indicated in patients with one spinal fracture.
- Consider CT angiography in the presence of a penetrating neck trauma close to the arterial blood supply.

Management

Establish airway (orotracheal intubation, cricothyroidotomy or tracheostomy), stop bleeding, stabilize the cervical spine until clearance can be definitively made.

SPINAL CORD TRAUMA

One of the most devastating trauma-related injuries. Most spinal cord trauma is caused by blunt trauma from a motor vehicle accident.

- **Symptoms/Exam:** Depends on the degree of injury, but may include flaccid paralysis and loss of sensation below the level of the lesion, urinary and fecal retention, loss of reflex activity, spastic paraplegia or quadriplegia, hyperreflexia and extensor plantar responses, priapism, paralytic ileus, vasomotor instability due to spinal neurogenic shock, loss of temperature and pain appreciation, or hypoventilation and hypoxia if above C5.

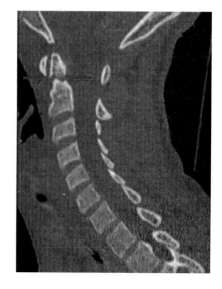

FIGURE 18.3. Cervical spine fracture. A sagittal reformation of a cervical spine CT shows a fracture through the base of the dens, a type 2 odontoid fracture (arrows). (Reproduced with permission from USMLE-Rx.com.)

- **Diagnosis:** Complete spinal series, portable CXR and pelvic radiograph, CT for evaluation of bony elements, MRI for evaluation of the spinal cord.
- **Management:** Prompt neurosurgical consultation, methylprednisolone 30 mg/kg within 8 hours of injury, anatomic realignment of the spinal cord, immobilization.
- **Complications:** Decubitus ulcers, aspiration PNA, depression, sensory deficits, incontinence, paralysis, death.

KEY FACT

Consult an ophthalmologist immediately for patients with:
- Red eye plus any of the following symptoms:
  - Severe pain
  - Photophobia
  - Acute changes in vision
  - Proptosis
  - Pupillary abnormalities
- Suspected acute angle close glaucoma, orbital cellulitis, or uveitis.

Ophthalmologic Trauma

Commonly manifests as orbital floor ("blowout") fractures resulting from blunt anteroposterior force directed against the eyeball. Other common consequences of ocular trauma necessitating immediate consultation include hyphema (postinjury accumulation of blood in the anterior chamber) and ruptured globe (disruption of the integrity of its outer membranes by blunt or penetrating trauma).

RED EYE EVALUATION

The red eye is a cardinal sign of ocular inflammation; caused by dilation of blood vessels in the eye. Although the differential diagnosis of red eye is large, most cases are benign and may be managed effectively by the patient's primary care clinician. Careful evaluation of red eye should be able to distinguish benign from severe and emergent cases.
- Always include visual acuity testing, extraocular movements, pupil shape and reactivity, eyelid inspection (evert lids to look for foreign body), fluorescein exam.
- Assess for photophobia, presence of pain, discharge.
- A thorough exam is best done after application of topical anesthetic drops.
- If available, slit-lamp examination of the cornea, anterior chamber (looking for cells), direct ophthalmoscopy (looking for optic nerve/cup, gross exam of fundus), and intraocular pressure measurement, to facilitate diagnosis.

ORBITAL FRACTURE

Fracture of any of the six facial bones composing the orbit: frontal bone, zygoma, maxilla, maxillary sinus, lacrimal bone, ethmoid bone and sphenoid bone. Blowout fractures occur when a blow to the eye ↑ pressure in the orbit, leading to a fracture of the weakest portion of the orbit, the thin orbital floor (maxilla), and lamina papyracea (ethmoid bone).
- **Symptoms/Exam:** ↓ visual acuity, enophthalmos, paresthesia of the cheek on the affected side, periorbital ecchymosis and edema, diplopia.
- **Diagnosis:**
  - Full ophthalmologic exam plus evaluation for facial asymmetry, tenderness or step-offs over the orbital bones, as well as for CSF leak (testing rhinorrhea) and septal hematoma.
  - CT of the face and sinus is the test of choice (Figure 18.4).
- **Management:** ABCs and trauma survey. Nasotracheal intubation may be contraindicated in severe facial injuries. Appropriate surgical referrals as indicated.
- **Complications:** Corneal abrasion, lens dislocation, traumatic iritis/uveitis, tears of the uveal tract, penetrating eye injury, foreign body, retinal detachment, hyphema, ocular muscle entrapment, globe rupture.

MNEMONIC

Causes of red eye:
GO SUCK

Glaucoma
Orbital disease
Scleritis
Uveitis
Conjunctivitis (viral, bacterial, allergic)
Keratitis (HSV)

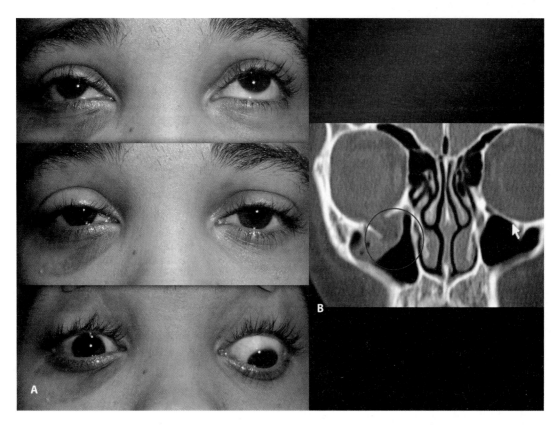

FIGURE 18.4. **Orbital blowout fracture.** (**A**) Clinical exam in this patient demonstrates periorbital ecchymosis and right inferior vertical gaze deficit. (**B**) Coronal reformat from a facial CT shows the fracture of the orbital floor (red circle) with herniation of orbital contents through the defect. (Reproduced with permission from USMLE-Rx.com.)

COMMON OCULAR EMERGENCIES

Orbital Cellulitis

A potentially devastating infection that can rapidly progress to blindness, meningitis, or death. Most cases develop from the direct spread of untreated sinusitis. Discussed in detail in the Infectious Diseases chapter.

Angle-Closure Glaucoma

A rare condition in which the iris blocks the aqueous humor outflow tract when the pupil is mid-dilated, causing an abrupt ↑ in intraocular pressure. Susceptible eyes have a shallow anterior chamber (more common in patients of East Asian origin). Also known as acute narrow-angle glaucoma. Can be precipitated by anticholinergic or sympathomimetic medications. See the Geriatric Medicine chapter for diagnosis and treatment.

Corneal Abrasion

Disruption of the integrity of the corneal epithelium, often as a result of external physical forces. Frequently caused by dry eye, foreign body, direct trauma, and contact lens wear. One of the most common, yet often overlooked, eye injuries.

- **Symptoms/Exam:** Eye pain, foreign body sensation, photophobia, tearing, history of traumatic injury or contact lens use. Can have normal or ↓ visual acuity.

> **KEY FACT**
>
> If concern for acute angle closure glaucoma, do **not** dilate the eye.

> **KEY FACT**
>
> Bacterial keratitis is an important complication of corneal abrasions in contact lens wearers. It is commonly caused by *Pseudomonas* species and has an aggressive course. Contact lens wearers with corneal abrasions should receive prophylactic topical antibiotics and close follow-up.

- **Diagnosis:** A defect in the corneal epithelium is seen with fluorescein staining and Wood's lamp. Slit-lamp examination is helpful but not necessary to diagnose corneal abrasions. Also characterized by bulbar conjunctival injection, and possible foreign body seen on eversion of the eyelids.
- **Management:**
  - Topical anesthetic for exam only; do not use for pain control after exam.
  - Topical antibiotic ointments/drops, and pain control with NSAIDs (systemic analgesics are preferred over local anesthetic drops because of the potential for causing inadvertent damage to an insensate cornea).
  - Monitor every 1 to 2 days until resolved.
  - Urgent ophthalmologic referral if a retained foreign body or corneal ulcer is suspected, markedly reduced visual acuity, or no improvement within 2 days.
  - Eye patching is no longer routinely recommended because of the ↑ risk of infection, especially among contact lens wearers.
- **Complications:** Usually minimal, although recurrent epithelial erosions or corneal ulcers may occur, leading to permanent loss of visual acuity.

Acute Uveitis

Inflammation of one or all parts of the uveal tract, including the iris and anterior chamber (iritis), ciliary body (iridocyclitis), and choroid (choroiditis or chorioretinitis). Can be infectious (HSV, VZV, toxoplasmosis, TB, syphilis, Lyme), HLA-B27 associated (IBD, ankylosing spondylitis, Reiter syndrome, Still disease), or medication related (rifabutin, moxifloxacin, cidofovir, IV bisphosphonates).

- **Symptoms/Exam:**
  - Unilateral, painful, aching red eye; blurred vision, tearing, photophobia, hyperemia at libus.
  - ↓ visual acuity, perilimbal injection ↑ toward the limbus (vs conjunctivitis), direct and consensual photophobia, constricted/unreactive pupil, normal or slightly ↓ intraocular pressure, keratitic precipitates, cells or flare on slit-lamp exam (rarely hypopyon, unless severe).
  - Presence of associated conjunctivitis, urethritis, and polyarthritis suggests Reiter syndrome.
- **Diagnosis:** No further workup is indicated for the first episode of simple acute uveitis, although bilateral, granulomatous or recurrent uveitis merits a workup (CBC, ESR, ANA, RPR, PPD, CXR, Lyme titer) to exclude less common etiologies.
- **Management:** Cycloplegics to ↓ pain and inflammation; ophthalmologic referral within 24 hours. Topical steroids should be initiated only by the consulting ophthalmologist. Treat underlying infection, when applicable.
- **Complications:** Acute ↑ in intraocular pressure can lead to optic nerve atrophy and permanent vision loss.

Maxillofacial Trauma

Injuries to any bony or fleshy structure of the face caused by physical force, foreign objects or burns. Maxillofacial trauma is most often due to athletic injuries, assaults or motor vehicle accidents, and should raise the question of intimate partner violence/ abuse.

Symptoms/Exam

- Pain, swelling, bleeding, ecchymosis, bony deformity, paresthesias, epistaxis, CSF rhinorrhea, difficulty breathing.
- A patient's description of malaligned teeth is a sensitive indicator that a mandibular or maxillary fracture is present.

Diagnosis

Can be clinical, but plain film radiographs and CT scans may help diagnose fractures.

Management

Depends on the type of injury, but may include establishment of an airway, realignment and immobilization of fractures, pain control and prompt referral to an otolaryngologist, a plastic surgeon or an oral and maxillofacial surgeon, as indicated.

Complications

Permanent facial deformity, chronic sinusitis, nonunion fractures, hemorrhage, scars, nerve damage, infection, airway compromise, chronic pain.

SEPTAL HEMATOMA

A blood-filled cavity between the cartilage and supporting perichondrium, resulting from nasal trauma. Left untreated, septal hematomas can easily become infected, causing necrosis of the underlying cartilage and permanent saddle nose deformity.

- **Symptoms/Exam:** History of nasal trauma, pain, progressive nasal obstruction and reddish-purple areas of fluctuance on one or both sides of the nasal septum, obstructing the nostril.
- **Differential:** Nasal polyps, deviated septum, enlarged nasal turbinates, sinusitis.
- **Diagnosis:** Usually made clinically (exam with nasal speculum, otoscope, gloved small finger); requires a high index of suspicion.
- **Management:** Aspiration ± placement of a sterile drain; splints applied to both sides of the septum to provide pressure and support.
- **Complications:** Avascular necrosis of the cartilage, infection or abscess formation, saddle nose deformity.

EPISTAXIS

An acute hemorrhage from the nostril, nasopharynx, or nasal cavity. May be due to anterior hemorrhage from the Kiesselbach plexus or from the anterior end of the inferior turbinate, or it may result from posterior hemorrhage from branches of the sphenopalatine artery in the posterior nasal cavity or nasopharynx.

Symptoms/Exam

- May report history of frequent epistaxis, anticoagulation use or coagulopathy, vascular abnormalities, or trauma.
- Bleeding from one or both nares.
- Visualize anterior epistaxis using a nasal speculum; posterior epistaxis usually presents with blood draining in the posterior pharynx.

Differential

Trauma, neoplasm, barotrauma, foreign bodies, hemophilia (or other coagulopathy), sinusitis, cocaine use, anticoagulation, hemoptysis, hematemesis.

Diagnosis

- Usually clinical, but a CT scan or nasopharyngoscopy may be indicated if a neoplasm is suspected.
- CBC, type and cross, bleeding time, and coagulation studies are warranted in cases of high volume or recurrent epistaxis, anticoagulation use, liver failure, suspected coagulopathy, neoplasm, or a platelet disorder.

 QUESTION

A woman presents with one day of moderate pain and redness in her right eye. She also has blurry vision, tearing, and photophobia. Exam shows conjunctival injection around the cornea and ↓ acuity. The cornea is constricted, intraocular pressure is normal. Slit exam reveals cells and flares in the chamber and deposits on the posterior corneal surface. What is the most likely diagnosis?

Management

- ABCs.
- Maintain continuous pressure over the entire nose for 10 minutes and you may also insert pledgets soaked with anesthetic-vasoconstrictor solution into the nasal cavity. Gently cauterize using silver nitrate if the bleeding site is easily identified. If pressure or cautery fails, apply nasal packing using a compressed sponge, Vaseline gauze or epistaxis balloons. Give empiric antibiotics with staphylococcal and streptococcal coverage if nasal packing is placed.
- ENT consultation and hospital admission are indicated in cases of posterior epistaxis that require packing.

Complications

Sinusitis, septal hematoma or perforation, aspiration, mucosal pressure necrosis, external nasal deformity.

Abdominal Trauma

A leading cause of morbidity and mortality among all age groups. Abdominal trauma may be due to blunt injuries, the majority of which are from motor vehicle accidents, or penetrating injuries, which are predominantly due to gunshot or stab wounds. Initial evaluation should be directed toward diagnosing hemorrhage, solid organ injury, or bowel rupture.

Symptoms/Exam

Lap-belt ecchymosis (with motor vehicle accidents), abdominal pain, tenderness over the ribs, referred pain to the left (splenic injury) or right (liver injury) shoulder, hypotension, gross hematuria, flank discoloration, acute abdomen.

Diagnosis

Physical exam, CXR, KUB, abdominal CT with contrast (Figure 18.5), FAST ultrasound (Figure 18.6), IV pyelogram, diagnostic peritoneal lavage (to detect the pres-

ANSWER

Anterior uveitis. The presence of eye pain with ↓ visual acuity and "ciliary flush" (redness around the cornea) is concerning for uveitis.

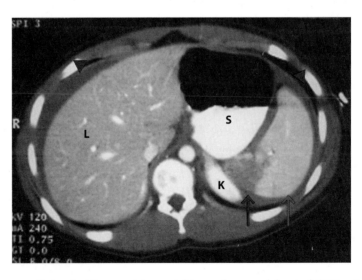

FIGURE 18.5. **Abdominal trauma.** A transaxial image from an abdominal CT in a trauma patient shows a splenic laceration (red arrow), which enhances less-than-normal splenic tissue (blue arrow), and hemoperitoneum (red arrowheads). L = liver; S = stomach; K = left kidney.
(Reproduced with permission from Stone CK, Humphries RL. *Current Diagnosis & Treatment: Emergency Medicine*, 6th ed. New York: McGraw-Hill, 2008, Fig. 23-2.)

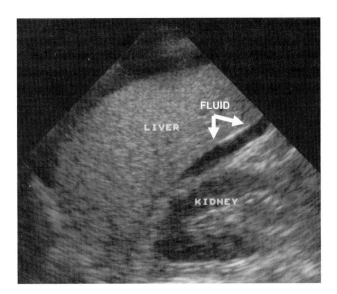

FIGURE 18.6.   FAST scan in abdominal trauma. Longitudinal image from a trauma FAST ultrasound shows hemoperitoneum (labeled "fluid") in the hepatorenal space. (Reproduced with permission from Brunicardi FC, et al. *Schwartz's Principles of Surgery*, 9th ed. New York: McGraw-Hill, 2010, Fig. 7-28A.)

ence of intraperitoneal blood), exploratory laparotomy, depending on clinical presentation and initial exam.

Management

Blood transfusions, pain control, fluid resuscitation, prompt surgical consultation, as indicated.

Complications

Intra-abdominal sepsis, hemorrhage or abscess formation, delayed rupture of solid organs, infection, death.

ABDOMINAL PAIN

A common complaint in emergency and urgent care, with a very broad differential (Table 18.3). Common pathologies are discussed below.

MESENTERIC ISCHEMIA

Caused by a ↓ in intestinal blood flow, usually from occlusion, vasospasm, or hypoperfusion. Categorized as acute or chronic based on the rapidity and degree to which blood flow is impaired. Consequences can be catastrophic, making rapid diagnosis and treatment imperative. Risk factors include: advanced age, atherosclerosis, low cardiac output states, cardiac arrhythmias, recent MI, severe cardiac valvular disease, and intra-abdominal malignancy.

Symptoms/Exam

- Rapid onset of severe periumbilical pain out of proportion to findings on the physical exam.
- Nausea, vomiting, anorexia, and diarrhea progressing to obstipation.
- Colonic (vs small bowel) ischemia is usually associated with hematochezia and less pain.
- Findings may initially be normal or reveal only mild abdominal distention or occult blood in the stool.

TABLE 18.3.   Differential Diagnosis of Abdominal Pain

GI
Appendicitis
Cholecystitis
Cholangitis
Diverticulitis
Enteritis
Gallstones
Gastritis/Dyspepsia/GERD
GI bleed
Hepatitis
Hernia
IBS/IBD
Pancreatitis
PUD

RENAL
Nephrolithiasis
Pyelonephritis
UTI

GU
Men:
Epididimitis
Prostatitis
Testicular torsion
Women:
Ectopic pregnancy
Endometriosis
Ovarian torsion
PID
Ruptured ovarian cyst

VASCULAR
ACS
Ischemic bowel
Mesenteric ischemia
Ruptured AAA

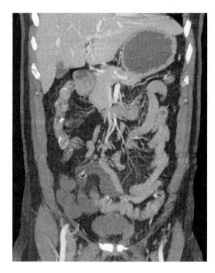

FIGURE 18.7. Mesenteric ischemia.
CT angiogram demonstrates reduced enhancement of the distal small intestine and right colon (arrow) compared to the rest of the bowel suspicious for bowel infarct. (Reproduced from El Hennawy HM, et al. Isolated ileocolic artery occlusion presented with segmental bowel infarction: a case report. *Cases J.* 2009;2:9153.)

- As ischemia progresses and infarction occurs, peritoneal signs develop and a feculent odor to the breath may be noted.

Differential

See Table 18.3.

Diagnosis

- High index of suspicion in patients with known risk factors, as early signs are nonspecific.
- Check CBC, ABG, lactate, CMP. Often associated with leukocytosis, metabolic acidosis.
- MRA, CT angiography (Figure 18.7), or duplex sonography.
- Angiography, although invasive, remains the gold standard.

Management

The goal is to restore intestinal blood flow as quickly as possible using the following measures:

- Aggressive hemodynamic monitoring and support, correction of metabolic acidosis, initiation of broad-spectrum antibiotics, and placement of an NG tube for gastric decompression.
- Systemic anticoagulation to prevent thrombus formation or propagation, unless contraindicated.
- Medical treatment with close observation may be considered for patients without peritoneal signs and with good mesenteric blood flow on angiography.
- Intra-arterial vasodilators or thrombolytic agents, angioplasty, stent placement, embolectomy, or exploratory laparotomy with resection of necrotic bowel may be necessary.

Complications

Bowel necrosis, septic shock, death.

RUPTURED ABDOMINAL AORTIC ANEURYSM

A degenerative process of the abdominal aorta due to atherosclerosis, leading to focal dilation with at least a 50% ↑ over normal arterial diameter. An estimated 65% of patients with ruptured abdominal aortic aneurysm (AAA) die of sudden cardiovascular collapse before arriving at a hospital. (See the Community and Preventive Medicine chapter for AAA screening in men.)

Symptoms/Exam

- Sudden onset of abdominal, back or flank pain, associated with hypotension, tachycardia or temporary loss of consciousness due to hypoperfusion.
- Symptoms may be mild if the rupture self-tamponades.
- Hypotension, tachycardia, abdominal bruit or pulsatile abdominal mass.

Differential

See Table 18.3.

Diagnosis

Abdominal CT (Figure 18.8) or MRI.

Management

Initial management includes hemodynamic support, blood transfusions, and immediate surgical consultation for repair.

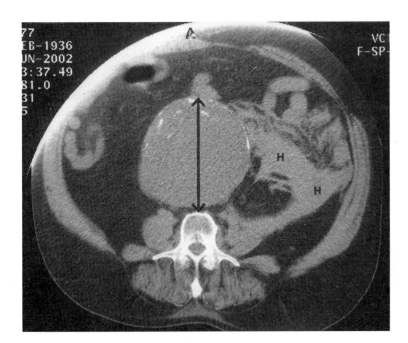

FIGURE 18.8. **Ruptured abdominal aortic aneurysm.** Transaxial image from noncontrast CT shows a very large abdominal aortic aneurysm (arrow) with hemorrhage (H) extending into the left retroperitoneum, indicating rupture. (Reproduced with permission from Tintinalli JE, et al. *Tintinalli's Emergency Medicine: A Comprehensive Study Guide*, 6th ed. New York: McGraw-Hill, 2004, Fig. 58-3.)

Complications

Hemorrhage; death from exsanguination. (See the Gastroenterology chapter for a discussion of other urgent and emergent etiologies of abdominal pain.)

GI BLEEDING

An important and common Emergency Medicine clinical scenario. Specific causes are covered in more detail in the Gastroenterology chapter. GI bleeding is typically divided into upper and lower tract sources (Table 18.4). Acute management and stabilization is discussed below.

TABLE 18.4.   Upper Versus Lower GI Bleeding

	CAUSES	SYMPTOMS/SIGNS
Upper GI bleed	Peptic ulcer disease (30%-50%)	Epigastric pain
	Mallory-Weiss tear (15%-20%)	Hematemesis (fresh blood or coffee-
	Varices (10%-20%)	ground emesis)
	Gastritis (10%-15%)	Melena or bright red blood per
	Esophagitis (5%-10%)	rectum if brisk bleeding
	Angiodysplasia (5%)	
	Cancer (1%-2%)	
Lower GI bleed	Diverticulosis (30%-40%)	Hematochezia, melena (depending
	Bowel ischemia (6%-18%)	on speed and location of bleed)
	Anorectal disease (6%-16%)	Abdominal pain
	Colon cancer (7%-11%)	Tenesmus
	Angiodysplasia (1%-3%)	Maroon-colored stools
	IBD (2%-4%)	Physical exam may reveal
	Infectious diarrhea	hemorrhoids, fissures, mass

KEY FACT

Lower GI bleeds tend to have a **more benign course** than upper GI bleeds, largely because there is less likelihood of hemodynamic compromise.

QUESTION

A 85-year-old woman with hyperlipidemia, diabetes, hypertension, CAD s/p 3-vessel CABG, and 50 pack-year smoking history presents with worsening abdominal pain and diarrhea for the last week. She denies blood in her stools, recent travel, changes in diet, and sick contacts. She is afebrile and mildly hypertensive, but not tachycardic. Her abdomen is mildly distended with hypoactive bowel sounds. She tolerates light touch to her abdomen in the periumbilical area. CBC is normal, BMP is notable for a mild metabolic acidosis, lactate is mildly elevated, there are no ketones in her urine, and KUB is normal. What is your diagnosis?

Goals of management are as follows:

- Resuscitate and stabilize:
  - NPO, discontinue aspirin (anti-platelets), NSAIDS, or other anticoagulants.
  - Two 18-guage IVs for aggressive fluid resuscitation.
  - Type and cross RBCs → consider transfusion with pRBCs, platelets or FFP.
  - NG tube for lavage both for diagnosis and therapy (decompress the stomach).
- Triage:
  - If low risk (slow, low volume chronic bleed without hemodynamic compromise), upper or lower endoscopy may be done in the outpatient setting.
  - If active, acute bleed, admit to the hospital and consider ICU for high-volume bleeds or those with significant comorbidities, such as liver disease, significantly elevated INR.

Chest Trauma

Present in one-half of all patients with trauma-related injuries. Approximately 25% of all trauma deaths are directly attributable to chest trauma. Table 18.5 lists immediately and potentially life-threatening thoracic injuries.

TABLE 18.5. Traumatic Chest Injuries

TYPE OF INJURY	PRESENTATION	TREATMENT
Flail chest	Paradoxical chest wall motion due to multiple fractured ribs, chest pain, tachypnea, shallow respirations, crepitus	Intubation if ventilation is compromised, supplemental O_2, pain control
Tension pneumothorax	↓ breath sounds, dyspnea, tracheal deviation, distended neck veins, chest pain, hypotension	Needle thoracostomy in the second intercostal space and midclavicular line, followed by chest tube placement at 4th intercostal space and midaxillary line
Open pneumothorax	↓ breath sounds, open thoracic wound, dyspnea, chest pain	Occlusive dressing taped on 3 sides, followed by chest tube placement and wound closure
Massive hemothorax	↓ breath sounds, dyspnea, chest pain, no midline shift, dullness to percussion on affected side	Chest tube placement, surgical repair, blood transfusion
Cardiac tamponade	JVD, muffled heart sounds, pulsus paradoxus, hypotension, tachycardia	Pericardiocentesis, fluid infusion
Myocardial contusion	Blunt trauma to the heart, causing episodes of chest pain, paroxysmal supraventricular tachycardia or self-limited ventricular tachycardia; abnormal ECG	Supportive care
Aortic rupture	Chest and back pain, dyspnea, hypotension, enlarged aortic knob, widened mediastinum, and rightward esophageal deviation on CXR	BP control, surgical repair

A significant source of morbidity and mortality in the United States, blunt injury to the chest includes chest wall fractures, dislocations, barotraumas, and injuries to the pleurae, lungs, digestive tract, heart, great vessels, or lymphatics. The most common cause of blunt chest trauma is a motor vehicle accident.

Symptoms/Exam

- Symptoms may range from minor pain to florid shock, depending on the mechanism of injury and the organ systems involved.
- Clinical findings depend on the organ systems affected. Rib fractures (particularly ribs 4-10) are the most common blunt thoracic injuries.

Diagnosis

Start with exam, ECG, CXR (aortic injury; see Figure 18.9) or chest CT, followed by more specific imaging depending on the suspected injury, such as TEE or TTE (cardiac injury), esophagoscopy (esophageal injury), bronchoscopy (tracheobronchial injury), aortography.

Management

- Most patients do not require surgery and can be treated with supportive measures and simple interventions, such as tube thoracostomy.
- Regardless of the type of injury, all patients require initial establishment of ABCs and a trauma survey.
- Immediate surgery is indicated for patients with loss of chest wall integrity, blunt diaphragmatic injuries, massive air leak following chest tube insertion, massive hemothorax, cardiac tamponade, pulmonary or cardiac emboli, or confirmed tracheal, major bronchial, esophageal or great vessel injury.

Complications

Wound infection, MI, arrhythmias, septal defects, valvular insufficiency, aneurysm formation, respiratory infections, hemothorax, fistula formation, stroke, DVT.

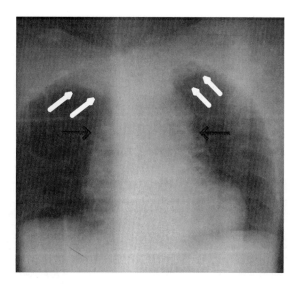

FIGURE 18.9. Aortic injury. A frontal CXR in a trauma patient shows widening of the superior mediastinum (red arrows), with bilateral "apical caps" (white arrows) corresponding to mediastinal bleeding extending into the extrapleural spaces above the lung apices. (Reproduced with permission from Brunicardi FC, et al. *Schwartz's Principles of Surgery*, 9th ed. New York: McGraw-Hill, 2010, Fig. 7-23A.)

Q QUESTION

A 74-year-old man with diabetes and hypertension is brought in by his wife for worsening, sudden-onset chest and upper back pain for the last 5 hours, and near syncopal episode. His vital signs are 38°C, BP 80/40 mm Hg in his right arm and 130/70 mm Hg in his left arm, HR 120 bpm. He is diaphoretic and cold to the touch, but A&Ox4. You note a diastolic murmur. Labs are pending. Portable CXR and ECG are unremarkable. What is the next appropriate step?

ANSWER

Chest CT angiogram. This man has a clinical picture consistent with aortic dissection. Only 50% to 60% of patients with dissection have widened mediastinum on chest radiography. Given low sensitivity of CXR, high clinical suspicion should lead you to more definitive imaging to not miss this deadly condition.

CHEST PAIN SYNDROMES

Aortic Dissection

Most common in men >60 years of age. Uncontrolled hypertension is the most important risk factor; less common associations include Marfan syndrome, congenital bicuspid aortic valves, aortic coarctation, pregnancy, cocaine use.

Symptoms/Exam

- Sudden, tearing pain in the anterior chest (ascending dissection) or posterior chest (descending dissection) that radiates to the neck, throat, or jaw.
- May be associated with syncope, focal neurologic deficits, signs of acute heart failure, acute MI, or abdominal pain.
- Exam may reveal hyper- or hypotension, asymmetrical pulses, asymmetrical BP, syncope, altered mental status, dyspnea, dysphagia, a new diastolic murmur from aortic regurgitation, and findings suggestive of cardiac tamponade (pericardial rub, pulsus paradoxus, elevated jugular venous pressure).

Differential

- CV: Acute coronary syndrome, pericarditis, aortic regurgitation, aortic aneurysm.
- Pulmonary: Embolus, pneumonia, pneumothorax.
- GI: Cholecystitis/choledocholithiasis, PUD, pancreatitis, esophageal spasm, gastritis, GERD, mesenteric ischemia, acute small bowel obstruction.
- Other: Musculoskeletal pain, mediastinal tumors, anxiety disorder.

Diagnosis

- Clinical symptoms, variation in pulses (absent pulse in a proximal extremity), BP difference of >20 mm Hg between the right and the left arm ± mediastinal widening on CXR. If clinical suspicion is high but CXR is normal, order a CT.
- Thoracic MRI or CT, transesophageal echocardiography (TEE), aortography (Figure 18.10).

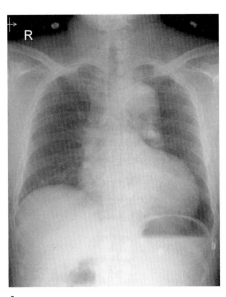

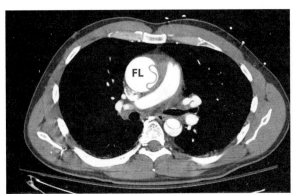

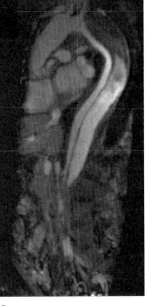

A **B** **C**

FIGURE 18.10. **Mediastinal widening on CXR and CT.** (A) Frontal CXR shows a widened mediastinum in a patient with an aortic dissection. (B) Transaxial contrast-enhanced CT shows a dissection involving the ascending and descending aorta (FL = false lumen). (C) Sagittal MRA image shows a dissection involving the descending aorta, with a thrombus (T) in the false lumen. (Images A and C reproduced with permission from USMLE-Rx.com; image B reproduced with permission from Doherty GM. *Current Diagnosis & Treatment: Surgery*, 13th ed. New York: McGraw-Hill, 2010, Fig. 19-17.)

Management

- Admit to the ICU and administer medications to ↓ cardiac contractility and control systemic arterial pressure (nitroprusside, β-blockers, calcium channel blockers).
- Treatment depends on the section of aorta involved:
  - Ascending (proximal to left subclavian, Stanford type A): Immediate surgical correction due to high risk of life-threatening complications (1%-2% mortality per hour after symptom onset) such as aortic regurgitation, tamponade, and MI.
  - Descending (distal to left subclavian, Stanford type B): Surgery indicated only in patients with early expansion, persistent pain, end-organ ischemia, or rupture.

Complications

MI, stroke, pericardial tamponade, claudication, compressive symptoms, acute aortic regurgitation, aortic rupture, aneurysmal dilation, mesenteric or renal ischemia, death.

Cardiac Ischemia/Acute Coronary Syndrome

Rapid development of myocardial necrosis caused by an imbalance between myocardial O_2 supply and demand. Usually results from plaque rupture with thrombus formation in a coronary vessel, but may also be from acute bleeding or vasospasm (eg, cocaine use). The acute coronary syndrome spectrum includes ST-segment elevation MI (STEMI), non-ST-segment elevation MI (NSTEMI), and unstable angina (see the Cardiology chapter).

Symptoms/Exam

- Presents with substernal pressure radiating to the arms or neck, often associated with nausea, vomiting, diaphoresis, dyspnea. Some patients, particularly women and diabetics may present atypically with only nausea, dyspnea, abdominal or neck pain.
- Exam may reveal diaphoresis, hypo- or hypertension, cool and clammy skin, systolic murmur (if valvular defects develop), S4 ± signs of CHF.

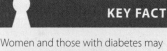

KEY FACT

Women and those with diabetes may present with **atypical symptoms of acute coronary syndrome** such as nausea, dyspnea, neck pain, and malaise.

Differential

- CV: Aortic dissection, pericarditis, aortic regurgitation, aortic aneurysm.
- Pulm: Pulmonary embolus, pneumonia, pneumothorax.
- GI: cholecystitis, PUD, pancreatitis, esophageal spasm, gastritis, GERD.
- Other: musculoskeletal pain (especially costrochondritis, myositis, rib fracture, myositis), mediastinal tumors, anxiety/panic disorder.

Diagnosis and Management

See the Cardiology chapter.

Complications

Arrhythmias, recurrent ischemia, CHF, cardiogenic shock, acute valvular abnormalities, acute pericarditis (1-4 days), late pericarditis (1-8 weeks), papillary muscle rupture (2-7 days), VSD (3-7 days), left ventricular free wall rupture (5-14 days), ventricular aneurysms (up to 6 weeks), mural thrombi, hypertension.

Note: See the Pulmonary chapter for a discussion of pulmonary embolism and the Cardiology chapter for a discussion of pericarditis, both are important causes of chest pain.

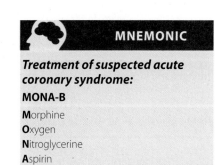

MNEMONIC

Treatment of suspected acute coronary syndrome:
MONA-B
Morphine
Oxygen
Nitroglycerine
Aspirin
β-blocker

Life Support

- For treatment of adult cardiopulmonary arrest from ventricular fibrillation, ventricular tachycardia; pulseless electrical activity, bradycardia, and asystole, use the Advanced Cardiovascular Life Support (ACLS) algorithms for each case.
- Unlike in adults, the main cause cardiopulmonary arrest in children is respiratory failure. A lone rescuer for an unresponsive child should begin with five cycles of 30 compressions and two breaths, and then activate the emergency medical services system. The ratio of compressions to breaths with two rescuers is 15:2, and the dose of defibrillation is 2 J/kg. Follow the Pediatric Advanced Life Support (PALS) algorithm.

AIRWAY MANAGEMENT

- Adequate ventilation and oxygenation are crucial. Start with proper airway opening techniques such as head tilt and chin lift, or jaw thrust if trauma is suspected.
- Start bag-mask ventilation immediately, with the use of oropharyngeal or nasopharyngeal airway adjuncts as necessary.
- If bag-mask ventilation is inadequate, consider an advanced airway (endotracheal tube, Combitube, or laryngeal mask airway). Confirm placement with both clinical assessment and confirmatory devices such as exhaled CO_2 detectors or esophageal detector devices as well as CXR.
- Rapid sequence intubation should be used only in patients in whom control of the airway is certain, as the patient will be paralyzed and unable to breathe. Indications include respiratory failure, acute intracranial lesions, drug overdoses, status epilepticus, and combative trauma patients.

Wound Care

Chronic wounds can arise from a number of causes, including: pressure (decubitus) ulcers, diabetic foot ulcers, venous stasis ulcers, arterial insufficiency ulcers, neoplasms, atheroembolic disease, pyoderma gangrenosum, anticoagulant-induced skin necrosis, radiation damage and various infections. Table 18.6 reviews wound care guidelines for common chronic wounds.

HAND INJURIES

Common injuries seen in the ED or urgent care setting, hand injuries may cause significant disability and include **soft tissue injuries,** nerve damage, sprains, dislocations, and fractures. Hand injuries may be isolated or part of multisystem trauma. (See the Sports Medicine and Musculoskeletal Disorders chapter for more details.)

Symptoms/Exam

- A full examination of the upper extremity is warranted, with special attention to symmetry, anatomic deformities, color change, range of motion against resistance, muscle strength, muscle wasting and sensory deficits.
- Patients with injuries to the dorsum of the hand should be questioned about the possibility of a closed-fist injury with a human bite. Exam reveals a small laceration over the dorsal MCP joint ± fracture of the fifth metacarpal bone (Figure 18.11).

Diagnosis

Plain film radiographs are indicated if fracture or occult foreign body is suspected; MRI may help detect tendon rupture, but not on an emergent basis.

KEY FACT

In patients with hand injuries, it is important to **test resistance when assessing tendon function** because up to 90% of a tendon can be lacerated with preservation of function.

KEY FACT

The combination of a **fifth metacarpal fracture and lacerations** over the dorsal MCP joints is a closed-fist injury until proven otherwise and should be **treated as a human bite wound.**

TABLE 18.6.   **Management of Common Wounds**

WOUND	HISTORY/PRESENTATION	TREATMENT
Animal bite	Type of animal and status, foreign body in wound, tendon or tendon sheath involvement, bone injury, joint space violation, neurovascular status	Irrigation, debridement, 1° closure if clean or facial wound (otherwise delayed 1° closure), tetanus ± rabies prophylaxis, antibiotics (amoxicillin-clavulanate) for cat bites or puncture wounds
Human bite	Tendon or tendon sheath involvement, crepitus, tissue loss, foreign body in wound	Irrigation, tetanus prophylaxis, fracture treatment if necessary, delayed closure, IV antibiotics (amoxicillin-clavulanate)
Pressure ulcer, stage 1	Nonblanchable erythema of intact skin	Transparent dressings
Pressure ulcer, stage 2	Partial-thickness skin loss of epidermis, dermis, or both, with superficial ulcer formation	Hydrocolloid or transparent dressings
Pressure ulcer, stage 3	Full-thickness skin loss involving damage to subcutaneous tissue and extending into, but not through, underlying fascia	Debridement, irrigation, hydrocolloid or transparent dressings
Pressure ulcer, stage 4	Full-thickness skin loss with extensive involvement of underlying tissues, including muscle, bone, or supportive structures	Surgical debridement, irrigation, advanced topical dressings ± antibiotics, flap closure to cover defect
Diabetic foot ulcer	Poor diabetes control, peripheral neuropathy, presence of Charcot foot deformity	Appropriate footwear and prevention, maintenance of moist wound environment, debridement, antibiotic therapy, blood glucose control, podiatry
Venous stasis ulcer	Due to ambulatory venous hypertension, brawny induration in extremities; shallow ulcer with weeping discharge	Compression, debridement, maintenance of moist wound environment ± skin grafting
Arterial insufficiency ulcer	Pulseless, cool skin, delayed capillary refill, atrophic skin, loss of hair, well-circumscribed punctate ulcers	Debridement, maintenance of moist wound environment, surgical or medical treatment to ↑ arterial circulation

Management

Depends on the type of injury, but may include laceration repair if the wound is <12 hours old, antibiotic prophylaxis in closed-fist injuries and cat and human bites, irrigation and debridement of open wounds, analgesics and anti-inflammatory agents, reduction of dislocations, splinting and prompt referral to a hand surgeon, as indicated.

Complications

Pain, joint stiffness, nonunion of fractures, infection, scar formation, loss of extremity use.

DERMATOLOGIC EMERGENCIES

Stevens-Johnson syndrome (SJS) and toxic epidermal necrolysis (TEN) are thought to be variants of the same disease spectrum, whose features include widespread distribution of skin and mucosal lesions. Commonly affected sites include the torso, face, palms, soles and extensor surfaces. SJS and TEN carry mortality rates of 5% and 40%, respectively (see Table 18.7 for a comparison of the two conditions).

- **SJS:** An immune complex–mediated hypersensitivity reaction involving the skin and mucous membranes (Figure 18.12). Also known as erythema multiforme major, SJS is a serious systemic illness that can cause significant morbidity and mortality.
- **TEN:** A rapidly evolving mucocutaneous reaction characterized by widespread erythema, necrosis and bullous detachment of the epidermis (Figure 18.13). More

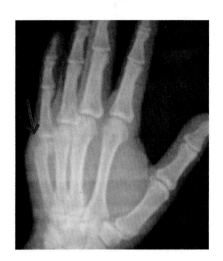

FIGURE 18.11.   Boxer fracture.
Hand radiograph shows fifth metacarpal head fracture (arrow) with overlying soft tissue swelling, compatible with a Boxer fracture. (Reproduced from Boussakri H, et al. Fractures of the neck of the fifth metacarpal bone, treated by percutaneous intramedullary nailing: surgical technique, radiological and clinical results study (28 cases). *Pan Afr Med J.* 2014;18:187.)

TABLE 18.7. **Stevens-Johnson Syndrome Versus Toxic Epidermal Necrolysis**

	STEVENS-JOHNSON SYNDROME	TOXIC EPIDERMAL NECROLYSIS
Symptoms	**Chief complaint:** Pain associated with a rash 1-14-day prodrome consisting of fever, sore throat, cough, malaise, arthralgias, chills, headache, vomiting and diarrhea Nonpruritic mucocutaneous lesions last 2-4 weeks	**Chief complaint:** Pain associated with a rash 2-3-day prodrome consisting of fever, sore throat, cough, malaise, arthralgias and anorexia 8-12-day acute phase consisting of persistent fevers, generalized epidermal sloughing and mucosal involvement
Exam	Nonpruritic macular rash, develops into papules, vesicles, bullae and confluent erythema with a characteristic target appearance <10% of body surface area (BSA) is affected Associated findings include fever, tachycardia, orthostasis, hypotension, altered mental status, epistaxis, conjunctivitis, erosive vulvovaginitis or balanitis, seizures, and coma	Erythematous maculopapular rash with bullae, erosions and targetlike lesions, rapidly leading to confluent blisters that easily slough off **More than 30% of BSA is affected** ⊕ Nikolsky sign—epidermis separation when pressure is applied laterally to the epidermal surface Same associated findings as SJS
History	Drug exposure (sulfa, phenytoin, allopurinol, and penicillin are most commonly implicated), malignancies, vaccinations, and infections	Same as for SJS, but drugs are almost always the cause of TEN
Differential	Chemical or thermal burns, exfoliative dermatitis, EM, pemphigus, cutaneous T-cell lymphoma, staphylococcal scalded skin syndrome, toxic shock syndrome	
Diagnosis	Skin biopsy shows subepidermal bullae ± epidermal cell necrosis and lymphocytic infiltration of perivascular areas	Skin biopsy shows full-thickness epidermal necrosis with little dermal and epidermal inflammation
Treatment	Supportive treatment with airway management, fluid replacement, electrolyte correction, wound care, and pain control; plasmapheresis or IVIG may also be indicated in TEN	
Complications	Depends on the organ system involved, but may include: infection, corneal ulceration, anterior uveitis, blindness, renal tubular necrosis, renal failure, vaginal or penile scarring, esophageal strictures, GI hemorrhage, respiratory failure, and cosmetic deformity	

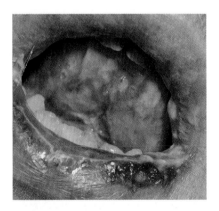

FIGURE 18.12. Stevens-Johnson syndrome involving the mucous membranes. (Reproduced with permission from Wolff K, et al. *Fitzpatrick's Dermatology in General Medicine*, 7th ed. New York: McGraw-Hill, 2008, Fig. 39-4A.)

often seen in adults, TEN is potentially life threatening and is a true dermatologic emergency requiring prompt diagnosis and treatment.

Altered Mental Status

Acute change in mental status; may range from mild confusion to severe delirium to coma (Table 18.8).

Symptoms/Exam

Presentation depends on underlying disorder, but almost all patients exhibit disorientation, confusion, irritability, fluctuating levels of consciousness, mental slowing, agitation and inattention. They may not present with overt vital sign abnormalities.

Diagnosis

- Generally diagnosed through comprehensive history and physical exam, including the Mini-Mental Status Exam to assess cognitive function and rule out dementia.
- If not obvious on history and physical exam, obtain blood glucose, lactate, CBC, CMP, UA, ECG, CXR, ABG, blood cultures, and toxicology screen. Consider additional workup based on likely diagnosis, which may include LP, head CT or MRI, and EEG.

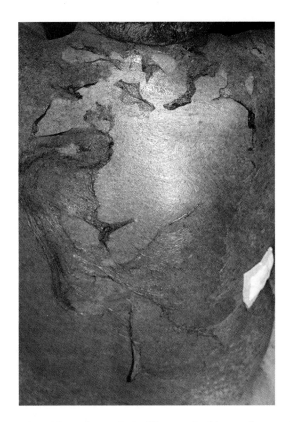

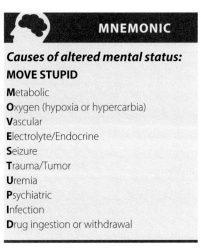

FIGURE 18.13.   Toxic epidermal necrolysis. Characterized by confluent rash with skin sloughing leading to extremely painful erosions. Patients with TEN have ↑ risk of infection and dehydration, much like burn patients. (Reproduced with permission from Wolff K, Johnson RA. *Fitzpatrick's Color Atlas and Synopsis of Clinical Dermatology*, 6th ed. New York: McGraw-Hill, 2009, Fig. 8-8.)

TABLE 18.8.   Causes of Altered Mental Status

	ETIOLOGIES	TREATMENT
Metabolic	1. Hypo-/hyperglycemia 2. Hepatic encephalopathy (HE) 3. Wernicke encephalopathy 4. Nutritional deficiencies: vitamin B$_1$ (beriberi) vitamin B$_{12}$ (pernicious anemia), folate, nicotinic acid (pellagra) 5. Hypo-/hyperthermia	1. Fluids, glucose, and thiamine/insulin 2. Lactulose (see Gastroenterology chapter on HE) 3. Thiamine 4. Correct nutritional deficiency 5. Return to euthermia
Oxygen	1. Hypercapnia (eg, asthma/COPD) 2. Hypoxia (eg, PNA)	1. Correct underlying cause (eg, bronchodilators); consider BIPAP, intubation (see Pulmonary chapter on COPD) 2. O$_2$ supplementation
Vascular	1. Hypertensive encephalopathy 2. Arrhythmias 3. Stroke/TIA 4. Thrombotic thrombocytopenic purpura 5. CNS vasculitis 6. Subarachnoid hemorrhage	1. BP control to DBP <100 mm Hg 2. Antiarrhythmic agents or cardioversion (see Cardiology chapter on Dysrhythmias) 3. Evaluate for embolic source ± anticoagulation (see Neurology chapter on Stroke) 4. Plasma exchange transfusion ± prednisone, immunosuppressants, aspirin 5. Glucocorticoids ± cyclophosphamide 6. Surgical drainage ± clipping

(continues)

TABLE 18.8. **Causes of Altered Mental Status** *(continued)*

	ETIOLOGIES	TREATMENT
Electrolyte/ Endocrine	1. Hypo-/hypernatremia 2. Hypercalcemia 3. Hypo-/hypermagnesemia 4. Thyroid dysfunction	1-3. Correct electrolyte disturbance 4. Replete thyroid hormone or treat hyperthyroid with cooling measures, propranolol, PTU; consider prednisone, iodine compounds
Seizure	1. Postictal state 2. Nonconvulsive status epilepticus	1-2. Anticonvulsant therapy
Trauma/Tumor	1. Tumors may be primary or metastatic, malignant or benign 2. Hydrocephalus 3. Subdural hematoma	1. Surgical decompression, radiation, chemotherapy; consider steroids for reduction of mass effect 2. Ventriculoperitoneal shunt 3. Craniotomy and evacuation
Uremia	Any cause of renal failure	Treat renal failure (see Nephrology chapter on CKD)
Psychiatric	1. Psychosis (due to schizophrenia, depression, bipolar, schizotypal, or other causes) 2. Alzheimer, parkinsonism, Huntington chorea, Pick disease, other dementias 3. Sundowning 4. ICU psychosis	1. Psychiatric medications 2. Neurologic medications, as indicated 3. Antipsychotics (eg, haloperidol) 4. Normal sleep–wake cycle, calm environment ± sedatives
Infection	1. Meningitis/encephalitis 2. Bacteremia, pyelonephritis, pneumonia 3. AIDS 4. Neurosyphillis 5. Toxoplasmosis; brain abscesses can present with focal neurologic findings	1-5. Treat underlying infection in all cases (see the Infectious Disease chapter)
Drugs	1. Ingestion 2. Withdrawal	1-2. See toxicology and intoxication/withdrawal sections

Management

- Begin with ABCs to stabilize the patient. Do not delay treatment while awaiting diagnosis.
- Discontinue medications that may exacerbate mental status; establish a comfortable, nonthreatening environment with adequate nursing; fluid resuscitation depending on etiology; and behavioral control with medications (haloperidol, risperidone) or physical restraints if patient threatening harm to self or others.
- Consider naloxone as both a diagnostic and therapeutic measure if any concern for opioid intoxication.

KEY FACT

Most shock tends to present with tachycardia, tachypnea, hypotension, and **altered mental status.** Distributive shock will generally also present with fever, diaphoresis, and warm extremities.

SHOCK

A physiologic state in which alterations in tissue perfusion lead to ↓ tissue O_2 delivery. Although initially reversible, untreated or refractory shock can cause permanent organ damage, failure of multiple organ systems, and eventually death. Shock can be classified into three categories: **hypovolemic, cardiogenic,** and **distributive** (Table 18.9).

TABLE 18.9. **Etiologies and Mechanisms of Shock**

TYPE	MECHANISM OF ACTION	COMMON ETIOLOGIES
Hypovolemic	Absolute or effective deficiency in intravascular blood volume caused by hemorrhage or fluid loss	▪ Blood loss: Trauma/fractures, GI or pulmonary bleeding, ruptured AAA ▪ Fluid loss: Diarrhea, vomiting, heat stroke, inadequate replacement of insensible losses, burns, "third spacing" (intestinal obstruction, pancreatitis and cirrhosis)
Cardiogenic	Impaired cardiac contractility	▪ Intrinsic cardiac: Ischemic and nonischemic cardiomyopathies, arrhythmias, valvular abnormalities ▪ Extracardiac/obstructive: Massive pulmonary embolus, tension pneumothorax, pericardial tamponade
Distributive (vasodilatory)	Inappropriate relaxation of peripheral vascular tone, often associated initially with ↑ cardiac output	Sepsis, anaphylaxis, neurologic injury, drug-related causes

KEY FACT

Types of shock:
▪ Hypovolemic: ↓ of blood **volume**
▪ Cardiogenic: Impaired blood **pump**
▪ Distributive: Abnormal blood **vessel**

Symptoms/Exam

Findings vary widely based on etiology and type of shock (see Table 18.9), but generally expect **altered mentation,** ranging from confusion to loss of consciousness. Almost all patients also have tachycardia, tachypnea, hypotension, and cool, clammy skin—except in distributive shock where you will have fever, diaphoresis, and warm extremities.

Diagnosis

- History is key to diagnosis. Look first for preexisting illness such as cardiac risk factors, hypercoagulable conditions such as pregnancy, estrogen use or malignancy, recent infections or immunocompromise, medication changes or allergies, or drug intoxication.
- Do **not** wait for results. Pinpoint diagnosis before initiating early resuscitation with fluids and antibiotics.
- If the etiology is undifferentiated from the history and physical exam, start a basic workup in stepwise fashion, first for infection (CBC with differential, UA, CXR, blood cultures prior to starting antibiotics) and metabolic derangements (complete metabolic panel, lipase, lactate).
- If the history and physical exam lead you to a clear diagnosis, focus on the lab(s), imaging, or consult that will confirm your diagnosis and direct treatment. For instance:
  - Cardiac lesion (eg, multiple cardiac risk factors concerning for ACS, recent viral illness concerning for pericarditis): ECG, cardiac enzymes, and/or echocardiography to visualize a pericardial effusion or valvular disease.
  - Pulmonary emboli (eg, high estrogen state, known or suspected malignancy): chest CT.
  - GI bleeding (hematemesis, melena, or bright-red blood per rectum): GI consult for colonoscopy or upper endoscopy.

Q QUESTION ▶

A 78-year-old woman with a history of dementia and DM is sent to the ED from her nursing home because of fever, lethargy, and hypotension. Her caregiver reports a recent history of foul-smelling urine, ↓ mentation, and urinary incontinence. In the ED, the patient's temperature is 39.2°C (102.5°F) and a BP of 72/35 mm Hg. What is her most likely diagnosis?

Management

- Do **not** delay resuscitation while evaluating exact etiology.
- Start with the **ABCs**:
  - **Airway** and **Breathing** compromise: Bag-mask ventilation, noninvasive ventilation, or intubation and mechanical ventilation to facilitate elimination of CO_2 and compensate for any coexisting metabolic acidosis.
  - **Circulation:** Aggressive volume resuscitation with isotonic fluids and blood products is generally the default unless you suspect heart failure, renal failure, or severe volume overload. In severe shock inadequately responsive to volume resuscitation, vasopressors or cardiac inotropic agents may be necessary.
- If sepsis is a concern, begin early coverage with empiric broad-spectrum IV antibiotics.
- Sodium bicarbonate may be indicated in patients with marked hypoperfusion causing lactic acidosis and a pH <7.1.

KEY FACT

In acute alcohol withdrawal, give thiamine before, or simultaneously with, glucose to prevent precipitating Wernicke-Korsakoff syndrome.

INTOXICATION/WITHDRAWAL

Drug use may be associated with addiction and can encompass a spectrum of symptoms, depending on the type, amount of drug used, and duration of usage. Tables 18.10 and 18.11 outline the intoxication and withdrawal syndromes of the most commonly used substances.

PSYCHIATRIC DISORDERS

Psychosis

Defined as an impaired sense of reality, leading to an inability to communicate, emotional turmoil, and impaired cognitive abilities. Not a diagnosis in itself, psychosis is often linked to schizophrenia, severe clinical depression, bipolar disorder, drug intoxication and withdrawal (in particular, cocaine, amphetamines, PCP and hallucinogens), SLE, dementia, traumatic brain injury, and electrolyte imbalances (particularly in the elderly patients).

- Laboratory testing (eg, CBC, UA, LFTs, chemistry panel, TFTs, VDRL, HIV and toxicology screen; heavy metal screen and ceruloplasmin level rarely indicated) and head imaging may be indicated to rule out organic causes of acute psychosis.
- **Management:**
  - Antipsychotics are given initially to manage acute symptoms, followed by hospitalization and long-term treatment directed toward the underlying etiology.
- Rapid tranquilization is necessary for violent, extremely agitated patients:
  - **Typical antipsychotics** (droperidol, haloperidol, chlorpromazine): Give with diphenhydramine or benztropine to prevent extrapyramidal reactions.
  - **Atypical antipsychotics** (olanzapine, risperidone).
  - **Benzodiazepines:** May be used as adjuncts to antipsychotics for sedative effects; treatment of choice for alcohol and benzodiazepine withdrawal.

KEY FACT

Evaluation of a patient who may be suicidal includes:
- Ideation: Content and duration, including any recent changes
- Intention and plan: Specific preparation, method, place, time and means

ANSWER

Distributive shock due to urosepsis. If diagnosed early, fluid resuscitation, prompt initiation of IV antibiotics, and pressor support may resolve her symptoms.

Suicidal Ideation

Risk factors associated with completed suicide include: male gender, white race, advanced age, widowed or divorced status, living alone, access to firearms, coexisting psychiatric disorders or substance use disorder, major life stressors, and a prior personal or family history of suicide attempt.

Symptoms/Exam

Anhedonia, hopelessness, insomnia, anxiety, impaired concentration, psychomotor agitation.

TABLE 18.10.   **Common Intoxication Syndromes**[a]

	OPIOID	SEDATIVE	STIMULANT	HALLUCINOGEN
Symptoms	Altered mental status, euphoria, drowsiness, pruritus, nausea, abdominal pain, constipation, vomiting, urinary retention	Altered mental status, slurred speech, ataxia, ↓ fine motor function, disinhibition, anxiety, drowsiness, hallucinations, coma	Altered mental status, paranoia, seizures, hypervigilance, euphoria, chest pain, agitation, flushing, stroke symptoms, epistaxis, cough with black sputum	Altered mental status, visual hallucinations, disorientation, sweating, mood lability, acute panic
Exam	Respiratory depression, miosis, hypoxia, pulmonary rales	Nystagmus, hypotonia, respiratory depression	Seizures, diaphoresis, hyperthermia, dyspnea, tachycardia, mydriasis, hypertension	Diaphoresis, tachycardia, mydriasis, tachypnea
Treatment	Airway management and supportive care; naloxone for reversal; activated charcoal if recent oral overdose	Airway management and supportive care; activated charcoal for acute benzodiazepine ingestion; flumazenil for benzodiazepine reversal	Airway management and supportive care; benzodiazepines for seizures and sedation; cooling measures; sedation; avoidance of nonselective β-blockers (eg, propranolol); activated charcoal for acute oral ingestion	Supportive care in a nonstimulating environment; benzodiazepines if needed for sedation; cooling measures
Complications	Pulmonary edema, hypotension, respiratory failure, death	**Benzodiazepines:** Aspiration pneumonia, respiratory failure, death **Alcohol:** Holiday heart, hypoglycemia, cardiomyopathy, liver failure, pancreatitis, hepatitis	MI, cardiomyopathy, hypertensive crisis, pulmonary edema, behavioral toxicity, death	Behavioral toxicity, hyperthermia, rarely respiratory arrest, coma

[a]Examples: opioids: morphine and heroin; sedatives: benzodiazepine and alcohol; stimulants: cocaine, amphetamine, "bath salts"; hallucinogens: LSD, mushrooms.

Diagnosis

Clinical through a thorough psychiatric history, including discussion of the following factors:

- **Extent of suicidal ideation:** When suicidal thoughts began, precipitating factors, frequency of thoughts, aggravating/alleviating factors, formulation of suicidal plan, ability to control suicidal thoughts, deterrents to carrying out plan.
- **Lethality of suicidal plan:** Access to firearms and harmful medications, recent changes in will or life insurance policy, prior attempts.

Management

- Immediate hospitalization is indicated for all patients with a plan, access to lethal means, recent social stressors, and symptoms indicative of a psychiatric disorder.
- Involuntary commitment may be made if a person poses an imminent danger to self or others, or displays an inability to care for self.
- Outpatient treatment may be an option if the patient displays good judgment and has adequate social support. Suicide contracts have not been shown to reduce suicide risk; they should not replace ongoing assessment and open discussion.

TABLE 18.11. Common Withdrawal Syndromes[a]

	OPIOID	SEDATIVE	STIMULANT	HALLUCINOGEN
Symptoms	Sneezing, yawning, lacrimation, leg and abdominal cramps, nausea, vomiting, diarrhea	Tremor, anxiety, nausea, disorientation, agitation, insomnia, hallucinations, sensory hyperacuity, seizures	Dysphoria, craving, sleep disturbances, hunger, depression	No true withdrawal state, but dysphoria may occur after discontinuation of chronic use
Exam	Rhinorrhea, mydriasis, tachycardia, tachypnea, hypertension, piloerection, hyperthermia	Tachypnea, tachycardia, diaphoresis, hyperthermia, hyperreflexia	Psychomotor retardation	
Treatment	Methadone, buprenorphine for withdrawal and maintenance; naltrexone can also be used for maintenance; clonidine can help tolerate taper	Benzodiazepines or barbiturates for withdrawal symptoms and seizures; dextrose, thiamine, β-blockers; maintenance options include: naltrexone, acamprosate, gabapentin, disulfuram	Psychosocial treatments are effective. No pharmacotherapies available	

[a]Examples of opioids include morphine and heroin; sedatives, benzodiazepine and alcohol; stimulants, cocaine, amphetamine, "bath salts"; and hallucinogens, LSD, mushrooms.

- Antidepressant therapy (in particular, SSRIs) and close monitoring are essential, as patients may be at ↑ risk for suicide in the weeks following SSRI initiation. MAOIs are contraindicated in suicidal ideation because of their lethal potential in the event of an overdose.

Homicidal Ideation

Associated with prior history of violence, coexisting psychiatric disorder, substance abuse, access to weapons.

Diagnosis

As with suicide, no clinician is able to predict what will happen. The goal is accurate risk assessment to develop a reasonable treatment plan and prevent injury.

Management

- Immediate hospitalization in all patients with a plan, access to lethal means and symptoms indicative of a psychiatric disorder.
- Involuntary commitment may be made if a person poses an imminent danger to self or others, or displays an inability to care for self.
- Initiation of appropriate psychiatric intervention, depending on the underlying diagnosis.

KEY FACT

When someone's life is in imminent danger, the physician is allowed (and is in fact obligated) to breach the patient's confidentiality if it is necessary to intervene.

KEY FACT

ACEI-induced angioedema is thought to be non-mast cell mediated. Anaphylaxis reactions, in contrast, are thought to be mast cell mediated. Thus, ACEI angioedema does not respond to epinephrine, antihistamines and corticosteroids, and should be avoided if non–mast cell mediated angioedema is suspected.

Anaphylaxis

Severe allergic reaction involving more than one organ system; caused by the release of inflammatory mediators from mast cell. Requires prior sensitization to an allergen with later reexposure. Symptoms can range from urticaria (hives) to angioedema with hypotension and bronchospasm (see Table 18.12 for common causes and their symptoms).

TABLE 18.12.   **Common Classes of Allergens Causing Anaphylaxis**

ALLERGEN	COMMON OFFENDERS	SYMPTOMS/DIAGNOSIS
Medications	Penicillin and cephalosporin antibiotics (most common); IV radiocontrast; aspirin and NSAIDs	May occur without a prior history of drug exposure Desensitization or prophylactic pretreatment protocols may be instituted if there is no alternative to the particular allergenic medication In the case of angioedema (see image), provide supportive therapy until resolution of symptoms and discontinue the medication. ARBs do not need to be avoided.
Foods	Tree nuts, legumes, fish, shellfish, milk, soy, eggs	Common and usually limited to mild GI symptoms, although full-blown anaphylaxis can occur
Bites/stings	Insect stings (*Hymenoptera* venom)	Local reactions and urticaria are much more common than full-blown anaphylactic reactions Consider referral to an allergist for desensitization or a treatment kit with epinephrine and oral antihistamines for patients with a history of anaphylaxis or generalized urticaria following insect stings
Latex	Surgical gloves, Foley catheters, condoms	Reactions are usually cutaneous or involve the mucous membranes, although anaphylactic reactions can occur

Symptoms/Exam

- Urticaria, flushing, conjunctival and/or cutaneous pruritus, nonpitting angioedema, warmth, nasal congestion, rhinorrhea, dyspnea, throat tightness and hoarseness, wheezing, weakness, dizziness, chest pain, palpitations, crampy abdominal pain, nausea and vomiting (not just in cases of food allergy), diarrhea. Depends on the severity of the attack.
- Symptoms usually begin within 5 to 30 minutes of allergen exposure, although in rare cases symptom onset can be delayed for several hours.
- Severe symptoms include hypoxia, tachycardia, hypotension, flushing, frank cardiovascular collapse, and respiratory arrest.

Differential

Angioedema, anxiety/panic, asthma, conversion disorder, carcinoid syndrome, epiglottitis, tracheal foreign bodies, MI, pulmonary embolism, idiopathic urticaria.

Diagnosis

- By clinical history and exam; does not rely on laboratory testing.
- Skin testing and/or in vitro IgE testing may help confirm clinical reactivity and guide preventative measures (eg, avoidance of triggers, desensitization therapy).

Management

- ABCs, stabilize the patient.
- Remove the antigen source, if possible, or place tourniquet on the extremity with the antigen source (do not leave in place >30 minutes) as close to exposure time as possible.
- IM epinephrine into an unaffected extremity.
- Adjuvant medications include: antihistamines (both H_1 and H_2 blockers), inhaled β-agonists, corticosteroids (to prevent late-phase reactions), and IV fluids for BP support.

- In cases of respiratory failure, endotracheal intubation, cricothyrotomy, or tracheotomy may be required.
- Discharge with an epinephrine pen and instructions for self-injection.

Toxic Exposures

COMMON INGESTIONS

Ingestions may be asymptomatic on initial presentation, depending on the time and the amount of ingestion. Timely consultation with a regional poison control center (1-800-222-1222), gut decontamination, and administration of an antidote (if available) can ↓ morbidity and mortality. Table 18.13 lists common ingestions and their treatment (which should all start with ABCs).

TABLE 18.13.   **Common Ingestions and Toxidromes**

INGESTION	SYMPTOMS/EXAM	DIAGNOSIS	TREATMENT	COMPLICATIONS
Acetaminophen	Nausea, vomiting, jaundice but may be asymptomatic HOURS after acute ingestion	History of overdose (>140 mg/kg) or chronic overuse (>4 g/day) ↑ liver enzymes; toxic serum level; PT/INR	Activated charcoal if within 4 hr of ingestion *N*-acetylcysteine (PO for 72 hrs or IV for 21 hr) if serum level is toxic or any evidence of hepatotoxicity	Anion gap metabolic acidosis, hepatic encephalopathy, fulminant hepatic failure, renal failure, death
Acids or alkalis (commonly found in household cleaners)	Throat pain, abdominal pain, bloody emesis or stools, nausea, vomiting, difficulty swallowing or breathing, discoloration of skin and oral mucosa	History of ingestion; prompt EGD within first 24 hours to determine the extent of injury; CXR and AXR to evaluate for esophageal or gastric perforation	Do **not** induce emesis or give neutralizing agents (neutralizing releases heat that may cause further tissue damage)	Respiratory failure, ARDS, local tissue necrosis, burns, strictures, death
Anticholinergics (atropine, scopolamine, belladonna alkaloids, antihistamines, antipsychotics)	Mydriasis, dry mucous membranes, urinary retention, flushing, altered mental status ("dry as a bone, red as a beet, mad as a hatter"), tactile hallucinations	History of ingestion	Activated charcoal Benzodiazepines for agitation Physostigmine in severe cases who are altered (may induce seizures, arrhythmias or bronchospasm due to cholinergic effect)	Status epilepticus, hyperthermia, hypertension, coma, respiratory failure, death
Carbon monoxide	Confusion, coma, seizures, headache, fatigue, nausea	History of exposure to furnace or car exhaust ↑ carboxyhemoglobin level; normal O_2 saturation	Give **100% O_2** (↓ half life of CO from 300 minutes to 90 minutes) or hyperbaric O_2 (↓ half life to 30 minutes) in patients with end-organ impairment, metabolic acidosis (pH<7.1), LOC or carboxyhemoglobin level >25%-30% (or lower in pregnant patients)	Arrhythmias, myocardial ischemia, rhabdomyolysis, delayed neuropsych changes, death

(continues)

TABLE 18.13.   Common Ingestions and Toxidromes *(continued)*

INGESTION	SYMPTOMS/EXAM	DIAGNOSIS	TREATMENT	COMPLICATIONS
Cholinergics (organophosphates, pilocarpine, carbamates)	DUMBELS (Defecation, Urination, Miosis, Bronchorrhea/ bronchospasm, emesis, lacrimation, salivation	Found in fertilizers; history of ingestion; farming or industrial work exposure; ↑ serum cholinesterase levels	Skin decontamination with alkaline soap, then ethanol Activated charcoal **Atropine** to dry secretions (may cause ileus) **Pralidoxime** to treat neuromuscular symptoms	Seizures; respiratory failure; cranial nerve palsies; impaired hearing, visual memory, reaction time, dexterity, and problem solving; delayed peripheral neuropathy; death
Iron	Nausea, vomiting, diarrhea, hypotension, acidosis, signs of liver failure	History of ingestion Serum levels >350-500 µg/dL	IV fluids, whole bowel irrigation Deferoxamine to chelate the iron	GI bleeding, metabolic acidosis, peritonitis, sepsis, fulminant hepatic failure, death
Lead	Colicky abdominal pain, join/ muscle aches, constipation, headache, irritability, seizures, motor neuropathy, learning disorders, microcytic anemia with basophilic stippling	History of chronic repeated exposure **Mild:** 10-50 µg/dL **Moderate:** 50-70 µg/dL **Severe:** 70-100 µg/dL	Edetate calcium disodium **(EDTA)** ± dimercaprol **(BAL)** for severe toxicity Dimercaptosuccinic acid **(DMSA)** or EDTA for chelation in mild to moderate toxicity	Learning disorders, motor neuropathy, anemia
Salicylates	Nausea, vomiting, hyperventilation, tachycardia, tinnitus, coma, seizures, anion-gap metabolic acidosis, hyperthermia	History of acute overdose (>200 mg/kg) or chronic overmedication Serum level >100 mg/dL in acute, 60-70 mg/dL in chronic	Activated charcoal, hemodialysis Sodium bicarbonate to treat metabolic acidosis and alkalinize the urine	Coma, cardiovascular collapse, pulmonary edema, death
Theophylline	Nausea, vomiting, tachycardia, tremulousness, hypotension, seizures, hypokalemia, hyperglycemia, metabolic acidosis	History of acute overdose or chronic overmedication Serum level >100 mg/dL in acute, 40-60 mg/dL in chronic	Activated charcoal, whole bowel irrigation, hemodialysis Benzodiazepines or barbiturates for seizure treatment	Ventricular arrhythmias, status epilepticus, death
Tricyclic antidepressants (TCAs)	Mydriasis, tachycardia, dry mouth, flushing, muscle twitching, ↓ peristalsis, QRS widening and QT prolongation, seizures, diaphoresis, hypotension	History of ingestion, **serum TCA concentrations do not guide therapy**	Do **not** induce emesis Activated charcoal Sodium bicarbonate boluses to reverse QRS prolonogation Treat seizure with benzos	Ventricular arrhythmias, hyperthermia, status epilepticus, death

Gut decontamination measures include the following:

- **Activated charcoal:** The treatment of choice for most ingestions, except metals that are poorly absorbed (ie, lead and iron). Best if used within the first hour of overdose, but may be administered in all ingestions unless the agent is nontoxic or not bound by activated charcoal. Usual dose is 50 g in adults and 10 to 25 g in pediatric patients.
- **Whole bowel irrigation:** May be useful after the ingestion of enteric-coated and timed-release medications, internal concealment of drugs of abuse (body packers) and metal ingestion. Usual dose is 3 to 8 L of GoLytely.

MNEMONIC

Anticholigeneric intoxication:
DUMBELS

Defectation
Urination
Miosis
Bronrchorrhea/bronchospasm
Emesis
Lacrimation
Salivation

- **Gastric lavage "stomach pumping": No longer recommended.** Avoid and if you must use, only in patients who are intubated or able to protect their airway.
- **Ipecac:** Not useful for gut decontamination and no longer recommended for ingestions.

FOOD POISONING

An acute illness caused by ingestion of food contaminated by bacteria, bacterial toxins, viruses, parasites, natural poisons, or harmful chemical substances. Characterized by an incubation period of hours up to 1 week, most cases of food poisoning are mild and improve with supportive care, antiperistaltic or antisecretory agents, absorbents, and volume repletion. Some patients, however, may have severe disease requiring hospitalization, aggressive rehydration therapy, antibiotic treatment and judicious use of antiperistaltic agents.

- **Symptoms/Exam:** Table 18.14 lists the common etiologies of food poisoning and associated symptoms. **Rapid onset** occurs with *Bacillus cereus, Clostridium, Listeria, Staphylococcus,* and *Cholera.*
- **Think about antibiotics if:**
  - Severe, systemic disease.
  - Immunocompromised patient.
  - High suspicion of invasive *Campylobacter jejuni, Giardia, Listeria, Salmonella, Shigella, Vibrio cholera.*
- **Management: Use antidiarrheals (eg, loperamide) with caution.** May prolong course, cause severe constipation, lead to toxic megacolon and ↑ risk of HUS; avoid in children.

Note: See the section on Gastroenteritis and Colitis in the Infectious Diseases chapter.

KEY FACT

Most cases of anthrax resolve without sequelae, but 10% to 20% of untreated cases of cutaneous anthrax are fatal.

TABLE 18.14. **Common Causes of Food Poisoning**

SUBSTANCE	FOODS	SYMPTOMS/EXAM	ONSET	TREATMENT
Bacillus cereus	Rice	Vomiting, diarrhea	1-6 hr	Supportive care
Ciguatera	Red snapper, grouper, warm-water fish	GI symptoms followed by perioral numbness, hot–cold reversal on the face, cranial nerve palsies, hallucinations and hypotension	Minutes to hours	Supportive care, gut decontamination, calcium gluconate or atropine as needed
Campylobacter jejuni	Untreated water, undercooked meat, milk, shellfish	Foul-smelling watery diarrhea, followed by bloody diarrhea, cramps, fever, and headache	2-5 days	Supportive care; erythromycin for invasive (bacteria invade intestinal mucosa cells and damage the tissue) disease
Clostridium perfringens	Undercooked meat or poultry	Watery diarrhea, nausea, cramps	6-12 hr	Supportive care
Clostridium botulinum	Improperly canned foods, honey	Diplopia, ptosis, descending weakness and paralysis, respiratory difficulties	4-72 hr	Supportive care, airway management, antitoxin

(continues)

TABLE 18.14.   **Common Causes of Food Poisoning** *(continued)*

SUBSTANCE	FOODS	SYMPTOMS/EXAM	ONSET	TREATMENT
Cryptosporidium	Contaminated water and food	Diarrhea, nausea, anorexia, malaiase, low-grade fever (30% asymptomatic) in immune-competent; systemic disease in immunocompromised	7-10 days	Supportive care in immune-competent; if severe or immunecompromised, nitazoxanide
Enterotoxic *E coli*	Contaminated water and food	Watery diarrhea, vomiting, cramps	1-3 days	Supportive care
E coli O157:H7	Untreated water, raw beef, unpasteurized milk	Cramps, bloody diarrhea, nausea, vomiting, fever	1-4 days	Supportive care; treatment of hemolytic-uremic syndrome if present
Giardia lamblia	Contaminated groundwater	Watery diarrhea ± bloody diarrhea, cramps, fatigue, bloating, weight loss	2-3 days	Supportive care, metronidazole
Hepatitis A virus	Contaminated food	Fatigue, fever, nausea, vomiting, cramps, anorexia, jaundice, darkened urine	14-50 days	Supportive care; prophylaxis with immunization; liver transplantation for liver failure
Listeria	Deli meats, hot dogs, unpasteurized soft cheese and milk	Fever, watery diarrhea, nausea, vomiting, joint/ muscle aches	6-24 hr	Supportive care, amoxicillin, TMP-SMX
Norovirus	Contaminated water and food	Vomiting predominance, diarrhea, "winter vomiting disease"	24-48 hr	Supportive care
Salmonella	Eggs, poultry	Bloody diarrhea, cramps, low-grade fever, vomiting	8-48 hr	Supportive care; antibiotics for systemic infection
Shigella	Undercooked food, egg salad	Nausea, vomiting, fever, bloody diarrhea, neurologic symptoms, tenesmus	36-72 hr	Supportive care; antibiotics for severe infection
Staphylococcus spp.	Improperly stored meats, dairy, bakery products	Vomiting, cramps, mild diarrhea	1-2 hr	Supportive care
Vibrio cholerae	Contaminated water and food	Profuse rice-water stools, cramps	8-24 hr	Supportive care, tetracycline

BIOTERRORISM

Bioterrorism refers to a spectrum of natural organisms or toxins that can be used to incapacitate, kill or otherwise harm individuals. Characterized by low visibility, high potency, substantial accessibility, and easy delivery, biological weapons can cause widespread destruction. Typical biological weapons and their syndromes are listed in Table 18.15.

KEY FACT

Postexposure antibiotic prophylaxis is recommended for anthrax or tularemia exposure; use doxycycline or ciprofloxacin. Postexposure vaccination should be utilized for smallpox exposure.

TABLE 18.15. Effects of Exposure to Biological Agents

AGENT	DESCRIPTION	SYMPTOMS/EXAM	DIAGNOSIS	TREATMENT
Anthrax (*Bacillus anthracis*)	Gram-positive, nonmotile, aerobic, spore-forming bacillus; spread by contact with domesticated/wild animals or via inhaled spores	Nonspecific illness (fever, malaise, nausea and vomiting); suppurative regional adenopathy **Cutaneous (>95% of cases):** Painless papule or vesicle that later turns into necrotic ulcer (Figure 18.14) **Pulmonary:** Woolsorter disease **GI:** Oral ulcer from ingestion of raw or undercooked meat from an infected animal	Gram stain or culture of cutaneous lesion, peripheral blood, pleural fluid; tissue biopsy for immunohistochemistry; mediastinal widening and pleural effusion on CXR are suggestive of inhalation infection	Ciprofloxacin or doxycycline + 1-2 other agents
Brucellosis (*Brucella* spp.)	Gram-negative, nonmotile, aerobic coccobacillus transmitted via skin abrasions, conjunctivae, GI or respiratory tract	Acute, systemic febrile illness, insidious chronic illness, or a localized inflammatory process Depression, headache, irritability, cough; focal pain in the bones, joints, or GU tract with localized infection	Tube agglutination test; Cultures of blood, bone marrow, or body fluid samples	Doxycycline + streptomycin or rifampin
Plague (*Yersinia pestis*)	Gram-negative nonmotile coccobacillus transmitted by flea bites from an infected animal (usually a rat) or inhalation of an infectious aerosol	**Bubonic (85%-90%):** High fevers, chills, headache, nausea, vomiting, painful lymphadenopathy (buboes), severe malaise, altered mental status, cough **Septicemic (10%-15%):** Fevers, chills, nausea, vomiting, diarrhea, DIC, acrocyanosis, purpura **Pneumonic (1%):** Cough with blood-tinged sputum; bilateral alveolar infiltrates on CXR	Cultures of blood, bubo aspirate, sputum, and CXR; fourfold rise in antibody titers	Droplet precautions; gentamycin, streptomycin ± chloramphenicol (add if meningitis or hemodynamic instability)

(continues)

TABLE 18.15. **Effects of Exposure to Biological Agents** (*continued*)

AGENT	DESCRIPTION	SYMPTOMS/EXAM	DIAGNOSIS	TREATMENT
Tularemia (*Francisella tularensis*)	Gram-negative, nonmotile, intracellular coccobacillus spread by tick bites from an infected animal (usually a rabbit)	**Ulceroglandular (75%):** Fever, localized skin or mucous membrane ulceration, regional lymphadenopathy >1 cm, cough, malaise **Typhoidal (25%):** Fever, cough, shortness of breath, malaise, hemoptysis	Cultures of blood, sputum, ulcers, pharyngeal and conjunctival swabs, gastric washings; ELISA or bacterial agglutination	Gentamycin, streptomycin
Q fever (*Coxiella burnetii*)	Rickettsia-like organism with main reservoir being the tick infecting exposed livestock and humans	Acute or insidious presentation Fever, chills, headache, diaphoresis, malaise, fatigue, anorexia, pneumonia, acute hepatitis, heart failure, acute endocarditis, clubbing, and splenomegaly	Serologic studies (ELISA is most sensitive method)	Tetracycline
Botulism (*Clostridium botulinum*)	Gram-negative, anaerobic spore-forming bacillus; toxins cause neuromuscular blockade. Spread via ingestion, dirty cut, inhalation	Diplopia, mydriasis, ptosis, dysphagia, dysphonia, muscle weakness, symmetric descending flaccid paralysis, cranial nerve palsies, respiratory failure	Isolation of toxin in serum, stool or food or culturing bacteria from wound	Trivalent antitoxin, supportive care, botulinum immunization
Smallpox)	Highly infectious poxvirus, spread in aerosol	High fever, headache, rigors, vomiting, malaise, abdominal pain, altered mental status, synchronous exanthem with a centrifugal distribution	Virions on electron microscopy of vesicular scrapings; silver stain or gel diffusion test	Respiratory isolation, supportive treatment
Ricin	Plant protein toxin derived from castor plant beans	Nausea, vomiting **Inhalation:** Sudden onset nasopharyngeal congestion, urticaria, chest tightness, respiratory distress **Ingestion:** Less toxic due to poor absorption; diarrhea, fever, cramps, hematochezia, shock	ELISA analysis of nasal swab sample; bilateral infiltrates on CXR	Supportive treatment; activated charcoal and gastric lavage for ingestion; decontaminate skin and clothing

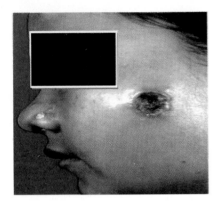

FIGURE 18.14. **Cutaneous anthrax.** Extensive edema of the cheek with a central black eschar typically develops over 2 to 7 days from first signs of illness. (Reproduced from Siddiqui MA, et al. Recent outbreak of cutaneous anthrax in Bangladesh: clinico-demographic profile and treatment outcome of cases attended at Rajshahi Medical College Hospital. *BMC Res Notes.* 2012;5:464.)

Hypertensive Disorders

- **Hypertensive urgency:** SBP >180 to 200 mm Hg or DBP >120 mm Hg, without acute signs of end-organ damage.
- **Hypertensive emergency:** SBP >180 mm Hg or DBP >120 mm Hg, with signs of acute end-organ effects with associated symptoms:
    - Brain, hypertensive encephalopathy (headache, confusion, and lethargy are concerning for cerebral edema or hemorrhage).
    - Eye (blurry vision, papilledema).
    - Heart (chest pain or SOB may indicate aortic dissection, ACS or pulmonary edema).
    - Kidney (oliguria, hematuria, or ↑ creatinine, concerning for ARF).
- **Malignant hypertension:** Hypertension with retinal hemorrhages, exudates, or papilledema, usually with DBP >120 mm Hg.

Diagnosis

Blood pressure, clinical symptoms and laboratory studies/additional testing demonstrating acute organ damage (eg, significant ↑ in creatinine above baseline, transaminitis, troponin elevation, ECG with ischemic changes, pulmonary edema on CXR).

Management

- Treat the underlying etiology (kidney disease, medications, renal artery stenosis, hyperthyroidism, intoxication).
- Lower BP over hours to days to avoid risk of stroke or MI when autoregulation cannot compensate quickly enough, leading to hypoperfusion.
- **Hypertensive urgency:** Restarting oral antihypertensive therapy is often adequate with proper outpatient follow-up.
- **Hypertensive emergency:** Potential medical therapies (largely dictated by local availability and route of administration as opposed to evidence) include short-acting antihypertensive agents such nitrates (nitroprusside, nitroglycerin), short-acting dihydropyridine calcium channel blockers (nicardipine, clevidipine), dopamine-1 agonist therapy (fenoldopam), adrenergic blockers (labetolol, esmolol), short-acting ACEIs (captopril), and arteriolar vasodilator therapy (hydralazine).
- Initiate long-term oral medications as short-acting parenteral ones are tapered off and discontinued.

Environmental Exposures

DEHYDRATION

A loss of free water disproportionate to the loss of sodium. Dehydration may exist ± volume depletion. Although dehydration can present in any age group, the highest rates of morbidity and mortality occur at age extremes (pediatric and geriatric), usually as a result of diarrheal illnesses, burns, and poor PO intake.

- Symptoms, diagnosis, and treatment are described in Table 18.16.
- Complications: Electrolyte imbalances, CNS sequelae from overly aggressive replacement of volume deficits, coma, death.

KEY FACT

Follow the "4-2-1 rule" for estimating maintenance fluid requirements:
- 4 mL/kg/hr for the first 10 kg of weight
- 2 mL/kg/hr for the second 10 kg of weight
- 1 mL/kg/hr for each additional kilogram thereafter

Maintenance rate for a 24-kg child is:
$(4 \times 10) + (2 \times 10) + (1 \times 4) = 64$ mL/hr

TABLE 18.16.   **Dehydration Findings and Treatment by Severity**

DEGREE OF DEHYDRATION	SYMPTOMS/EXAM	DIAGNOSIS	TREATMENT
Mild to moderate	Tachycardia 10%-15% above baseline; dry mucous membranes, thirst, headache, concentrated urine	Clinical, but if labs drawn, may see BUN:CR >20	Oral rehydration therapy given at doses of 50-100 mL/kg over 4 hr
Severe	Tachycardia, tachypnea, hypotension, delayed cap refill; cold/mottled skin, ↓ skin turgor, dizziness, lethargy/coma, oliguria, sunken eyeballs, sunken anterior fontanelle (in infants)	↑ urine specific gravity, ↑ serum osmolarity, ↓ arterial pH	IV rehydration (with calculation of electrolyte and free water deficits, maintenance requirements, and replacement of ongoing losses) Begin with isotonic fluids in 20 mL/kg boluses. "4-2-1" rule for children

HYPOTHERMIA

Decline in core temperature <35°C (95°F) due to either accidental exposure to cold (primary hypothermia) or a failure of thermoregulatory function (secondary hypothermia). Most cases in the United States occur in an urban setting and are related to homelessness, coexisting psychiatric illness, trauma, substance use or advanced age.

Symptoms/Exam

Table 18.17 lists the symptoms and exam findings for the different degrees of hypothermia. To ensure appropriate diagnosis, a true core temperature should be measured using a low-reading temperature probe in the bladder, esophagus or rectum.

Differential

Stroke, drug toxicity, hypothyroidism, hypopituitarism, frostbite, alcoholism, septic or hemorrhagic shock, delirium, anorexia nervosa, spinal cord injury, MI, CNS trauma.

TABLE 18.17.   **Symptoms and Exam Findings of Hypothermia**

DEGREE OF HYPOTHERMIA	SYMPTOMS	EXAM
Mild 32°-35°C (89.6°-95°F)	Lethargy, confusion, shivering, loss of fine motor coordination	Shivering, altered mental status, tachypnea, tachycardia, vasoconstriction, dysarthria, ataxia, lethargy
Moderate 28°-32°C (82.4°-89.6°F)	Delirium, slowed reflexes	Bradycardia (Figure 18.15), cessation of shivering, stupor, dilated pupils, arrhythmias
Severe <28°C (82.4°F)	Unresponsiveness, coma, respiratory difficulties	Rigidity, apnea, hypotension, very cold skin, areflexia, fixed pupils, unresponsiveness, ventricular fibrillation

    QUESTION 1

A 51-year-old man with chronic hypertension comes into urgent care for treatment of cellulitis. His BP is 190/100 mm Hg, which you confirm with a manual cuff. He denies any headaches, shortness of breath, or chest pain. He says he ran out of his BP medications. What is your next step in evaluation?

QUESTION 2

A 33-year-old man who uses IV heroin daily presents to the ED after being brought in by ambulance for fever, malaise, and ↑ difficulty in walking. His temperature is 39.4°C, P100 and BP is 110/75 mm Hg. He is disheveled and appears older than stated age. He has multiple track marks with mild erythema in right antecubital fossa. Heart and lungs are clear. Speech is dysarthric. He has bilateral ptosis, ↓ sensation of his face and symmetric 4/5 strength in proximal extremities but 5/5 strength in distal extremities. You are concerned about cellulitis and what other organism of infection?

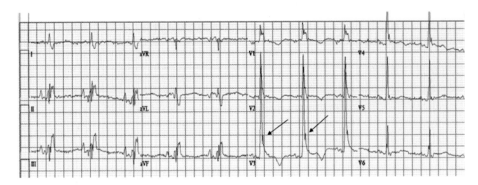

FIGURE 18.15. **Osborn (J) waves on ECG (arrows).** Positive deflection at the J point (Reproduced from Serafi SW, et al. Osborn waves in a hypothermic patient. *J Community Hosp Intern Med Perspect.* 2011;1(4):10.3402/jchimp.v1i4.10742.)

Diagnosis

- Labs: ↑ hematocrit (↑ 2% for each 1°C drop in core temperature) due to volume contraction; electrolyte abnormalities; hypo- or hyperglycemia; ↑ pH and ↓ Pao_2 and $Paco_2$ on ABG; prolonged bleeding time.
- ECG: PR, QRS, and QTc prolongation and Osborn (J) waves (see Figure 18.15).

Management

Rewarming: Remove wet clothing; apply heat packs or warmed blankets to the axillae, groin and abdomen; warmed, humidified O_2 and heated IV saline; warmed gastric, thoracic and/or peritoneal lavage; warm water immersion; initiation of CPR as needed; hemodialysis; cardiopulmonary bypass.

Complications

Cardiac arrhythmias, hypotension due to marked vasodilation during rewarming, aspiration pneumonia, pulmonary edema, peritonitis, acute tubular necrosis, metabolic acidosis, rhabdomyolysis, gangrene, compartment syndrome, death.

HYPERTHERMIA

Represents a continuum of illness ranging from heat exhaustion to heat stroke. Heat exhaustion, the most common heat-related illness, involves mild to moderate dysfunction of temperature control caused by ↑ ambient temperatures and/or strenuous exercise, leading to dehydration and salt depletion. Heat stroke, which is associated with a systemic inflammatory response, is extreme hyperthermia (>41.1°C [106°F]) leading to end-organ damage and significant morbidity and mortality.

Symptoms

Depends on the degree of heat illness, but may include: fatigue, weakness, nausea and vomiting, headache, muscle cramps, irritability, altered mental status, coma, sweating, anhidrosis (late finding).

Exam

↑ temperature (usually >41°C [105.8°F]), tachycardia, orthostatic pulse and BP changes, piloerection, tachypnea, hyperventilation, CNS dysfunction, muscle tenderness, signs of DIC, and GU symptoms (hematuria, oliguria, or anuria), which may be due to concurrent acute renal failure.

Differential

Delirium, DKA, DTs, hepatic or uremic encephalopathy, hyperthyroidism, encephalitis, meningitis, neuroleptic malignant syndrome, serotonin syndrome, tetanus, status

KEY FACT

Patients with hypothermia are not considered dead until they are warm and dead. Severely hypothermic patients may appear dead on presentation.

ANSWER 1

Check labs (eg, lactate, troponin, CBC, CMP) to rule out end-organ damage. If no end-organ damage, the patient has hypertensive urgency. If lab workup reveals end-organ damage, then he has hypertensive emergency. Restart oral hypertensive agents and have the patient follow-up with his primary care doctor in the next few days with strict return precautions.

ANSWER 2

Clostridium botulinum, known to be used in bioterrorism attacks, more commonly infect people in other ways. Those with wound botulism may have a history of an injury with contaminated soil or chronic IV drug use, particularly black tar heroin. Symptoms are similar, but notably GI symptoms are lacking and the wound may be benign-appearing.

epilepticus, septic shock, cerebral malaria, drug toxicity (especially cocaine, amphetamine, phencyclidine, salicylates, anticholinergics and MAOIs).

Diagnosis

- **Labs** to detect end-organ damage: CBC, coagulation panel (abnormal when concurrent DIC), metabolic panel, UA, hepatic enzymes (almost universally ↑ in heat stroke), ↑ CK, serum glucose (reveals hypoglycemia), and ABG (reveals respiratory alkalosis and/or metabolic acidosis).
- **Imaging:** CXR, head CT to rule out other causes of altered mental status.

Management

- **Heat stroke is a medical emergency** requiring rapid reduction of core body temperature, as the duration of hyperthermia is the main determinant of outcome.
- Goal rate for ↓ core temperature is 0.2°C/min; target temp is 39°C (102.2°F).
- Rapid cooling measures include removal of clothing, covering the patient with ice water–soaked sheets or ice packs, ice water immersion and evaporative techniques (running a fan over patient).
- Supportive measures include: IV $D_{50}W$ to prevent/treat hypoglycemia, NG tube to monitor for GI bleeding and fluid losses, constant monitoring of core temperature, Foley catheter to monitor urine output, Swan-Ganz catheter to guide fluid management, and mechanical ventilation if indicated.
- Useful adjunctive medications include benzodiazepines to stop agitation, shivering (caused by cooling measures) and seizures, as well as barbiturates for refractory seizures.
- Avoid anticholinergics, α-adrenergic agonists, and antipyretics.

Complications

Seizures, neurologic deficits, rhabdomyolysis, acute renal failure, hepatic failure, DIC, ARDS, pulmonary edema, respiratory alkalosis, electrolyte imbalances, death.

ALTITUDE SICKNESS

One of a group of syndromes resulting from altitude-induced hypoxia. Acute mountain sickness or altitude sickness is from hypoxia related to both the ascent rate and maximum altitude achieved, and represents the mildest and most common form of altitude illness. Other diseases in the spectrum include high-altitude pulmonary edema (HAPE) and high-altitude cerebral edema (HACE), which generally occur at elevations of 3500-5500 meters (11,000-18,000 feet).

- **Symptoms/Exam:** Headache, anorexia, nausea, vomiting, weakness, lightheadedness, fluid retention with ↓ urination, dyspnea, cough. No characteristic physical findings.
  - HACE: Ataxia and altered mental status.
  - HAPE: Cough, rales or wheezing, dyspnea, tachypnea, tachycardia and low-grade fevers.
- **Differential:** Anxiety, asthma, COPD, dehydration, MI, pneumonia, pulmonary embolism, viral illness.
- **Diagnosis:** Usually made by clinical history and exam, but ↓ arterial O_2 saturation and a CXR showing unilateral or bilateral fluffy infiltrates are characteristic of HAPE.
- **Management:**
  - For HAPE and HACE, definitive treatment is descent, but supplemental O_2, nifedipine and portable hyperbaric chambers may be useful adjunctive treatments.
  - For AMS, slow, gradual ascent with time for acclimatization, supplemental O_2, acetazolamide and dexamethasone help both to prevent and treat symptoms.

QUESTION

A 21-year-old medical student visiting Cusco, Peru (about 11,000 ft above sea level) awakens one morning with a severe headache. She feels lethargic and nauseated and vomits twice during the day. Her symptoms resolve the following day. What is the most likely diagnosis?

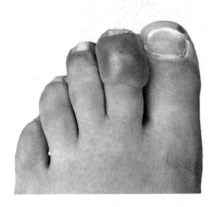

FIGURE 18.16.   Frostbite. Affected toes of a mountain climber. (Reproduced from Wikimedia Commons.)

FROSTBITE

Cold-related injury due to formation of ice crystals within tissues and cellular death. Common sites of injury include the hands, feet and exposed tissue, such as the ears, nose, and lips.

Symptoms/Exam

- Cold, numbness, clumsiness; throbbing or burning pain on rewarming.
- Findings depend on the degree of injury, but all injuries may cause joint pain, excessive sweating, white/bluish discoloration, hyperemia, skin necrosis or gangrene (Figure 18.16).
- Severity of frostbite is distinguished as follows:
  - **First degree:** Insensate white plaque with surrounding hyperemia, edema, erythema.
  - **Second degree:** Clear blisters with surrounding erythema within 24 hours of injury.
  - **Third degree:** Hemorrhagic blisters followed by eschar formation over several weeks.
  - **Fourth degree:** Focal necrosis with tissue loss. Can affect muscle/bone in children, and can result gangrene.

Diagnosis

No routine lab tests or radiographs are indicated, but technetium scintigraphy or MRI/MRA may help visualize nonviable tissue earlier than clinical examination.

Management

- Rapid rewarming of affected parts (as long as it can be maintained) in circulating warm water at 40° to 42°C (104°-108°F) for 15 to 30 minutes until thawing is complete.
- Blisters may need to be drained, debrided or aspirated but management is controversial.
- Topical application of aloe vera to debrided clear blisters and intact hemorrhagic blisters, elevation of affected parts to ↓ edema, tetanus prophylaxis, analgesia as needed, daily hydrotherapy for range of motion.
- Growing evidence supports use of IV thrombolytics to ↓ amputation rates.
- Optional antibiotic coverage to prevent infection.
- Surgical debridement should be delayed for 3 to 4 weeks to prevent removal of viable tissue, but consult surgery early for management guidance.

Complications

Sensory deficits, hyperhidrosis or anhidrosis, abnormal color changes, autoamputation, phantom pain of amputated extremities, cold sensitivity (with ↑ risk of frostbite), atrophy of muscle/bone/nerves/tendons, arthritis/joint pains, wound infection, tetanus, gangrene, death.

BURNS

May be classified by etiology into thermal, chemical, or radiation burns. Thermal burns are most common and occur when soft tissue is exposed to temperatures >45.5°C (114°F). Regardless of the mechanism of thermal burn (scald, contact, steam, flame, gas, flash or electrical), the injury involves ↑ capillary permeability, fluid loss and ↑ plasma viscosity, leading to microthrombus formation.

ANSWER

Acute mountain sickness. Gradual acclimatization and adjuvant treatment with acetazolamide result in timely resolution of symptoms.

Symptoms/Exam

As with frostbite, findings depend on the degree of injury:

- **First degree:** Red, warm, painful tissue involving the epidermis; blanches with pressure.
- **Second degree:** Red, wet, painful tissue, ± blisters involving the epidermis and portions of the dermis.
- **Third degree:** Dry, insensate, waxy, leathery tissue ± overlying blisters involving the epidermis, dermis; may underlie subcutaneous fat tissue, muscle and bone.

Diagnosis

- Evaluation of the extent (in BSA) and depth is crucial for appropriate fluid management.
- Extent of injury in adults may be estimated using the "rule of 9s" (Figure 18.17).
- Severe burns necessitate CBC, CMP, ABG with carboxyhemoglobin, coagulation panel, UA, type and screen, creatinine kinase and urine myoglobin (in electrical burns), and CXR for suspected inhalational injuries.

Management

- Superficial burns may be managed in an outpatient setting with wound cleansing, pain control, topical dressing, and appropriate follow-up care.
- Deeper, more extensive burns should be managed in an inpatient setting (preferably a burn center) with attention to the ABCs, fluid resuscitation using isotonic crystalloid solution for the first 24 hours (may use modified Brooke or Parkland formulas to calculate fluid deficit based on calculated BSA), wound excision and grafting if necessary, and rehabilitation.
- Topical medications include silver sulfadiazine, aqueous 0.5% silver nitrate, petrolatum, debriding enzymes and topical antibiotic ointments.

Complications

Scarring, cosmetic deformity, burn infections, ARDS, sepsis, death.

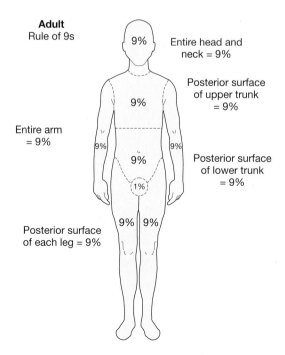

FIGURE 18.17. Adult "rule of 9s" for burn evaluation. (Reproduced with permission McPhee SJ, Papadakis MA. *Current Medical Diagnosis and Treatment*, 49th ed. New York: McGraw-Hill, 2010, Fig. 37-2.)

NOTES

Index

HHS (hyperosmolar hyperglycemic state), 66, 69
HHV-6 (human herpesvirus-6), 314-315, 321-322
HHV-7 (human herpesvirus-7), 321-322
Hib (*Haemophilus influenzae* type B) vaccine, 421
Hidradenitis suppurativa, 326, 327
High-altitude cerebral edema (HACE), 657
High-altitude pulmonary edema (HAPE), 657
Hip
developmental dysplasia of the, 398
imaging of, 577
snapping, 595
Hip dislocation, 594
Hip fractures, 595-596
in older patients, 491
Hip injuries, 594-596
Hip pain, 594
HIPAA (Health Insurance Portability and Accountability Act), 31-32
Hirschsprung disease, 431, 433
Hirsutism due to polycystic ovarian syndrome, 554
Histoplasma spp, 199
HIT (heparin-induced thrombocytopenia), 214
HIV. *See* Human immunodeficiency virus (HIV)
HMB (beta-hydroxy-beta-methylbutyrate) as sports supplement, 607
H1N1 virus, 158
Hodgkin lymphoma, 231-232
Holosystolic murmur, 35
Homicidal ideation, emergency care for, 646
Hormonal agents, chemotherapeutic, 240
Hormone replacement therapy (HRT) for menopause, 558-559
Horner syndrome, 359-360
Horse chestnut, 19
Hospice care, 495
Hospital-acquired pneumonia (HAP), 161, 164
Hot flashes, 558
HPV (human papillomavirus), 541, 543
HPV (human papillomavirus) vaccine, 9
for adolescents, 444
HRT (hormone replacement therapy) for menopause, 558-559
HSV. *See* Herpes simplex virus (HSV)
HTN. *See* Hypertension (HTN)
Human bite, 183, 638, 639
Human granulocytic anaplasmosis, 195
Human growth hormone as sports supplement, 608
Human herpesvirus-6 (HHV-6), 314-315, 321-322
Human herpesvirus-7 (HHV-7), 321-322
Human immunodeficiency virus (HIV), 187-193, 542
AIDS and opportunistic infections due to, 191-193
chronic infection with, 188
diagnosis of, 188, 189
diarrhea with, 171
differential diagnosis of, 188
epidemiology of, 187
etiology and pathogenesis of, 187
management of, 188-190, 191
perinatal, 399
during pregnancy, 531
preventive services for, 12
prevention of, 11, 190
primary infection with, 188
symptoms/exam for, 188
Human monocytic ehrlichiosis, 195
Human papillomavirus (HPV), 541, 543
Human papillomavirus (HPV) vaccine, 9
for adolescents, 444
Huntington disease, 355-356

HUS (hemolytic-uremic syndrome), 213
acute kidney injury due to, 287
Hyaline casts, 285
Hyaline membrane disease, 403
Hydatidiform molar pregnancy, 504-505
Hydatidiform mole, 548
Hydralazine for heart failure, 53-54
Hydration in end-of-life care, 496
Hydrocele, 566-567
Hydrocephalus, normal pressure, 484
Hydrocortisone for adrenal insufficiency, 90
Hydronephrosis, 283, 284
Hydrops fetalis, 209
Hyperaldosteronism, 90-91
Hyperbilirubinemia, neonatal, 400-401
Hypercalcemia, 82-85
ECG findings in, 45
of malignancy, 245-246
Hyperchloremic metabolic acidosis, 303
Hyperemesis gravidarum, 501-502
Hyperkalemia, 300-301
ECG findings in, 45, 301
pseudo-, 300
Hyperlipidemia, 45-48
management of, 48
risk factors with, 47-48
screening guidelines for, 47
Hypermagnesemia, ECG findings in, 45
Hypernatremia, 299-300
Hyperosmolar hyperglycemic state (HHS), 66, 69
Hyperoxia test, 427
Hyperparathyroidism, 85
Hyperprolactinemia, 77
Hypersensitivity pneumonitis, 23
Hypertension (HTN), 44-46, 47
defined, 44
diagnosis of, 45-46
essential, 46
idiopathic intracranial, 343
malignant, 46, 654
management of, 46, 47
preventive services for, 11
pulmonary artery, 275-276
secondary, 46
severe, 46
stages of, 46
symptoms/exam for, 45, 46
transient gestational, 513-514
types of, 45, 46
Hypertensive disorders
emergency care for, 654
of pregnancy, 512-515
eclampsia as, 514
HELLP syndrome as, 515
preeclampsia as, 514
transient gestational hypertension as, 513-514
Hypertensive emergency, 46, 654
Hypertensive encephalopathy, 46
Hypertensive urgency, 46, 654
Hyperthermia, 656-657
Hyperthyroidism, 78-80
Hypertonic hyponatremia, 297, 298
Hypertrophic cardiomyopathy, 59
Hypertrophic obstructive cardiomyopathy in children, 425
Hyperuricemia, 613, 614, 615
Hypervigilance in posttraumatic stress disorder, 457
Hypoactive sexual desire disorder, 559
Hypocalcemia, 85-86
ECG findings in, 45
Hypochondriasis, 469
Hypoglycemia, 68
Hypokalemia, 301
ECG findings in, 45

Hypomagnesemia
ECG findings in, 45
hypocalcemia due to, 86
with hypokalemia, 301
Hypomania, 451
Hyponatremia, 296-298
Hypoparathyroidism, hypocalcemia due to, 86
Hypopituitarism, 73-74
Hypoplastic right heart, 427
Hypopnea, 258
Hypothalamic-pituitary endocrine system, 71, 72
Hypothalamic-pituitary hormone regulation, 77
Hypothermia, 655-656
Hypothesis testing, 29
Hypothyroidism, 80-81
Hypotonic hyponatremia, 297
Hypoventilation, 250
Hypovolemic shock, 642, 643
Hypoxemia, 250-251
Hypoxia, 250
altitude-induced, 657
during birth, 400

I

IBD (inflammatory bowel disease), 110-112
IBD (inflammatory bowel disease)–associated arthritis, 613
IBS (irritable bowel syndrome), 112-113
and fibromyalgia, 618
IC (inspiratory capacity), 248
ICD (implantable cardioverter-defibrillator), 55
ICH (intracerebral hemorrhage), 345
ICP (intracranial pressure), increased in children, 423
IDA (iron deficiency anemia), 204-205
Idiopathic intracranial hypertension, 343
Idiopathic thrombocytopenic purpura, 213-214
IgA (immunoglobulin A) nephropathy, 293
ILD (interstitial lung disease), 268-269
Ileus
gallstone, 126
meconium, 431
Iliotibial band (ITB)–related pathology, 594-595
Iliotibial band (ITB) syndrome, 595
Imaging of musculoskeletal disorders, 577-579, 580, 581
Immunizations
adolescent, 444
adult, 8, 9
for children, 415
contraindications to, 415
for influenza, 9, 159, 160
during pregnancy, 501
before travel, 21
Immunoglobulin A (IgA) nephropathy, 293
Immunologic diseases of skin, 331-332
Immunotherapeutic agents, 240
Impairment, 24
Impetigo, 182, 183, 326
Implanon (contraceptive implants), 537
Implantable cardioverter-defibrillator (ICD), 55
Inborn errors of metabolism, 406
Incidence, 26
Incidentalomas, adrenal, 92-93
Incisional hernia, 383, 384
Inclusion body myositis, 368
Incomplete emptying in older patients, 489
Incontinence
fecal, 114-115
urinary in older patients, 486-489
incomplete emptying or overflow, 489
due to pelvic organ prolapse, 488-489
stress, 487-488
urge, 486-487
Indirect inguinal hernia, 383, 384
Induction of labor, 523-524

About the Authors

Tao Le, MD, MHS

Tao developed a passion for medical education as a medical student. He currently edits more than 15 titles in the *First Aid* series. In addition, he is Founder and Chief Education Officer of USMLE-Rx for exam preparation and ScholarRx for undergraduate medical education. As a medical student, he was editor-in-chief of the University of California, San Francisco (UCSF) *Synapse*, a university newspaper with a weekly circulation of 9000. Tao earned his medical degree from UCSF in 1996 and completed his residency training in internal medicine at Yale University and fellowship training at Johns Hopkins University. Tao subsequently went on to cofound Medsn, a medical education technology venture, and served as its chief medical officer. He is currently chief of adult allergy and immunology at the University of Louisville.

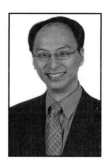

Michael D. Mendoza, MD, MPH, MS, FAAFP

Mike is commissioner of public health for the Monroe County Health Department, Monroe County, NY, and associate professor in the Departments of Family Medicine, Public Health Sciences, and Nursing at the University of Rochester. His education interests include teaching residents about quality improvement, primary care practice innovation, and public health. Previously, he worked closely with medical students as a community preceptor on the South Side of Chicago. His teaching there earned him recognition as Teacher of the Year from the Illinois Academy of Family Physicians. Mike earned his medical degree from the University of Chicago, his master's degree in public health from the University of Illinois at Chicago, and his master's degree in business administration from the University of Rochester. He completed his residency training and served an additional year as chief resident in family and community medicine at the University of California, San Francisco, and San Francisco General Hospital. Mike devotes his free time to his family, photography, and running.

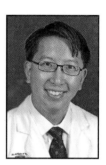

Diana Coffa, MD

Diana is an associate professor in the Department of Family and Community Medicine at UCSF and the residency program director at the UCSF Family and Community Medicine Residency Program at San Francisco General Hospital. In addition to practicing primary care and hospital care with underserved populations, Diana specializes in the treatment of chronic pain and substance use disorders. She has dedicated her career to building learning environments where future leaders in Family Medicine can find their voice. In her free time, she can be found playing dress-up with her toddler and running the hills of San Francisco.

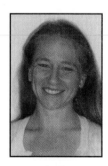

Lamercie Saint-Hilaire, MD

Lamercie is an assistant clinical professor in the Department of Family and Community Medicine at UCSF. After graduating from the University of Central Florida, she attended Meharry Medical College where she studied social determinants of health and health policy. She trained at UCSF Family and Community Medicine Residency Program at ZSFG and served as a chief resident. She now provides primary care at Tom Waddell Urban Health Clinic and is a John A. Watson Faculty Scholar at UCSF. In addition to providing care to her amazing patients, she specializes in unconscious bias and allyship, and is dedicated to efforts around diversity and inclusion. Outside of health care, Lamercie enjoys spending time with family and friends, cooking, and the arts.

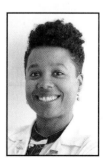